NURSE'S 5-MINUTE CLINICAL CONSULT

Treatments

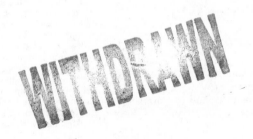

Lippincott Williams & Wilkins
a Wolters Kluwer business
Philadelphia • Baltimore • New York • London
Buenos Aires • Hong Kong • Sydney • Tokyo

STAFF

Executive Publisher
Judith A. Schilling McCann, RN, MSN

Editorial Director
H. Nancy Holmes

Clinical Director
Joan M. Robinson, RN, MSN

Senior Art Director
Arlene Putterman

Art Director
Elaine Kasmer

Editorial Project Manager
Jennifer Kowalak

Clinical Project Manager
Carol A. Saunderson, RN, BA, BS

Editors
Naina D. Chohan, Julie Munden

Clinical Editors
Joanne M. Bartelmo, RN, MSN; Collette
Bishop Hendler, RN, BS, CCRN; Jennifer
Meyering, RN, MS, CCRN; Kate McGovern
Stout, RN, MSN, CCRN; Beverly Ann
Tscheschlog, RN, BS

Copy Editors
Kimberly Bilotta (supervisor), Scotti Cohn,
Tom DeZego, Heather Ditch, Amy Furman,
Pamela Wingrod

Designers
Jan Greenberg (project manager), BJ Crim,
Joseph John Clark

Digital Composition Services
Diane Paluba (manager), Joyce Rossi Biletz,
Donald G. Knauss, Donna S. Morris

Manufacturing
Beth J. Welsh

Editorial Assistants
Megan L. Aldinger, Karen J. Kirk,
Linda K. Ruhf

Indexer
Barbara Hodgson

Library of Congress
Cataloging-in-Publication Data

Nurse's 5-minute clinical consult treatments.
   p. ; cm.
  Includes bibliographical references and index.
  1. Nursing—Handbooks, manuals, etc. 2.
Clinical medicine—Handbooks, manuals, etc. I.
Lippincott Williams & Wilkins. II. Title: Nurse's
five-minute clinical consult treatments.
  [DNLM: 1. Nursing Care—methods—Handbooks. 2. Clinical Medicine—Handbooks. 3.
Therapeutics—Handbooks. WY 49 N972955
2007]
RT51.N87 2007
610.73—dc22
ISBN 1-58255-512-5 (alk. paper)   2006017482

Contents

Contributors and consultants

Lillian Craig, RN, MSN, FNP-C
Instructor
Oklahoma Panhandle State University
Goodwell

Colleen Davenport, RN,C, MSN
Consultant
Renton, Wash.

Vivian Gamblian, RN, MSN
Professor of Nursing
Collin County Community College
District
McKinney, Tex.

Timothy Hudson, RN, BSN, MS, MEd
Chief Nurse, 274th Forward Surgical Team
U.S. Army
Fort Bragg, N.C.

Julia A. Isen, RN, MS, FNP-C
Nurse Practitioner (primary care)
Assistant Clinical Professor
University of California
San Francisco

Patricia Lemelle-Wright, RN, MS
Staff Nurse/Clinical Instructor-Educator
University of Chicago Hospital and
Malcolm X Community College

Ann S. McQueen, RNC, MSN, CRNP
Family Nurse Practitioner
Health Link Medical Center
Southampton, Pa.

Noel C. Piano, RN, MS
Instructor Lafayette School of Practical
Nursing
Adjunct Faculty
Thomas Nelson Community College
Williamsburg, Va.

Kendra S. Seiler, RN, MSN
Nursing Instructor
Rio Hondo College
Whittier, Calif.

Kelley Straub, RN, BSN, CCRN, RCIS
Critical Care Nurse
Intelistaff
Bala Cynwyd, Pa.

Allison J. Terry, RN, MSN, PhD
Director, Center for Nursing
Alabama Board of Nursing
Montgomery

Brenda Williams, MSN
Director of Student Health/Assistant
Professor
Albany (Ga.) State University

Treatments

Abdominal aortic aneurysm repair or resection

OVERVIEW

- Abdominal aortic aneurysm (AAA): abnormal widening of the distal descending part of the aorta; descending aorta subdivided into thoracic (above diaphragm) and abdominal (below diaphragm down to iliac arteries)
- May be saccular (outpouching), fusiform (spindle shaped), or dissecting in form
- 95% of AAAs caused by pattern of inflammatory changes within the arterial walls with weakening of the muscular architecture (which can resemble atherosclerotic changes); remaining AAAs the result of congenital cystic medial necrosis, trauma, syphilis, or other inflammatory or infectious disease processes
- Mortality greatly reduced by repair and resection techniques, which can be performed by open surgery or minimally invasive (endovascular) surgery

INDICATIONS

- Large (greater than 4 cm diameter) or symptomatic aneurysms (symptoms may be result of aneurysmal infection, adherence to or bleeding into nearby abdominal organs, or slow or rapid leaking into the abdominal cavity)

PROCEDURE

OPEN SURGICAL REPAIR

- AAAs usually require resection and replacement of the aortic section with a vascular (patient's or donor vein) or polymer (polytetrafluoroethylene, Dacron, Teflon, or Gore-Tex) synthetic graft.
- Surgery requires general anesthesia.
- Abdominal incision is made to expose the aneurysm site, and clamps are applied to the aorta above and below the aneurysm.
- The aneurysm sac is opened and the aneurysm is resected.
- A prosthetic graft is sewn into place and carefully tested for leakage.

ENDOVASCULAR REPAIR

- Uncomplicated AAAs beginning below the left renal artery may be repaired endovascular grafting.
- This procedure is performed under fluoroscopy with a local or regional anesthetic.
- The access site in the femoral or iliac artery is prepared.
- A delivery catheter with an attached compressed graft is inserted over a guide wire.
- The delivery catheter is advanced to the aorta, where it's positioned across the aneurysm.
- A balloon inside the graft expands the aortic and right femoral segments and affixes them to the vessel walls where they're sewn in place. (See *Repairing an AAA with endovascular grafting.*)
- Before elective surgery, such medications as I.V. nitroprusside (Nitropress) to maintain blood pressure at 100 to 120 mm Hg systolic and an analgesic to relieve pain may be required.

COMPLICATIONS

- Hemorrhage and shock from aneurysm repair or rupture

   ⚠ **WARNING** *Rupture of an AAA is a medical emergency requiring prompt surgical intervention. Other emergency procedures initiated before or during surgery are replacement of fluid and blood and possible administration of I.V. propranolol (Inderal) to reduce myocardial contractility. An arterial line and indwelling urinary catheter are also placed.*

- Left-sided heart failure
- Arrhythmias
- Myocardial infarction
- Renal failure
- Acute tubular necrosis
- Ileus or bowel rupture
- Pancreatitis
- Ischemia of the left colon
- Paralysis due to spinal cord ischemia
- Lower-extremity ischemia or embolization
- Infection such as peritonitis, catheter insertion site
- Aortic dissection or perforation
- Endovascular graft migration

Repairing an AAA with endovascular grafting

Endovascular grafting (shown below) is a minimally invasive procedure for the patient who requires repair of an abdominal aortic aneurysm (AAA).

   The patient is instructed to walk the first day after surgery and is discharged from the hospital in 1 to 3 days.

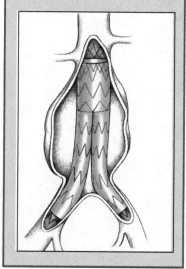

NURSING DIAGNOSES

- Acute pain
- Ineffective tissue perfusion: Peripheral
- Risk for infection

EXPECTED OUTCOMES
The patient will:
- express feelings of comfort and relief from pain
- maintain present and strong peripheral pulses without skin color or temperature change
- show no evidence of infection.

PRETREATMENT CARE

- Explain the treatment and preparation to the patient and his family. On admission to the critical care unit, help ease their fears about this type of care, the threat of impending rupture, and planned surgery. Take time to provide appropriate explanations and to answer questions.
- Verify that the patient has signed an appropriate consent form.
- Assess the patient's vital signs, especially blood pressure, every 2 to 4 hours or more frequently, depending on the severity of his condition.
- Monitor blood pressure and pulses in the extremities, and compare findings bilaterally. If the difference in systolic blood pressure exceeds 10 mm Hg, notify the physician immediately.
- Assess heart rate and rhythm frequently via telemetry; obtain 12-lead electrocardiogram results and cardiac enzyme levels.
- Monitor kidney function by obtaining blood urea nitrogen, creatinine, and electrolyte levels and measuring intake and output regularly.
- Monitor complete blood count for evidence of blood loss as indicated by a decrease in hemoglobin level, hematocrit, and red blood cell count.
- Monitor liver function test results for signs of impaired perfusion.
- Obtain an arterial sample for arterial blood gas analysis as ordered.

- Insert an arterial line to allow for continuous blood pressure monitoring.
- Assist with insertion of a pulmonary artery catheter to assess hemodynamic balance if ordered.
- Observe the patient for signs of rupture, including decreasing blood pressure; increasing pulse and respiratory rates; cool, clammy skin; restlessness; and decreased sensorium.
- Prepare the patient for preoperative abdominal computed tomography scan, magnetic resonance imaging, or angiography to assist the surgeon in locating landmarks and involvement of other nearby tissues.
- Administer ordered medications to prevent aneurysm progression. Provide an analgesic to relieve pain, if present.
- If rupture occurs, insert a large-bore I.V. catheter, begin fluid resuscitation, and administer propranolol I.V. to reduce left ventricular ejection velocity as ordered. Expect to administer additional doses every 4 to 6 hours until oral medications can be used.
- Prepare the patient for elective surgery, as indicated, or emergency surgery if rupture occurs.

POSTTREATMENT CARE

- Perform pulmonary hygiene measures, including suctioning, chest physiotherapy, and deep-breathing exercises.
- Provide continuous cardiac monitoring.
- Assess urine output hourly.
- Maintain nasogastric tube patency to ensure gastric decompression.
- Assist with serial Doppler examination of extremities to ensure that the vascular area is healing properly and that no emboli are present.
- Monitor the patient for signs and symptoms of poor arterial perfusion, such as pain, paresthesia, pallor, pulselessness, paralysis, and coldness.

PATIENT TEACHING

GENERAL
- Provide psychological support for the patient and his family.
- Reinforce instructions for controlling hypertension; stress the importance of medication and diet therapy and the need for smoking cessation.
- Instruct the patient to take all medications as prescribed and to carry a list of them at all times in case of an emergency.
- Advise the patient about activity restrictions, such as no pushing, pulling, or lifting heavy objects, until the physician allows him to do so.

RESOURCES
Organizations
American College of Surgeons: *www.facs.org*
Society of Vascular Surgery: *www.vascularweb.org*

Selected references
Kukreja, N. "Randomized Clinical Trial of Vertical or Transverse Laparotomy for Abdominal Aortic Aneurysm Repair," *British Journal of Surgery* 93(2):251, February 2006.
Kunihara, T., et al. "The Less Incisional Retroperitoneal Approach for Abdominal Aortic Aneurysm Repair to Prevent Postoperative Flank Bulge," *Journal of Cardiovascular Surgery (Torino)* 46(6):527-31, December 2005.
Nano, G., et al. "Sac Enlargement Due to Seroma After Endovascular Abdominal Aortic Aneurysm Repair with the Endologix PowerLink Device," *Journal of Vascular Surgery* 43(1):169-71, January 2006.

Abdominal myomectomy

- Surgery to remove large or symptomatic uterine leiomyomas—tumors composed of smooth muscle that usually occur in the uterine body, although may appear on the cervix or on the round or broad ligament; also called *fibroids, myomas,* and *fibromyomas* and are classified according to location
- Location and removal of fibroids:
- Submucosal: inner surface of the uterus; usually removed hysteroscopically (vaginally with a resectoscope)
- Subserosal: outer surface of the uterus; may be pedunculated (stemmed; on a stalk), commonly removed laparoscopically, through several small incisions in the abdomen
- Intramural: deep within the muscular wall of the uterus; generally removed by abdominal myomectomy; for the patient not concerned about future childbearing, hysteroscopic myomectomy (alternative surgery) performed vaginally (see *Understanding hysteroscopic myomectomy*)
- Preserves uterus for future childbearing as opposed to hysterectomy for fibroids

AGE FACTOR *Uterine fibroids may cause complications, including spontaneous abortion, preterm labor, malposition of the uterus, and secondary infertility (rare), in a woman of childbearing age.*

- Patients usually discharged from hospital within 48 hours of surgery
- Recovery varied; women whose work doesn't require heavy lifting can return to work in 4 to 6 weeks

INDICATIONS

- Abnormal and extensive uterine bleeding
- Abdominal pressure and impingement on adjacent viscera resulting in mild hydronephrosis, bladder compression, or bowel obstruction
- Abdominal pain associated with torsion of a pedunculated subserous fibroid or a fibroid undergoing degeneration
- Anemia secondary to excessive bleeding
- Infection (if tumor protrudes out of the vaginal opening)

- A low horizontal ("bikini") incision is made in the abdomen, and the uterus is lifted through it.
- The uterus is palpated to identify fibroids deep inside that may not be visible.
- A vasoconstrictive drug is injected into the uterus to shrink the blood vessels, and then a laser is used to incise the uterus so the fibroids can be removed.
- Each fibroid is carefully dissected from the muscular portion of the uterus (myometrium) until the blood supply to the fibroid can be identified. Special care is taken in tying, cauterizing, and suturing these vessels to prevent bleeding.
- The uterine walls are sutured together with dissolving sutures. This is done in many layers to ensure greater strength of the repair.
- A special nonadhesive cloth barrier to prevent adhesions is wrapped around the uterus. This material disintegrates in about 2 weeks, when sufficient healing has occurred to prevent most adhesions.
- The uterus is replaced into the abdomen and the incision is closed.

COMPLICATIONS

- Excessive bleeding and hemorrhage
- Ruptured uterus during pregnancy if inadequate surgical closing (increased risk with laparoscopic procedure)
- Accidental laceration or perforation of nearby organs
- Smaller fibroids, which may likely be left behind if a laparoscopic approach is used
- Adhesion formation
- Ureter damage from laceration, inadvertent ligation of the ureter, compression, or puncture (rare)
- Blood clot formation
- Continued menorrhagia despite treatment
- Infertility
- Infection

Understanding hysteroscopic myomectomy

Submucosal (and some intramural) myomas can be removed by inserting a resectoscope, a special type of hysteroscope, through the vagina and cervix and into the uterus. The resectoscope has a wire loop or a roller-type tip that directs high-frequency electrical energy to ablate the fibroid. The fibroid tissue can be seen through the resectoscope's telescopic-like lens.

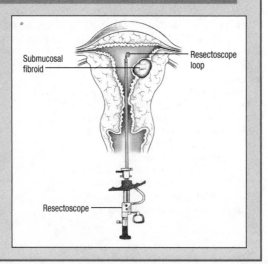

Submucosal fibroid

Resectoscope loop

Resectoscope

NURSING DIAGNOSES

- Acute pain
- Deficient knowledge (disorder and treatment)
- Risk for deficient fluid volume

EXPECTED OUTCOMES

The patient will:
- report increased comfort and decreased pain
- verbalize an understanding of the disorder and its treatment
- maintain normal blood pressure and heart rate, intake and output, and adequate peripheral pulses.

PRETREATMENT CARE

- Explain the treatment and preparation to the patient and her family.
- Verify that the patient has signed an appropriate consent form.
- Send a blood sample for type and cross-matching because blood transfusions may be necessary.
- Administer a gonadotropin-releasing hormone agonist to suppress pituitary gonadotropin release, reducing the size of the uterine fibroid if ordered.
- Reinforce teaching about the procedure and posttreatment care.

POSTTREATMENT CARE

- Monitor the patient for signs of bleeding.
- Monitor laboratory results, especially hemoglobin level and hematocrit.
- Administer an analgesic, as ordered, for pain.
- Maintain patency of I.V. line. Record intake and output, and monitor hydration.
- Monitor the patient's vital signs, and report changes in trends.

PATIENT TEACHING

GENERAL

- Be sure to cover the importance of reporting abnormal bleeding or pelvic pain immediately, and the importance of receiving regular gynecologic examinations.
- Reassure the patient that abdominal myomectomy doesn't cause premature menopause because the ovaries are left intact.
- Review prescribed medications with her, including dosage and possible adverse effects; in a patient with severe anemia from excessive bleeding, an iron supplement may be administered.
- Reassure women of childbearing age that pregnancy may still be possible if desired. Explain, however, that a cesarean delivery may be necessary.
- Advise the patient about complications of blood transfusions.

RESOURCES
Organizations
American College of Obstetrics and Gynecology: *www.acog.org*
Obstetrics, Gynecology, Infertility, and Women's Health: *www.obgyn.net*

Selected references
Damiani, A., et al. "Laparoscopic Myomectomy for Very Large Myomas Using an Isobaric (Gasless) Technique," *Journal of the Society of Laparoendoscopic Surgeons* 9(4):434-38, October-December 2005.
Huang, J.Y., et al. "Failure of Uterine Fibroid Embolization," *Fertility and Sterility* 85(1):30-35, January 2006.
West, S., et al. "Abdominal Myomectomy in Women with Very Large Uterine Size," *Fertility and Sterility* 85(1):36-39, January 2006.

Ablation therapy for arrhythmias

OVERVIEW

◆ Destroys (ablates) heart tissue that's creating a heart beat originating outside the sinoatrial node (an ectopic foci) or permitting conduction of such foci (see *Types of cardiac ablation*)

◆ Type of ablation performed dependent on the type of arrhythmia and the presence of other heart disease

(see *Types of cardiac ablation*)

INDICATIONS

◆ Atrial fibrillation
◆ Atrial flutter
◆ Supraventricular tachycardia, including atrioventricular (AV) nodal reentry and Wolff-Parkinson-White syndrome, and certain types of ventricular tachycardia

PROCEDURE

◆ The procedure is typically performed under conscious sedation with an I.V. tranquilizer and opioid. General anesthesia is used in children and selected adults undergoing surgical ablation.

◆ A nonsurgical procedure generally takes place in the electrophysiology laboratory. The patient's groin area is shaved and his neck, upper chest, arm, and groin are cleaned with antiseptic. Sterile drapes are placed over the patient.

◆ The physician numbs the insertion site with an anesthetic.

◆ Two to five electrode catheters are inserted via the femoral or internal jugular vein into the left side of the heart, the right side of the heart, or both. The coronary sinus may also be entered to evaluate for left-sided abnormal conduction.

◆ Anticoagulation with I.V. heparin is used to reduce the risk of thromboembolism.

◆ The patient is connected to monitors for electrocardiography, heart rate, blood pressure, pulse oximetry and, possibly, hemodynamic monitoring.

◆ After the catheters are in place, the heart's conduction system is assessed and present rhythm confirmed.

◆ During traditional ablation, the physician uses a pacemaker to initiate the arrhythmia. Then the physician moves the catheters around the heart to determine the area of origin. When the physician finds the area, energy is applied to ablate the source.

⚡ **WARNING** *The patient may feel some discomfort or a burning sensation in the chest when the tissue is being destroyed, which may provoke anxiety; determine if the patient would like extra pain medication. Also remind him that the discomfort is normal and ask him to lie quietly and avoid taking deep breaths.*

◆ Atrial fibrillation is commonly treated with pulmonary vein ablation where the tissue circling each entrance to the four pulmonary veins is

---

Types of cardiac ablation

Cardiac ablation therapy depends on the specific ablative method and type of medical procedure required. Here's a list of common types of cardiac ablation:

◆ *Surgical ablation:* This term is generally used to specify that the patient will be undergoing surgical opening of the chest. It can refer to open heart with cardiopulmonary bypass or any of the newer techniques for open chest or minimally invasive chest procedures. The ablation technique itself may not involve direct surgical incision of the heart.

◆ *Minimally invasive ablation:* Although this term can be used as above, it generally means a procedure where peripheral access (femoral, brachial, subclavian) to a vein is obtained followed by placement of several specialized catheters that provide intracardiac rhythm monitoring and a source of energy for ablation of the cardiac tissue. This procedure generally takes place in the electrophysiology laboratory instead of the operating suite.

◆ *The Maze or Cox-Maze III procedure:* The gold standard for arrhythmia treatment, including atrial fibrillation, this procedure was originally only done during open heart surgery with cardiopulmonary bypass. The procedure can now be done in some patients via minimally invasive access to the beating heart through a smaller chest incision where endoscopes guide the surgical treatment. However, not all arrhythmias can be treated with this more limited access.

The surgeon makes several small, specifically located cuts in the heart muscle where abnormal impulses are originating based on intracardiac monitoring leads, leaving the normal conduction pathways open. The cut areas form scar tissue that then prevents the abnormal impulses from being conducted through the heart.

◆ *Radiofrequency ablation:* Instead of surgical incisions, radio waves are directed to the ectopic foci in the heart muscle, obliterating small portions of abnormal tissue by heat. These areas also scar, permanently blocking abnormal conduction. Newer radiofrequency ablation equipment comes with the capacity to direct cooled saline to the area to reduce excessive heat production, making the procedure more comfortable and safer. Most of these procedures are carried out with minimally invasive techniques through peripheral access sites, but can be done during other cardiac surgery as well.

◆ *Microwave and ultrasound techniques:* Microwave and high-frequency sound waves are being used in several research hospitals to determine if either of these methods of tissue destruction reduce the risks of ablation, such as damage to adjacent tissues or stenosing of veins or arteries proximal to the ectopic tissue. These procedures are primarily done via peripheral access sites and specialized catheters and monitoring leads.

◆ *Laser ablation:* The increased technology of laser use has made delicate procedures, such as cardiac ablation, possible with small, very focused laser beams. The essential goals of the procedure remain the same. There's hope that this technique will be particularly useful for atrial fibrillation by reducing the risk of pulmonary vein stenosis. The procedure can be done by peripheral access or during cardiac surgery.

◆ *Cryoablation:* This technique uses a special extremely cold catheter tip to freeze and destroy tiny amounts of abnormally conducting cardiac tissue. Still being studied extensively, preliminary results show equal results compared to the Maze procedure, and equal complication rates. Cryoablation has been done by peripheral access and during other cardiac surgical procedures.

---

ablated. Other ectopic foci for atrial fibrillation are also ablated.

◆ To facilitate the ablation process, three-dimensional electroanatomical mapping systems are projected on monitors. Intracardiac echocardiography may also be used.

◆ When the ablation is complete, the physician monitors the electrocardiogram (ECG) to verify correction of the arrhythmic trigger.

◆ The physician removes the catheters from the groin and pressure is applied to the site.

COMPLICATIONS

◆ Death (rare)
◆ Cardiac complications: high-grade AV block, cardiac tamponade, coronary artery spasm or thrombosis, pericarditis
◆ Retroperitoneal bleeding
◆ Hematoma
◆ Vascular injury
◆ Thromboembolism
◆ Hypotension
◆ Transient ischemic attack or stroke
◆ Pulmonary hypertension from stenosis of the treated pulmonary veins
◆ Pneumothorax
◆ Left atrial-esophageal fistula
◆ Acute pyloric spasm or gastric hypomotility
◆ Phrenic nerve paralysis
◆ Infection at access site
◆ New or recurrent arrhythmias

NURSING DIAGNOSES

◆ Activity intolerance
◆ Decreased cardiac output
◆ Ineffective tissue perfusion: Cardiopulmonary

EXPECTED OUTCOMES
The patient will:
◆ carry out activities of daily living without excess fatigue or decreased energy
◆ maintain adequate cardiac output
◆ maintain normal blood pressure, heart and respiratory rate, and clear lung sounds.

PRETREATMENT CARE

◆ Explain the treatment and preparation to the patient and his family.
◆ Verify that the patient has signed an appropriate consent form.
◆ Obtain a 12-lead ECG, blood samples for complete blood count, laboratory studies, and complete chemistry panel if not done before admission. Other tests, such as an echocardiogram, exercise stress testing, or cardiac catheterization, may have been done before admission to assist the physician in diagnosis and treatment planning.
◆ Confirm that cardiac drugs with electrophysiologic effects, such as beta-adrenergic blockers, calcium channel blockers, digoxin, and class I and III antiarrhythmics, were reduced or discontinued as instructed. Verify that warfarin (Coumadin) therapy has also been stopped as ordered, and obtain serum coagulation testing.
◆ Ask the woman of childbearing age if it's possible that she could be pregnant, and notify the physician of results because exposure to radiation should be avoided.
◆ Confirm that the patient has had no food or fluids since 12 a.m. the day of the procedure.

⚡ **WARNING** *Left atrial ablation and ablation for persistent atrial flutter are contraindicated if an atrial thrombus is present. Left ventricular ablation is contraindicated if a left ventricular thrombus is found. Ablation catheters usually aren't inserted through a mechanical prosthetic heart.*

POSTTREATMENT CARE

◆ Enforce bed rest for 1 to 6 hours, as ordered, with the operative leg extended during this time to prevent bleeding.
◆ Monitor telemetry for arrhythmias, as indicated.
◆ Initiate aspirin therapy to prevent thromboembolic aftereffects.

PATIENT TEACHING

GENERAL

◆ Review insertion site care with the patient. Emphasize the importance of keeping the area clean and dry.
◆ Tell the patient to call the physician if redness, swelling, or drainage at the incision site occurs.
◆ Instruct the patient to report signs and symptoms indicating that his arrhythmia is recurring. Inform him that healing after ablation may take 6 to 8 weeks.
◆ Review with the patient his prescribed medications, including dosage and possible adverse effects.
◆ Review with the patient how to take his pulse and keep a record for the physician.
◆ Teach the patient with ablation along the tricuspid or mitral valve annulus, that antibiotics to prevent endocarditis may be recommended for up to 12 weeks postablation.

RESOURCES
Organizations
American College of Cardiology: *www.acc.org*
American Medical Association: *www.ama-assn.org*

Selected references
Chen, M.C., et al. "Clinical Determinants of Sinus Conversion by Radiofrequency Maze Procedure for Persistent Atrial Fibrillation in Patients Undergoing Concomitant Mitral Valvular Surgery," *American Journal of Cardiology* 96(11):1553-557, December 2005.

Nattel, S., and Opie, L.H. "Controversies in Atrial Fibrillation," *Lancet* 367(9506): 262-72, January 2006.

Rao, B.H., et al. "Successful Radiofrequency Catheter Ablation of Recurrent Atrial Fibrillation Due to Left Inferior Pulmonary Vein Tachycardia," *Indian Heart Journal* 57(4):339-42, July-August 2005.

Adrenalectomy

- Involves surgical removal of one or both adrenal glands, partially or completely
- Surgery done laparoscopically or through abdominal incision
- Laparoscopic approach not used for malignant tumors or tumors larger than 4″ (10 cm) in diameter

INDICATIONS
- Adrenal hyperfunction
- Hyperaldosteronism
- Benign or malignant adrenal tumor
- Secondary treatment of neoplasms or corticotropin oversecretion
- Pheochromocytoma

PROCEDURE
- After the patient is anesthetized, an anterior (transperitoneal) or a posterior (lumbar) approach is used.
- The adrenal gland is identified and dissected free from the upper pole of the kidney.
- Wound closure follows.
- If adrenalectomy is done because of a tumor, the glands are explored first, and then the tumor is resected or one or both glands is removed.
- In pheochromocytoma, the affected adrenal gland is excised, and the abdominal organs are palpated for other tumors.

COMPLICATIONS
- Acute life-threatening adrenal crisis with hypoglycemia and electrolyte disturbances
- Hemorrhage
- Poor wound healing
- Pancreatic injury
- Hypotension (with gland removal) or hypertension (with gland manipulation)

NURSING DIAGNOSES
- Decreased cardiac output
- Ineffective tissue perfusion: Cardiopulmonary
- Risk for infection

EXPECTED OUTCOMES
The patient will:
- maintain adequate cardiac output
- maintain normal heart rate and blood pressure
- remain free from infection.

PRETREATMENT CARE
- Explain the treatment and preparation to the patient and his family.
- Verify that the patient has signed an appropriate consent form.
- Administer ordered drugs to control edema, diabetes, cardiovascular symptoms, and as prophylaxis against infection.
- Administer an aldosterone antagonist to control hypertension and supplemental potassium as ordered.
- Give a glucocorticoid on the morning of surgery as ordered.
- Draw blood samples for laboratory tests as ordered.

FOR PATIENT WITH PHEOCHROMOCYTOMA
- Between 1 and 2 weeks before surgery, administer an alpha-adrenergic blocker, as ordered, followed by a beta-adrenergic blocker (when stable) to control hypertension and tachycardia.
- Monitor the patient for arrhythmias, palpitations, severe headache, hypertension, hyperglycemia, nausea, vomiting, diaphoresis, and vision disturbances.

POSTTREATMENT CARE

TO COUNTERACT SHOCK
- Administer an I.V. vasopressor; adjust the dosage based on the patient's blood pressure response as ordered.
- Increase the I.V. fluid rate as ordered.
- Administer an I.V. glucocorticoid as ordered.
- Administer an analgesic as ordered.

MONITORING
- Monitor the patient's vital signs and intake and output, and report changes.
- Monitor invasive arterial pressure for signs of hemorrhage, acute adrenal crisis, or adrenal hypofunction (hypotension).
- Administer glucocorticoids and mineralocorticoids as ordered.
- Report trends in serum electrolyte levels and glucose levels; administer glucose and electrolytes as ordered.
- Assess and provide care for the surgical wound and dressings.
- Monitor the patient for abdominal distention and return of bowel sounds.
- Keep the patient's room cool.

GENERAL

- Review the prescribed medications, including the dosage and possible adverse effects.
- Teach the patient not to stop steroid therapy abruptly.
- Review potential complications, including adrenal insufficiency, with the patient and when to notify the practitioner.
- Tell the patient that an increase in the steroid dosage may be necessary during stress or illness. (See *Preventing adrenal crisis.*)
- Tell the patient treated for adrenal hyperfunction to expect improvement of signs and symptoms within a few months.
- Provide wound assessment and care instructions and review signs and symptoms of infection.
- Teach the patient about stress-reduction techniques if appropriate.
- Reiterate the importance of wearing medical identification.

RESOURCES
Organizations
American College of Surgeons: *www.facs.org*
National Adrenal Diseases Foundation: *www.medhelp.org/nadf*

Selected references
Hara, I., et al. "Clinical Outcomes of Laparoscopic Adrenalectomy According to Tumor Size," *International Journal of Urology* 12(12):1022-1027, December 2005.
Li, H., et al. "Role of Adrenalectomy in Ectopic ACTH Syndrome," *Endocrine Journal* 52(6):721-26, December 2005.

 PATIENT-TEACHING AID

Preventing adrenal crisis

Dear Patient,

Even though you follow your treatment plan carefully, unexpected situations can create stress and worsen your condition. Because your adrenal glands can't respond to increased demands, you'll need to prepare for stressful situations and know what to do to prevent adrenal crisis.

TAKE PRECAUTIONS

- Always wear or carry medical identification with your name, the name of your disorder, and the phone numbers of your health care provider and a responsible person.
- Always carry a clearly labeled emergency kit, especially when you travel. Double-check to make sure that the kit contains a syringe and needle, 100 milligrams of hydrocortisone, and instructions for use.

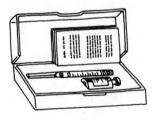

- Avoid physical activity in hot, humid weather. If you begin to perspire heavily, drink more fluids and add salt to your food.

- Follow your health care provider's directions for increasing your daily doses of prescribed streroids during stressful times — emotional crisis, overexertion, infection, illness, or injury.

WATCH YOUR DIET AND GET ADEQUATE REST

- Eat regularly. Don't skip meals or go for a long time without food.
- Be sure to follow a high-carbohydrate, high-protein diet with up to 8 grams of salt (sodium) daily—more if you perspire a lot.
- Balance active periods with rest.

RECOGNIZE WARNING SIGNS

Notify your health care provider immediately (or go directly to the nearest hospital emergency department) if you have any of the warning signs of adrenal crisis:

- apathy or restlessness, apprehensiveness, confusion, dizziness, headache

- pallor or cool, clammy skin
- fever
- increased breathing and pulse rates
- unusual fatigue or weakness
- loss of appetite, stomach cramps, diarrhea, nausea, and vomiting
- dehydration or reduced urine output.

If you can't reach your health care provider or get to a hospital at once, give yourself a subcutaneous injection of 100 milligrams of hydrocortisone. Then seek medical help.

PLAN AHEAD

Instruct a family member or friend to give you a subcutaneous injection of 100 milligrams of hydrocortisone if he finds you unconscious or physically unable to take your medicine by mouth. He should then seek medical help immediately.

Amniocentesis, therapeutic

OVERVIEW

- Needle aspiration of amniotic fluid (also called *amnioreduction);* used when placental blood flow is compromised in multiple gestational pregnancy

INDICATIONS
- Twin-to-twin transfusion syndrome (TTTS):
- occurring when twin or multiple fetuses share a single placenta that develops abnormal anastamoses between each fatal circulatory system despite each fetus developing in a separate amniotic sac
- resulting in a pressure gradient between the two circulatory systems resulting in one fetus having too much amniotic fluid and blood volume and one not enough
- removing excess amniotic fluid from the enlarged sac allows pressure to normalize and increases blood flow to the fetus with insufficient blood supply and amniotic fluid
- generally done repeatedly throughout the pregnancy

PROCEDURE

- Ultrasonography is performed to locate the fetuses, the placenta, and the amniotic sacs.
- Maintaining sterility, the patient's abdominal skin is cleaned with an antiseptic solution, and the physician administers a local anesthetic to the appropriate site.
- The physician, guided by continued ultrasonographic imaging, inserts the needle and stylet through the abdomen and uterine wall into the amniotic sac. The stylet is removed and the presence of amniotic fluid is confirmed. Amniotic fluid is then aspirated by a syringe.
- If specimens are needed for study, fluid is transferred to appropriate tubes.
- Monitoring for signs and symptoms of supine hypotension (light-headedness, nausea, diaphoresis, low blood pressure) is done throughout the process. Fetal heart rates (FHRs) are also monitored.
- The needle is withdrawn; an adhesive bandage is placed over the insertion site.

COMPLICATIONS
- Amniotic fluid embolism
- Hemorrhage or infection
- Premature labor or birth
- Abruptio placentae
- Placental or umbilical cord trauma
- Bladder or intestinal puncture
- Rh isoimmunization
- Intrauterine fetal death
- Amnionitis
- Amniotic fluid leakage
- Fetal bleeding
- Spontaneous abortion
- Merging of the two amniotic sacs together, increasing the risk of cord entanglement and fetal death

NURSING DIAGNOSES

- Anxiety
- Risk for imbalanced fluid volume
- Risk for injury

EXPECTED OUTCOMES
The patient will:
- express feelings of reduced anxiety
- exhibit no signs or symptoms of maternal or fetal bleeding
- exhibit no signs of maternal or fetal injury.

PRETREATMENT CARE

- Explain the procedure to the patient, and verify that a consent form has been signed.
- Assist the patient when she voids to reduce the risk of bladder puncture.
- Place the patient in a supine position.
- Obtain baseline maternal vital signs and FHRs.

POSTTREATMENT CARE

- Assist the patient who is in the third trimester to lie on her side to avoid hypotension from pressure of the gravid uterus on the vena cava.
- Assess maternal vital signs every 15 minutes for 30 minutes and regularly thereafter to detect changes from baseline.
- Continuously monitor the patient electronically for uterine irritability until discharge.
- Monitor FHRs electronically for a few hours after the procedure to allow early intervention if complications occur.

WARNING *Changes in FHR, such as tachycardia and bradycardia, signal distress. If these signs appear, notify the physician and continue to monitor the FHRs.*

PATIENT TEACHING

GENERAL

- Instruct the patient to report signs and symptoms of complications: vaginal discharge (fluid or blood), decreased fetal movement, contractions, or fever and chills.
- Review with the patient the high protein supplements and bed rest requirements associated with TTTS.
- Instruct the patient to report a rapid increase in uterine size and weight gain or difficulty breathing to the physician promptly.

RESOURCES

Organizations

Obstetrics, Gynecology, Infertility and Women's Health: *www.obgyn.net*

The Twin to Twin Transfusion Syndrome Foundation: *www.tttsfoundation.org*

Selected references

Galea, P.T., et al. "Insights into the Pathophysiology of Twin-Twin Transfusion Syndrome," *Prenatal Diagnosis* 25(9): 777-85, September 2005.

Harkness, U.F., and Crombleholme, T.M. "Twin-Twin Transfusion Syndrome: Where Do We Go From Here?" *Seminars in Perinatology* 29(5):296-304, October 2005.

Quintero, R.A., et al. "Management of Twin-twin Transfusion Syndrome in Pregnancies with Iatrogenic Detachment of Membranes Following Therapeutic Amniocentesis and the Role of Interim Amniopatch," *Ultrasound in Obstetrics & Gynecology* 26(6):628-33, November 2005.

Amputation

OVERVIEW

- Involves surgical removal of an extremity
- In closed amputation: skin flaps used to cover the bone end
- In guillotine (open) amputation: tissue and bone cut flush and wound is left open to be repaired in a second operation

INDICATIONS

- Preservation of the function of a remaining part
- Severe trauma
- Gangrene
- Cancer
- Vascular disease
- Congenital deformity
- Thermal injury

PROCEDURE

- The patient receives general or local anesthesia.

CLOSED AMPUTATION

- Tissue is excised to the bone, leaving sufficient skin to cover the limb end.
- Bleeding is controlled by tying off the bleeding vessels above the site.
- The bone (or joint) is sawed and filed, with the periosteum removed about $1/4''$ (0.5 cm) from the bone end.
- All vessels are ligated and the nerves divided.
- Opposing muscles are sutured over the bone end and periosteum.
- Skin flaps are closed and an incision drain may be placed.
- Soft dressings are applied; rigid dressings may be used in below-the-knee amputation. An elastic shrinker may be applied to reduce edema and pain.

GUILLOTINE AMPUTATION

- A perpendicular incision is made through the bone and all tissue.
- The wound isn't sutured closed.
- A large, bulky dressing is applied.

COMPLICATIONS

- Infection
- Contractures
- Skin breakdown, necrosis, or hematoma formation
- Phantom pain in the residual limb
- Chest pain, myocardial infarction, or stroke

NURSING DIAGNOSES

- Acute pain
- Impaired physical mobility
- Ineffective tissue perfusion: Peripheral

EXPECTED OUTCOMES

The patient will:
- express feelings of increased comfort
- attain the highest degree of mobility possible within the confines of injury
- exhibit adequate tissue perfusion and pulses proximal to the amputation, with no evidence of skin breakdown.

PRETREATMENT CARE

- Explain the treatment and preparation to the patient and his family.
- Verify that the patient or a family member has signed an appropriate consent form.
- Provide emotional support.
- If possible, arrange for the patient to meet with someone else who has undergone amputation and has adjusted well to the life changes that it brings.
- Demonstrate prescribed exercises.
- Administer a broad-spectrum antibiotic as ordered.

POSTTREATMENT CARE

- Elevate the affected limb as ordered.
- Provide an analgesic as ordered and comfort measures for pain.
- Keep the residual limb wrapped properly with elastic compression bandages or an elastic shrinker as ordered.
- Provide cast care if a rigid plaster dressing has been applied.
- Maintain the patient in proper body alignment.
- Reinforce physical therapy instructions and activities.
- Encourage frequent ambulation, as appropriate.
- Encourage active or passive range-of-motion exercises.
- Help the patient with turning and positioning without propping the limb on a pillow.
- Monitor the patient's vital signs and intake and output, and report changes.
- Observe the surgical wound, and reinforce or change dressings as ordered.
- Monitor and record amount of bleeding, patency of drains, and amount and type of drainage.
- Provide emotional support.
- Encourage the patient to stop smoking, if appropriate.

PATIENT TEACHING

GENERAL

- Review with the patient prescribed medications, including the dosage and possible adverse effects.
- Review postoperative care and rehabilitation.
- Review use and care of the prosthesis and phantom limb sensation.
- Reiterate the importance of daily examination of the distal limb and describe daily limb care and dressings as well as daily care after healing is complete.
- Review signs and symptoms of infection and skin breakdown.
- Review complications, and tell the patient when to notify the physician.
- Review use of elastic bandages or a limb shrinker. (See *Wrapping your residual limb*.)
- Teach proper use of crutches as appropriate.
- Review activities to strengthen the residual limb and toughen the skin.
- Emphasize the importance of follow-up care.

◆ Assist the patient with finding a local support group or obtaining a referral for psychological counseling.

RESOURCES

Organizations

American College of Emergency Physicians: *www.acep.org*

Amputation Coalition of America: *www.amputee-coalition.org*

Selected references

Poljak-Guberina, R., et al. "The Amputees and Quality of Life," *Collegium Antropologicum* 29(2):603-609, December 2005.

Walker, J.L., et al. "Femoral Lengthening after Transfemoral Amputation," *Orthopedics* 29(1):53-59, January 2006.

Wang, J.N., et al. "Salvage of Amputated Upper Extremities with Temporary Ectopic Implantation Followed by Replantation at a Second Stage," *Journal of Reconstructive Microsurgery* 22(1):15-20, January 2006.

PATIENT-TEACHING AID

Wrapping your residual limb

Dear Patient,

Wrapping your residual limb with an elastic bandage will promote healing and provide a comfortable fit for your prosthesis.

BEFORE YOU START

1. Assemble the supplies you'll need — skin care articles, 6″ (15-centimeter) wide elastic bandage (you may need two rolls), and fasteners (adhesive tape, safety pins, or clips).

Now do the skin care you learned in the hospital. For comfort, wear only lightweight or no underclothing while applying the bandage.

2. Have an elastic bandage ready. Sit in a chair with your one foot resting flat on the floor. Now raise your limb about 6″ off the seat. Starting at the top front, wrap the bandage diagonally toward the lower inside of your residual limb.

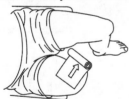

3. Wrap the bandage around the back. Then bring it diagonally upward and across the front and center of your limb. Be sure to secure the end of the bandage.

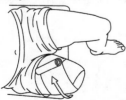

4. Now bring the bandage around the back again. Keep it as close to your groin as you can.

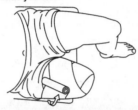

5. Next, place the bandage toward the lower inside surface of your limb — slightly to one side of the last wrap. Continue around to the back, wrapping diagonally downward.

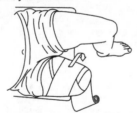

6. Bring the bandage forward just below the last wrap, then up and across to the opposite hip.

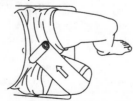

7. Take the bandage around your back at waist level, and bring it around to the front of your body. The bandage should make an "X" over your thigh.

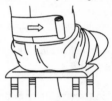

8. Now bring the bandage down toward the inside surface of your residual limb once again and around the back in an upward diagonal. Continue wrapping diagonally until your limb is covered. Secure the bandage with clips, pins, or tape.

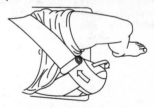

INSPECTING THE BANDAGE

Make sure that all limb areas are covered, the bandage is wrinkle-free, and every turn is diagonal. The bandage should appear smooth and rounded and fit snugly at the bottom of the residual limb. If the bandage fails your inspection, you may need to re-wrap it.

Angioplasty, percutaneous transluminal coronary

- Nonsurgical alternative to coronary artery bypass surgery
- Uses a tiny balloon catheter to dilate a coronary artery that's been narrowed by atherosclerotic plaque; usually includes atherectomy
- May include placement of a regular or drug-eluting stent

INDICATIONS

- Documented myocardial ischemia and angina
- Proximal lesion in a single coronary artery
- Acute myocardial infarction
- Postthrombolytic therapy with high-grade stenosis
- Previous coronary artery bypass surgery
- Poor surgical candidate for coronary artery bypass surgery
- Stenosis that narrows the arterial lumen by 70% or more

PROCEDURE

- The catheter insertion site, usually femoral, is prepared and anesthetized.
- A guide wire is inserted into the femoral artery using a percutaneous or cutdown approach, and the catheter is guided fluoroscopically.
- The lesion is confirmed using angiography.
- A small, double-lumen, balloon-tipped catheter with or without a stent over the balloon is inserted over the guide wire and positioned properly, and the balloon is inflated repeatedly with normal saline solution and contrast medium for 15 to 30 seconds, to a pressure of 6 atmospheres. Atherectomy may be performed before balloon insertion.
- The expanding balloon compresses the plaque, expanding the arterial lumen and pressure gradients across the stenotic area.
- The balloon is inflated repeatedly until the residual gradient decreases to about 20% or until the pressure gradient measures less than 16 mm Hg. The stent is fixed to the vessel wall during this procedure.
- Angiography is repeated.
- The catheter may be left in place or removed, and the patient is taken to the intensive care unit or to a post-anesthesia care unit for monitoring. (See *Relieving occlusions with angioplasty*.)

COMPLICATIONS

- Arterial dissection
- Coronary artery rupture
- Cardiac tamponade
- Myocardial ischemia or infarction

Relieving occlusions with angioplasty

Percutaneous transluminal coronary angioplasty can open an occluded coronary without opening the chest—an important advantage over bypass surgery. First, the physician confirms the presence and location of the arterial occlusion using coronary angiography. Then the physician threads a guide catheter through the patient's femoral artery into the coronary artery under fluoroscopic guidance (shown below left).

When angiography shows the guide catheter positioned at the occlusion site, the phyisician carefully inserts a smaller double-lumen balloon catheter through the guide catheter and directs the balloon through the occlusion (shown below center). A marked pressure gradient will be obvious.

The physician alternately inflates and deflates the balloon until an angiogram verifies successful arterial dilation (shown below right) and the pressure gradient has decreased.

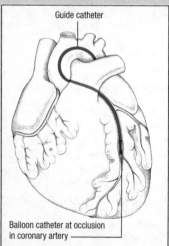

Guide catheter

Balloon catheter at occlusion in coronary artery

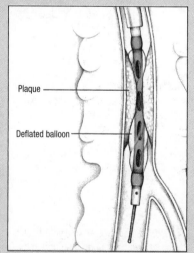

Plaque

Deflated balloon

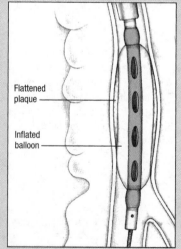

Flattened plaque

Inflated balloon

- Abrupt reclosure of the affected artery (occurring within a few hours of the procedure)
- Restenosis (usually occurring within 30 days to 6 months)
- Coronary artery spasm
- Arrhythmias
- Bleeding
- Hematoma
- Thromboembolism
- Adverse reactions to the contrast medium

NURSING DIAGNOSES

- Activity intolerance
- Decreased cardiac output
- Ineffective tissue perfusion: Cardiopulmonary

EXPECTED OUTCOMES
The patient will:
- carry out activities of daily living without excess fatigue or decreased energy
- maintain adequate cardiac output
- maintain normal blood pressure, heart and respiratory rate, and clear lung sounds.

PRETREATMENT CARE

- Explain the treatment and preparation and verify that an appropriate consent form is signed.
- Tell the patient that contrast medium injection may cause a flushing sensation or transient nausea. Ask him whether he has had reactions to shellfish, iodine, or contrast medium in the past. Also determine if he has had a reaction to aspirin products or antiplatelet drugs. Notify the surgeon if the patient reports a reaction to any of these items.
- Restrict food and fluid intake for at least 6 hours before the procedure.
- Obtain results of coagulation studies, complete blood count, serum electrolyte levels, blood urea nitrogen and creatinine levels, and blood typing and crossmatching, as ordered.
- Obtain the patient's weight.

- Insert I.V. line and arterial line if ordered; apply electrocardiogram (ECG) monitoring leads, automatic blood pressure cuff, and pulse oximetry monitor.
- Locate, mark, and record the amplitude of bilateral distal pulses.
- Administer a sedative as ordered.
- Instruct the patient to tell the surgical team immediately if he has breathing difficulties, sweating, numbness, itching, nausea, vomiting, chills, or heart palpitations during the procedure.

POSTTREATMENT CARE

- Administer an anticoagulant, I.V. nitroglycerin, and I.V. fluids as ordered.
- Keep the affected extremity straight, and elevate the head of the bed no more than 15 degrees as ordered.
- If an expanding ecchymosis appears, mark the area, and obtain hemoglobin and hematocrit samples as ordered.
- Monitor for hematoma formation, ecchymosis, or bleeding at the catheter insertion site. Report bleeding sites to the surgeon and apply direct pressure to them.
- After the sheath is removed, apply direct pressure to the insertion site until hemostasis occurs. Apply a pressure dressing as ordered.
- Monitor the patient's vital signs and intake and output, and report changes.
- Continually monitor heart rate and rhythm, invasive arterial pressures if ordered, peripheral pulses, and neurovascular status of extremities as indicated.
- Report ECG monitoring and 12-lead ECG results, particularly changes in ST segments indicating ischemia or infarction.
- Provide analgesia as needed.

⚡ **WARNING** *Immediately report signs and symptoms of angina (including chest pain), infection, fluid overload (tachycardia, dyspnea, edema), and abrupt arterial reclosure (chest pain, ECG changes).*

PATIENT TEACHING

GENERAL
- Review with the patient the prescribed medications, such as antiplatelets, including the dosage and possible adverse effects.
- Discuss with the patient puncture site care, activity restrictions if applicable, and follow-up care and testing.
- Tell the patient to report signs and symptoms of bleeding, infection, restenosis, or complications, and when to notify the physician.
- Teach the patient that a low cholesterol diet and regular exercise plus stress reduction and smoking cessation if appropriate reduces the risk of recurrence.

RESOURCES
Organizations
American College of Cardiology: *www.acc.org*
American Heart Association: *www.americanheart.org*
American Medical Association: *www.ama-assn.org*

Selected references
Marret, E., et al. "Thrombosis after Implantation of Drug-Eluting Stents," *JAMA* 295(1):36, January 2006.
Mitka, M. "Progress in Percutaneous Heart Procedures Leads to Update in Clinical Guidelines," *JAMA* 295(3): 263-64, January 2006.
Oliver, B., et al. "Open New Care Pathways With Drug-Eluting Stents," *Nursing Management* 37(2):33-39, February 2006.

Appendectomy

- Involves surgical removal of an inflamed vermiform appendix to prevent imminent rupture or perforation of the organ
- Laparoscopy: may be used to help diagnose the condition

INDICATIONS
- Acute appendicitis

- The patient receives general anesthesia.
- The surgeon makes an incision in the right lower abdominal quadrant to expose the appendix.
- In laparoscopic appendectomy, three or four small abdominal incisions are made.
- The base of the appendix is ligated.
- A purse-string suture is placed in the cecum.
- Excess fluid or tissue debris is removed from the abdominal cavity.
- The incision is closed.
- If perforation occurs, one or more Penrose drains or abdominal sump tubes, or both, are placed and the incision may or may not be closed.

COMPLICATIONS
- Infection
- Paralytic ileus

With perforation
- Local or general peritonitis
- Paralytic ileus
- Intestinal obstruction
- Abscess

- Acute pain
- Imbalanced nutrition: Less than body requirements
- Ineffective tissue perfusion: GI

EXPECTED OUTCOMES
The patient will:
- express feelings of comfort
- resume a normal diet by discharge
- have normal bowel sounds and function by discharge.

PRETREATMENT CARE

- Explain the treatment and preparation to the patient and his family.
- Verify that the patient has signed an appropriate consent form.
- Administer a prophylactic antibiotic as ordered.
- Administer I.V. fluids as ordered.
- Insert a nasogastric (NG) tube as ordered.
- Place the patient in Fowler's position.
- Avoid giving an analgesic, a cathartic, or an enema, and avoid applying heat to the abdomen.
- Provide reassurance.

POSTTREATMENT CARE

- Place the patient in Fowler's position after the anesthesia wears off.
- Maintain patency of drainage catheters and tubes.
- Encourage the patient to ambulate as soon as possible.
- Encourage the patient to cough, breathe deeply, and change positions frequently.
- Auscultate for bowel sounds in all four quadrants.
- Help the patient gradually resume oral intake after NG tube removal.
- Assist with emergency treatment of peritonitis if needed.
- Monitor the patient's vital signs and intake and output, and report changes.
- Monitor surgical wounds and dressings.
- Report signs or symptoms of peritonitis or other complications.
- Record the type and amount of drainage.

PATIENT TEACHING

GENERAL

- Review with the patient prescribed medications and possible adverse effects.
- Review with the patient signs and symptoms of infection and intestinal obstruction and when to notify the physician.
- Teach the patient about wound care and activity restrictions.
- Emphasize the importance of follow-up care.

RESOURCES
Organizations
American Academy of Pediatrics: *www.aap.org*
American College of Gastroenterology: *www.acg.gi.org*
Harold D. Portnoy, MD, editor: *www.yoursurgery.com*

Selected references
Acosta, R., et al. "CT Can Reduce Hospitalization for Observation in Children with Suspected Appendicitis," *Pediatric Radiology* 35(5):495-500, May 2005.

Bristow, N. "Treatment and Management of Acute Appendicitis," *Nursing Times* 100(43):34-36, October-November, 2004.

Dalal, I., et al. "Serum and Peritoneal Inflammatory Mediators in Children with Suspected Acute Appendicitis," *Archives of Surgery* 140(2):169-73, February 2005.

Filewood, F. "Improving Diagnosis and Treatment for Appendicitis," *Nursing Times* 101(17):41, April-May, 2005.

Arthrocentesis

- Procedure in which a sterile needle and syringe are used to drain fluid from the joint; also called *joint aspiration*
- Although any joint in the body may be aspirated, arthrocentesis more commonly performed on larger ones, such as the knees and shoulders
- Typically performed as an office procedure or at the bedside of hospitalized patients
- Possible injection of cortisone into the joint during the aspiration to rapidly relieve joint inflammation and further reduce symptoms

INDICATIONS

- Joint swelling and pain (removal of fluid removes the white blood cells that are sources of enzymes that can be destructive to the joint)

PROCEDURE

- The skin over the joint is sterilized using a liquid iodine solution or another antiseptic.
- Local anesthetic is used in the area of the joint, either by injection, topical liquid freezing, or both.
- A needle with a syringe attached is inserted into the affected joint; fluid is then aspirated back into the syringe. For certain conditions, the physician will also inject cortisone into the joint after fluid removal.
- The needle is then removed and an adhesive dressing is applied over the entry point. (See *Using arthrocentesis to obtain fluid from a joint.*)

COMPLICATIONS

- Local bruising
- Minor bleeding into the joint
- Loss of pigment in the skin entered by the needle
- Infection of the joint (septic arthritis)
  If a cortisone medication (a corticosteroid) is injected into the joint, additional complications include:
- inflammation in the joint as a result of the medication crystallizing
- increased blood glucose level (rare)
- aggravation of preexisting infection elsewhere in the body.

Using arthrocentesis to obtain fluid from a joint

Arthrocentesis is aspiration of the fluid from an affected joint. It's commonly used as a diagnostic procedure, but it's also performed to remove fluid from the joint as a treatment.

Bone

Ligament

Fibrous capsule

Synovial cavity containing synovial fluid

Synovial membrane

Ligament

Bone

NURSING DIAGNOSES

- ◆ Acute pain
- ◆ Impaired physical mobility
- ◆ Risk for infection

EXPECTED OUTCOMES
The patient will:
- ◆ express feelings of increased comfort
- ◆ attain the highest degree of mobility possible within the confines of the injury
- ◆ experience no fever, reddening, heat, recurrent swelling, increased pain, or drainage at the puncture site in the joint.

PRETREATMENT CARE

- ◆ Review the procedure with the patient and review his medical history.
- ◆ Assess the patient for reactions to steroids or current usage of steroids systemically.

  ⚡ **WARNING** *Before arthrocentesis, check the patient's history for a preexisting bleeding disorder, use of an anticoagulant with poorly controlled blood levels, and allergic reaction to local anesthetic to avoid further complications.*

- ◆ Diagnostic studies may include an X-ray of the joint or magnetic resonance imaging to confirm diagnosis and presence of joint fluid.

POSTTREATMENT CARE

- ◆ Ice may be applied to the joint for 20 to 30 minutes every 3 to 4 hours for the first 24 hours after treatment.
- ◆ The physician may apply an elastic bandage to help support the joint.

PATIENT TEACHING

GENERAL
- ◆ Review with the patient the prescribed pain medications, including the dosage and possible adverse effects.
- ◆ Tell the patient to avoid stressing the joint; activities may be resumed according to the physician's orders. Activities are usually restricted to allow time for the joint to rest, as determined by the physician.
- ◆ Review the need for follow-up care.
- ◆ Tell the patient to report signs and symptoms of complications: recurrence of joint fluid, swelling, drainage from the puncture area, fever, increasing pain even though an analgesic is taken, and signs and symptoms of joint infection (redness and warmth).

RESOURCES
Organizations
American Academy of Orthopedic Surgeons:*www.aaos.org*
American College of Rheumatology: *www.rheumatology.org*
Arthritis Foundation: *www.arthritis.org*

Selected references
Ostergaard, M., et al. "Magnetic Resonance Imaging in Rheumatoid Arthritis Advances and Research Priorities," *Journal of Rheumatology* 32(12):2462-464, December 2005.
Sharp, J.T., et al. "Measurement of Joint Space Width and Erosion Size," *Journal of Rheumatology* 32(12):2456-461, December 2005.
Tanaka, N., et al. "Volume of a Wash and the Other Conditions for Maximum Therapeutic Effect of Arthroscopic Lavage in Rheumatoid Knees," *Clinical Rheumatology* 25(1):65-69, February 2006.

Biliopancreatic diversion

OVERVIEW

- Procedure that restricts both food intake and the amount of calories and nutrients the body absorbs to achieve long-term, major weight loss in individuals weighing more than 100 lb (45 kg) over their ideal body weight
- Stomach capacity: 4 to 5 oz after biliopancreatic diversion (BPD), compared with 1 oz after standard gastric bypass operation, making it a less restrictive option
- Two types of BPD surgery:
  - in *BPD*, the stomach is removed just below the esophagus forming a small pouch. The remaining pouch is connected to the ileum, restricting absorption of fats and other nutrients. The freed duodenal and jejunal limbs of the small intestine are then connected to the lower end of the ileum, allowing the biliary and pancreatic digestive juices to mix with food just before entering the colon to permit digestion of some fats, vitamins, and minerals. (See *Understanding biliopancreatic diversion.*)
  - in *BPD with duodenal switch* (BPD/DS), less of the stomach is removed, and the pyloric valve and a small segment of the duodenum are retained, maintaining some digestion in the stomach as well as the normal flow of food through the pyloric sphincter. This duodenal area is then connected to the ileum. However, the remaining portion of the stomach, duodenum, and jejunum are reconnected to the lower end of the ileum, permitting gastric juices as well as bile salts and pancreatic digestive enzymes to aid absorption of more fats and other nutrients than in BPD alone.
- Ghrelin, a hormone secreted by the stomach and responsible for the sensation of hunger, along with the reduced capacity to hold food, giving the patient a feeling of fullness after eating 1 cup of food
- Removal of the gallbladder may be done prophylactically

INDICATIONS

- Obesity for at least 5 years without a history of alcohol abuse, untreated depression, or another major psychiatric disorder
- Body mass index (BMI) 40 or higher despite repeated attempts to lose weight
- BMI 35 to 40 and presence of a life-threatening or disabling condition related to weight

PROCEDURE

BPD

- The patient is placed under general anesthesia. If he's undergoing an open procedure, a large incision is made in the abdomen. Alternatively, if a laparoscopic approach is being used, several small incisions are made, carbon dioxide gas is insufflated into the abdomen to separate the organs from each other, and smaller instruments and a camera are used to guide the surgery.
- All but a portion of the stomach is removed.
- The stomach pouch is connected directly to the ileum, through an opening made in the mesothelium.
- The bypassed portions of the intestine are anastomosed to the final 2 to 4' (1.2 m) of ileum, forming a common channel before entering the colon.
- The newly anastomosed sites are checked for leakage by being filled with sterile saline solution.

BPD/DS

- In BPD/DS, the pyloric valve and about 2" (5 cm) of the proximal duodenum is preserved, as a large portion of the stomach is excised, parallel to the greater curvature.
- An opening in the mesothelium is created and the ileum is attached to the residual duodenum.
- The detached stomach, duodenum, and jejunum are connected to the final 2' to 4' (0.6 to 1.2 m) of the distal ileum, as in BPD, and similarly checked for leakage.

COMPLICATIONS

- Loose stools or dumping syndrome (mainly with BPD)
- Malodorous gas
- Serious deficiencies in protein, fat, calcium, iron, or vitamins B_{12}, A, D, E, and K due to malabsorption
- Paralytic ileus
- Stomal ulcers (rare with BPD/DS)
- Anemia
- Infection or poor wound healing at the incision site

Understanding biliopancreatic diversion

In a biliopancreatic diversion, a portion of the stomach is removed and the remainder is connected to the lower portion of the small intestine. The food bypasses much of the small intestine, resulting in fewer calories absorbed and weight loss.

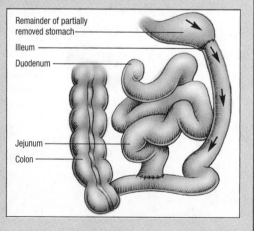

Remainder of partially removed stomach

Illeum

Duodenum

Jejunum

Colon

- Peritonitis
- Embolization of the large bowel or lungs
- Gallstones due to rapid weight loss
- Osteoporosis
- Coagulopathy due to reduced vitamin K absorption
- Death (rare)

NURSING DIAGNOSES

- Acute pain
- Imbalanced nutrition: Less than body requirements
- Ineffective tissue perfusion: GI

EXPECTED OUTCOMES
The patient will:
- express feelings of comfort
- have laboratory values within normal parameters and verbalize an understanding of the need for nutritional supplementation for life
- show no signs of peritonitis or bowel obstruction.

PRETREATMENT CARE

- Verify that the patient has signed an informed consent form.
- Instruct the patient not to have anything to eat or drink after midnight before the surgery.
- Insert an I.V. access device
- Check that preoperative testing results are available.
- Verify that the patient completed preoperative bowel cleansing and administer an antibiotic, as ordered.
- Explain the treatment, preparation, and postoperative care to the patient and his family.
- Tell the patient that a nasogastric (NG) tube will be in place after surgery and will be removed in a few days.
- Prepare the patient for early postoperative ambulation.
- Tell the patient to expect to have an I.V. line and possibly abdominal drains after surgery.

POSTTREATMENT CARE

- Maintain I.V. replacement therapy as ordered.
- Keep the NG tube patent, but don't reposition it.
- Monitor drainage from incisions and provide care of incisions and skin folds, as indicated.
- Encourage regular coughing and deep-breathing exercises.
- Teach the patient to splint the incision site as necessary.
- Monitor the patient's vital signs, intake and output, and daily weight.
- Assist with early ambulation.

⚡ **WARNING** *Monitor the patient for and immediately report signs and symptoms of anastomotic leakage, including low-grade fever, malaise, slight leukocytosis, abdominal distention, tenderness, hemorrhage, hypovolemic shock, bloody stool, and wound drainage.*

- Administer medications as ordered.
- Assess the patient for abdominal pain or cramps and shoulder pain. Explain that bloating or abdominal fullness from laparoscopy will subside as the infused gas is absorbed. Administer analgesics as required.
- Provide comfort measures.

PATIENT TEACHING

GENERAL
- Tell the patient to avoid abdominal straining and lifting until the practitioner approves.
- Tell the patient to return to activities as directed, usually within 3 to 5 weeks.
- Tell the patient to keep follow-up appointments with the surgeon.
- Discuss dumping syndrome and how to minimize it:
– occurs when food moves too quickly through the GI, tract causing nausea, weakness, sweating, faintness and, possibly, diarrhea soon after eating
– commonly triggered by eating highly refined, high-calorie carbohydrates.

- Reinforce the lifestyle changes that are needed, such as consuming only small portions of food high in protein, vitamins, and minerals and minimizing carbohydrates. Remind the patient that initially his appetite is suppressd so he may have to schedule meals.
- Tell the patient that his taste and tolerance for different foods may completely change.
- Tell the patient that because part of the intestine is bypassed, deficiencies may occur in iron, calcium, magnesium, or vitamins. Inform the patient that lifelong fat-soluble (A, D, E, K) vitamin supplementation is necessary to prevent severe anemia, bone loss, and nerve problems and that he may need to work with a dietitian to plan meals.
- Emphasize the need for repeated laboratory studies, such as measuring protein stores. Oral protein supplementation may be necessary.
- Be sure to review the prescribed medications, including dosage and possible adverse effects; incision site care; signs and symptoms of infection; complications; and when to notify the practitioner.

RESOURCES
Organizations
American College of Gastroenterology: *www.acg.gi.org*
American College of Surgeons: *www.facs.org*
American Society for Bariatric Surgery: *www.asbs.org*

Selected references
Crookes, P.F. "Surgical Treatment of Morbid Obesity," *Annual Review of Medicine* 57:243-64, February 2006.
Parikh, M.S., et al. "Objective Comparison of Complications Resulting from Laparoscopic Bariatric Procedures," *Journal of the American College of Surgeons* 202(2):252-61, February 2006.
Vaidya, V. (ed.) "Health and Treatment Strategies in Obesity," *Advances in Psychosomatic Medicine* 27:1-93, 2006.

Bladder and bowel retraining

- May be needed to treat such elimination problems as bladder and fecal incontinence (especially in elderly patients)
- Incontinence: can have serious psychosocial effects and threaten a patient's ability to live independently

INDICATIONS
- Loss or impairment of urinary or anal sphincter control
- Age- or disease-related changes in genitourinary (GU) or GI system function or, less commonly, in other body systems, such as the musculoskeletal and nervous systems
- Fecal stasis and impaction

BLADDER RETRAINING
- Make sure that the patient maintains adequate daily fluid intake.
- Frequently assess the patient's mental and functional status.
- Encourage or assist the patient to void every 2 hours (or more frequently to maintain dryness between voidings).
- Respond to patient calls promptly, and help him get to the bathroom as quickly as possible.
- Implement an exercise program for strengthening pelvic floor muscles such as Kegel exercises.
- Suggest biofeedback to reinforce pelvic muscle contraction as needed.
- When the patient can stay dry for 2 hours, increase the time between voidings by 30 minutes each day until a 3- to 4-hour voiding schedule is achieved.
- Have the patient empty his bladder completely before bedtime.

BOWEL RETRAINING
- Remind or help the patient to get to the toilet or commode 15 to 20 minutes before his usual bowel movement time.
- Ask the patient if the bowel movement felt complete, allowing more time if needed and tolerated.
- Encourage the patient to alternately contract and release his abdominal muscles, sway back and forth on the toilet, or take a large breath, hold briefly while bearing down, and then release it to stimulate peristalsis.

  AGE FACTOR Stay with a patient who has dementia and reinforce the need to remain on the toilet.
- Encourage a fiber-rich diet that includes raw, leafy vegetables, unpeeled fruits, and whole grains, such as bran cereals.
- Encourage adequate daily fluid intake.
- Promote regular exercise.

COMPLICATIONS
- Skin breakdown
- Infection

- Bowel incontinence
- Risk for situational low self-esteem
- Total urinary incontinence

EXPECTED OUTCOMES
The patient will:
- demonstrate bowel continence with a schedule
- demonstrate urinary continence with a schedule
- express feelings of positive self-worth about continence issues.

♦ Explain the treatment and preparation to the patient and his family.
♦ Perform careful assessment of diet, fluid status, dentition and swallowing, usual bowel and bladder patterns in the past and presently, laxative use, ability to comprehend and follow instructions, and abdominal physical findings.
♦ Assess the patient for signs and symptoms of urinary tract infection (UTI).
♦ Provide support and help the patient deal with feelings of shame, embarrassment, or powerlessness caused by loss of control.
♦ Monitor the patient's vital signs, fluid intake and output, and diet patterns to determine baseline values.
♦ Assess the patient for signs of infection or incomplete elimination.
♦ Refer the patient for dental, GU, physical, and speech therapy (for swallowing), as needed to improve contributing factors and proper intake before initiating the therapy program.

♦ Praise the patient's successful efforts.
♦ Encourage persistence, tolerance, and a positive attitude.
♦ Be sensitive to the patient's feelings of embarrassment and low self-confidence.
♦ Maximize the patient's independence while minimizing risks to his self-esteem.
♦ Regularly reassess food and fluid intake, character and patterns of voiding, and mental capacity to respond to the treatment program.

GENERAL

♦ Teach the patient and caregiver how to manage the steps of retraining. (See *Retraining your bladder,* pages 24 and 25.)
♦ Explain that periodic incontinence doesn't mean program failure.
♦ Explain the need for gradual elimination of laxative use, if necessary, and how to transition to the use of natural laxatives, such as prunes or prune juice.
♦ Review medications, such as antibiotics for UTI, and potential adverse reactions.
♦ Review signs and symptoms of infection and when to notify the physician.
♦ Emphasize the importance of follow-up care.

RESOURCES
Organizations
American Association of Clinical Urologists: *www.aacuweb.org*
American Society of Colon and Rectal Surgeons: *www.fascrs.org*
National Association for Continence: *www.nafc.org*

Selected references
Bharucha, A.E. "Update of Tests of Colon and Rectal Structure and Function," *Journal of Clinical Gastroenterology* 40(2):96-103, February 2006.
Jumadilova, Z., et al. "Urinary Incontinence in the Nursing Home: Resident Characteristics and Prevalence of Drug Treatment," *American Journal of Managed Care* 11(Suppl 4):S112-120, July 2005.
Karon, S. "A Team Approach to Bladder Retraining: A Pilot Study," *Urological Nursing* 25(4):269-76, August 2005.

(continued)

Retraining your bladder

Dear Patient,

You can "retrain" your bladder — and correct or manage incontinence — by reestablishing a normal urination pattern.

First you'll keep a careful record of your fluid intake and urination pattern. Then you'll schedule urination at regular intervals and increase the time between urinations gradually. Your goal will be to urinate no more than once every 3 to 4 hours.

STEP 1: KEEPING A RECORD

Do your accidental urinations follow a pattern? You'll know at a glance by recording your fluid intake, how you urinated (intentionally or by accident), and why you think an accident occurred. Keep a chart (like the one shown) throughout your retraining program. Record exact times and amounts. Make notations.

After a few days, your chart will show when you're most likely to become incontinent — for example, after meals or during the night. Your chart will also help your health care provider evaluate your progress and adjust your treatment, if necessary.

DATE				
TIME	FLUID INTAKE	URINATE IN TOILET	SMALL OR LARGE ACCIDENT	REASON FOR ACCIDENT, IF KNOWN
6 to 8 a.m.				
8 to 10 a.m.				
10 a.m. to noon				
Noon to 2 p.m.				
2 to 4 p.m.				
4 to 6 p.m.				
6 to 8 p.m.				
8 to 10 p.m.				
10 p.m. to midnight				
Midnight to 2 a.m.				
2 to 4 a.m.				
4 to 6 a.m.				

STEP 2: SCHEDULING URINATION

Next, schedule specific times to urinate. Practice this technique at home, where you're relaxed and close to the bathroom. Start by urinating every 1½ to 2 hours, whether or not you feel the need. If you have the need to urinate sooner, practice "holding" it by relaxing, concentrating, and taking three slow, deep breaths until the urge decreases or goes away. Wait 5 minutes. Then go to the bathroom and urinate — even if the urge has passed. Otherwise, your next urge may be very strong and difficult to control.

If you have an accident before the 5 minutes have passed, shorten your next waiting time to 3 minutes. After a week of training, if waiting 5 minutes is easy, increase your waiting time to 10 minutes. Using the method above, gradually increse the intervals between urinations. Strive for 3- or 4-hour intervals. Don't get discouraged if you have an accident.

TIPS FOR SUCCESS

◆ Set an alarm clock to remind you when to use the toilet, including once or twice during the night.
◆ Make sure that you can reach the bathroom or portable toilet easily.
◆ Walk to the bathroom slowly.
◆ Always urinate just before bedtime.
◆ Ask your nurse to teach you Kegel exercises, which help increase bladder tone.
◆ Avoid drinks that contan caffeine or alcohol.
◆ Drink between eight and ten 8-ounce (240-milliliter) glasses of fluid every day. This helps prevent urinary tract infection and constipation, which also can cause incontinence. To prevent nighttime accidents, drink most of your fluids before 6 p.m. Remember to count foods containing mostly liquid (such as ice cream, soup, and gelatin) as fluids.

Blood and plasma product transfusion

- Whole blood: blood with all blood components intact
- Packed red blood cells (RBCs): whole blood with 80% of the plasma removed; volume usually 250 ml
- Leukocyte-poor RBCs: same as packed RBCs with about 95% of the leukocytes removed; volume about 200 ml
- Each unit of whole blood or RBCs: contains enough hemoglobin (Hb) to raise the Hb level in an average-size adult by 1 g/dl (by about 3%)
- White blood cells (WBCs or leukocytes): whole blood with all RBCs and about 80% of the plasma removed; volume usually 150 ml
- Platelets: platelet sediment from RBCs or plasma; volume 35 to 50 ml/unit; 1 unit of platelets equal to 10^7 of platelets
- Above products requiring the patient's blood to be identified by ABO and Rh type and crossmatched for antibodies so a matching product can be given
- Fresh frozen plasma (FFP): uncoagulated plasma separated from RBCs and rich in coagulation factors V, VIII, and IX; volume 200 to 250 ml
- Albumin 5% (buffered saline) and albumin 25% (salt-poor saline): small plasma protein prepared by fractionating pooled plasma; volume of 5%, 12.5 g/250 ml; volume of 25%, 12.5 g/50 ml
- Factor VIII: insoluble portion of plasma recovered from FFP; volume about 30 ml (freeze-dried)
- Factors II, VII, IX, and X complex (prothrombin complex): lyophilized, commercially prepared solutions drawn from pooled plasma

- To prevent errors and a potentially fatal reaction, two nurses or practitioners required (per the Joint Commission on Accreditation of Healthcare Organization standards and most facility policies) to identify the patient by two criteria and to double check the blood product compatibility before transfusion
- If the patient is a Jehovah's Witness, special written permission required
- Alternatives to blood transfusions when specific blood components are adequate but volume has been lost: normal saline or lactated Ringer's solution, albumin or purified protein fractions, hydroxyethyl starch or dextrans

INDICATIONS

- Whole blood (rarely used) to rapidly restore blood volume and oxygen-carrying capability of blood as from hemorrhage
- Packed RBCs to maintain or boost oxygen-carrying capability of the blood, such as from blood loss from GI bleeding or surgery or RBC destruction from chemotherapy
- Packed RBCs by exchange transfusion every 3 to 4 weeks in high-risk children with sickle cell anemia to keep sickled hemoglobin below 30% and reduce incidence of stroke
- Leukocyte-poor RBCs for the patient who has had a febrile, nonhemolytic transfusion reaction, caused by WBC antigens reacting with the patient's WBC antibodies or platelets
- WBCs used to treat sepsis unresponsive to antibiotics (especially if the patient has positive blood cultures or a persistent fever exceeding 101° F [38.3° C] and granulocytopenia [granulocyte count usually less than 500/μl])

- Platelets to treat thrombocytopenia caused by decreased platelet production, increased platelet destruction, or massive transfusion of stored blood; to treat acute leukemia and marrow aplasia; and to improve platelet count preoperatively in a patient whose count is 100,000/μl or less
- FFP to correct an undetermined coagulation factor deficiency; to replace a specific factor when it isn't available; and to correct factor deficiencies resulting from hepatic disease

> **WARNING** FFP is no longer indicated for use as a volume expander due to its high load of clotting factors. It's also contraindicated as prophylaxis after cardiopulmonary bypass surgery or with massive blood transfusions.

- Albumin to replace volume lost because of shock from burns, trauma, surgery, or infections; to replace volume and prevent marked hemoconcentration; and to treat hypoproteinemia (with or without edema)
- Factor VIII to treat hemophilia A; to control bleeding associated with factor VIII deficiency; and to replace fibrinogen or deficient factor VIII
- Factors II, VII, IX, and X complex to treat a congenital factor V deficiency and other bleeding disorders resulting from an acquired deficiency of factors II, VII, IX, and X

> **WARNING** Factors II, VII, IX, and X complex transfusions are contraindicated in patients who have hepatic disease resulting in fibrinolysis and in patients who have disseminated intravascular coagulation and aren't undergoing heparin therapy.

◆ Put on gloves, a gown, and a face shield as appropriate.

◆ If the patient doesn't have an I.V. line in place, perform a venipuncture using a 20G or larger-diameter catheter.

AGE FACTOR *Pediatric and elderly patients require a smaller-diameter catheter, such as 20G, to transfuse RBCs because they have smaller veins.*

◆ Prepare a bag of normal saline solution to flush the line before and after transfusion or keep the vein open during a reaction or between transfusions.

◆ Obtain an infusion pump suitable for administering blood per facility policy. Obtain a blood warmer, if ordered, to prevent hypothermia from rapid infusion of large volumes of blood.

WARNING *Only normal saline solution is compatible with blood and plasma products. Never start a transfusion in an I.V. line that has been used for another infusion without flushing the line completely with saline.*

◆ Give whole blood or packed RBCs through a Y-type I.V. set with a 170-micron filter unless a 20- to 40-micron filter (for microaggregates from degenerating platelets and fibrin strands) is ordered.

◆ Administer leukocyte-poor RBCs with a straight-line or Y-type I.V. set to infuse blood over 1½ to 4 hours. Use a 40-micron filter suitable for hard-spun, leukocyte-poor RBCs.

◆ Administer WBCs using a straight-line I.V. set with a standard in-line blood filter to provide 1 unit daily for 5 days or until the infection resolves.

◆ Because a WBC infusion induces fever and chills, administer an antipyretic if fever occurs. Don't discontinue the transfusion; instead, reduce the flow rate, as ordered, for patient comfort.

◆ Agitate the WBC container to prevent settling, thus preventing the delivery of a bolus infusion of WBCs.

◆ Platelets require a component drip administration set to infuse 100 ml over 15 minutes. As prescribed, premedicate with an antipyretic and an antihistamine if the patient's history includes a platelet transfusion reaction. If the patient has a fever before administration, notify the practitioner for probable delay of the transfusion.

◆ For FFP, use a straight-line I.V. set, and administer the infusion rapidly.

◆ For albumin, use a straight-line I.V. set with rate and volume dictated by the patient's condition and response.

◆ For factor VIII, use the administration set supplied by the manufacturer. Administer with a filter; the standard dose recommended for the treatment of acute bleeding episodes in patients with hemophilia is 15 to 20 units/kg.

◆ Factors II, VII, IX, and X complex are administered with a straight-line I.V. set, basing the dose on the desired factor level and the patient's weight.

◆ Adjust the flow rate as appropriate for the component transfusion; remain with the patient and reassess his vital signs and blood pressure, facial color, and any complaints frequently for the initial 15 minutes, according to facility policy.

WARNING *If signs of a reaction develop, stop the transfusion and record the patient's vital signs. Infuse normal saline solution through a new I.V. line at a moderately slow infusion rate, and notify the physician. Save the blood product bag for return to the blood bank. Obtain a urine and blood sample and send them to the laboratory.*

◆ If no signs of a reaction appear within 15 minutes, adjust the flow to the ordered infusion rate, which should be as rapid as the circulatory system can tolerate.

COMPLICATIONS

◆ Transfusion reaction
◆ Infectious disease transmission
◆ Hepatitis C
◆ Circulatory overload
◆ Hemolytic reactions
◆ Coagulation disturbances
◆ Citrate intoxication
◆ Hyperkalemia
◆ Acid-base imbalance
◆ Allergic, febrile, and pyogenic reactions
◆ Hypothermia

(continued)

NURSING DIAGNOSES

- Activity intolerance
- Deficient fluid volume
- Ineffective tissue perfusion: Renal, cerebral, cardiopulmonary

EXPECTED OUTCOMES

The patient will:
- demonstrate increased ability to perform activities of daily living
- maintain adequate fluid volume
- maintain adequate intake and output, vital signs, and blood pressure without deterioration in his level of consciousness.

PRETREATMENT CARE

- Explain the procedure to the patient and verify that he has signed the appropriate consent form.
- Record the patient's baseline vital signs.
- Obtain the blood product from the blood bank no more than 30 minutes before starting the transfusion.
- Check the expiration date on the component bag, and watch for abnormal color, clumping, gas bubbles, and extraneous material.
- Return outdated or abnormal components to the blood bank.
- Compare the name and medical record number on the patient's wrist band with those on the component bag label.
- Check the component bag identification number, ABO blood group, and Rh compatibility, as appropriate.
- Compare the patient's blood bank identification number, if present, with the number on the blood bag.

⚡ **WARNING** *ABO incompatibility from mistakes in blood product labeling or patient identification is the major cause of fatal hemolytic transfusion reactions.*

- Identification of blood and blood products is performed at the patient's bedside by two licensed professionals, according to policy.
- When administering WBCs, premedicate with diphenhydramine (Benadryl) as prescribed.

⚡ **WARNING** *Keep in mind that albumin is contraindicated in patients with severe anemia and administered cautiously to those with cardiac or pulmonary disease due to the risk of heart failure from circulatory overload.*

- Draw blood for a coagulation assay before administration of factors II, VII, IX, and X complex and at suitable intervals during treatment.

POSTTREATMENT CARE

- After completing the transfusion, put on gloves and remove and discard the used infusion equipment in the biohazard material receptacle. Reconnect the original I.V. fluid, if necessary, or discontinue the I.V. infusion.
- Return the empty component bag to the blood bank, if facility policy dictates.
- Record the patient's vital signs.
- Prepare to draw blood for a platelet count, as ordered, 1 hour after platelet administration to determine platelet transfusion increments.
- Large-volume transfusions of FFP may require correction for hypocalcemia because citric acid in FFP binds calcium.
- The half-life of factor VII is 8 to 10 hours, which necessitates repeated transfusions at specified intervals to maintain normal levels.

PATIENT TEACHING

GENERAL

◆ Teach the patient to immediately report the following complaints to the nurse:
- flushing, feverish feeling, chills, nausea, and headache (transfusion reaction)
- palpitations (with hypotension, arrhythmia, and shaking chills; may be sign of hypothermia)
- difficulty swallowing or breathing (possible anaphylaxis)
- tingling in the fingers, muscle cramps, nausea and vomiting, faintness (with hypotension, arrhythmia, and seizures; may signal hypocalcemia from citrate toxicity or liver impairment)
- intestinal colic, diarrhea, muscle weakness (with irritability, oliguria, T-wave changes on the electrocardiogram, and bradycardia; may signal hyperkalemia from large-volume transfusions).

RESOURCES
Organizations

American College of Emergency Physicians: *www.acep.org*
American Medical Association: *www.ama-assn.org*
National Heart, Lung, and Blood Institute, National Institutes of Health: *www.nhlbi.nih.gov*

Selected references

Blajchman, M.A. "The Clinical Benefits of the Leukoreduction of Blood Products," *The Journal of Trauma* 60(Suppl 6):S83-90, June 2006.

Newman, B.H., and Roth, A.J. "Estimating the Probability of a Blood Donation Adverse Event Based on 1000 Interviewed Whole-Blood Donors," *Transfusion* 45(11):1715-721, November 2005.

Sapatnekar, S., et al. "Acute Hemolytic Transfusion Reaction in a Pediatric Patient Following Transfusion of Apheresis Platelets," *Journal of Clinical Apheresis* 20(4):225-29, December 2005.

Bone grafting

- Refers to many surgical methods augmenting or stimulating the formation of new bone where needed
- Used during orthopedic procedures to stimulate the bone to heal and to provide support to the skeleton by filling in gaps between two bones
- A portion of bone graft placed into a space helps support the structure, holding the bones apart while the body grows to the bone graft at either end; over time, the entire piece of bone that was grafted is "remodeled" and replaced with new bone
- Bone taken from the patient's body known as an *autograft* or an *autogenous bone graft;* bone graft taken from someone else's body, such as an organ donor, known as an *allograft;* some major spine fusions need a lot of bone graft, so the surgeon may mix allografts with autografts
- When donated bone tissue is crushed into powder and placed around a fracture or fusion site, chemicals in the bone tissue stimulate healing; with an autograft, living bone cells (called *osteocytes*) survive after transfer to a new location and continue making new bone
- Artificial bone graft materials have been developed, such as sea coral harvested from the ocean; successfully used as the basis for a structural bone replacement
- Demineralized bone matrix (a type of allograft) has been developed from cadaver bones in a bone bank; the bone (with calcium removed) can be made into a putty, sheet, or gel and then added to a graft site to improve fusion (Bone morphogenetic protein is an additional chemical that's added to bone graft and enhances bone growth when added to a fusion site.)
- Minimally invasive bone grafting (when bone marrow or other graft materials are delivered by injection) available; however, most methods require open implantation to ensure adequate space and proper positioning of graft material and allow for removal of scar tissue and dead or poorly vascularized tissue from graft site that might interfere with healing

INDICATIONS

- Stimulation of healing for fractures that are fresh or those that have failed to heal after an initial treatment attempt
- Stimulation of healing between two bones across a diseased joint (arthrodesis or fusion)
- Regeneration of bone that's lost or missing as a result of trauma, infection, or disease
- Improvement of bone healing response and regeneration of bone tissue around surgically implanted devices (artificial joint replacements or plates and screws)

PROCEDURE

- In an autogenous bone graft, the surgeon makes a separate incision and takes a small piece of bone from another area of the body (such as the pelvis or iliac crest). The surgeon transfers the bone graft to the graft site with a needle or by open, incisional surgery. (See *Autogenous bone grafting.*)
- As an alternative, biological products, such as bone graft extenders or bone graft replacements, may be used. An allograft is bone harvested from a cadaver or an organ donor. The bone may be demineralized in which some of the proteins that stimulate bone formation are extracted and readily used as an extender to the patient's own bone.
- Other options include ceramics, calcium phosphates, and other synthetic materials, which have similar biomechanical properties and structure to that of cadaver bone; however, these substances aren't biologically active, nor do they stimulate a spinal fusion by themselves. Although adding the patient's bone marrow cells to these compounds can give them more biological activity, this approach is still being tested.
- Platelet gels may be used because they're easily removed from the patient's blood with few complications. The major disadvantages are that they don't contain osteoinductive proteins and they aren't powerful

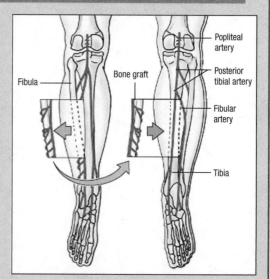

Autogenous bone grafting

During an autogenous bone graft, bone is harvested from the patient's own body such as the iliac crest. Sometimes the blood vessels supplying the bone graft are kept with it and attached to the blood vessels surrounding the recipient site. (The fibula is commonly a source of vascularized bone grafts.) The graft is then placed into the surgical site required.

Fibula

Bone graft

Popliteal artery

Posterior tibial artery

Fibular artery

Tibia

enough stimulants to induce bone formation. They can be used as graft extenders but not graft replacements.

◆ Bone morphogenetic proteins have been produced, concentrated, and placed in the body in areas where bone formation is needed. They're powerful enough to stimulate bone formation without the patient's bone. Several of these proteins are found naturally in the body and play a role in bone formation. The most promising ones are BMP-2 and BMP-7.

COMPLICATIONS

◆ Nerve injury
◆ Infection
◆ Bleeding
◆ Stiffness
◆ Pain and soreness that last well after the surgery, and increased blood loss (autografts)
◆ Graft rejection (allografts)

NURSING DIAGNOSES

◆ Acute pain
◆ Impaired physical mobility
◆ Ineffective tissue perfusion: Peripheral

EXPECTED OUTCOMES

The patient will:
◆ express feelings of increased comfort
◆ attain the highest degree of mobility possible within the confines of the injury
◆ exhibit adequate tissue perfusion and pulses distally.

PRETREATMENT CARE

◆ Explain the treatment and patient preparation.
◆ Verify that the patient has signed the appropriate consent form.
◆ Make sure that prescribed preoperative tests and laboratory work have been completed.
◆ Tell the patient to refrain from taking aspirin and nonsteroidal anti-inflammatory drugs (NSAIDs) 1 week before surgery.

◆ Instruct the patient not to eat or drink anything after midnight.
◆ Have the patient remove all jewelry, body piercings, makeup, nail polish, hairpins, and contact lenses before surgery.
◆ Start an I.V. line and administer fluids as ordered.
◆ Administer medications, such as a prophylactic antiemetic, as ordered.

POSTTREATMENT CARE

◆ Monitor the patient's vital signs and intake and output.
◆ Report laboratory results.
◆ Assess the patient for such complications as infection, hemorrhage, and graft-versus-host disease, as indicated.
◆ Assist with electrical current as indicated; this is known to stimulate bone growth, so many surgeons use electrical stimulation devices during the first weeks after surgery to speed up a fusion.
◆ Elevate the patient's upper body as ordered.
◆ Administer an analgesic, as ordered, for pain.
◆ Provide cast care, as indicated. Monitor the patient for adequate circulation distally, signs of bleeding, compartment syndrome, and infection.
◆ Apply heat to the injured area, as ordered, to improve blood circulation and promote healing.
◆ After the cast is removed, massage the injured area with ice.

PATIENT TEACHING

GENERAL

◆ Tell the patient to follow a nutritious diet and exercise the nonaffected muscle groups to maintain overall health during the recovery process.
◆ Advise the patient to avoid smoking, because nicotine can inhibit fracture healing. The patient should also avoid radiation therapy, chemotherapy, NSAIDs, and systemic corticosteroids because all of these treatments are known to slow bone healing.
◆ Tell the patient that the physician will use an X-ray to determine whether the fracture has fully healed.
◆ Advise and provide instructions about weight bearing as ordered. Activity at home depends on instructions as ordered.

RESOURCES
Organizations
American Academy of Orthopedic Surgeons: *www.aaos.org*
American Medical Association: *www.ama-assn.org*

Selected references
Chougle, A., et al. "Long-Term Survival of the Acetabular Component after Total Hip Arthroplasty With Cement in Patients with Developmental Dysplasia of the Hip," *The Journal of Bone and Joint Surgery* 88(1):71-79, January 2006.

Phipatanakul, W.P., and Norris, T.R. "Treatment of Glenoid Loosening and Bone Loss due to Osteolysis with Glenoid Bone Grafting," *The Journal of Shoulder and Elbow Surgery* 15(1):84-87, January-February 2006.

Yen, C.Y., et al. "Osteonecrosis of the Femoral Head: Comparison of Clinical Results for Vascularized Iliac and Fibula Bone Grafting," *Journal of Reconstructive Microsurgery* 22(1):21-24, January 2006.

Bone growth stimulation, electrical

- Initiates or accelerates the healing process in a fractured bone that fails to heal properly
- Failure to heal: occurs in about 1 in 20 fractures as a result of infection, insufficient reduction or fixation, pseudarthrosis, or severe tissue trauma around the fracture
- Stimulates osteogenesis by imitating the body's natural electrical forces
- Three electrical stimulation techniques: fully implantable direct current stimulation, semi-invasive percutaneous stimulation, and noninvasive electromagnetic coil stimulation (see *Stimulating bone growth with electric current*)
- Choice of technique dependent on the fracture type and location, the physician's preference, or the patient's ability and willingness to comply with the treatment
- Fully implantable device requiring little or no patient management
- Semi-invasive and noninvasive techniques requiring patient to manage his own treatment schedule and maintain the equipment
- Treatment time averaging 3 to 6 months

INDICATIONS

- Treating spinal fusions
- Promoting healing of fractures

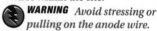 **WARNING** *Electromagnetic coils are contraindicated in pregnant patients, patients with tumors, and patients with arm fractures who also have a pacemaker. Percutaneous electrical bone stimulation is contraindicated if the patient has any kind of inflammation. Use caution in patients sensitive to nickel or chromium because both are present in the electrical bone stimulation system.*

PROCEDURE

DIRECT CURRENT STIMULATION

- Implantation is performed with the patient under general anesthesia.
- A small generator and leadwires that connect to a titanium cathode wire surgically implanted into a nonunited bone site are used.
- The physician may apply a cast or external fixator to immobilize the limb.
- The patient is usually hospitalized for 2 to 3 days after implantation.

PERCUTANEOUS STIMULATION

- Remove excessive hair from the injury site.
- An external anode skin pad is applied with a leadwire and lithium battery pack. The surgeon implants 1 to 4 Teflon-coated stainless steel cathode wires within the site.

WARNING *Avoid stressing or pulling on the anode wire.*

ELECTROMAGNETIC STIMULATION

- A generator is plugged into a standard 110-volt outlet.
- Two strong electromagnetic coils are placed on either side of the injured area. The coils can be incorporated into a cast, cuff, or orthotic device.

COMPLICATIONS

- Infection (with direct current electrical bone stimulation equipment)
- Local irritation or skin ulceration around cathode pin sites (with percutaneous devices)
- No known complications with electromagnetic coils

Stimulating bone growth with electric current

Stimulating bone growth with electric current can be invasive or noninvasive.

INVASIVE SYSTEM

An invasive system involves placing a spiral cathode inside the bone at the fracture site. A wire leads from the cathode to a battery-powered generator, also implanted in local tissues. The patient's body completes the circuit.

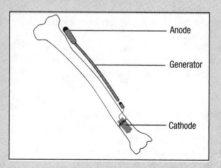

Anode

Generator

Cathode

NONINVASIVE SYSTEM

A noninvasive system may include a cufflike transducer or fitted ring that wraps around the patient's limb at the level of the injury. Electric current penetrates the limb.

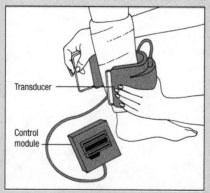

Transducer

Control module

NURSING DIAGNOSES

- Acute pain
- Impaired physical mobility
- Ineffective tissue perfusion: Peripheral

EXPECTED OUTCOMES
The patient will:
- express feelings of increased comfort
- attain the highest degree of mobility possible within the confines of the injury
- exhibit adequate tissue perfusion and pulses distally.

PRETREATMENT CARE

- Follow instructions provided by the manufacturer.
- Make sure that all parts are included and sterilized according to facility policy and procedure.
- Discuss with the patient the use of anesthetics.

POSTTREATMENT CARE

DIRECT CURRENT STIMULATION
- Weight bearing may be ordered as tolerated.
- After the bone fragments join, the generator and leadwire can be removed while the patient is under local anesthesia. The titanium cathode remains implanted.

⚡ **WARNING** *A patient with direct current electrical bone stimulation shouldn't undergo electrocauterization, diathermy, or magnetic resonance imaging (MRI). Electrocautery may "short" the system. Diathermy may potentiate the electrical current, possibly causing tissue damage. MRI will interfere with or stop the current.*

PERCUTANEOUS STIMULATION
- Instruct the patient to change the anode pad every 48 hours.
- Tell the patient to report local pain to his physician and not to bear weight on the limb for the duration of treatment.

ELECTROMAGNETIC STIMULATION
- Show the patient where to place the coils, and tell him to apply them for 3 to 10 hours each day or as ordered.
- Many patients find it most convenient to perform the procedure at night.
- Advise the patient not to interrupt the treatments for more than 10 minutes at a time.
- Teach the patient how to use and care for the generator.
- Restate the physician's instructions for weight bearing. The physician usually advises against bearing weight until evidence of healing appears on X-rays.

PATIENT TEACHING

GENERAL
- Teach the patient how to care for his cast or external fixation devices.
- Tell the patient how to care for the electrical generator.
- Urge the patient to follow treatment instructions.
- Tell the patient to report increasing discomfort from the procedure as well as signs of infection or circulatory compromise.
- Review activity restrictions with the patient.
- Teach the patient with a direct current implant to inform all health care providers of the implant, and not to have MRI testing or diathermy treatments, or any procedure where blood vessels might be treated electrically.

RESOURCES
Organizations
American Academy of Orthopedic Surgeons: *www.aaos.org*
American Medical Association: *www.ama-assn.org*

Selected references
Cowan, C.M., et al. "Nell-1 Induced Bone Formation within the Distracted Intermaxillary Suture," *Bone* 38(1):48-58, January 2006.
Harle, J., et al. "Effects of Ultrasound on Transforming Growth Factor-Beta Genes in Bone Cells," *European Cells & Materials* (electronic resource) 10:70-76; discussion 76, December 2005.
Weinraub, G.M. "Orthobiologics: A Survey of Materials and Techniques," *Clinics in Podiatric Medicine and Surgery of North America* 22(4):509-19, v. Review, October 2005.

Bowel resection

- In bowel resection with ostomy: diseased bowel excised and stoma created on the outer abdominal wall for feces elimination; laparoscopic approach possible for standard colostomy and end-ileostomy
- In bowel resection with anastomosis: diseased intestinal tissue surgically resected and remaining segments connected or anastomosed (preferred surgical technique for treating localized bowel cancer)

INDICATIONS
Bowel resection with ostomy
- Inflammatory bowel disease
- Familial adenomatous polyposis
- Diverticulitis
- Advanced colorectal cancer

Bowel resection with anastomosis
- Localized obstructive disorders secondary to diverticulitis, intestinal polyps, adhesions, or malignant or benign intestinal lesions

- All procedures are performed under general anesthesia

BOWEL RESECTION WITH OSTOMY
- The surgeon makes an incision in the abdominal wall. (The location depends on the bowel area to be resected and type of ostomy required.)
- The diseased bowel segment is resected, possibly along with several more inches of bowel.
- The surgeon creates a stoma.

Abdominoperineal resection
- A low abdominal incision is made and the sigmoid colon is divided.
- The proximal end of the colon is brought out through another, smaller abdominal incision to create an end stoma.
- A wide perineal incision is made and the anus, rectum, and distal portion of the sigmoid colon are resected.
- The abdominal wound is closed and abdominal drains are placed.
- The perineal wound may be left open, packed with gauze, or closed; several Penrose drains are placed.

Ileostomy
- The surgeon resects all or part of the colon and rectum (proctocolectomy).
- A permanent ileostomy is created by bringing the end of the ileum out through a small abdominal incision in the right lower quadrant to create a stoma.

Ileoanal reservoir
- A colectomy is performed and an ileal loop or the distal ileum is used to create a stoma for a temporary ileostomy.
- The rectal mucosal layer is removed and an internal pouch is made with a portion of the ileum.
- A pouch-anal anastomosis is performed.
- The temporary ileostomy is usually closed after 3 to 4 months.

Kock ileostomy
- The surgeon removes the colon, rectum, and anus, and closes the anus.
- A reservoir is constructed from a loop of the terminal ileum.
- A portion of the ileum is intussuscepted to form a nipple valve.
- The upper part of the sutured and cut ileum is pulled down and sutured to form a pouch.
- The nipple valve is used to create a stoma by pulling it through the abdominal wall and suturing it flush with the skin. A catheter is placed in the stoma.

BOWEL RESECTION WITH ANASTOMOSIS
- An abdominal incision is made, depending on location of the lesion.
- The diseased area is resected, along with a wide margin of surrounding normal tissue.
- Remaining bowel segments are anastomosed end-to-end or side-to-side.
- The incision is closed.
- A sterile dressing is applied.

COMPLICATIONS
- Hemorrhage
- Sepsis
- Ileus
- Fluid and electrolyte imbalance
- Skin excoriation
- Pelvic abscess
- Incompetent nipple valve (with a Kock ileostomy)
- Bleeding or leakage from the anastomosis site
- Peritonitis, postresection obstruction, wound infection, or atelectasis
- Psychological problems

- Acute pain
- Anxiety
- Ineffective tissue perfusion: GI

EXPECTED OUTCOMES
The patient will:
- demonstrate or express feelings of increased comfort
- verbalize and show signs of decreased anxiety
- regain regular bowel movements.

PRETREATMENT CARE

- Explain preoperative and postoperative procedures and equipment to the patient and his family.
- Discuss postoperative analgesia.
- Verify that the patient has signed the appropriate consent form.
- Tell the patient what to expect for fecal drainage and bowel movement control for the type of ostomy performed.
- Provide total parenteral nutrition as ordered.
- Administer an antibiotic and other medications as ordered.
- Monitor the patient's vital signs, nutritional status, fluid and electrolyte status, intake and output, and daily weight.

POSTTREATMENT CARE

- Provide meticulous wound care.
- Administer an analgesic as ordered.
- Maintain I.V. replacement therapy as ordered.
- Keep the nasogastric tube patent, but don't reposition it.
- After an abdominoperineal resection, irrigate the perineal area as ordered.
- If the patient has a Kock pouch with a catheter inserted in the stoma:
– Connect the catheter to low intermittent suction or to straight drainage as ordered.

– Check catheter patency regularly, and irrigate with 20 to 30 ml of normal saline solution as ordered.
– Assess pouch drainage and advance the patient's diet as ordered.
– Clamp and unclamp the pouch catheter to increase its capacity as ordered.
- Encourage the patient to express feelings and concerns.
- Arrange for a consultation with an enterostomal therapist as appropriate.
- Arrange for the patient to meet with a well-adjusted ostomy patient if possible.
- Monitor the patient's vital signs and intake and output.
- Assess the patient for dehydration and electrolyte imbalance.
- Assess stoma appearance and drainage. Look for skin irritation and excoriation.
- Monitor the patient for signs of infection, peritonitis, and sepsis.

⚡ **WARNING** *Immediately report excessive blood or mucus draining from the stoma, which could indicate hemorrhage or infection.*

- Encourage deep-breathing and coughing exercises. Encourage splinting of the incision site as necessary.
- For anastomosis patients, encourage oral fluid intake and give stool softeners and laxatives as ordered.

⚡ **WARNING** *Monitor for and immediately report signs and symptoms of anastomotic leakage, including low-grade fever, malaise, slight leukocytosis, abdominal distention, tenderness, hemorrhage, hypovolemic shock, and bloody stool or wound drainage.*

GENERAL
- Review prescribed medications, including the dosage and possible adverse effects.
- Explain ostomy type and function and review care of ostomy appliances.
- Discuss resumption of sexual intercourse.
- Review stoma and skin care.
- Explain dietary restrictions and emphasize the importance of a high fluid intake.
- Explain the need for avoidance of alcohol, laxatives, and diuretics (unless approved by the physician).
- Review bowel retraining for appropriate ostomy patients.
- Review the use of sitz baths (after abdominoperineal resection).
- Review the signs and symptoms of inflammation and infection and when to notify the physician.
- Emphasize the need for follow-up care.

RESOURCES
Organizations
American College of Gastroenterology: *www.acg.gi.org*
American College of Surgeons: *www.facs.org*

Selected references
Chan, K.Y., et al. "Chylous Ascites after Anterior Resection for Rectal Carcinoma: A Rare but Significant Incident," *Asian Journal of Surgery* 29(1):46-48, January 2006.
Chang, R.W., et al. "Serial Transverse Enteroplasty Enhances Intestinal Function in a Model of Short Bowel Syndrome," *Annals of Surgery* 243(2):223-28, February 2006.
O'Keefe, S.J., et al. "Short Bowel Syndrome and Intestinal Failure: Consensus Definitions and Overview," *Clinical Gastroenterology and Hepatology* 4(1):6-10, January 2006.

Breast reconstruction

OVERVIEW

- One of several methods used to rebuild the breast after mastectomy, depending on the patient's needs; method of surgery also dependent on choice of a flap (or expander) and implant
- With breast reconstruction under the skin: breast tissue removed but skin and nipple preserved; implant then placed beneath skin to replace lost breast tissue (suitable only for women with fairly small breasts)
- With breast reconstruction under the muscle: implant placed beneath the muscles covering the chest; approach suitable only for women with fairly small breasts and impossible if the patient underwent radical mastectomy, in which the chest muscle has been taken away or if the patient has received radiotherapy, in which the muscles and skin are unlikely to stretch
- Breast reconstruction involving tissue expansion: makes use of the ability of the skin and muscle to stretch through the use of an expandable implant with a valve for filling it; expansion takes place over a few months by injecting a sterile saline solution into the implant through a valve that's just under the skin of the armpit; process continues until size is slightly larger than the remaining breast, thus permitting insertion of a permanent implant
- Another option: using areas of muscle and skin (known as *flaps*) that are taken from the back (latissimus dorsi) or abdomen (rectus abdominis) (These areas of the body contain very large muscles, providing enough skin, fat, and muscle with a good blood supply to create the shape of a breast on the chest wall. It's appropriate when tissue expansion is unsuitable because a lot of skin and muscle needs to be removed—or has been removed—from the breast. It's also useful where previous radiotherapy has made the skin unsuitable for tissue expansion or when reconstructing large breasts.)

INDICATIONS

- To rebuild the breast after mastectomy

PROCEDURE

SKIN EXPANSION

- Following mastectomy, the surgeon inserts a balloon expander beneath the skin and chest muscle.
- Through a tiny valve mechanism buried beneath the skin, the physician periodically injects saline solution to gradually fill the expander over several weeks or months.
- After the skin has stretched enough, the expander is removed in a second operation and a more permanent implant is inserted. Some expanders are designed to be left in place as the final implant.
- The nipple and the areola are reconstructed in a subsequent procedure.
- Some patients don't require preliminary tissue expansion before receiving an implant. Instead, the surgeon inserts an implant as the first step.

FLAP RECONSTRUCTION

- In one type of flap surgery, the tissue remains attached to its original site, retaining its blood supply. The flap, consisting of the skin, fat, and muscle with its blood supply, is tunneled beneath the skin to the chest by the surgeon, creating a pocket for an implant. It can also be made to create the breast mound itself, without the need for an implant.
- Another flap technique uses tissue that's surgically removed from the abdomen, thighs, or buttocks and then transplanted to the chest by reconnecting the blood vessels to new ones in that region. This procedure requires the skill of a plastic surgeon who's experienced in microvascular surgery as well. (See *Reconstructing the breast with a flap*.)

FOLLOW-UP PROCEDURE

- Follow-up surgery may be required to replace a tissue expander with an implant or to reconstruct the nipple and areola.

Reconstructing the breast with a flap

Flaps may be taken from large muscles of the body. In this breast reconstruction, the latissimus dorsi muscle is taken and moved to its new location.

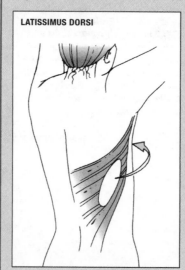

LATISSIMUS DORSI

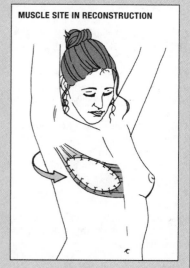

MUSCLE SITE IN RECONSTRUCTION

- Many surgeons recommend an additional operation to enlarge, reduce, or lift the natural breast to match the reconstructed breast.

COMPLICATIONS
- Bleeding
- Fluid collection and swelling
- Bruising
- Excessive scar tissue
- Numbness or change in feeling
- Infection from the implant (the implant may need to be removed for several months until the infection clears; a new implant can later be inserted)
- Capsular contracture (the scar or capsule around the implant begins to tighten)
- Complications with flap source site (limited movement)

NURSING DIAGNOSES

- Acute pain
- Impaired tissue integrity
- Risk for infection

EXPECTED OUTCOMES
The patient will:
- verbalize or demonstrate feelings of comfort
- demonstrate healing of wounds
- show no signs of infection.

PRETREATMENT CARE

- Women with other health conditions, such as obesity, high blood pressure, or smoking, may be advised to wait until these conditions are under control.
- Explain the treatment and preparation to the patient and her family.
- Verify that the patient has signed the appropriate consent form
- Explain postoperative care.
- Provide emotional support.

POSTTREATMENT CARE

- Monitor the patient's vital signs and intake and output.
- Monitor drainage from the wound and provide skin care.
- Assess the patient for pain and provide an analgesic as ordered.
- Monitor the patient for infection, hemorrhage, and other signs of complications.
- Elevate the patient's arm on a pillow; position it to facilitate drainage, ensuring also that the patient is comfortable.
- Initiate flexion and extension arm exercises as ordered.
- Place a sign in the patient's room indicating that no blood pressure readings, injections, or venipunctures should be performed on the affected arm.

PATIENT TEACHING

GENERAL
- Advise the patient to stop smoking; nicotine can delay healing, resulting in conspicuous scars and prolonged recovery. Occasionally, these complications are severe enough to require a second operation.
- Tell the patient that the surgical drain to remove excess fluids from the site is removed within the first week or two after surgery. Most stitches are removed in 7 to 10 days.
- Review the prescribed medications, including the dosage and possible adverse effects.
- Tell the patient which signs and symptoms she should report to the physician, such as infection or increasing pain.
- Review exercises, as ordered, and care of the operative site.
- Tell the patient to have venipunctures, injections, and blood pressure measurements in the unaffected arm only.

RESOURCES
Organizations
American Cancer Society: *www.cancer.org*
American College of Surgeons: *www.facs.org*
American Society of Plastic Surgeons: *www.plasticsurgery.org*

Selected references
Chan, L.K., et al. "Smoking and Wound Healing Problems in Reduction Mammaplasty: Is the Introduction of Urine Nicotine Testing Justified?" *Annals of Plastic Surgery* 56(2):111-15, February 2006.
Christian, C.K., et al. "A Multi-Institutional Analysis of the Socioeconomic Determinants of Breast Reconstruction: A Study of the National Comprehensive Cancer Network," *Annals of Surgery* 243(2):241-49, February 2006.
Shafir, R., and Gur, E. "Defining the 'Gold Standard' in Breast Reconstruction with Abdominal Tissue," *Plastic Reconstructive Surgery* 117(1):315-17, January 2006.

Bronchoscopy

- Involves direct visualization of the larynx, trachea, and bronchi using a rigid or fiber-optic bronchoscope
- Flexible fiber-optic bronchoscope: allows a better view of the segmental and subsegmental bronchi with less risk of trauma
- Large, rigid bronchoscope: used to remove foreign objects, excise endobronchial lesions, and control massive hemoptysis (requires general anesthesia)

INDICATIONS

- Visual examination of tumors, obstructions, secretions, or foreign bodies in the tracheobronchial tree
- Diagnosis of bronchogenic carcinoma, tuberculosis, interstitial pulmonary disease, and fungal or parasitic pulmonary infections
- Specimens for microbiological and cytologic examination
- Bleeding sites in the tracheobronchial tree
- Removal of foreign bodies, malignant or benign tumors, mucus plugs, and excessive secretions from the tracheobronchial tree

- The patient is properly positioned and given supplemental oxygen if ordered.
- Pulse oximetry, vital signs, and cardiac rhythm are monitored.
- Local anesthetic is sprayed into the mouth and throat.
- The bronchoscope is inserted through the mouth or nose; a bite block is placed in the mouth if using the oral approach.
- When the bronchoscope is just above the vocal cords, 3 to 4 ml of 2% to 4% lidocaine is flushed through the inner channel to the vocal cords.
- A fiber-optic camera is used to take photographs for documentation.
- Tissue specimens are obtained from suspect areas.
- A suction apparatus may remove foreign bodies or mucus plugs.
- Bronchoalveolar lavage may remove thickened secretions or may aid in the diagnosis of infectious causes of infiltrates.
- Specimens are properly prepared and immediately sent to the laboratory.

COMPLICATIONS

- Subcutaneous crepitus, which may indicate tracheal or bronchial perforation or pneumothorax
- Laryngeal edema or laryngospasm causing stridor and dyspnea
- Hypoxemia
- Cardiac arrhythmias
- Bleeding
- Infection
- Bronchospasm

- Impaired gas exchange
- Ineffective breathing pattern
- Ineffective tissue perfusion: Cardiopulmonary

EXPECTED OUTCOMES
The patient will:
- maintain adequate ventilation
- exhibit normal breathing pattern
- maintain normal heart and respiratory rates, blood pressure, and have pink nail beds and mucosa.

PRETREATMENT CARE

- Review with the patient the purpose of the test and how it's performed, including who will perform it and where.
- Reassure the patient that the airway isn't blocked during the test.
- Verify that the patient has signed the appropriate consent form and note any allergies.
- Instruct the patient to fast for 6 to 12 hours before the test.
- Obtain the patient's vital signs and results of preprocedure studies. Report abnormal results.
- Administer an I.V. sedative as ordered.
- Remove the patient's dentures.
- Inform the patient that his airway won't be blocked and that hoarseness, loss of voice, hemoptysis, and sore throat may occur.

POSTTREATMENT CARE

- If the patient is conscious, position him in semi-Fowler's position. If the patient is unconscious, position him on one side with the head of his bed slightly elevated.
- Instruct the patient to spit out saliva rather than swallow it.
- Observe the patient for bleeding.
- Maintain nothing-by-mouth status until the gag reflex returns.
- Help the patient resume his usual diet, beginning with sips of clear liquid or ice chips, when the gag reflex returns.
- Provide lozenges or a soothing liquid gargle to ease discomfort when the gag reflex returns.
- Check the follow-up chest X-ray for pneumothorax.
- Monitor the patient's vital signs, sputum characteristics, and respiratory status.

  WARNING *Immediately report subcutaneous crepitus around the patient's face, neck, or chest because these may indicate tracheal or bronchial perforation or pneumothorax.*

  WARNING *Watch for and immediately report signs and symptoms of respiratory difficulty associated with laryngeal edema or laryngospasm, such as laryngeal stridor and dyspnea.*

PATIENT TEACHING

GENERAL

- Tell the patient that hoarseness, loss of voice, hemoptysis, and sore throat may occur.

RESOURCES

Organizations

American College of Chest Physicians: *www.chestnet.org*

American College of Emergency Physicians: *www.acep.org*

American Medical Association: *www.ama-assn.org*

Selected references

Kvale, P.A. "Chronic Cough Due to Lung Tumors: ACCP Evidence-Based Clinical Practice Guidelines," *Chest* 129(Suppl 1):147S-153S, January 2006.

Moorthy, S.S., et al. "Management of Airway in Patients with Laryngeal Tumors," *Journal of Clinical Anesthesia* 17(8):604-609, December 2005.

Tomaske, M., et al. "Anesthesia and Peri-interventional Morbidity of Rigid Bronchoscopy for Tracheobronchial Foreign Body Diagnosis and Removal," *Paediatric Anaesthesia* 16(2):123-29, February 2006.

Cardiomyoplasty

OVERVIEW

- Surgical procedure in which the patient's skeletal muscle—usually the latissimus dorsi—is wrapped around weakened heart muscle to provide support
- After wrapping: a pulse generator implanted near the abdomen stimulates the implanted muscle to contract simultaneously with the heart; skeletal muscle eventually becoming resistant to fatigue
- Still considered experimental (left ventricular assist devices usually used); performed only at a few well-established heart centers in the country, with variable results
- In some patients, produces a small increase in left ventricular ejection fraction, thus a reduction of symptoms for a few months after surgery; however, latissimus dorsi muscle may not be able to sustain beneficial effect over time
- Also known as *cardiac wrap* and *muscle-flap procedure*

INDICATIONS

- Advanced heart failure
- Ischemic or dilated cardiomyopathy

PROCEDURE

- The surgeon dissects a portion of the left latissimus dorsi muscle from its surrounding tissues, leaving the neurovascular supply intact.
- Two stimulation electrodes are attached to the muscle flap.
- The muscle flap is then transposed into the left thoracic cavity through a window created by a partial resection of the second rib.
- A median sternotomy is performed to open the pericardium and access the heart. Sensing electrodes are then implanted into the right and left ventricles.
- The muscle flap is then rotated inward and wrapped around the ventricular surface of the heart and is then attached to the pericardium with sutures.
- The pacing and sending electrodes are then attached to a special pacemaker that's implanted in an epigastric pocket.
- After a 2-week postoperative period, to allow for adhesion between the latissimus dorsi and the heart, the skeletal muscle is electrostimulated and conditioned to pace synchronously with the heart.

  WARNING *Cardiomyoplasty requires the use of a unique pacemaker manufactured by Medtronic (the Transform Cardiomyostimulator); however, to date, it hasn't yet received Food and Drug Administration (FDA) approval. Therefore, the procedure is offered only in an FDA investigational device exemption trial; clinical trials are ongoing.*

COMPLICATIONS

- Infection
- Cardiac tamponade
- Failure of graft procedure and return of heart failure symptoms
- Hemothorax, pneumothorax
- Arrhythmias

NURSING DIAGNOSES

- Activity intolerance
- Decreased cardiac output
- Ineffective tissue perfusion: Cardiopulmonary

EXPECTED OUTCOMES

The patient will:

- carry out activities of daily living without excess fatigue or decreased energy
- maintain adequate cardiac output
- maintain adequate tissue perfusion.

PRETREATMENT CARE

- Review the procedure with the patient, and verify that he has signed a consent form.
- Monitor the patient's vital signs, intake and output, and hemodynamic status.
- Obtain laboratory results and notify the surgeon of the results.

POSTTREATMENT CARE

- Monitor the patient's vital signs and mental status.
- Monitor hemodynamic status and report changes in trends.
- Monitor for signs of complications and report symptoms as indicated.
- Monitor the electrocardiogram for new-onset arrhythmias and report as indicated.
- Monitor intake and output.
- Monitor the patient for and report abnormal heart and breath sounds immediately.
- Monitor results of laboratory studies.
- Maintain patency of I.V. lines and maintain fluids as ordered.
- Maintain patency of chest tubes and monitor drainage; report signs of bleeding or alterations in pulmonary status.
- Provide wound care and assess dressings as indicated.
- Maintain oxygenation status, and suction as indicated.
- Monitor for pain and effects of pain medication as ordered.

PATIENT TEACHING

GENERAL

- Inform the patient about the signs and symptoms of heart failure and when to notify the practitioner.
- Refer the patient for follow-up care.

RESOURCES

Organizations

American College of Cardiology:
www.acc.org
American Medical Association:
www.ama-assn.org
HeartCenterOnline:
www.heartcenteronline.com

Selected references

Bosen, D.M. "New Strategies for Treating Patients with Heart Failure," *Nursing* 33(12):44-47, December 2003.

Egerod, I., and Hansen, G.M. "Evidence-Based Practice among Danish Cardiac Nurses: A National Survey," *Journal of Advanced Nursing* 51(5):465-73, September 2005.

Nesher, N., et al. "Thermo-Wrap Technology Preserves Normothermia Better than Routine Thermal Care in Patients Undergoing Off-Pump Coronary Artery Bypass and is Associated with Lower Immune Response and Lesser Myocardial Damage," *Journal of Thoracic and Cardiovascular Surgery* 129(6):1371-78, June 2005.

Odim, J., et al. "Results of Aortic Valve-Sparing and Restoration with Autologous Pericardial Leaflet Extensions in Congenital Heart Disease," *Annals of Thoracic Surgery* 80(2):647-53, August 2005.

Olearchyk, A.S. "Congenital Bicuspid Aortic Valve and an Aneurysm of the Ascending Aorta," *Journal of Cardiovascular Surgery* 19(5):462-63, September-October 2004.

Cardioversion, synchronized

- Used to treat tachyarrhythmias; delivers an electric charge to the myocardium at the peak of the R wave, which causes immediate depolarization, interrupting reentry circuits and allowing the sinoatrial node to resume control
- Also treatment of choice for arrhythmias that don't respond to vagal maneuvers or drug therapy, such as atrial tachycardia, atrial flutter, atrial fibrillation, and symptomatic monomorphic ventricular tachycardia
- Synchronizes electric charge with R wave to ensure that current won't be delivered on the vulnerable T wave and, thus, disrupt repolarization
- May be an elective or urgent procedure, depending on how well the patient tolerates the arrhythmia; for example, with hemodynamically unstable patient, immediate cardioversion needed

INDICATIONS

- Unstable supraventricular tachycardia due to reentry
- Atrial fibrillation
- Atrial flutter
- Unstable monomorphic ventricular tachycardia

PROCEDURE

- Verify the patient's identity using two patient identifiers according to facility policy.
- Consider administering oxygen for 5 to 10 minutes before the cardioversion to promote myocardial oxygenation.
- Connect the patient to a pulse oximeter and automatic blood pressure cuff, if available.

⚡ **WARNING** *Remember that when preparing for cardioversion, the patient's condition can deteriorate quickly, necessitating immediate defibrillation.*

- If the patient wears dentures, evaluate whether they support his airway or may cause an airway obstruction. If they may cause an obstruction, remove them.
- Place the patient in the supine position and assess his vital signs, level of consciousness (LOC), cardiac rhythm, and peripheral pulses.
- Remove any oxygen delivery device just before cardioversion to avoid possible combustion.
- Have emergency cardiac medications at the patient's bedside.
- Make sure that the resuscitation bag is at the patient's bedside.
- Administer a sedative as ordered. The patient should be sedated but still able to breathe adequately.
- Carefully monitor the patient's blood pressure and respiratory rate until he recovers from the sedation.
- Press the POWER button to turn on the defibrillator.
- Push the SYNC button to synchronize the machine with the patient's QRS complexes. Make sure that the SYNC button flashes with each of the patient's QRS complexes. You should also see a marker on the monitor to signify correct synchronization.
- Turn the ENERGY SELECT dial to the ordered amount of energy. Advanced cardiac life support protocols call for an initial monophasic energy dose of 50 to 100 joules for a patient with unstable supraventricular tachycardia, 100 to 200 joules for a patient with atrial fibrillation, 50 to 100 joules for a patient with atrial flutter, and 100 joules for a patient who has ventricular tachycardia with a pulse (or clinically equivalent biphasic energy dose). Increase the second and subsequent shock doses as needed.
- Remove the paddles from the machine, and prepare them as you would if you were defibrillating the patient.
- Place the conductive gel pads or paddles in the same positions as you would to defibrillate.

⚡ **WARNING** *To prevent damage to an implanted pacemaker, avoid placing the paddles directly over the pacemaker.*

- Make sure that everyone stands away from the bed, and move equipment that's touching the bed or patient.
- Discharge the current by pushing the DISCHARGE buttons of both paddles simultaneously or pressing the SHOCK button on the mahcine; don't remove the paddles from the patient's chest until the device discharges. (Unlike in defibrillation, the discharge won't occur immediately; you'll notice a slight delay while the machine synchronizes with the R wave.)
- Hold the paddles in place and wait for the energy to be discharged — the machine has to synchronize the discharge with the QRS complex.
- Check the waveform on the monitor.
- If the arrhythmia fails to convert, repeat the procedure. Gradually increase the energy level to a maximum of 360 joules with each additional countershock.

⚡ **WARNING** *Be aware that improper synchronization may result if the patient's electrocardiogram (ECG) tracing contains artifact-like spikes, such as peaked T waves or bundle-branch heart blocks when the R' wave may be taller than the R wave.*

COMPLICATIONS

- Transient, harmless arrhythmias, such as atrial, ventricular, and junctional premature beats
- Serious ventricular arrhythmias such as ventricular fibrillation

⚡ **WARNING** *Ventricular fibrillation is more likely to result from high amounts of electrical energy, digoxin toxicity, severe heart disease, electrolyte imbalance, or improper synchronization with the R wave.*

NURSING DIAGNOSES

◆ Decreased cardiac output
◆ Impaired gas exchange
◆ Ineffective tissue perfusion: Cardio-pulmonary, cerebral, peripheral

EXPECTED OUTCOMES
The patient will:
◆ demonstrate hemodynamic stability
◆ maintain adequate oxygenation and perfusion
◆ maintain adequate blood pressure, heart rate, and peripheral pulses.

PRETREATMENT CARE

◆ Explain the procedure to the patient, reinforce the practitioner's explanation of the procedure, and verify that the patient has signed a consent form.
◆ Check the patient's recent serum potassium and magnesium levels, arterial blood gas levels, and recent digoxin levels.

⚡ **WARNING** *If the patient takes digoxin, reduce or withhold the dose on the day of the procedure to avoid induction of ventricular arrhythmias.*

◆ Withhold food and fluids for 6 to 12 hours before the procedure.
◆ If the cardioversion is urgent, withhold the previous meal.
◆ Obtain a 12-lead ECG to serve as a baseline.
◆ Check to see if the practitioner has ordered administration of any cardiac drugs before the procedure.
◆ Verify that the patient has a patent I.V. site in case drug administration becomes necessary.

POSTTREATMENT CARE

◆ After the cardioversion, frequently assess the patient's LOC and respiratory status, including airway patency, respiratory rate and depth, and the need for supplemental oxygen.

⚡ **WARNING** *Because the patient is sedated, he may require airway support.*

◆ Record a postcardioversion 12-lead ECG, and monitor the patient's ECG rhythm.
◆ Check the patient's chest for electrical burns.

PATIENT TEACHING

GENERAL
◆ Review with the patient how to take his pulse and record it for the practitioner to review on follow-up visits.
◆ Review signs and symptoms to report (recurrence of previous rhythm).

RESOURCES
Organizations
American College of Cardiology:
www.acc.org
American Medical Association:
www.ama-assn.org
HeartCenterOnline:
www.heartcenteronline.com

Selected references
"Critical Care: Ablation Helps Some Patients with Atrial Fibrillation and Heart Failure," *Nursing 2005* 35(1):32cc8-32cc8, January 2005.
Frodsham R. "Cardiac Resynchronisation Therapy for Patients with Heart Failure," *Nursing Standard: Official Newspaper of the Royal College of Nursing* 19(45):46-50, July 2005.
Quinn T. "The Role of Nurses in Improving Emergency Cardiac Care," *Nursing Standard: Official Newspaper of the Royal College of Nursing* 19(48):41-48, August 2005.
Thompson, E.J. "Radiofrequency Ablation in the Pulmonary Veins for Paroxysmal, Drug-Resistant Atrial Fibrillation," *Dimensions of Critical Care Nursing* 23(6):255-63, November-December 2004.
Wickliffe, A.C., and Leon, A.R. "Pacing and Heart Failure: Should all Patients Receive a Biventricular Device?" *Current Heart Failure Report* 2(1):35-59, March 2005.

Carpal tunnel release

OVERVIEW

- Carpal tunnel syndrome: most common nerve entrapment syndrome; results from compression of the median nerve in the wrist where it passes though the carpal tunnel, causing loss of movement and sensation in the wrist, hand, and fingers (see *Locating the carpal tunnel*)

- Surgery to decompress the median nerve that relieves pain and restores function in the wrist and hand (see *Relieving symptoms of carpal tunnel syndrome*)

INDICATIONS

- Carpal tunnel syndrome unrelieved by splinting or medication

PROCEDURE

- The procedure may be performed as outpatient surgery using local anesthesia.
- The surgeon can choose from several approaches to perform carpal tunnel release. However, entire transverse carpal tunnel ligament must be transected to ensure adequate decompression of the median nerve.
- The surgeon makes an incision around the thenar eminence to expose the flexor retinaculum, which he then transects to relieve pressure on the median nerve. Depending on the extent of nerve compression, he may perform neurolysis to free flattened nerve fibers. Neurolysis involves stretching the nerve, which relieves tension and loosens surrounding adhesions.
- Decompression of the median nerve can also be accomplished through a small incision in a puncture site via endoscopic carpal tunnel release. In the endoscopic procedure, which may be single portal or double portal, the carpal tunnel is approached through small incisions that allow the passage of the endoscope along the ulnar border of the transverse carpal ligament. The ligament is sharply divided after transverse fibers are well visualized. The antebrachial fascia proximally is divided under direct vision.

  ⚡ **WARNING** *Contraindications to the procedure include rheumatoid arthritis, mass lesions, and repeat surgery.*

COMPLICATIONS
- Hematoma formation
- Infection
- Painful scar formation
- Tenosynovitis
- Nerve damage

Locating the carpal tunnel

The carpal tunnel lies between the longitudinal tendons of the hand-flexing forearm muscles (not shown) and the transverse carpal ligament. Note the median nerve and flexor tendons passing through the tunnel on their way from the forearm to the hand.

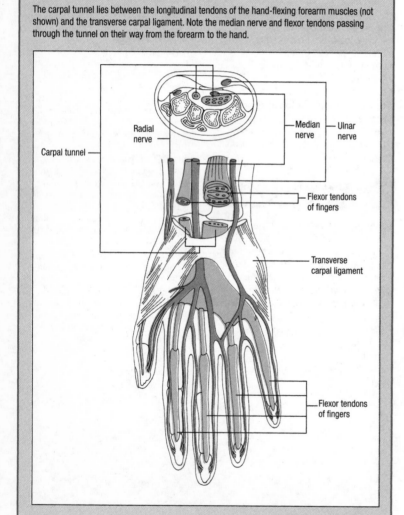

Radial nerve

Carpal tunnel

Median nerve

Ulnar nerve

Flexor tendons of fingers

Transverse carpal ligament

Flexor tendons of fingers

Relieving symptoms of carpal tunnel syndrome

Dear Patient,

If you're having symptoms of carpal tunnel syndrome, you know how disabling they can be. You know, too, that strain on your wrist nerve triggers your discomfort. To get relief and prevent permanent damage, you need to *stop* or *cut back* on the activity producing the strain.

    Of course, that's easier said than done. If the activities that produce strain are related to your job or hobbies, stopping or decreasing them takes careful planning. Use the following suggestions to help.

MAKE CHANGES AT WORK

Modify your work habits and work area. If you work on an assembly line, do piecework, or have a repetitive job, ask your supervisor to help you change or eliminate activities that strain your wrist. For example:

◆ Make sure that the tools you use fit your hand correctly so you don't need to twist your wrist too much when turning, gripping, or squeezing objects.

◆ If you must lift and move objects, use both hands rather than the hand with carpal tunnel syndrome.

◆ Install a padded armrest at your workstation to relieve stress on your hands, wrists, and shoulders.

◆ Arrange to rotate your duties, or find a different technique for doing your job that puts less stress on your wrist.

◆ If you work at a typewriter, computer, or another type of terminal, try lowering the height of your work table to decrease the angle of wrist flexion.

◆ Raise your chair or sit on a pillow if you can't adjust your work table. Just be sure to support your feet to promote good posture and good circulation in your lower legs.

WEAR A RESTRAINING DEVICE

Wear a splint or a specially designed glove when you perform repetitive activities—or all the time, if your health care provider advises. These devices are available by prescription from medical supply stores.

SLOW DOWN

Slow down when performing repetitive activities with your hands. For example, if knitting causes symptoms, you can knit at a slower pace. But if you do piecework or if you work on an assembly line and a machine paces your work, discuss the problem with your supervisor or union representative.

DO HAND EXERCISES

Your health care provider will teach you special exercises to strengthen all your hand and wrist muscles. If all your muscles are strong, you'll put less strain on one particular muscle or group of muscles.

REDUCE SWELLING

If fluid retention aggravates your symptoms, ask your health care provider about taking diuretics to relieve some of the swelling in the carpal tunnel. Or drink plenty of fluids. Coffee or tea are natural diuretics (increasing urination). Elevating your hand may also help relieve swelling temporarily.

(continued)

- Acute pain
- Disturbed sensory perception (tactile)
- Impaired physical mobility

EXPECTED OUTCOMES
The patient will:
- verbalize relief from pain
- exhibit improved or normal sensory perception
- demonstrate stability or improvement in mobility.

- Reinforce the purpose of the planned surgery. Tell the patient that the procedure should relieve pain in his wrist and help him regain full use of his hand.
- Outline the steps of surgery, tailoring your explanation to the particular procedure the surgeon has chosen as well as to the patient's level of understanding.
- Explain to the patient that before surgery, the affected arm will be shaved and cleaned and that he'll be given a local anesthetic. Reassure him that although he may feel some pressure, the anesthetic will ensure a pain-free operation.
- Discuss postoperative care measures. Point out that he'll have a dressing wrapped around his hand and lower arm, which usually will remain in place for 1 or 2 days after surgery. Explain that although he may experience pain when the anesthetic wears off, analgesics will be available.
- Teach the patient the rehabilitative exercises that he'll be asked to do during the recovery period: gentle range-of-motion exercises with the wrist and fingers to prevent muscle atrophy. Demonstrate these exercises, and have him perform a return demonstration. However, be aware that severe pain may prevent him from doing so.

- After the patient returns from surgery, monitor his vital signs and carefully assess circulation and sensory and motor function in the affected arm and hand.
- Keep the hand elevated to reduce swelling and discomfort.
- Check the dressing often for unusual drainage or bleeding, which may indicate infection.
- Assess for pain and provide analgesics as needed.

    WARNING *Report severe, persistent pain or tenderness, which may indicate tenosynovitis or formation of a hematoma.*

- Encourage the patient to perform his wrist and finger exercises daily to improve circulation and enhance muscle tone. If these exercises are painful, have him perform them with his wrist and hand immersed in warm water. (Have him wear a surgical glove if his dressing is still in place.)
- Assess the need for home care and follow-up with activities of daily living, especially if the patient lives alone.

    WARNING *Patients who had very numb fingers or wasting of the thumb muscles before surgery will probably never regain full nerve function. Recovery can be slow (6 to 12 months). As the nerves grow back, the fingers can actually feel tingly or even unpleasant.*

GENERAL

◆ Discuss the medication prescribed, dosage, and adverse effects.
◆ Emphasize the importance of follow-up care.
◆ Refer the patient for resource and support services.
◆ Inform the patient about caring for the incision site. Tell him to keep the incision site clean and dry, and to cover it with a surgical or rubber glove when immersing it in water for exercise or when taking a bath or shower.
◆ Teach the patient how to change the dressing; instruct him to do so once daily until healing is complete.
◆ Tell the patient to notify the surgeon if redness, swelling, pain, or excessive drainage persists at the operative site.
◆ Encourage the patient to continue daily wrist and finger exercises. Warn him against overusing the affected wrist or lifting an object heavier than a thin magazine.
◆ If the patient's condition is job related, suggest that he seek occupational counseling to help him find more suitable employment.
◆ Inform the patient that keeping the hand elevated is important to prevent swelling and stiffness of the fingers. Remind the patient not to walk with the hand dangling or to sit with the hand held in the lap.

RESOURCES
Organizations
American Academy of Orthopedic Surgeons: *www.aaos.org*
American Medical Association: *www.ama-assn.org*
Carpal Tunnel Syndrome: *www.carpaltunnel.com*

Selected references
Bland, J.D. "Carpal Tunnel Syndrome," *Current Opinions in Neurology* 18(5):581-85, October 2005.
Dunn, D. "Preventing Perioperative Complications in Special Populations," *Nursing2005* 35(11):36-43, November 2005.
Eskandari, M.M., et al. "Effect of Patient Age and Symptom Duration on Subjective and Objective Outcomes of Carpal Tunnel Surgery," *Orthopedics* 28(6):600-602, June 2005.
Hopp, P.T. "Carpal Tunnel Syndrome— The Role of Psychosocial Factors in Recovery," *JAAOHN* 52(11):458-60, November 2004.

Casting

OVERVIEW

◆ Defined as a hard mold that encases a body part, usually an extremity, to provide immobilization of bones and surrounding tissue

◆ Can be used to treat injuries (including fractures), correct orthopedic conditions (such as deformities), or promote healing after general or plastic surgery, amputation, or nerve and vascular repair (see *Types of cylindrical casts*)

◆ May be constructed of plaster, Fiberglas, or other synthetic materials

◆ Plaster (commonly used): inexpensive, nontoxic, nonflammable, easy to mold, and rarely causes allergic reactions or skin irritation

◆ Fiberglas: lighter, stronger, and more resilient than plaster; dries rapidly, thus is more difficult to mold, but can bear body weight immediately, if necessary

◆ Practitioner applies cast; nurse prepares patient and equipment and assists during the procedure (although nurse may apply or change standard cast *after* fracture reduced and set by orthopedist)

⚡ *WARNING Contraindications include skin diseases, peripheral vascular disease, diabetes mellitus, open or draining wounds, overwhelming edema, and susceptibility to skin irritations. However, these aren't strict contraindications; the practitioner must weigh the potential risks and benefits for each patient.*

INDICATIONS
◆ Fractures

PROCEDURE

◆ Begin preparing the equipment by gently squeezing the packaged casting material to make that sure the envelopes don't have air leaks. Humid air can enter leaks and cause plaster to become stale, which could make it set too quickly, form lumps, fail to bond with lower layers, or set as a soft, friable mass.

◆ Follow the manufacturer's directions for water temperature when preparing plaster.

◆ Usually, room temperature or slightly warmer water is best because it allows the cast to set in about 7 minutes without excessive exothermia. Cold water slows the rate of setting and may be used to facilitate difficult molding; warm water speeds the rate

---

Types of cylindrical casts

Made of plaster, Fiberglas, or synthetic material, casts may be applied almost anywhere on the body — to support a single finger or the entire body. Common casts are shown below.

HANGING ARM CAST

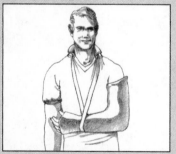

SHOULDER SPICA

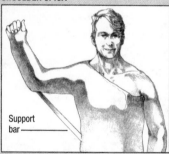

Support bar

SHORT ARM CAST

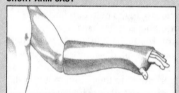

ONE AND ONE-HALF HIP SPICA

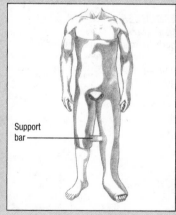

Support bar

LONG LEG CAST

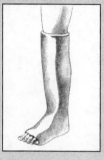

SHORT LEG CAST

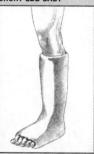

SINGLE HIP CAST

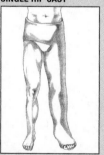

of setting and raises skin temperature under the cast.

- Help the practitioner position the limb as ordered; it's usually immobilized in the neutral position.
- Support the limb in the prescribed position while the practitioner applies the tubular stockinette and sheet wadding.
- The stockinette, if used, should extend beyond the ends of the cast to pad the edges. If the patient has an open wound or a severe contusion, the practitioner may decide to not use the stockinette.
- The practitioner then wraps the limb in sheet wadding, starting at the distal end, and applies extra wadding to the distal and proximal ends of the cast area as well as any points of prominence.
- Check for wrinkles as the practitioner applies the sheet wadding.
- Prepare the various cast materials as ordered.

PREPARING A PLASTER CAST

- Place a roll of plaster casting on its end in the bucket of water, immersing it completely.
- When air bubbles stop rising from the roll, remove it, gently squeeze out the excess water, and hand the casting material to the practitioner, who will begin applying it to the extremity. As he applies the first roll, prepare a second roll in the same manner. Stay at least one roll ahead of the practitioner during the procedure.
- After the practitioner applies each roll, he'll smooth it to remove wrinkles, spread the plaster into the cloth webbing, and empty air pockets. If he's using plaster splints, he'll apply them in the middle layers of the cast.
- Before wrapping the last roll, he'll pull the ends of the tubular stockinette over the cast edges to create padded ends, prevent cast crumbling, and reduce skin irritation.
- The practitioner will then use the final roll to keep the ends of the stockinette in place.

PREPARING A COTTON AND POLYESTER CAST

WARNING *Open these casting materials one roll at a time because cotton and polyester casting must be applied within 3 minutes— before humidity in the air hardens the tape.*

- Immerse the roll in cold water, and squeeze it four times to ensure uniform wetness.
- Remove the dripping wet material from the bucket.
- Tell the patient that it will be applied immediately. Forewarn him that the material will feel warm and give off heat as it sets.

PREPARING A FIBERGLAS CAST

- If you're using water-activated Fiberglas, immerse the tape rolls in tepid water for 10 to 15 minutes to initiate the chemical reaction that causes the cast to harden.
- Open one roll at a time. Avoid squeezing out excess water before application. If you're using light-cured Fiberglas, you can unroll the material more slowly. It remains soft and malleable until it's exposed to ultraviolet light, which sets it.

COMPLICATIONS

- Compartment syndrome
- Palsy
- Paresthesia
- Ischemia
- Ischemic myositis
- Pressure necrosis
- Misalignment or nonunion of fractured bones

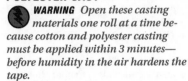
NURSING DIAGNOSES

- Acute pain
- Impaired physical mobility
- Ineffective tissue perfusion: Peripheral

EXPECTED OUTCOMES
The patient will:
- express feelings of increased comfort
- attain the highest degree of mobility possible within the confines of injury
- exhibit adequate tissue perfusion and pulses distally.

PRETREATMENT CARE

- Explain the procedure to the patient.
- If plaster is being used, make sure that the patient understands that heat will build under the cast because of a chemical reaction between the water and plaster.
- Also begin explaining aspects of proper cast care to prepare him for patient teaching and to assess his knowledge level.
- Cover the appropriate parts of the patient's bedding and gown with a linen-saver pad.
- If the cast is applied to the wrist or arm, remove rings that may interfere with circulation in the fingers.
- Assess the condition of the skin in the affected area, noting redness, contusions, or open wounds. This will make it easier to evaluate any complaints the patient may have after the cast is applied.
- If the patient has an open wound, prepare him for a local anesthetic if the practitioner will administer one.
- Clean the wound.
- Assist the practitioner as he closes the wound and applies a dressing.
- To establish baseline measurements, assess the patient's neurovascular status. Palpate the distal pulses; assess the color, temperature, and capillary refill of the appropriate fingers or toes; and check neurologic function, including sensation and motion in the affected and unaffected extremities.

(continued)

COMPLETING THE CAST

- As necessary, "petal" the cast's edges to reduce roughness and to cushion pressure points.
- Use a cast stand or your palm to support the cast in the therapeutic position until it becomes firm to the touch (usually 6 to 8 minutes) to prevent indentations in the cast.
- Place the cast on a firm, smooth surface to continue drying.
- Place pillows under joints to maintain flexion, if necessary.
- To check circulation in the casted limb, palpate the distal pulse and assess the color, temperature, and capillary refill of the fingers or toes. Determine neurologic status by asking the patient if he's experiencing paresthesia in the extremity or decreased motion of the extremity's uncovered joints. Assess the unaffected extremity in the same manner and compare findings.

- Elevate the limb above heart level with pillows or bath blankets, as ordered, to facilitate venous return and reduce edema.
- The practitioner will then send the patient for X-rays to ensure proper positioning.
- Instruct the patient to notify the practitioner if any pain, foul odor, drainage, or burning sensation under the cast occurs.
- After the cast hardens, the practitioner may cut a window in it to inspect the painful or burning area.
- Dispose of materials appropriately; pour water from the plaster bucket into a sink containing a plaster trap.

⚡ **WARNING** *Don't use a regular sink because plaster will block the plumbing.*

- Care consists of monitoring for changes in the drainage pattern, preventing skin breakdown near the cast, and averting the complications of immobility.
- Never use the bed or a table to support the cast as it sets because mold-

ing can result, causing pressure necrosis of underlying tissue.
- Also, don't use rubber- or plastic-covered pillows before the cast hardens because they can trap heat under the cast.
- If a cast is applied after surgery or traumatic injury, remember that the most accurate way to assess for bleeding is to monitor the patient's vital signs.

⚡ **WARNING** *A visible blood spot on the cast can be misleading: One drop of blood can produce a circle 3″ (7.6 cm) in diameter.*

- Casts may need to be opened to assess underlying skin or pulses or to relieve pressure in a specific area.
- In a windowed cast, a specific area is cut out to allow inspection of underlying skin or to relieve pressure.
- A bivalved cast is split medially and laterally, creating anterior and posterior sections. One of the sections may be removed to relieve pressure while the remaining section maintains immobilization. (See *Removing a plaster cast.*)

Removing a plaster cast

Typically, a cast is removed when a fracture heals or requires further manipulation. Less common indications include cast damage, a pressure ulcer under the cast, excessive drainage or bleeding, and a constrictive cast.

Explain the procedure to the patient. Tell him he'll feel some heat and vibration as the cast is split with the cast saw. If the patient is a child, tell him that the saw is very noisy but won't cut the skin beneath. Warn the patient that when the padding is cut, he'll see discolored skin and signs of poor muscle tone. Reassure him that you'll stay with him. The illustrations below show how a plaster cast is removed.

The practitioner cuts one side of the cast, then the other. As he does so, closely monitor the patient's anxiety level.

Next, the practitioner opens the cast pieces with a spreader.

Finally, using cast scissors, the practitioner cuts through the cast padding.

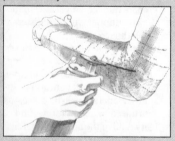
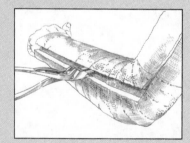
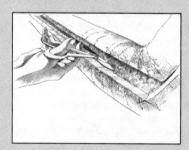

When the cast is removed, provide skin care to remove accumulated dead skin and to begin restoring the extremity's normal appearance.

GENERAL

- Tell the patient that a Fiberglas cast dries immediately after application; a plaster extremity cast dries in about 24 to 48 hours; and a plaster spica or body cast in 48 to 72 hours.
- During this drying period, tell the patient that the cast must be properly positioned to prevent a surface depression that could cause pressure areas or dependent edema.
- Instruct the patient on how to monitor his neurovascular status, drainage, and condition of the cast.
- Inform the patient that after the cast dries completely, it looks white and shiny and no longer feels damp or soft.
- Tell the patient that the practitioner usually removes the cast at the appropriate time, with the assistance of a nurse.
- Tell the patient that when the cast is removed, his casted limb will appear thinner and flabbier than the uncasted limb and his skin will appear yellowish or gray from the accumulated dead skin and oils from the glands near the skin surface.
- Reassure the patient that with exercise and good skin care, his limb will return to normal.
- Before the patient is discharged, teach him how to care for his cast. Tell him to keep the casted limb elevated above heart level to minimize swelling. Raise a casted leg by having the patient lie in a supine position with his leg on top of pillows. Prop a casted arm so that the hand and elbow are higher than the shoulder. (See *Caring for your cast*, pages 52 and 53.)

⚡ **WARNING** *Instruct the patient to call the practitioner if he can't move his fingers or toes, has numbness or tingling in the affected limb, or if he has symptoms of infection, such as a fever, unusual pain, or a foul odor from the cast.*

- Advise the patient to maintain muscle strength by continuing recommended exercises.
- Tell the patient to notify the practitioner if the cast needs repair (if it loosens, cracks, or breaks) or if he has questions about caring for the cast.
- Warn the patient not to get the cast wet because moisture will weaken or destroy it. If the practitioner approves, have the patient cover the cast with a plastic bag or cast cover for showering or bathing.
- Urge the patient not to insert anything (such as a back scratcher or powder) into the cast to relieve itching because it can damage the skin and cause an infection.
- Tell the patient that he can apply alcohol on the skin at the cast edges.

⚡ **WARNING** *Warn the patient not to chip, crush, cut, or otherwise break any area of the cast and not to bear weight on the cast unless instructed to do so by the practitioner.*

- Tell the patient who needs crutches to have throw rugs removed from the floor and have furniture rearranged to reduce the risk of tripping or falling.
- Inform the patient who has a cast on his dominant arm that he may need help with bathing, toileting, eating, and dressing.

RESOURCES
Organizations
American Academy of Orthopedic Surgeons: *www.aaos.org*
American Medical Association: *www.ama-assn.org*

Selected references
Altizer L. "Casting for Immobilization," *Orthopedic Nursing* 23(2):136-41, March-April 2004.

Berkowitz, M.J., and Kim, D.H. "Process and Tubercle Fractures of the Hindfoot," *Journal of the American Academy of Orthopedic Surgery* 13(8):492-502, December 2005.

Faulks, S., and Luther, B. "Changing Paradigm for the Treatment of Clubfeet," *Orthopedic Nursing* 24(1):25-30, January-February 2005.

(continued)

Caring for your cast

Dear Patient,

Think of your new cast as a temporary body part—one that needs the same attentive care as the rest of you. While you wear your cast, follow these guidelines.

SPEEDING UP DRYING TIME

Your health care provider may apply a cast made of plaster, Fiberglas, or a synthetic material. The wet material must dry thoroughly and evenly for the cast to support your broken bone properly. (At first, your wet cast will feel heavy and warm, but don't worry—it will get lighter as it dries.)

To speed drying, keep the cast exposed to the air. (Fiberglas and synthetic casts dry soon after application, but plaster casts don't. A plaster arm or leg cast dries in about 24 to 48 hours.)

When you raise the cast with pillows, make sure that the pillows have rubber or plastic covers under the linen case. Use a thin towel placed between the cast and the pillows to absorb moisture. Never place a wet cast directly onto plastic.

DRYING EVENLY

To make sure that the cast dries evenly, change its position on the pillows every 2 hours—using your palms, not your fingertips. You can have someone else move the cast for you.

To avoid creating bumps inside the cast—bumps that could cause skin irritation or sores—don't poke at the cast with your fingers while it's wet. Also, be careful not to dent the cast while it's still wet.

KEEPING YOUR CAST CLEAN

After your cast dries, you can remove dirt and stains with a damp cloth and powdered kitchen cleaner. Use as little water as possible, and wipe off moisture that remains when you're done.

PROTECTING YOUR CAST

Avoid knocking your cast against a hard surface. To protect the foot of a leg cast from breakage, scrapes, and dirt, place a piece of used carpet (or a carpet square) over the bottom of the cast. Slash or cut a "V" shape at the back so the carpet fits around the heel when you bring it up toward the ankle.

Hold the carpet in place with a large sock or slipper sock. Extending the carpet out beyond the toes a little will also help prevent bumped or stubbed toes.

PREVENTING SNAGS

To keep an arm cast from snagging clothing and furniture, make a cast cover from an old nylon stocking. Cut off the stocking's toe, and cut a hole in the heel.

Then pull the stocking over the cast to cover it.

Extend your fingers through the cut-off toe end, and poke your thumb through the hole you cut in the heel. Trim the other end of the stocking to about 1½" (4 cm) longer than the cast, and tuck the ends of the stocking under the cast's edges.

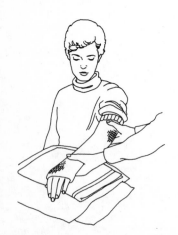

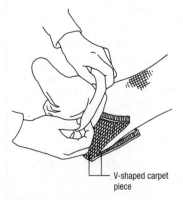

V-shaped carpet piece

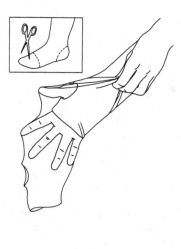

CARING FOR YOUR SKIN

Wash the skin along the cast's edges every day, using a mild soap. Before you begin, protect the cast's edges with plastic wrap. Then use a washcloth wrung out in soapy water to clean the skin at the cast's edges and as far as you can reach inside the cast. Avoid getting the cast wet. Afterward, dry the skin thoroughly with a towel. Then massage the skin at and beneath the cast's edges with a towel or pad saturated with rubbing alcohol. This helps toughen the skin. To help prevent skin irritation, remove loose plaster particles you can reach inside the cast.

RELIEVING ITCHING

No matter how itchy the skin under your cast may feel, never try to relieve the itch by inserting a sharp or pointed object into the cast. This could damage your skin and lead to infection. Also, don't put powder or lotion in your cast or stuff cotton or toilet tissue under the cast's edges. This may reduce your circulation.

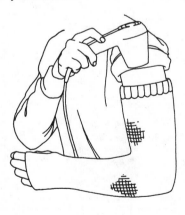

Here's a safe technique to relieve itching. Set a handheld blow-dryer on "cool," and aim it at the problem area.

STAYING DRY

If you have a plaster cast, you'll need to cover it with a plastic bag before you shower, swim, or go out in wet weather. You can use a garbage bag or a cast shower bag, which you can buy at a drugstore or medical supply store. Above all, *don't get a plaster cast wet.* Moisture will weaken or even destroy it. If the cast gets a little wet, let it dry naturally, such as by sitting in the sun.

Don't cover the cast until it's dry. If you have a Fiberglas or synthetic cast, check with your health care provider to find out if you may bathe, shower, or swim. If he does allow you to swim, he'll probably tell you to flush the cast with cool tap water after swimming in a chlorinated pool or a lake. Make sure that no foreign material remains trapped inside the cast. To dry a Fiberglas or synthetic cast, first wrap the cast in a towel. Then prop it on a pad of towels to absorb remaining water. The cast will air-dry in 3 to 4 hours; to speed dry it, use a handheld blow-dryer.

SIGNING THE CAST

Family members and friends may want to sign their names or draw pictures on the cast. That's okay, but don't let them paint over large cast areas because this could make those areas nonporous and damage the skin underneath.

Cataract extraction

- Lens opacities—*cataracts*—removed by intracapsular cataract extraction (ICCE) or extracapsular cataract extraction (ECCE)
- ICCE: entire lens removed, most commonly with a cryoprobe
- ECCE: anterior capsule, cortex, and nucleus removed and posterior capsule left intact; technique possibly done by manual extraction, irrigation and aspiration, or phacoemulsification

🌸 *AGE FACTOR ECCE is the primary treatment for congenital and traumatic cataracts. It's characteristically used to treat children and young adults because the posterior capsule adheres to the vitreous until about age 20. By leaving the posterior capsule undisturbed, ECCE avoids disruption and loss of vitreous.*

- Immediately after removal of natural lens, many patients implanted with intraocular lens

INDICATIONS

- Loss of vision or visual abnormalities due to the presence of cataracts

PROCEDURE

- The patient may receive a local or general anesthetic.

🌸 *AGE FACTOR Children are typically given general anesthesia to keep them in a deep sleep and pain-free; adults usually are awake but sedated and pain-free with local anesthesia.*

- For a review of cataract removal procedures, see *Comparing methods of cataract removal.*
- After cataract removal, the surgeon may insert a lens implant. After enlarging the incision, he'll implant the lens into the capsular sac.

Comparing methods of cataract removal

Cataracts can be removed by intracapsular or extracapsular techniques.

INTRACAPSULAR CATARACT EXTRACTION

When performing intracapsular cataract extraction, the surgeon makes a partial incision at the superior limbus arc. He then removes the lens using specially designed forceps or a cryoprobe, which freezes and adheres to the lens to facilitate its removal.

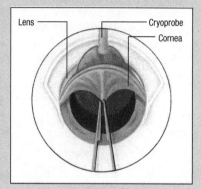

EXTRACAPSULAR CATARACT EXTRACTION

When performing extracapsular cataract extraction, the surgeon may use irrigation and aspiration or phacoemulsification. If he uses irrigation and aspiration, he makes an incision at the limbus, opens the anterior lens capsule with a cystotome, and exerts pressure from below to express the lens. He then irrigates and suctions the remaining lens cortex.

During phacoemulsification, the surgeon uses an ultrasonic probe to break the lens into minute particles, which are aspirated by the probe.

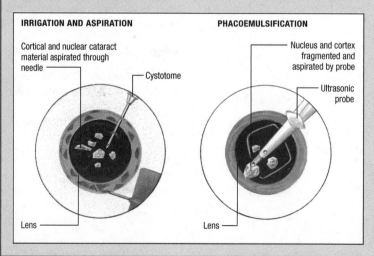

- If he implants the lens without sutures, he'll administer miotic agents, such as pilocarpine (Pilocar), to prevent the iris from dilating too widely and causing the lens to slip.
- In ICCE and ECCE, the surgeon may also perform a peripheral iridectomy to reduce intraocular pressure (IOP) and may briefly instill alpha-chymotrypsin, a proteolytic enzyme, in the anterior chamber to dissolve resistant zonular fibers.
- After the procedure, the surgeon closes the sutures, instills antibiotic drops or ointment, and patches and shields the eye.

COMPLICATIONS
- Papillary block
- Corneal decompensation
- Vitreous loss
- Hemorrhage
- Cystoid macular edema
- Lens dislocation
- Secondary membrane opacification
- Retinal detachment

NURSING DIAGNOSES

- Acute pain
- Disturbed sensory perception (visual)
- Risk for infection

EXPECTED OUTCOMES
The patient will:
- express feelings of comfort
- demonstrate improved visual function
- demonstrate intact tissue without signs of infection.

PRETREATMENT CARE

- Explain the planned surgical technique to the patient. Tell him that he'll receive mydriatics and cycloplegics to dilate the eye and facilitate cataract removal, that he'll receive osmotics and antibiotics to reduce the risk of infection, and that he may receive a sedative to help him relax.
- Inform the patient that after surgery he'll have to wear an eye patch temporarily to prevent traumatic injury and infection.
- Explain that he'll temporarily experience loss of depth perception and decreased peripheral vision on the operative side.
- Perform an antiseptic facial scrub to reduce the risk of infection, if ordered.
- Verufy that the patient has signed a consent form.

POSTTREATMENT CARE

- After the patient returns to his room, notify the surgeon if severe pain, bleeding, increased drainage, or fever occurs.
- Because of the change in the patient's depth perception, keep the side rails of his bed raised, assist him with ambulation, and observe other safety precautions.
- Maintain the eye patch, and have the patient wear an eye shield, especially when sleeping. Tell him to continue wearing the shield during sleep for several weeks as ordered.

PATIENT TEACHING

GENERAL
- Instruct the patient to immediately contact the surgeon if sudden eye pain, red or watery eyes, photophobia, or sudden visual changes occur.
- Tell the patient to avoid activities that raise IOP, including heavy lifting, bending, straining during defecation, or vigorous coughing and sneezing. Tell him not to exercise strenuously for 6 to 10 weeks.
- Explain that follow-up appointments are needed to monitor the results of the surgery and to detect any complications.
- Teach the patient or a family member how to instill eyedrops and ointments and how to change the eye patch. (See *Eye care after cataract surgery,* pages 56 and 57.)
- Suggest that the patient wear dark glasses to relieve glare because photophobia is common after eye surgery.
- Explain that changes in the patient's vision can present safety hazards if he'll be wearing eyeglasses. To compensate for loss of depth perception, show him how to use up-and-down head movements to judge distances. To overcome the loss of peripheral vision on the operative side, teach him to turn his head fully in that direction to view objects to his side.
- Remind the patient that although his vision may not stabilize for several weeks following surgery, visual acuity will increase as the affected eye heals.

RESOURCES
Organizations
American Academy of Ophthalmology: *www.aao.org*
American Medical Association: *www.ama-assn.org*

Selected references
Dunn, D. "Preventing Perioperative Complications in Special Populations," *Nursing2005* 35(11):36-43, November 2005.

(continued)

Khng, C., and Snyder, M.E., "Iris Reconstruction with a Multipiece Endocapsular Prosthesis in Iridocorneal Endothelial Syndrome," *Journal of Cataract and Refractive Surgery* 31(11):2051-54, November 2005.

Kuo, I.C., et al. "Excimer Laser Surgery for Correction of Ametropia after Cataract Surgery," *Journal of Cataract and Refractive Surgery* 31(11):2104-10, November 2005.

Marsden, J. "Cataract: The Role of Nurses in Diagnosis, Surgery and Aftercare," *Nursing Times* 100(7):36-40, February 2004.

PATIENT-TEACHING AID

Eye care after cataract surgery

Dear Patient,

Your eye surgeon wants you to remove the eye shield and eye patch from the surgery 24 hours after the procedure. You have been given one or two eye medications to use, and a schedule for their administration. At bedtime for the next 4 to 6 weeks, or anytime you lay down, you should reapply the eye shield. This will prevent rubbing or bumping your eye during sleep.

REMOVING THE SHIELD AND PATCH

1. Wash your hands thoroughly with soap and water.
2. Use a downward motion to peel the tape off your forehead. Gently remove the shield and patch from your eye and continue to peel the tape downward to your cheek. Next, remove the tape from the shield and discard the patch.
3. You may very gently soak away any dried drainage with a warm moist clean cloth, but don't rub or press on the eye.

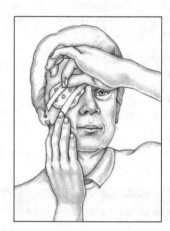

INSTILLING EYEDROPS

1. Wash your hands thoroughly with soap and water.
2. Stand in front of a mirror.
3. Pull your lower lid down gently with a finger or the thumb of your nondominant hand to make a pocket.

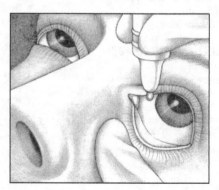

INSTILLING EYEDROPS (continued)

4. Rest your dominant hand with the bottle on your forehead to help steady it.

5. Look upward and slightly away from the bottle tip.

6. Squeeze the appropriate number of drops into the eye pocket.

7. Close your eye and press gently where the nose meets the inner eye for 2 or 3 minutes, without pinching.

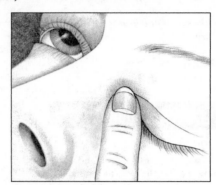

8. With your eye closed, gently wipe away any unabsorbed drops and tears.

9. Wait 3 to 5 minutes before instilling another medication.

10. Wash your hands with soap and water when you are done.

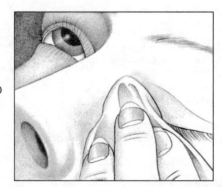

APPLYING THE SHIELD

1. Wash your hands thoroughly with soap and water.

2. Place the shield over the affected eye.

3. Secure it with two parallel strips of hypoallergenic tape, taping from the middle of your forehead to your cheekbone. Make sure that you leave a space between the strips of tape so that you can see through the shield.

4. When you get up, carefully remove the shield. Wash it with soap and water as needed. Keep it in a convenient place ready to apply again.

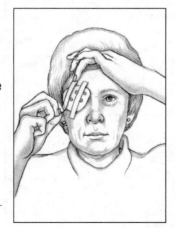

Cerebral aneurysm repair

- Surgical repair: clipping the aneurysm neck with at least one titanium clip
- Endovascular repair: use of electrically detachable platinum coils that promote electrothrombosis within the aneurysm
- Decision of neurosurgeon and endovascular radiologists whether to obliterate an aneurysm surgically through a craniotomy and clipping or to use endovascular methods based on the patient's condition

> **AGE FACTOR** *Treatment depends on the patient's age and the location of the aneurysm. Younger patients commonly undergo surgical clipping because coiling has a high recurrence rate. However, posterior fossa aneurysms (especially the basilar artery tip) tend to be treated using the coil procedure. In most major aneurysm centers, many cases are still obliterated by surgical clipping, although coiling is being used more frequently.*

- Cerebral aneurysms: usually arise at the arterial junction in the circle of Willis (see *Common sites of cerebral aneurysm*)

> **AGE FACTOR** *The prognosis is always guarded, but is affected by the patient's age and neurologic condition, the presence of other diseases, and the extent and location of the aneurysm.*

INDICATIONS

- Cerebral aneurysm

CLIPPING

- General anesthesia is used and the area of the skull where the craniotomy will occur is shaved. The exact position of the opening depends on the approach that the neurosurgeon will use to reach the aneurysm.
- The bone flap is removed and the various layers of tissue are cut away to expose the brain.
- Brain tissue is gently retracted back to expose the area containing the aneurysm.
- Surgical techniques performed through a microscope are then used to dissect the aneurysm away from the vessels feeding the aneurysm and expose the neck to receive the clip, which is usually made of titanium.
- The clip is placed on the neck of the aneurysm to stop the flow of blood into the aneurysm, causing it to deflate or obliterate. (See *Clipping a cerebral aneurysm.*)
- The brain tissue is carefully lowered back into place, the various layers sutured closed, and the bone flap is reseated for healing.
- The skin and other outer layers are also sutured closed.

COILING

- A specially trained radiologist called a *neurointerventionist* performs the procedure using fluoroscopic angiography. A microcatheter is threaded from the patient's femoral artery to the aneurysm. The catheter is used to place small platinum coils within the aneurysm using a delivery wire.
- Once the coil has been maneuvered into place, an electrical charge is sent through the delivery wire that disintegrates the stainless steel of the coil, separating it from the delivery wire, which is then removed from the body.
- Several coils may be necessary to block the neck of the aneurysm from the normal circulation and obliterate it, as with the clip procedure.
- The coils act as a thrombogenic agent, causing blood to coagulate in the aneurysm, decreasing the risk of rupture.

> **WARNING** *Coil treatment is contraindicated if the patient has a cerebral hematoma (which precludes anticoagulation during the procedure) or an aneurysm with a wide opening. The coil mass could lapse into the parent artery, partially or completely occluding it and causing a stroke.*

Common sites of cerebral aneurysm

Cerebral aneurysms usually arise at the arterial bifurcation in the circle of Willis and its branches. This illustration shows the most common sites around this circle.

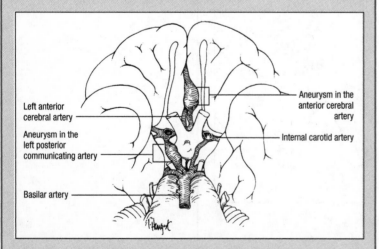

Left anterior cerebral artery

Aneurysm in the left posterior communicating artery

Basilar artery

Aneurysm in the anterior cerebral artery

Internal carotid artery

COMPLICATIONS
◆ Infection
◆ Rebleeding of cerebral aneurysm
◆ Vasospasm
◆ Neurologic damage
◆ Hypothermia

NURSING DIAGNOSES

◆ Ineffective tissue perfusion: Cerebral
◆ Risk for infection
◆ Risk for injury

EXPECTED OUTCOMES
The patient will:
◆ demonstrate normal neurologic functioning
◆ remain free from infection
◆ remain free from injury.

PRETREATMENT CARE

◆ Check laboratory values, electrocardiogram, and chest X-rays as ordered; notify the surgeon or radiologist of any abnormalities.
◆ Explain the planned surgical technique to the patient and his family, reinforcing the surgeon's explanations as necessary.
◆ Explain all tests, neurologic examinations, treatments, and procedures to the patient and his family.
◆ Perform a neurologic examination.

◆ Verify that the patient has signed a consent form.

POSTTREATMENT CARE

◆ A postoperative magnetic resonance angiogram may be performed to confirm good clip placement, total obliteration of the aneurysm, and continued blood flow through the neighboring vessels.
◆ Treatments for vasospasm include medications to relax the smooth muscles in vessel walls or to increase blood pressure, or I.V. fluids to increase blood volume.
◆ Carefully monitor blood pressure and notify the surgeon of a significant increase, especially in the systolic pressure.
◆ Because aneurysms can re-form, patients are followed by angiography, skull X-rays, or magnetic resonance angiography.
◆ Administer oxygen as indicated; suction and turn the patient.
◆ Apply elastic stockings or compression boots to reduce the risk of deep vein thrombosis.
◆ Administer I.V. fluids as ordered.
◆ Assess the patient's neurologic status and report changes in trends; monitor him for increased intracranial pressure.

◆ Monitor laboratory values and intake and output.
◆ Monitor the femoral puncture site for bleeding or hematoma and the leg for signs of ischemia.

⚡ **WARNING** *Notify the surgeon immediately if you notice pain, pallor, pulselessness, poikilothermia (cool to touch), or paresthesia.*

◆ Patients who received a coil are usually on a heparin infusion postoperatively and then on aspirin indefinitely.

PATIENT TEACHING

GENERAL
◆ Review signs of rebleeding to report, such as headache, nausea, vomiting, and changes in level of consciousness.
◆ Refer the patient to a home health care service or rehabilitation center before he's discharged, as needed.

RESOURCES
Organizations
American Academy of Neurology: *www.aan.com*
American Medical Association: *www.ama-assn.org*

Selected references
Dunn, D. "Preventing Perioperative Complications in Special Populations," *Nursing* 35(11):36-43, November 2005.
Feng, L., et al. "Healing of Intracranial Aneurysms with Bioactive Coils," *Neurosurgical Clinics of North America* 16(3):487-99, July 2005.
Wagner, M., and Stenger, K. "Unruptured Intracranial Aneurysms: Using Evidence and Outcomes to Guide Patient Teaching," *Critical Care Nursing Quarterly* 28(4):341-54, October-December 2005.

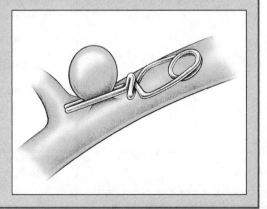

Clipping a cerebral aneurysm

The clip, which is made of materials that won't affect metal detectors and that will not rust, is placed at the base of the aneurysm to stop the blood supply. The clip remains in place permanently.

Cerebrospinal fluid drainage

- Aims to reduce cerebrospinal fluid (CSF) pressure to desired level and then to maintain it at that level
- Fluid withdrawn from lateral ventricle (ventriculostomy) or lumbar subarachnoid space, depending on indication and desired outcome
- To place the ventricular drain: practitioner inserts a ventricular catheter through a burr hole in the patient's skull; usually done in the operating room, with the patient under general anesthesia
- To place the lumbar subarachnoid drain: practitioner may administer a local spinal anesthetic at the bedside or in the operating room (see *Using a cerebrospinal fluid drainage system*)

INDICATIONS

- Ventricular drainage to reduce increased intracranial pressure (ICP); lumbar drainage, to aid healing of the dura mater
- External CSF drainage, to manage increased ICP and to facilitate spinal or cerebral dural healing after traumatic injury or surgery

PROCEDURE

- Open all equipment using sterile technique. Check all packaging for breaks in seals and for expiration dates.
- Label all medications, medication containers, and other solutions on and off the sterile field.

INSERTING A VENTRICULAR DRAIN

- Place the patient in the supine position.
- Place the equipment tray on the overbed table, and unwrap the tray.
- Adjust the height of the bed so that the practitioner can perform the procedure comfortably.
- Illuminate the area of the catheter insertion site.

- The practitioner will shave the hair from the area of the insertion site, clean the insertion site, and administer a local anesthetic.
- The practitioner will put on sterile gloves and drape the insertion site.
- To insert the drain, the practitioner will request a ventriculostomy tray with a twist drill.
- After completing the ventriculostomy, he'll connect the drainage system and suture the ventriculostomy in place.
- The practitioner will then cover the insertion site with a sterile dressing.

INSERTING A LUMBAR SUBARACHNOID DRAIN

- Position the patient in a side-lying position with his chin tucked to his chest and knees drawn up to his abdomen (as for a lumbar puncture).
- Urge the patient to remain still during the procedure.
- An alternate position for the patient would be sitting up at the bedside, leaning forward over a bedside table.
- To insert the drain, the practitioner attaches a Tuohy needle (or spinal needle) to the whistle-tip catheter.
- After the practitioner removes the needle, he connects the drainage system, sutures or tapes the catheter securely in place, and covers it with a sterile dressing.
- After the practitioner places the catheter, connect it to the external drainage system tubing.
- CSF is drained by a catheter or ventriculostomy tube in a sterile, closed drainage collection system.
- Secure connection points with tape or a connector.
- Place the collection system, including the drip chamber and collection bag, on an I.V. pole.

COMPLICATIONS

- Excessive CSF drainage
- Acute overdrainage that may result in collapsed ventricles, tonsillar herniation, and medullary compression
- Cessation of drainage due to clot formation

Using a cerebrospinal fluid drainage system

Cerebrospinal fluid drainage aims to control intracranial pressure (ICP) during treatment for traumatic injury or other conditions that cause a rise in ICP.

VENTRICULAR DRAIN

For a ventricular drain, the practitioner makes a burr hole in the patient's skull and inserts the catheter into the ventricle. The distal end of the catheter is connected to a closed drainage system.

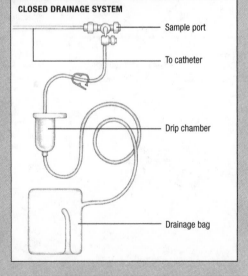

CLOSED DRAINAGE SYSTEM

- Sample port
- To catheter
- Drip chamber
- Drainage bag

NURSING DIAGNOSES

◆ Disturbed sensory perception (all)
◆ Ineffective tissue perfusion: Cerebral
◆ Risk for infection

EXPECTED OUTCOMES
The patient will:
◆ exhibit improved or normal sensory functions
◆ maintain normal neurologic status
◆ exhibit no signs of infection.

PRETREATMENT CARE

◆ Explain the procedure to the patient and his family.
◆ Verify that the patient has signed a consent form.
◆ Wash your hands thoroughly.
◆ Perform a baseline neurologic assessment, including vital signs, to help detect alterations or signs of deterioration.

POSTTREATMENT CARE

◆ Check the patient's neurologic vital signs regularly for signs of deteriorating level of consciousness from acute overdrainage.
◆ Assess for signs of excessive drainage, which may include headache, tachycardia, diaphoresis, and nausea. Reassure the patient that this isn't unusual; administer analgesics as appropriate.
◆ Maintain a continuous hourly output of CSF by raising or lowering the drainage system drip chamber.
◆ Make sure the drip chamber is slightly lower than or at the level of the lumbar drain insertion site.
◆ For ventricular drains, make sure that the flow chamber of the ICP monitoring setup remains positioned as ordered.
◆ Correlate changes in ICP readings to the drainage.
◆ Drain CSF as ordered, maintaining sterile technique.
◆ Document the time and the amount of CSF obtained.
◆ Check the dressing frequently for drainage, which could indicate leakage of CSF.
◆ Check the tubing for patency by watching the CSF drops in the drip chamber.
◆ Observe CSF for color, clarity, amount, blood, and sediment.
◆ Obtain CSF specimens for laboratory analysis from the collection port attached to the tubing and not from the collection bag.
◆ Change the collection bag when it's full or every 24 hours, according to your facility's policy.

> **WARNING** *Never empty the drainage bag. Instead, replace it when full using sterile technique.*

◆ Record and monitor hourly output of CSF.
◆ Check for kinked tubing, catheter displacement, and drip chamber placement.
◆ Be aware that raising or lowering the head of the bed can affect the CSF flow rate.
◆ When changing the patient's position, reposition the drip chamber.

The patient with a lumbar drain is generally kept in a flat position, especially if the drain is placed for a spinal dural tear.
◆ Be aware that the patient may experience chronic headache during continuous CSF drainage.

PATIENT TEACHING

GENERAL
◆ Instruct the patient and his family not to change the head of the bed or patient position without nursing assistance and approval as it may affect the results of treatment.
◆ Tell the patient and his family to promptly report changes in vision, hearing, thinking, alertness, breathing, extremity movement or sensation, or discomfort levels.
◆ Inform the patient and his family that the drainage system will be removed when ICP has stabilized, per the practitioner's assessment and further diagnostic testing.

RESOURCES
Organizations
American Academy of Neurology: *www.aan.com*
American Medical Association: *www.ama-assn.org*

Selected references
Matsumoto, J., et al. "A Long-Term Ventricular Drainage for Patients With Germ Cell Tumors or Medulloblastoma," *Surgical Neurology* 65(1):74-80, January 2006.
Norlela, S. "Syndrome of Inappropriate Antidiuretic Hormone Caused by Continuous Lumbar Spinal Fluid Drainage after Transphenoidal Surgery," *Singapore Medical Journal* 47(1):75-76, January 2006.
Overstreet, M. "How Do I Manage a Lumbar Drain?" *Nursing2003* 33(3):74-75, March 2003.
Thiex, R., and Mull, M. "Basilar Megadolicho Trunk Causing Obstructive Hydrocephalus at the Foramina of Monro," *Surgical Neurology* 65(2):199-201, February 2006.

Chemotherapy

- Chemotherapeutic drugs: may be administered through several routes; may be administered by specially trained nurses or practitioners
- Used to destroy or suppress the growth of cancer cells
- May be used alone or as an adjunct to surgery or radiation therapy

- I.V. route (using peripheral or central veins) most commonly used, although also may be given orally, subcutaneously, intramuscularly, intraarterially, into a body cavity, through a central venous (CV) catheter, or through an Ommaya reservoir into the spinal canal
- Other routes: an artery, peritoneal cavity, or pleural space (see *Intraperitoneal chemotherapy: An alternative approach*)

- Administration route dependent on drug's pharmacodynamics and tumor's characteristics; for example, if malignant tumor is confined to one area, drug may be administered through localized, or regional, method
- Regional administration: allows delivery of a high dose directly to the tumor, which is advantageous because many solid tumors don't respond to drug levels that are safe for systemic administration
- Adjuvant chemotherapy: may be administered to a patient whose cancer is believed to have been eradicated through surgery or radiation therapy; helps to ensure that no undetectable metastasis exists
- Induction chemotherapy (or neoadjuvant or synchronous chemotherapy): may be administered before surgery or radiation therapy; helps improve survival rates by shrinking a tumor before surgical excision or radiation therapy
- Although proven to be more effective when given in higher doses, adverse effects usually limit dosage; methotrexate (MTX) being the exception, which is particularly effective against rapidly growing tumors but toxic to normal tissues that are growing and dividing rapidly (However, oncologists have learned that they can give a large dose of methotrexate to destroy cancer cells and then, before the drug can permanently damage vital organs, give a dose of folinic acid antidote, which stops the effects of methotrexate and, thus, preserves normal tissue.)

Intraperitoneal chemotherapy: An alternative approach

Administering chemotherapeutic drugs into the peritoneal cavity has several benefits for the patient with malignant ascites or ovarian cancer that has spread to the peritoneum. Intraperitoneal chemotherapy passes drugs directly to the tumor in the peritoneal cavity, exposing malignant cells to high concentrations of chemotherapy—up to 1,000 times the amount that can be safely given systemically. Furthermore, the semipermeable peritoneal membrane permits prolonged exposure of malignant cells to the drug.

Typically, this technique is performed using a peritoneal dialysis kit, but drugs can also be administered directly to the peritoneal cavity by using a Tenckhoff catheter (as shown here). This method can be performed on an outpatient basis, if necessary; it uses equipment that's readily available on most units with oncology patients.

In this method, the chemotherapy bag is connected directly to the Tenckhoff catheter with a length of I.V. tubing, the solution is infused, and the catheter and I.V. tubing are clamped. Then the patient is asked to change positions every 10 to 15 minutes for 1 hour to move the solution around in the peritoneal cavity.

After the prescribed dwell time, the chemotherapeutic drugs are drained into an I.V. bag. The patient is encouraged to change positions to facilitate drainage. Then the I.V. tubing and catheter are clamped, the I.V. tubing is removed, and a new intermittent infusion cap is fitted to the catheter. Finally, the catheter is flushed with a syringe of heparin flush solution.

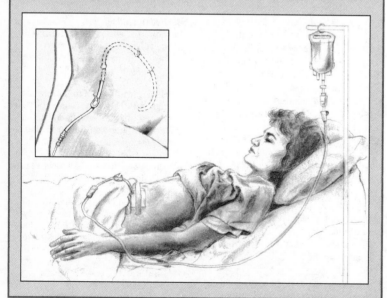

INDICATIONS

Alkylating agents
- Chronic and acute leukemias
- Non-Hodgkin's lymphoma
- Multiple myeloma
- Myeloma
- Sarcoma
- Breast, ovarian, and uterine cancers
- Testes, bladder, and prostate cancers
- Lung cancer
- Brain cancer
- Stomach cancer

Antimetabolites
- Acute leukemia
- Breast cancer
- GI tract adenocarcinomas
- Non-Hodgkin's lymphoma
- Squamous cell carcinomas of the head, neck, and cervix

Antibiotic antineoplastic agents
- Sarcomas
- Lymphomas
- Acute nonlymphoblastic leukemia
- Nonlymphocytic leukemia
- Breast cancer

Hormonal antineoplastic agents
- Hormone-dependent tumors
- Cancers of the prostate, breast, and endometrium

Tubulin-interactive agents
- Lymphomas
- Leukemias
- Sarcomas
- Breast and ovarian cancers

PROCEDURE

- Assess the patient's physical condition, and review his medical history.
- Make sure that you understand what needs to be given and by what route, and provide the necessary teaching and support to the patient and his family.
- Determine the best site to administer the drug. When selecting the site, consider drug compatibilities, frequency of administration, and the vesicant potential of the drug. (See *Classifying chemotherapeutic drugs.*) For example, if the oncologist has ordered the intermittent administration of a vesicant drug, give it by either instilling the drug into the side port of an infusing I.V. line or by direct I.V. push.
- If the vesicant drug is to be infused continuously, administer it only through a CV line or a vascular access device.
- Nonvesicant agents (including irritants) may be given by direct I.V. push, through the side port of an infusing I.V. line, or as a continuous infusion.

Classifying chemotherapeutic drugs

Chemotherapeutic drugs may be classified as irritants, vesicants, or nonvesicants.

IRRITANTS
- Carmustine
- Dacarbazine
- Etoposide
- Ifosfamide
- Streptozocin
- Topotecan

VESICANTS
- Dactinomycin
- Daunorubicin
- Doxorubicin
- Mechlorethamine
- Mitomycin-C
- Mitoxantrone
- Paclitaxel
- Vinblastine
- Vincristine

NONVESICANTS
- Asparaginase
- Bleomycin
- Carboplatin
- Cisplatin (if > 20 ml of 0.5 mg/ml, it is considered a vesicant)
- Cyclophosphamide
- Cytarabine
- Floxuridine
- Fluorouracil

- Check your facility's policy before administering a vesicant. Because vein integrity decreases with time, some facilities require that vesicants be administered before other drugs. Conversely, because vesicants increase vein fragility, other facilities require that vesicants be given after other drugs.
- Evaluate the patient's condition, paying attention to recent laboratory test results, specifically the complete blood count, blood urea nitrogen level, platelet count, urine creatinine level, and liver function studies.
- Determine whether the patient has received chemotherapy before, and note the severity of any adverse reactions.
- Check the patient's drug history for medications that might interact with chemotherapy.

⚡ **WARNING** *As a rule, you shoul not mix chemotherapeutic drugs with other medications. If you have questions or concerns about giving the chemotherapeutic drug, talk with the oncologist or pharmacist before you give it.*

- Double-check the patient's chart for the complete chemotherapy protocol order, including the patient's name, drug's name and dosage, and the route, rate, and frequency of administration.
- See if the drug's dosage depends on certain laboratory values.
- Know that some facilities require two nurses to read the dosage order and to check the drug and the amount being administered.
- Check to see whether the oncologist has ordered an antiemetic, fluids, a diuretic, or electrolyte supplements to be given before, during, or after chemotherapy administration.
- Verify the patient's identity using two patient identifiers according to facility policy.
- Evaluate the patient's and his family's understanding of chemotherapy, and make sure that the patient or a responsible family member has signed the consent form.
- Put on gloves. Keep them on through all stages of handling the drug, in-

(continued)

cluding preparation, priming the I.V. tubing, and administration.

- Before administering the drug, perform a new venipuncture proximal to the old site.
- To identify an administration site, examine the patient's veins, starting with his hand and proceeding to his forearm.
- When an appropriate line is in place, infuse 10 to 20 ml of normal saline solution to test vein patency.

⚡ **WARNING** *Never test vein patency with a chemotherapeutic drug.*

- Next, administer the drug as appropriate: nonvesicants by I.V. push or admixed in a bag of I.V. fluid; vesicants by I.V. push through a piggyback set connected to a rapidly infusing I.V. line.
- During I.V. administration, closely monitor the patient for signs of a hypersensitivity reaction or extravasation.
- During infusion, some drugs need protection from direct sunlight to avoid possible drug breakdown. If this is happens, cover the vial with a brown paper bag or aluminum foil.
- If indicated, use an infusion pump or controller to ensure drug delivery within the prescribed time and rate.
- Check for adequate blood return after 5 ml of the drug has been infused or according to your facility's guidelines.
- After infusion of the medication, infuse 20 ml of normal saline solution. Do this between administrations of different chemotherapeutic drugs and before discontinuing the I.V. line.

COMPLICATIONS
- Nausea and vomiting
- Bone marrow suppression
- Intestinal irritation
- Stomatitis
- Pulmonary fibrosis
- Cardiotoxicity
- Nephrotoxicity
- Neurotoxicity
- Hearing loss
- Anemia
- Alopecia (see *Caring for your hair and scalp during cancer treatment*)

- Urticaria
- Anorexia
- Esophagitis
- Diarrhea
- Constipation
- Psychological problems, including depression and altered body image
- Extravasation, causing inflammation, ulceration, necrosis, and loss of vein patency

NURSING DIAGNOSES

- Fatigue
- Imbalanced nutrition: Less than body requirements
- Risk for infection

EXPECTED OUTCOMES
The patient will:
- maintain energy level to perform daily activities
- maintain normal body weight
- exhibit no signs of infection.

PRETREATMENT CARE

- Explain the treatment and preparation to the patient and his family.
- Verify that the patient has signed an appropriate consent form.
- Provide emotional support to the patient and his family.
- Obtain the patient's medical and drug history, and perform a physical assessment.
- Review laboratory test results.
- Assess the patient's nutritional status, rehabilitation needs, and ability to self-care.
- Develop a care plan for managing symptoms.
- Instruct the patient to report adverse reactions during chemotherapy.
- If administering a vesicant agent, avoid sites in the wrist or dorsum of the hand.
- Verify the drug, dosage, and administration route by checking the medication record against the oncologist's order.
- Make sure you know the immediate and delayed adverse effects of the ordered drug.
- Administer pretreatment medications.

POSTTREATMENT CARE

- Dispose of used needles and syringes carefully.
- To prevent aerosol dispersion of chemotherapeutic drugs, don't clip needles. Place them intact in an impervious container for incineration.
- Dispose of I.V. bags, bottles, gloves, and tubing in a properly labeled and covered trash container.
- Wash your hands thoroughly with soap and warm water after giving any chemotherapeutic drug, even though you have worn gloves.
- Observe the I.V. site frequently for signs of extravasation and allergic reaction (such as swelling, redness, and urticaria).

  WARNING *If you suspect extravasation, stop the infusion immediately. Leave the I.V. catheter in place, and notify the oncologist. A conservative method for treating extravasation involves aspirating any residual drug from the tubing and I.V. catheter, instilling an I.V. antidote, and then removing the I.V. catheter. Afterward, you may apply heat or cold to the site and elevate the affected limb.*
- Observe the patient for adverse reactions.
- Maintain a list of the types and amounts of drugs the patient has received, especially if he has received drugs that have a cumulative effect and that can be toxic to organs, such as the heart or kidneys.
- For 48 hours after drug administration, wear latex gloves when handling items contaminated with the patient's excreta.

Caring for your hair and scalp during cancer treatment

Dear Patient,

Some hair loss is inevitable during chemotherapy or radiation therapy. But sometimes you can help minimize hair loss by keeping your hair and scalp clean and treating them gently. Just follow these suggestions.

IF YOU'RE HAVING CHEMOTHERAPY

- Shampoo regularly—every 2 to 4 days. (Shampooing every day may be too harsh.)
- Use a mild *protein-based* shampoo—for example, Appearance, an apple pectin shampoo. (Baby shampoo isn't necessarily mild.) You may want to talk with a hairdresser to determine which shampoo is best for you.

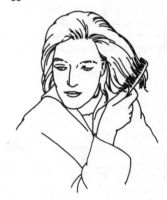

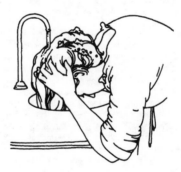

- Use a conditioner after shampooing.
- Gently pat your hair dry.
- If your scalp is very dry and flaky, try massaging it with mineral oil, castor oil, or vitamin A and D ointment after shampooing and rinsing your hair.
- Brush and comb your hair very gently, using a soft-bristled brush and a pliable, wide-toothed comb.

- Avoid harsh chemicals, permanents, and dyes. Also avoid tight curls or braids. Don't use a curling iron, hair dryer, or hot rollers. And don't sleep with curlers in your hair.
- To minimize friction on your hair, try sleeping on a satin pillowcase. And to keep your hair from shedding, try using a hair net.
- Wear a hat to protect your scalp from sunburn.

IF YOU'RE HAVING RADIATION THERAPY

- Don't use anything on your scalp except Eucerin or Aquaphor cream. You can buy these products at your local pharmacy without a prescription.
- When your hair starts to grow back, follow the hair and scalp care instructions listed above.

(continued)

GENERAL

- Review the medications and adverse reactions with the patient.
- Discuss the management of adverse reactions with the patient. (See *Managing common adverse effects of chemotherapy*.)
- Review the signs and symptoms of abnormal bleeding, infection, or bone marrow suppression.
- Advise the patient when to contact the practitioner.
- Emphasize follow-up care.

- Refer the patient to local resources or a home health care agency.

RESOURCES

Organizations

American College of Surgeons Oncology Group: *www.acosog.org*
American Medical Association: *www.ama-assn.org*
National Cancer Institute: *www.cancer.gov*

Selected references

Cao, M.G., et al. "Biochemotherapy with Temozolomide, Cisplatin, Vinblastine, Subcutaneous Interleukin-2 and Interferon-alpha in Patients with Metastatic Melanoma," *Melanoma Research* 16(1):59-64, February 2006.

Koppe, M.J., et al. "Peritoneal Carcinomatosis of Colorectal Origin: Incidence and Current Treatment Strategies," *Annals of Surgery* 243(2): 212-22, February 2006.

Sarela, A.I., et al. "Clinical Outcomes with Laparoscopic Stage M1, Unresected Gastric Adenocarcinoma," *Annals of Surgery* 243(2):189-95, February 2006.

Slack, S.M., et al. "Shared Decision Making: Empowering the Bedside Nurse," *Clinical Journal of Oncological Nursing* 9(6):725-27, December 2005.

Managing common adverse effects of chemotherapy

ADVERSE EFFECT	NURSING ACTIONS	HOME CARE INSTRUCTIONS
Bone marrow depression (leukopenia, thrombocytopenia, anemia)	• Establish baseline white blood cell (WBC) and platelet counts, hemoglobin level, and hematocrit before therapy begins. Monitor laboratory studies during therapy. • If WBC count drops suddenly or falls to < 2,000/mm^3, stop the drug and notify the practitioner. Initiate reverse isolation if absolute granulocyte count falls to < 1,000/mm^3. Report a platelet count < 100,000/mm^3. If necessary, assist with transfusion. • Monitor temperature orally every 4 hours, and regularly inspect the skin and body orifices for signs of infection. Observe for petechiae, easy bruising, and bleeding. Check for hematuria and monitor the patient's blood pressure. Be alert for signs of anemia. • Limit subQ and I.M. injections. If these are necessary, apply pressure for 3 to 5 minutes after injection to prevent leakage or hematoma. Report unusual bleeding after injection. • Take precautions to prevent bleeding. Use extra care with razors, nail trimmers, dental floss, toothbrushes, and other sharp or abrasive objects. • Give vitamin and iron supplements as ordered. Provide a diet high in iron.	• Instruct the patient to immediately report fever, chills, sore throat, lethargy, unusual fatigue, or pallor. • Warn the patient to avoid exposure to persons with infections during chemotherapy and for several months after the treatments have ended. • Explain that the patient shouldn't receive immunizations during or shortly after chemotherapy because an exaggerated reaction may occur. • Tell the patient to avoid activities that could cause traumatic injury and bleeding. Advise him to report episodes of bleeding or bruising to the practitioner. • Tell the patient to eat high-iron foods, such as liver and spinach. • Stress the importance of follow-up blood studies after completion of treatment.
Anorexia	• Assess the patient's nutritional status before and during chemotherapy. Weigh him weekly or as ordered. • Explain the need for adequate nutrition despite the loss of appetite.	• Encourage the patient's family to supply favorite foods to help him maintain adequate nutrition. • Suggest that the patient eat small, frequent meals.
Nausea and vomiting	• Before chemotherapy begins, administer antiemetics, as ordered, to reduce the severity of these reactions. • Monitor and record the frequency, character, and amount of vomitus. • Monitor serum electrolyte levels, and provide total parenteral nutrition, if necessary.	• Teach the patient and his family how to insert antiemetic suppositories. • Tell the patient to take the drug on an empty stomach, with meals, or at bedtime. GI upset indicates that the drug is working. Instruct him to report vomiting to the practitioner. • Tell the patient to follow a high-protein diet.

Managing common adverse effects of chemotherapy *(continued)*

ADVERSE EFFECT	NURSING ACTIONS	HOME CARE INSTRUCTIONS
Diarrhea and abdominal cramps	◆ Assess the frequency, color, consistency, and amount of diarrhea. Give antidiarrheals as ordered. ◆ Assess the severity of cramps, and observe for signs of dehydration and acidosis, which may indicate electrolyte imbalance. ◆ Encourage fluids and, if ordered, give I.V. fluids and potassium supplements. ◆ Provide good skin care, especially to the perianal area.	◆ Teach the patient how to use antidiarrheals, and instruct him to report diarrhea to the practitioner. ◆ Encourage the patient to maintain adequate fluid intake and to follow a bland, low-fiber diet. ◆ Explain that good perianal hygiene can help prevent skin breakdown and infection.
Stomatitis	◆ Before drug administration, observe for dry mouth, erythema, and white patchy areas on the oral mucosa. Stay alert for bleeding gums or complaints of a burning sensation when drinking acidic liquids. ◆ Emphasize the principles of good mouth care with the patient and his family. ◆ Provide mouth care every 4 to 6 hours with normal saline solution or half-strength hydrogen peroxide. Coat the oral mucosa with milk of magnesia. Avoid lemon-glycerin swabs because they tend to reduce saliva and change mouth pH. ◆ To make eating more comfortable, apply a topical viscous anesthetic, such as lidocaine, before meals. Administer special mouthwashes as ordered. ◆ Consult the dietitian to provide bland foods at medium temperatures. ◆ Treat cracked or burning lips with petroleum jelly.	◆ Teach the patient good mouth care. Instruct him to rinse his mouth with 1 tsp of salt dissolved in 8 oz (237 ml) of warm water or hydrogen peroxide diluted to half strength with water. ◆ Advise the patient to avoid acidic, spicy, or extremely hot or cold foods. ◆ Instruct the patient to report stomatitis to the practitioner, who may order a change in medication.
Alopecia	◆ Reassure the patient that alopecia is usually temporary. ◆ Inform the patient that he may experience discomfort before hair loss starts.	◆ Suggest that the patient have his hair cut short to make thinning hair less noticeable. ◆ Advise the patient to wash his hair with a mild shampoo and avoid frequent brushing or combing. ◆ Suggest that the patient wear a hat, scarf, toupee, or wig.

Chemotherapy infusion and chemoembolization of liver

- Primary liver cancer (also known as *hepatoma* or *hepatocellular carcinoma*): derives its blood exclusively from the hepatic artery; very vascular tumor
- Chemotherapy infusion: delivers chemotherapeutic agents through hepatic artery directly to the tumor; higher concentrations may be delivered to tumors without systemic toxicity
- Arterial chemotherapy infusion of the liver and chemoembolization of the liver (transarterial chemoembolization or TACE): involve chemotherapy injected into the hepatic artery supplying the liver tumor; however, with chemoembolization, additional injected material blocks the small branches of the hepatic artery
- Provide relief or lessen the severity of disease; however, not curative and produces less than 50% decrease in tumor size
- Can be used only in patients with relatively preserved liver function

INDICATIONS

- Hepatoma or hepatocellular carcinoma

ARTERIAL CHEMOTHERAPY INFUSION

- An interventional radiologist works closely with an oncologist, who determines the amount of chemotherapy that the patient receives at each session. Some patients may undergo repeat sessions at 6- to 12-week intervals.
- Under fluoroscopy imaging, a catheter is inserted into the femoral artery in the groin, threaded into the aorta, and advanced into the hepatic artery.
- When the branches of the hepatic artery that feed the liver cancer are identified, the chemotherapy is infused.
- The procedure takes 1 to 2 hours, and then the catheter is removed and a compression device is placed over the puncture site.

CHEMOEMBOLIZATION

- TACE is similar to intra-arterial infusion of chemotherapy; in TACE, however, there's an additional step of embolizing the small blood vessels with different types of compounds, such as gelfoam or small metal coils.

COMPLICATIONS

- Systemic chemotherapeutic adverse effects
- Inflammation of the gallbladder (cholecystitis)
- Intestinal and stomach ulcers
- Inflammation of the pancreas (pancreatitis)
- Liver failure
- Blocking of the feeding vessels to the tumor with chemoembolization possibly making future attempts at intra-arterial infusions impossible

- Deficient fluid volume
- Impaired nutrition: Less than body requirements
- Risk for infection

EXPECTED OUTCOMES

The patient will:
- maintain adequate fluid volume
- maintain normal weight
- remain free from infection.

PRETREATMENT CARE

◆ Review the procedure with the patient and emphasize the importance of remaining still during the procedure. Also review possible adverse reactions of the treatment with the patient.
◆ Monitor laboratory results as ordered, and notify the practitioner of results.
◆ Monitor the patient's vital signs and intake and output.
◆ Provide pretreatment medications as ordered.
◆ Check for patient allergies.
◆ Verify that the patient has signed an informed consent form.

POSTTREATMENT CARE

ARTERIAL CHEMOTHERAPY INFUSION

◆ Maintain sandbag or other compression device over the puncture site.
◆ Monitor for signs of bleeding from the femoral artery puncture.
◆ Monitor pulses in the affected extremity.
◆ Monitor laboratory test results. Generally, liver tests increase (get worse) during the 2 or 3 days after the procedure. This worsening of the liver tests is actually due to death of the tumor (and some nontumor) cells.
◆ Monitor for postprocedure abdominal pain and low-grade fever. Severe abdominal pain and vomiting suggests serious complications.
◆ Monitor the patient for adverse effects.
◆ Administer analgesics as ordered.
◆ Provide emotional support.

PATIENT TEACHING

GENERAL

◆ Refer the patient and his family to support services available in the community.
◆ Tell the patient that imaging studies of the liver are repeated in 6 to 12 weeks to assess the size of the tumor in response to the treatment.

RESOURCES

Organizations

American College of Surgeons Oncology Group: *www.acosog.org*
American Medical Association: *www.ama-assn.org*
National Cancer Institute: *www.cancer.gov*

Selected references

Fisher, R.A., et al. "Non-resective Ablation Therapy for Hepatocellular Carcinoma: Effectiveness Measured by Intention-to-Treat and Dropout from Liver Transplant Waiting List," *Clinical Transplant* 18(5):502-12, October 2004.
Luo, B.M., et al. "Percutaneous Ethanol Injection, Radiofrequency and their Combination in Treatment of Hepatocellular Carcinoma," *World Journal of Gastroenterology* 11(40):6277-80, October 2005.
Park, H.S., et al. "Postbiopsy Arterioportal Fistula in Patients with Hepatocellular Carcinoma: Clinical Significance in Transarterial Chemoembolization," *American Journal of Roentgenology* 186(2):556-61, February 2006.
Slack, S.M., et al. "Shared Decision Making: Empowering the Bedside Nurse," *Clinical Journal of Oncological Nursing* 9(6):725-27, December 2005.

Chest drainage

- Uses gravity and suction to remove material (air, blood, pus, chyle, other serous fluids, or blood clots) that collects in the pleural cavity, thus restoring negative pressure and reexpanding a partially or totally collapsed lung
- Underwater seal: allows air and fluid to escape from the pleural cavity but doesn't allow air to reenter

INDICATIONS

- Hemothorax
- Pneumothorax
- Pleural effusion

- Open the packaged system, and place it on the floor; after prepared, hang it from the side of the bed.
- Remove the plastic connector from the short tube attached to the water-seal chamber, using a 50-ml, catheter-tip syringe. Instill sterile distilled water into the water-seal chamber until it reaches the 2-cm mark or the mark specified by the manufacturer.
- Water may need to be added to help detect air leaks with some systems.
- Replace the plastic connector.
- If suction is ordered, remove the cap (also called the muffler or atmosphere vent cover) on the suction-control chamber to open the vent.
- Next, instill sterile distilled water until it reaches the 20-cm mark or the ordered level, and recap the suction-control chamber.
- Using the long tube, connect the chest tube to the closed drainage collection chamber and secure with tape.
- Connect the short tube to the suction source, and turn on the suction. Gentle bubbling should begin.

COMPLICATIONS

- Tension pneumothorax
- Bleeding
- Infection

- Acute pain
- Impaired physical mobility
- Ineffective breathing pattern

EXPECTED OUTCOMES
The patient will:
- have adequate pain control
- maintain physical mobility after analgesic administration
- display easy, unlabored respirations.

- Explain the procedure to the patient, and wash your hands.
- Maintain sterile technique throughout the procedure and when you make changes in the system or alter connections.

◆ Note character, consistency, and amount of drainage; mark level in the drainage collection chamber; and note time and date at the drainage level on the chamber every 8 hours (more often if a large amount of drainage).

◆ Check water level in the water-seal chamber every 8 hours. If necessary, add sterile distilled water until the level reaches the 2-cm mark.

◆ Check for fluctuation in the water-seal chamber as the patient breathes.

◆ To check for fluctuation with a suction system, momentarily disconnect the suction system so the air vent is opened, and observe for fluctuation.

◆ Check for intermittent bubbling in the water-seal chamber. Absence of bubbling may indicate that the pleural space has sealed.

◆ Check the water level in the suction-control chamber. Detach the chamber from the suction source; when bubbling ceases, observe the water level. If needed, add sterile distilled water to bring the level to the 20-cm line or as ordered.

⚡ **WARNING** *Occlusion of the air vent results in buildup of pressure in the system that could cause a tension pneumothorax.*

◆ Coil the system's tubing and secure it to the edge of the bed. Make sure that tubing remains at the level of the patient. Avoid dependent loops, kinks, or pressure on the tubing. Avoid lifting the system above the patient's chest; fluid may flow back into the pleural space.

◆ Keep two rubber-tipped clamps at the bedside to clamp the chest tube if the system cracks or to locate an air leak in the system.

◆ Check rate and quality of respirations; auscultate lungs to assess air exchange. Diminished or absent breath sounds indicates nonexpansion.

◆ When clots are visible, milk the tubing depending on your facility's policy. Milk in direction of the drainage chamber as needed.

◆ Check chest tube dressing at least every 8 hours according to facility policy.

◆ Give ordered pain medication for comfort and to help with deep-breathing, coughing, and range-of-motion exercises.

◆ If excessive continuous bubbling occurs, especially with suction, rule out a leak in the system. Locate by clamping the tube momentarily at various points along its length, beginning at the proximal end and working down to the drainage system. If a connection is loose, push it together and tape securely. Bubbling will stop when a clamp is placed between the air leak and the water seal. If you clamp along the tube's entire length and bubbling doesn't stop, the drainage unit may be cracked and need replacement.

◆ If the drainage collection chamber fills, replace it. Double-clamp the tube close to the insertion site (use two clamps facing in opposite directions), exchange the system, remove the clamps, and retape the connection.

⚡ **WARNING** *Never leave tubes clamped for more than 1 minute to prevent tension pneumothorax.*

◆ If the system cracks, clamp the chest tube momentarily with the two rubber-tipped clamps placed close to each other near the insertion site facing opposite directions. Observe for altered respirations while the tube is clamped. Replace the damaged equipment. (Prepare the new unit before clamping.)

◆ Instead of clamping the tube, submerge the distal end of the tube in a container of normal saline solution to create a temporary water seal while you replace the drainage system. Check your facility's policy for the proper procedure.

GENERAL

◆ Encourage the patient to cough frequently and breathe deeply.

◆ Instruct the patient to sit upright and to splint the insertion site while coughing to minimize pain.

⚡ **WARNING** *Tell the patient to report breathing difficulty immediately. Notify the practitioner immediately if cyanosis, rapid or shallow breathing, subcutaneous emphysema, chest pain, or excessive bleeding occurs.*

◆ Remind the ambulatory patient to keep the drainage system below chest level and to be careful not to disconnect the tubing to maintain the water seal.

RESOURCES
Organizations

American College of Emergency Physicians: *www.acep.org*
American Medical Association: *www.ama-assn.org*

Selected references

Allibone, L. "Principles for Inserting and Managing Chest Drains," *Nursing Times* 101(42):45-49, October 2005.

Carroll, P. "Keeping Up with Mobile Chest Drains," *RN* 68(10):26-31, October 2005.

Clubley, L., and Harper, L. "Using Negative Pressure Therapy for Healing of a Sternal Wound," *Nursing Times* 101(16):44-46, April 2005.

Lehwaldt, D., and Timmins, F. "Nurses' Knowledge of Chest Drain Care: An Exploratory Descriptive Survey," *Nursing Critical Care* 10(4):192-200, July-August 2005.

Chest physiotherapy

- Includes postural drainage, chest percussion and vibration, and coughing and deep-breathing exercises; techniques mobilize and eliminate secretions, reexpand lung tissue, and promote efficient use of respiratory muscles
- Postural drainage: encourages peripheral pulmonary secretions to empty by gravity into the major bronchi or trachea; accomplished by sequential repositioning of the patient
- Best drainage achieved with patient positioned so that the bronchi are perpendicular to the floor
- Lower and middle lobe bronchi: usually empty best with patient in the head-down position; upper lobe bronchi, in the head-up position
- Percussing the chest with cupped hands: mechanically dislodges thick, tenacious secretions from the bronchial walls
- Can use vibration with percussion or as an alternative in a patient who's frail, in pain, or recovering from thoracic surgery or trauma
- Hasn't proven effective in treating patients with status asthmaticus, lobar pneumonia, or acute exacerbations of chronic bronchitis when the patient has scant secretions and is being mechanically ventilated
- Has little value for treating patients with stable, chronic bronchitis

INDICATIONS
- Bedridden patient to mobilize secretions
- Atelectasis
- Pneumonia
- Patients who expectorate large amounts of sputum, such as those with bronchiectasis or cystic fibrosis

 WARNING *Contraindications to chest physiotherapy include:*
- *active pulmonary bleeding with hemoptysis and the immediate posthemorrhage stage*
- *fractured ribs*
- *unstable chest wall*
- *lung contusions*
- *pulmonary tuberculosis*
- *untreated pneumothorax*
- *acute asthma*
- *bronchospasm*
- *lung abscess*
- *tumor*
- *bony metastasis*
- *head injury*
- *recent myocardial infarction.*

- Explain the procedure to the patient, provide privacy, and wash your hands.
- Auscultate the patient's lungs to determine baseline respiratory status.
- Position the patient as ordered. In generalized disease, drainage usually begins with the lower lobes, continues with the middle lobes, and ends with the upper lobes.
- In localized disease, drainage begins with the affected lobes and then proceeds to the other lobes to avoid spreading the disease to uninvolved areas.
- Instruct the patient to remain in each position for 10 to 15 minutes.
- During this time, perform percussion and vibration as ordered. (See *Performing percussion and vibration.*)

Performing percussion and vibration

Instruct the patient to breathe slowly and deeply, using the diaphragm, to promote relaxation. Percuss each segment with a cupped hand for 1 or 2 minutes. Listen for a hollow sound on percussion to verify correct performance of technique.

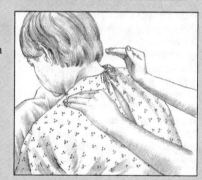

To perform vibration, ask him to inhale deeply, and then exhale slowly. During exhalation, firmly press your hands against the chest wall. Tense the muscles of your arms and shoulders in an isometric contraction to send fine vibrations through the chest wall. Do this during five exhalations over each chest segment.

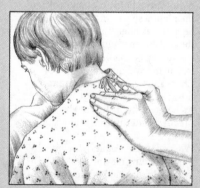

- For optimal effectiveness and safety, modify chest physiotherapy based on the patient's condition: for example, initiate or increase the flow of supplemental oxygen, if indicated.
- Also, suction the patient who has an ineffective cough reflex.
- If the patient tires quickly during therapy, shorten the sessions because fatigue leads to shallow respirations and increased hypoxia.
- Refrain from percussing over the spine, liver, kidneys, or spleen to avoid injury to the spine or internal organs. Also avoid performing percussion on bare skin or the female patient's breasts.
- Percuss over soft clothing (but not over buttons, snaps, or zippers), or place a thin towel over the chest wall.

COMPLICATIONS
- Impaired excursion leading to hypoxia or orthostatic hypertension that may occur during postural drainage (in the head-down position due to abdominal contents placing pressure on the diaphragm)
- Increased intracranial pressure (in the head-down position, precluding the patient with acute neurologic impairment)
- Rib fracture due to vigorous percussion or vibration, especially in a patient with osteoporosis
- Pneumothorax due to coughing in an emphysematous patient with blebs

NURSING DIAGNOSES
- Anxiety
- Impaired gas exchange
- Ineffective airway clearance

EXPECTED OUTCOMES
The patient will:
- express feelings of comfort and demonstrate decreased anxiety
- maintain adequate ventilation and oxygenation
- maintain airway patency.

PRETREATMENT CARE
- Gather the equipment at the patient's bedside.
- Set up suction equipment and test its function.
- Maintain adequate hydration in the patient to prevent mucus dehydration and promote easier mobilization.
- Avoid performing postural drainage immediately before or within 1 to 2 hours after meals to avoid nausea, vomiting, and aspiration of food or vomitus.
- Because chest percussion can induce bronchospasm, adjunct treatment (for example, intermittent positive-pressure breathing, aerosol, or nebulizer therapy) should precede chest physiotherapy.
- Explain deep-breathing and coughing exercises so that the patient can practice them preoperatively.
- Remove jewelry that might scratch or bruise the patient.

POSTTREATMENT CARE
- After postural drainage, percussion, or vibration, instruct the patient to cough to remove loosened secretions.
- First, tell him to inhale deeply through his nose and then exhale in three short huffs.
- Then have him inhale deeply again and cough through a slightly open mouth.
- Three consecutive coughs are highly effective.
- An effective cough sounds deep, low, and hollow; an ineffective one, high-pitched.
- Have the patient perform exercises for about 1 minute and then rest for 2 minutes; gradually progress to a 10-minute exercise period four times daily.
- Provide oral hygiene because secretions may have a foul taste or a stale odor.
- Auscultate the patient's lungs to evaluate the effectiveness of therapy.

PATIENT TEACHING
- Teach the patient how to splint his incision to minimize pain during coughing.

RESOURCES
Organizations
American College of Chest Surgeons: *www.chestnet.org*
American Medical Association: *www.ama-assn.org*

Selected references
Bradley, J.M., et al. "Evidence for Physical Therapies (Airway Clearance and Physical Training) in Cystic Fibrosis: An Overview of Five Cochrane Systematic Reviews," *Respiratory Medicine* 100(2):191-201, February 2006.

McCool, F.D., and Rosen, M.J. "Nonpharmacologic Airway Clearance Therapies: ACCP Evidence-Based Clinical Practice Guidelines," *Chest* 129(Suppl 1):250S-259S, January 2006.

Rosen, M.J. "Chronic Cough due to Bronchiectasis: ACCP Evidence-Based Clinical Practice Guidelines," *Chest* 129(Suppl 1):122S-131S, January 2006.

Varela, G., et al. "Cost-Effectiveness Analysis of Prophylactic Respiratory Physiotherapy in Pulmonary Lobectomy," *European Journal of Cardiothoracic Surgery* 29(2):216-20, February 2006.

Cholecystectomy

- Surgical removal of the gallbladder
- May be performed as an open abdominal surgical procedure or as a laparoscopic procedure

INDICATIONS

- Gallbladder or biliary duct disease refractory to drug therapy, dietary changes, and other supportive treatments

PROCEDURE

- The open abdominal and laparoscopic approaches require general anesthesia.

ABDOMINAL CHOLECYSTECTOMY

- A right subcostal or paramedial incision is made.
- The surgeon surveys the abdomen.
- Laparotomy packs are used to isolate the gallbladder from the surrounding organs.
- After biliary tract structures are identified, cholangiography or ultrasonography may be used to identify gallstones.
- The bile ducts are visualized using a choledochoscope.
- The ducts are cleared of stones after insertion of a Fogarty balloon-tipped catheter.
- The surgeon ligates and divides the cystic duct and artery and removes the entire gallbladder.
- A choledochotomy may be performed, with a T tube inserted into the common bile duct.
- A Penrose drain may be placed into the ducts.
- The incision is closed and a dressing is applied.

LAPAROSCOPIC CHOLECYSTECTOMY

- A small incision is made just above the umbilicus.
- A trocar, connected to an insufflator, is inserted through the incision.
- Carbon dioxide or nitrous oxide is injected into the abdominal cavity.
- A laparoscope is passed through the trocar to view the intra-abdominal contents.
- The patient is placed in a 30-degree, reverse Trendelenburg's position and tilted slightly to the left.
- With laparoscopic guidance, the surgeon makes three incisions in the right upper quadrant: one below the xiphoid process in the midline; one below the right costal margin in the midclavicular line; and one in the anterior axillary line at the umbilical level.
- Using the laparoscope, the surgeon passes instruments through the three incisions to clamp and tie off the cystic duct and excise the gallbladder.
- The gallbladder is removed through the umbilical opening.
- The surgeon sutures all four incisions and places a dressing over each.

COMPLICATIONS

- Peritonitis
- Postcholecystectomy syndrome
- Atelectasis
- Bile duct injury
- Small bowel injury
- Wound infection
- Ileus
- Urine retention
- Retained gallstones

NURSING DIAGNOSES

◆ Acute pain
◆ Ineffective breathing pattern
◆ Risk for infection

EXPECTED OUTCOMES
The patient will:
◆ express feelings of comfort
◆ maintain a normal breathing pattern
◆ remain free from infection.

PRETREATMENT CARE

◆ Explain the treatment and preparation to the patient and his family.
◆ Verify that the patient has signed an appropriate consent form.
◆ Withhold oral intake as ordered.
◆ Administer preoperative medications as ordered.

ABDOMINAL APPROACH
◆ Tell the patient that:
– a nasogastric (NG) tube will be in place for 1 or 2 days and an abdominal drain will be in place for 3 to 5 days after surgery
– a T tube may remain in place for up to 2 weeks
– he may be discharged with the T tube in place.

LAPAROSCOPIC APPROACH
◆ Tell the patient that:
– an indwelling urinary catheter will be inserted into the bladder
– an NG tube will be placed in the stomach
– the tube is usually removed in the postanesthesia room
– three small incisions will be covered with a small sterile dressing
– discharge may occur on the day of surgery or 1 day after.

POSTTREATMENT CARE

◆ Administer medications as ordered.
◆ Place the patient in low Fowler's position.
◆ Attach the NG tube to low intermittent suction as ordered.
◆ Report drainage greater than 500 ml after 48 hours.
◆ Provide meticulous skin care, especially around drainage tube insertion sites.
◆ After the NG tube is removed, introduce foods as ordered.
◆ Clamp the T tube before and after each meal as ordered.
◆ After laparoscopic cholecystectomy, start clear liquids as ordered when the patient has fully recovered from anesthesia.
◆ Assist the patient with early ambulation.
◆ Encourage coughing and deep-breathing exercises.
◆ Encourage incentive spirometry use.
◆ Provide analgesics as ordered.
◆ Monitor the patient's vital signs and intake and output.
◆ Observe the patient for signs of complications and postcholecystectomy syndrome.
◆ Monitor the patient's respiratory status.
◆ Record the amount and characteristics of drainage.
◆ Monitor surgical dressings and provide wound care as ordered.
◆ Maintain the position and patency of drainage tubes.

PATIENT TEACHING

GENERAL
◆ Review the medications and possible adverse reactions with the patient.
◆ Instruct the patient about coughing and deep-breathing exercises.
◆ Teach the patient about T tube home care, if applicable. (See *Caring for your T tube*, pages 76 and 77.)
◆ Tell the patient about the signs and symptoms of biliary obstruction.
◆ Inform the patient about the signs and symptoms of infection.
◆ Review the possible complications of the procedure with the patient.
◆ Emphasize follow-up care.

RESOURCES
Organizations
American College of Gastroenterology: *www.acg.gi.org*
American Gastroenterological Association: *www.gastro.org*
American Medical Association: *www.ama-assn.org*

Selected references
Dalton, S.J., et al. "Routine Magnetic Resonance Cholangiopancreatography and Intra-operative Cholangiogram in the Evaluation of Common Bile Duct Stones," *Annals of the Royal College of Surgeons of England* 87(6):469-70, November 2005.
Dunn, D. "Preventing Perioperative Complications in Special Populations," *Nursing2005* 35(11):36-43, November 2005.
Madsen, D., et al. "Listening to Bowel Sounds: An Evidence-Based Practice Project," *AJN* 105(12):40-49, December 2005.

(continued)

Caring for your T tube

Dear Patient,

Here are instructions for taking care of your T tube at home. You'll have this tube for 10 to 14 days. During that time, it will drain excess bile so that your incision will heal faster. The tube will also allow passage of retained gallstones.

Caring for your T tube isn't difficult, but it takes time and planning. Set aside about 20 uninterrupted minutes per day to empty your drainage bag and care for your incision. To help prevent infection and promote healing, carefully follow these directions.

GATHERING YOUR SUPPLIES

First, assemble these supplies on a table or countertop: a large measuring container, toilet paper, soap, a clean towel, a paper bag, a sterile paper cloth, five sterile 4″ × 4″ gauze pads, alcohol, normal saline solution, hydrogen peroxide, povidone-iodine solution (Betadine), sterile gloves, povidone-iodine ointment, scissors, and adhesive tape.

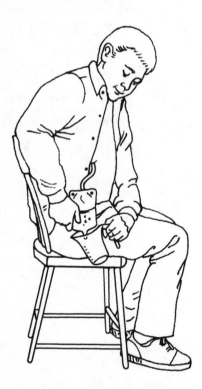

EMPTYING THE DRAINAGE BAG

Empty your drainage bag at about the same time each day or when it's two-thirds full. First, place the large measuring container within easy reach.

1. Sit on a chair, and remove the Velcro belt that secures the drainage bag and connecting tubing to your abdomen. Uncoil the tubing and position the spout at the bottom of the drainage bag over the measuring container. Don't pull on the connecting tubing, and don't place too much tension on it— you may dislodge the T tube.

2. To empty the drainage bag, release the clamp on the drainage spout so that the bile flows freely into the measuring container. When the bag is empty, clean the drainage spout with toilet paper. To reseal the drainage bag, close the clamp.

3. Gently coil the connecting tubing. Then position the drainage bag and tubing below the incision site. Secure the bag and tubing with the Velcro belt. Never place the drainage bag and connecting tubing higher than your incision. This could cause the draining bile to back up into the common bile duct.

4. Finally, note the amount, color, and odor of drainage. Contact your health care provider if you notice significant increases or decreases in the drainage amount or changes in the color or odor. These may signal complications, such as an infection or a T-tube obstruction.

CARING FOR YOUR INCISION

After you empty and resecure your drainage bag, you're ready to clean and redress the incision site. Just follow these steps:

1. Wash your hands with soap and water, and dry them with a fresh, clean towel. Carefully remove the soiled dressing and discard it in the paper bag. Then wash and dry your hands again.

2. Open the package containing the sterile paper cloth. Unfold the cloth and spread it on a table or countertop. Don't touch the top surface of the cloth.

3. Open the five sterile gauze pads and drop them on the sterile cloth.

4. Open the packets of alcohol, normal saline solution, hydrogen peroxide, and povidone-iodine solution, and place them on the table.

5. Put on the sterile gloves. Then pick up a sterile gauze pad with your dominant hand (your "sterile" hand).

6. Pick up the saline solution with your other hand and thoroughly soak the gauze pad.

7. Clean the incision area with the soaked pad. Wipe outward away from the tube in a 3″ (7.5 cm) circular area.

Using a clean pad, repeat this with the hydrogen peroxide and the povidone-iodine solution, again wiping outward.

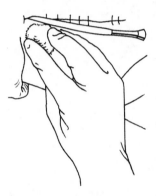

8. Soak a clean gauze pad with alcohol and use it to wipe the first 6″ (15 cm) of the tube. Start at the incision and wipe toward the drainage bag.

9. Apply a nickel-size drop of povidone-iodine ointment over the wound site. Cover the ointment with the remaining sterile gauze pad. Be sure to apply the pad so that the slit end faces up and slides under your tube. Next, tape the pad securely to your abdomen.

10. Finally, tape a small segment of the T tube to your abdomen so you won't accidentally dislodge the tube. Discard used supplies in a paper bag.

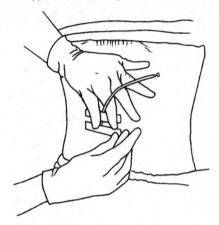

WATCHING FOR COMPLICATIONS

Report the following signs of infection when you're caring for your tubing and incision:
- redness, swelling, or pain
- puslike drainage.
   Also contact your health care provider if you have:
- fever
- nausea
- clay-colored stools.

Circumcision

- Removes about one-third of the penile skin (sensitive inner and outer preputial layers), including the peripenic dartos muscle, the frenar band, and part of the frenulum

INDICATIONS

- Primarily cultural, religious, or personal reasons

- If performed on a child, Velcro straps are used to restrain the arms and legs.
- The area is prepared with an antiseptic, such as iodine liquid, and a surgical drape is placed over the site.
- Some practitioners will use local anesthesia, but injections will cause the penis to swell, causing pain and making the surgery more difficult. An anesthetic cream may be applied.
- The foreskin is grasped with forceps and the opening widened.

  AGE FACTOR *The foreskin is normally attached to the glans by a membrane called the synechia. The glans and inner lining of the foreskin are still developing in the young child. During circumcision, the synechia must be torn apart.*

- The foreskin is clamped and a slit is made in the dorsal side of the foreskin.
- The slit is separated and the foreskin is laid back, exposing the glans.
- A PlastiBell device of appropriate size is slipped over the glans, and the foreskin is laid over it. A ligature is tied in the ridge of the bell, as tightly as possible around the foreskin.
- After 1 or 2 minutes, the foreskin is sliced off at the distal edge of the ligature using a knife or scissors. The surgeon trims as much tissue as possible to reduce the amount of necrotic tissue and the possibility of infection.
- The handle of the bell is snapped off at this time. The rim of tissue will become necrotic and separate with the bell in 5 to 10 days.
- Occasionally, edema will trap the plastic ring on the shaft of the penis and the ring will need to be removed using a guide and ring cutter. Application of ice sometimes reduces edema enough to remove the ring.
- Impregnated gauze may be applied to the site.

COMPLICATIONS

- Bleeding
- Infection
- Injury to the glans
- Complications from anesthesia, if used
- Surgical error, including removal of too much skin
- Meatal stenosis (narrowing of the urethral opening due to infection and subsequent scarring, that occurs almost exclusively in circumcised boys)
- Extensive scarring of the penile shaft
- Skin tags and skin bridges
- Curvature of the penis
- Tight, painful erections
- Psychological and psychosexual problems

- Acute pain
- Impaired tissue integrity
- Risk for infection

EXPECTED OUTCOMES
The patient will:
- exhibit signs of comfort
- demonstrate skin that's intact and healing
- show no signs of infection.

- Verify that an informed consent has been signed by the patient or his parents.
- Explain the procedure the patient and his parents, and answer any questions that they may have.
- Note any patient allergies.

- Monitor the patient's vital signs.
- Monitor for excessive drainage and for signs of infection.
- Keep the wound area clean, and apply antibiotic ointment as ordered.

GENERAL
- Review the care of the circumcised penis.
- Tell the patient or parents to notify the practitioner if infection or excessive bleeding occurs.
- Review follow-up care.

RESOURCES
Organizations
American Association of Clinical Urologists: *www.aacuweb.org*
American College of Obstetrics and Gynecology: *www.acog.org*

Selected references
Atashili, J. "Adult Male Circumcision to Prevent HIV?" *International Journal of Infectious Diseases* 10(3):202-205, May 2006.

Tanne, J.H. "Ultra-Orthodox Jews Criticised over Circumcision Practice," *British Medical Journal* 332(7534):137, January 2006.

Van Howe, R.S. "Incidence of Meatal Stenosis Following Neonatal Circumcision in a Primary Care Setting," *Clinical Pediatrics* 45(1):49-54, January-February 2006.

Weise, K.L., and Nahata, M.C. "EMLA for Painful Procedures in Infants," *Journal of Pediatric Health Care* 19(1):42-47, January-February 2005.

Clitoral therapy device

- Promotes greater clitoral and genital engorgement, increased vaginal lubrication, enhanced ability to achieve orgasm, and improved overall sexual satisfaction
- Consists of a small, soft, plastic vacuum cup attached by a tube to a palm-sized, battery-operated vacuum pump; cup placed over the clitoris before sex, with the pump drawing blood into the clitoris through gentle suction, thus causing engorgement and sexual arousal

INDICATIONS
- Diminished vaginal lubrication
- Diminished clitoral sensation
- Reduced ability to achieve orgasm
- Lowered sexual satisfaction

- The patient places the clitoral therapy device over her clitoris.
- When the device is turned on, a gentle vacuum is created, increasing blood flow to the genitalia, causing the clitoris to become engorged.
- Increased blood flow to the genitalia results in increased vaginal lubrication, enhanced ability to achieve orgasm, and increased clitoral and genital sensitivity.

COMPLICATIONS
- None known

- Anxiety
- Deficient knowledge (disorder and treatment)
- Sexual dysfunction

EXPECTED OUTCOMES
The patient will:
- express reduced anxiety
- verbalize understanding of the disorder and treatment regimen
- have improved sexual experience.

PRETREATMENT CARE

◆ Review the patient's medical history, especially previous sexual difficulty (such as painful intercourse or vaginal dryness), genital trauma (such as genital body piercings), diabetes, heart disease, hypertension, high cholesterol, or spinal injuries.

◆ Note any drug interactions that may influence the patient's condition, such as hormone medication (estrogen and progestin), phentolamine (Vasomax), prostaglandins, or vaginal lubricants. Some drugs can cause sexual problems in the female. Prescription and nonprescription medication, such as antidepressants (amitriptyline [Elavil] or fluoxetine [Prozac]) and beta-adrenergic blockers (metoprolol [Toprol] or propranolol [Inderal]), can also affect sexual response.

◆ Review the device and manual that comes with the product.

POSTTREATMENT CARE

◆ Tell the patient that the device may be used before having intercourse or without intercourse to condition and restore sexual responses.

◆ Inform the patient that it should be used three to four times per week to achieve the maximum benefits.

PATIENT TEACHING

GENERAL

◆ Review instructions regarding the use of the device with the patient.

◆ Inform the patient that it may take up to several weeks of recommended use to see an improvement in overall sexual function.

◆ Tell the patient that some women may notice changes immediately, whereas others may take longer to note results.

RESOURCES
Organizations
American Association of Clinical Urologists: *www.aacuweb.org*
American College of Obstetrics and Gynecology: *www.acog.org*
MedicineNet: *www.medicinenet.com*

Selected references
Archer, S.L., et al. "Aetiology and Management of Male Erectile Dysfunction and Female Sexual Dysfunction in Patients with Cardiovascular Disease," *Drugs and Aging* 22(10):823-44, October 2005.

Hockel, M., and Dornhofer, N. "Anatomical Reconstruction after Vulvectomy," *Obstetrics and Gynecology* 103(5 Pt 2):1125-28, May 2004.

Schroder, M., et al. "Clitoral Therapy Device for Treatment of Sexual Dysfunction in Irradiated Cervical Cancer Patients," *International Journal of Radiation Oncology, Biology, Physics* 61(4):1078-86, May 2005.

Cochlear implantation

- Auditory prosthetic device that improves auditory awareness; may improve hearing so that the patient can understand conversation
- Works by directly stimulating the auditory nerve that transmits impulses to the brain's hearing center (see *Cochlear implant: A closer look*)

INDICATIONS

- Deafness secondary to sensorineural hearing loss

- The surgeon implants the internal component of the device complete with one or more electrodes into the cochlea.
- A receiver is implanted behind the top of the auricle.
- On postoperative day 10 to 15, when wound healing is complete, the patient wears an external component consisting of a small microphone with an ear hook over the ear.
- The external component is connected to a speech processor and a transmitter coil with a magnet that keeps it in place over the receiver stimulator.

- The device picks up sound through the microphone and sends it to the processor, where it's broken down and stored.
- The converted sound information is transferred to the external device, further processed, and sent through any surviving nerve cells to the brain's hearing center, allowing the patient to hear.

COMPLICATIONS

- Infection
- Facial nerve paralysis
- Facial numbness
- Tinnitus

Cochlear implant: A closer look

A cochlear implant has an internal coil with a stranded electrode lead that's surgically inserted into the scala tympani of the cochlea (as shown). The external coil (the transmitter) aligns with the internal coil (the receiver) by a magnet.

When the microphone receives sound, the stimulator wires receive the signal after it's been filtered. This filtering allows the sound to transmit comfortably for the patient. Sound is then passed by the external transmitter to the inner coil receiver by magnetic conduction and is finally carried by the electrode to the cochlea.

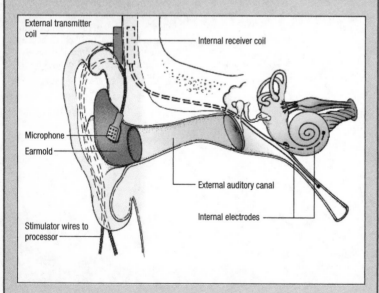

External transmitter coil · Internal receiver coil · Microphone · Earmold · External auditory canal · Internal electrodes · Stimulator wires to processor

---

NURSING DIAGNOSES

- Acute pain
- Anxiety
- Disturbed sensory perception (auditory)

EXPECTED OUTCOMES
The patient will:
- express feelings of comfort
- express his feelings and concerns
- regain hearing function.

PRETREATMENT CARE

- Explain the treatment and preparation to the patient and his family.
- Verify that the patient has signed a consent form.
- When addressing the patient, speak slowly in a clear, loud voice. Give the patient time to process the information and respond.
- Develop alternative communication methods.

POSTTREATMENT CARE

- Report incisional redness, swelling, or drainage.
- Administer analgesics as ordered.
- Monitor the patient's vital signs.
- Monitor the incision site for signs of drainage or infection.

PATIENT TEACHING

GENERAL
- Share information about sensorineural hearing loss with the patient.
- Inform the patient that hearing won't return to preloss level.
- Stress the importance of learning how to interpret sounds produced by the device.
- Review possible complications with the patient.
- Emphasize follow-up care.

RESOURCES
Organizations
American Academy of Neurology:
www.aan.com
American Medical Association:
www.ama-assn.org

Selected references
Ahmad, R.L., and Lokman, S. "Cochlear Implantation in Congenital Cochlear Abnormalities," *Medical Journal of Malaysia* 60(3):379-82, August 2005.

Dunn, D. "Preventing Perioperative Complications in Special Populations," *Nursing2005* 35(11):36-43, November 2005.

Higgins, M.B., et al. "Speech and Voice Physiology of Children who are Hard of Hearing," *Ear and Hearing* 26(6):546-58, December 2005.

Jin, Y., et al. "Vestibular-Evoked Myogenic Potentials in Cochlear Implant Children," *Acta Oto-laryngologica* 126(2):164-69, February 2006.

Colporrhaphy

- Surgical repair of a defect in the vaginal wall

  AGE FACTOR *Factors that are linked to pelvic organ prolapse include age, repeated childbirth, hormone deficiency, ongoing physical activity, and prior hysterectomy.*
- Reserved for more severe cases; mild cases may be treated by Kegel exercises (strengthens the pelvic floor and may help prevent urinary incontinence) or a pessary (device inserted into the vagina to help support the pelvic organs); hormone replacement therapy may be prescribed to a postmenopausal woman to improve quality of supporting pelvic tissues

INDICATIONS

- Cystocele
- Rectocele
- Urethrocele

- Colporrhaphy may be performed on the anterior or posterior walls of the vagina. An anterior colporrhaphy treats a cystocele or urethrocele, whereas a posterior colporrhaphy treats a rectocele.
- General, regional, or local anesthesia is administered.
- A speculum is inserted into the vagina to hold it open during the procedure.
- An incision is made into the vaginal skin and the defect in the underlying fascia is identified.
- The vaginal skin is separated from the fascia and the defect is folded over and sutured. Excess vaginal skin is removed and the incision is closed with stitches.

COMPLICATIONS

- Anesthesia-associated complications
- Infection
- Bleeding
- Injury to other pelvic structures
- Dyspareunia (painful sexual intercourse)
- Recurrent prolapse
- Fistula between the vagina and bladder or the vagina and rectum

- Acute pain
- Impaired body image
- Impaired urinary elimination

EXPECTED OUTCOMES

The patient will:
- verbalize or demonstrate relief from pain
- have a positive body image
- demonstrate normal elimination patterns.

PRETREATMENT CARE

◆ Physical examination is most commonly used to diagnose prolapse of the pelvic organs; a cystogram may also be used to determine the extent of a cystocele.
◆ Review the procedure with the patient and verify that an informed consent form has been signed.
◆ Instruct the patient to refrain from eating or drinking after midnight on the day of the procedure.
◆ If posterior colporrhaphy is to be performed, inform the patient if an enema will be administered the night before the procedure.
◆ A indwelling urinary catheter is inserted before surgery.

POSTTREATMENT CARE

◆ Monitor the patient's vital signs and amount and type of vaginal bleeding.
◆ Administer analgesics and monitor for effect.
◆ Apply a sequential compression device.
◆ Perform perineal care as ordered.
◆ Resume diet; usually a liquid diet is given until normal bowel function returns.
◆ Assist with deep-breathing and coughing exercises.
◆ Encourage ambulation.
◆ Monitor for complications.
◆ Provide catheter care, informing the patient that the indwelling catheter will be removed 1 to 2 days after surgery.

PATIENT TEACHING

GENERAL

◆ Inform the patient of activities that cause strain on the surgical site are usually restricted for several weeks, including lifting, coughing, long periods of standing, sneezing, straining with bowel movements, and sexual intercourse. She can resume normal activities, including sexual intercourse, about 4 weeks after the procedure.
◆ Instruct the patient on the use of the incentive spirometer and coughing and deep-breathing exercises.
◆ Tell the patient that after successful colporrhaphy, the symptoms associated with cystocele or rectocele will recede.

RESOURCES
Organizations
American College of Obstetrics and Gynecology: *www.acog.org*
American Medical Association: *www.ama-assn.org*

Selected references
Jordaan, D.J. "Posterior Intravaginal Slingplasty for Vaginal Prolapse," *International Urogynecology Journal and Pelvic Floor Dysfunction* 27:1-4, September 2005.
Lapitan, M.C., et al. "Open Retropubic Colposuspension for Urinary Incontinence in Women," *Cochrane Database of Systematic Review* 20(3):CD002912, July 2005.
Madsen, D., et al. "Listening to Bowel Sounds: An Evidence-Based Practice Project," *AJN* 105(12):40-49, December 2005.
Tunuguntla, H.S., and Gousse, A.E. "Female Sexual Dysfunction Following Vaginal Surgery: A Review," *Journal of Urology* 175(2):439-46, February 2006.

Conization

OVERVIEW

- Removal of a cone of tissue; most commonly refers to excision of the entire transformation zone and endocervical canal
- Uncommon procedure; has been replaced by colposcopy for diagnostic purposes

INDICATIONS
- Microinvasive cervical cancer
- Abnormal Papanicolaou test

PROCEDURE

- The patient receives a general or local anesthetic.
- The surgeon uses carbon dioxide, a large hot loop, a scalpel, or a laser to cut a circular incision around the external os of the cervix.
- A cone-shaped piece of tissue is removed.
- Biopsies are taken at the apex of the cone.
- The cervix is sutured.
- Dilatation and curettage may be performed.

COMPLICATIONS
- Uterine perforation
- Bleeding
- Infection
- Cervical stenosis
- Infertility
- Decreased cervical mucus
- Cervical incompetence

NURSING DIAGNOSES

- Anxiety
- Impaired tissue integrity
- Risk for infection

EXPECTED OUTCOMES
The patient will:
- express feelings of decreased anxiety
- remain free from discomfort
- remain free from signs of infection.

PRETREATMENT CARE

- Explain the treatment and preparation to the patient and her family. (See *Understanding conization*.)
- Verify that the patient has signed an appropriate consent form.
- Provide emotional support.
- Obtain results of diagnostic studies, medical history, and physical examination; notify the practitioner of any abnormalities.
- Make sure that the patient has fasted and used an enema preoperatively.
- Administer I.V. fluids as ordered.

POSTTREATMENT CARE

- Administer analgesics as ordered.
- Administer fluids as ordered.
- Provide the ordered diet as tolerated.
- Institute safety precautions.
- ⚡ **WARNING** *Be sure to report continuous, sharp abdominal pain that doesn't respond to analgesics, which indicates a possible symptom of uterine perforation, a potentially life-threatening complication.*
- Monitor the patient's vital signs and intake and output.
- Monitor the type and amount of vaginal drainage, and observe for signs of infection.

PATIENT TEACHING

GENERAL
- Discuss the medications and possible adverse reactions with the patient.
- Advise the patient about the possibility of postoperative abdominal cramping and pain in the pelvis and lower back.
- Inform the patient that postoperative vaginal drainage may occur.
- Inform the patient that abnormal bleeding may occur and to report such signs to the practitioner.
- Review the signs and symptoms of infection.
- Inform the patient about possible complications.

- Tell the patient that her menses may be heavier than normal for the first two or three menstrual cycles after the procedure.
- Emphasize follow-up care.

RESOURCES
Organizations
American College of Obstetrics and Gynecology: *www.acog.org*
American Medical Association: *www.ama-assn.org*

Selected references
Robova, H., et al. "Squamous Intraepithelial Lesion-Microinvasive Carcinoma of the Cervix during Pregnancy," *European Journal of Gynaecology and Oncology* 26(6):611-14, 2005.
Song, S.H., et al. "Persistent HPV Infection after Conization in Patients with Negative Margins," *Gynecologic and Oncology* 101(3):418-22, June 2006.
Ueda, M., et al. "Diagnostic and Therapeutic Laser Conization for Cervical Intraepithelial Neoplasia," *Gynecologic Oncology* 101(1):143-46, April 2006.

Understanding conization

Dear Patient,

You're scheduled to undergo a conization. This procedure involves removing a small piece of tissue from your cervix for microscopic study. Your health care provider may order a conization if previous tests show abnormal cells in your cervix.

The procedure takes less than 30 minutes. It's usually done in the hospital with either a local or spinal anesthetic. Make sure that you follow any preoperative instructions.

DURING THE PROCEDURE

If you're having a spinal anesthetic, you'll receive it before the procedure begins. Then you'll lie on your back on an examination table with your feet in stirrups, just as you would for an internal pelvic examination. The health care provider will insert a speculum into your vagina. This instrument will widen your vaginal canal to provide a clear view of your cervix.

If you're having a local anesthetic, you'll receive it at the time of the procedure. The health care provider will then remove a small, cone-shaped tissue sample from your cervix for analysis in the hospital laboratory.

If cancer is suspected in your uterus, a dilatation and curettage may be done to check for cancer cells. This will be discussed with you beforehand.

After these procedures, the speculum will be removed.

AFTER THE PROCEDURE

You can go home as soon as the anesthetic wears off, usually in about 30 to 60 minutes. Arrange to have someone transport you in case you feel unsteady.

Expect to feel some mild adverse effects from the conization. These may include abdominal cramping, some bleeding, and a feeling of fullness in your pelvis—especially if temporary vaginal packing has been inserted to control bleeding.

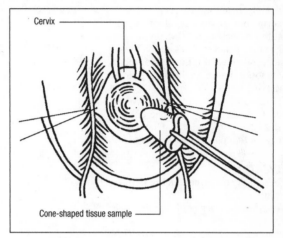

Cervix

Cone-shaped tissue sample

Also expect your next two or three menstrual periods to be heavier or longer than usual.

Immediately report these symptoms:
- heavy bleeding
- severe or persistent pain
- foul-smelling vaginal discharge
- fever.

Continuous passive motion

- Postoperative treatment that moves patient's joint—through full range of motion (ROM)—without using muscles, aiding in recovery after joint surgery
- Improves or maintains joint mobility and helps prevent contractures
- Motorized device: gradually moves the joint resulting in accelerated recovery time by decreasing soft-tissue stiffness, increasing ROM, promoting healing of joint surfaces and soft tissue, and preventing the development of motion-limiting adhesions (scar tissue)
- Continuous passive motion (CPM) devices available for the knee, ankle, shoulder, elbow, wrist, and hand (see *Continuous passive motion machine*)

INDICATIONS

- Temporary or permanent loss of mobility
- Total knee replacement
- Anterior cruciate ligament reconstruction
- Tendon repair
- Joint manipulation under anesthesia
- Arthroscopic debridement of adhesions
- Open reduction and internal fixation (stabilization) of intra-articular fractures
- Rotator cuff repair
- Articular cartilage microfracture
- Articular cartilage transplantation

PROCEDURE

- The device is applied to the joint needing continuous motion.
- The machine moves a joint through a defined ROM for an extended period.
- The practitioner determines how the CPM unit should be used by the patient (such as speed, duration of usage, amount of motion, and rate of increase of motion); the calibrations are set by the company or physical therapy department.
- Specialty CPM machines (hand, elbow, shoulder, ankle, and great toe) are available; these entail a more involved setup, and a therapist is usually needed for calibration and setup.

COMPLICATIONS

- Increased pain
- Intolerance of the procedure

Continuous passive motion machine

Postoperatively, a continuous passive motion machine may be used to aid in exercising the patient's affected joint. This is an illustration of one such device used for the lower leg.

NURSING DIAGNOSES

- Acute pain
- Impaired physical mobility
- Ineffective tissue perfusion: Peripheral

EXPECTED OUTCOMES

The patient will:
- express feelings of increased comfort
- attain the highest degree of mobility possible within the confines of the injury
- exhibit adequate tissue perfusion and pulses distally.

PRETREATMENT CARE

- Review the procedure with the patient.
- Make sure the settings on the device are as ordered by the practitioner and physical therapy department and that it's in working order.
- Inform the patient about the purpose of the device and that the joint can be moved through a ROM for an extended period. Tell him that CPM machine use can significantly reduce the recovery time, promote healing, reduce the development of adhesions and scar tissue, and decrease stiffness.

POSTTREATMENT CARE

- Keep the patient as comfortable as possible.
- Give analgesics as ordered and monitor for adverse effects.
- Maintain proper body alignment.
- Use splints or braces as ordered.
- Elevate the affected area and apply ice as tolerated when the patient's joint isn't in motion.
- Monitor the patient's vital signs.
- Monitor laboratory test results.
- Assess mobility and ROM.
- Monitor the patient for complications.

PATIENT TEACHING

GENERAL

- Stress the importance of follow-up examination.
- Advise the patient about activity restrictions and lifestyle changes.
- Review the use of the device and make sure that he can use it appropriately on discharge.
- Refer the patient for follow-up care.
- Refer the patient for physical and occupational therapy as indicated.

RESOURCES
Organizations
American College of Surgeons: *www.facs.org*
American Medical Association: *www.ama-assn.org*

Selected references
Friemert, B., et al. "Benefits of Active Motion for Joint Position Sense," *Knee Surgery, Sports Traumatology, and Arthroscopy* 23:1-7, November 2005.
Lynch, D., et al. "Continuous Passive Motion Improves Shoulder Joint Integrity Following Stroke," *Clinical Rehabilitation* 19(6):594-99, September 2005.
Zeifang, F., et al. "Continuous Passive Motion Versus Immobilisation in a Cast after Surgical Treatment of Idiopathic Club Foot in Infants: A Prospective, Blinded, Randomised, Clinical Study," *The Journal of Bone and Joint Surgery* 87(12):1663-65, December 2005.

Continuous renal replacement therapy

- Given round the clock, providing patients with continuous therapy and sparing them the destabilizing hemodynamic and electrolyte changes characteristic of intermittent hemodialysis (IHD)
- Slow continuous ultrafiltration: uses arteriovenous access and the patient's blood pressure to circulate blood through a hemofilter; the patient doesn't receive any fluids
- Continuous arteriovenous hemofiltration (CAVH): uses the patient's blood pressure and arteriovenous access to circulate blood through a flow resistance hemofilter; the patient receives replacement fluids to maintain filter patency and systemic blood pressure
- Continuous arteriovenous hemodialysis (CAVH-D): combines hemodialysis with hemofiltration; infusion pump moves dialysate solution concurrent to blood flow, adding the ability to continuously remove solute while removing fluid; like CAVH, may also be performed in patients with hypotension and fluid overload
- Continuous venovenous hemofiltration (CVVH): similar to CAVH except that a vein provides access that's channeled through the "arterial" lumen of a dual-lumen catheter and then mechanically pumped to the hemofilter
- Continuous venovenous hemodialysis: similar to CAVH-D, except that a vein provides access while a pump is used to move dialysate solution concurrent with blood flow

INDICATIONS

- Acute renal failure
- Patients unable to tolerate traditional hemodialysis such as those with hypotension

- If necessary, assist with inserting the catheters into the femoral artery and vein, using strict sterile technique. An internal arteriovenous fistula or external arteriovenous shunt may sometimes be used instead of the femoral route. If ordered, flush both catheters with the heparin flush solution to prevent clotting.
- Apply occlusive dressings to the insertion sites, and mark the dressings with the date and time. Secure the tubing and connections with tape.
- Put on sterile gloves and mask. Prepare the connection sites by cleaning them with gauze pads soaked in povidone-iodine solution, and then connect them to the exit port of each catheter.
- Turn on the hemofilter and monitor the blood-flow rate through the circuit. The flow rate is typically 500 to 900 ml/hour.
- Inspect the ultrafiltrate during the procedure. It should remain clear yellow, with no gross blood. Pink-tinged or blood ultrafiltrate may signal a membrane leak in the hemofilter, which permits bacterial contamination. If a leak occurs, notify the practitioner so that the hemofilter can be replaced.
- If the ultrafiltrate flow rate decreases, raise the bed to increase the distance between the collection device and the hemofilter. Lower the bed to decrease the flow rate.

WARNING *Clamping the ultrafiltrate line is contraindicated with some types of hemofilters because pressure may build up in the filter, clotting it and collapsing the blood compartment.*

- Calculate the amount of filtration replacement fluid every hour, as ordered, or according to your facility's policy. Infuse the prescribed amount and type of replacement fluid through the infusion pump into the arterial side of the circuit.

WARNING *When calculating the amount of replacement fluid, total the amount of fluid in the collection device from the previous hour with other fluid losses the patient may have (such as blood loss, emesis, or nasogastric tube drainage). From this total, subtract the patient's fluid intake for the past hour and the net fluid loss prescribed by the practitioner.*

- Assess hemodynamic parameters, including pulmonary artery pressure, central venous pressure, pulmonary arter wedge pressure, and blood pressure hourly, or more frequently if indicated.

WARNING *Stay alert for indications of hypovolemia, such as falling blood pressure and a decrease in hemodynamic pressures, from too-rapid removal of ultrafiltrate, or of hypervolemia due to excessive fluid replacement with a decrease in ultrafiltrate.*

- Institute continuous cardiac monitoring as indicated for arrhythmias (may indicate electrolyte imbalance).
- If the patient is receiving CVVH and the pressure alarm sounds, check the catheter for kinks, disconnections, or other problems. Determine whether the arterial or venous pressure alarm sounded; if it's the arterial pressure alarm, check the arterial lumen and if it's the venous pressure alarm, check the venous lumen. A sudden rise in pressure indicates blockage in the catheter or tubing, whereas a significant drop in pressure suggests a disconnection or opening of a port.
- Because blood flows through an extracorporeal circuit during CAVH and CVVH, the blood in the hemofilter may need to be anticoagulated. To do this, infuse heparin in low doses (usually starting at 500 units/hour) into an infusion port on the arterial side of the setup. Measure thrombin clotting time or the activated clotting time. This ensures that the circuit, not the patient, is anticoagulated. A normal value for activated clotting time is 100 seconds; during continu-

ous renal replacement therapy (CRRT) it's kept between 100 and 300 seconds, depending on the patient's clotting times. If the value is too high or low, the practitioner adjusts the heparin dose accordingly.

COMPLICATIONS
◆ Bleeding
◆ Hemorrhage
◆ Hemofilter occlusion
◆ Infection
◆ Hypotension
◆ Thrombosis (see *Preventing complications of CRRT*)
◆ Hypothermia
◆ Air embolism

◆ Deficient fluid volume
◆ Impaired gas exchange
◆ Risk for infection

EXPECTED OUTCOMES
The patient will:
◆ maintain adequate fluid volume
◆ maintain patent airway and adequate oxygenation
◆ remain free from infection.

◆ Prime the hemofilter and tubing according to the manufacturer's instructions.
◆ Wash your hands. Assemble the equipment at the patient's bedside according to the manufacturer's recommendations and your facility's policy, and explain the procedure to the patient. (See *Setup for CAVH and CVVH,* page 92.)
◆ If a catheter will be inserted, have the patient sign a consent form.
◆ Weigh the patient, take baseline vital signs, and make sure that all necessary laboratory studies have been done (such as electrolyte levels, coagulation factors, complete blood count, blood urea nitrogen, and creatinine studies). Monitor the patient's weight and vital signs hourly or as indicated.

◆ Assess the leg for signs of obstructed blood flow, such as coolness, pallor, and weak pulse. Check the groin area on the affected side for signs of hematoma. Ask the patient whether he has pain at the insertion sites.
◆ If possible, infuse medications or blood through another line rather than the venous line to prevent clotting in the hemofilter.
◆ Assess all pulses (dorsalis pedis, posterior tibial, popliteal, and femoral) in the affected leg every hour for the first 4 hours, then every 2 hours.
◆ To help prevent clots in the hemofilter, and also to prevent kinks in the catheter, make sure the patient doesn't bend the affected leg more than 30 degrees at the hip.
◆ Perform skin care at the catheter insertion sites every 48 hours, using sterile technique to prevent infection. Cover the site with an occlusive dressing.

Preventing complications of CRRT

Measures to avoid complications of continuous renal replacement therapy (CRRT) are listed here.

COMPLICATION	NURSING INTERVENTIONS
Hypotension	◆ Monitor blood pressure. ◆ Temporarily decrease the blood pump's speed for transient hypotension. ◆ Increase the vasopressor support.
Hypothermia	◆ Use an in-line fluid warmer placed on the blood return line to the patient or an external warming blanket.
Fluid and electrolyte imbalances	◆ Monitor the patient's fluid levels every 4 to 6 hours. ◆ Monitor the patient's sodium, lactate, potassium, and calcium levels and replace as necessary.
Acid-base imbalances	◆ Monitor the patient's bicarbonate and arterial blood gas levels.
Air embolism	◆ Observe for air in the system. ◆ Use luer-lock devices on catheter openings.
Hemorrhage	◆ Check all connections and keep the dialysis lines visible.
Infection	◆ Perform sterile dressing changes.

(continued)

Continuous renal replacement therapy is frequently performed using one of the two systems described here.

CONTINUOUS ARTERIOVENOUS HEMOFILTRATION

In continuous arteriovenous hemofiltration (CAVH), the physician inserts two large-bore, single-lumen catheters (as shown at right). One catheter is inserted into an artery—most commonly, the femoral artery. The other catheter is inserted into a vein, usually the femoral, subclavian, or internal jugular vein. During CAVH, the patient's arterial blood pressure serves as a natural pump, driving blood through the arterial line. A hemofilter removes water and toxic solutes (ultrafiltrate) from the blood. Replacement fluid is infused into a port on the arterial side. The same port can be used to infuse heparin. The venous line carries the replacement fluid and purified blood to the patient.

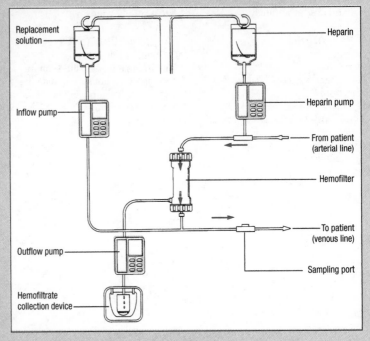

CONTINUOUS VENOVENOUS HEMOFILTRATION

In continuous venovenous hemofiltration (CVVH), the physician inserts a special double-lumen catheter into a large vein, commonly the subclavian, femoral, or internal jugular vein (as shown at right). Because the catheter is in a vein, an external pump is used to move blood through the system. The patient's venous blood moves through the "arterial" lumen to the pump, which then pushes the blood through the catheter to the hemofilter. Here, water and toxic solutes (ultrafiltrate) are removed from the patient's blood and drain into a collection device. Blood cells aren't removed because they're too large to pass through the filter. As the blood exits the hemofilter, it's then pumped through the "venous" lumen back to the patient.

Several components of the pump provide safety mechanisms. Pressure monitors on the pump maintain the flow of blood through the circuit at a constant rate. An air detector traps air bubbles before the blood returns to the patient. A venous trap collects blood clots that may be in the blood. A blood leak detector signals when blood is found in the ultrafiltrate; a venous clamp operates if air is detected in the circuit or if there's a disconnection in the blood line.

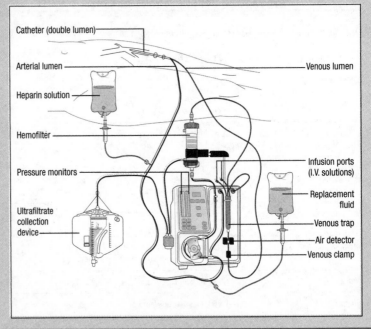

◆ Obtain serum electrolyte levels every 4 to 6 hours or as ordered; anticipate adjustments in replacement fluid or dialysate based on the results.
◆ Inspect the site dressing every 4 to 8 hours for infection and bleeding. To prevent infection, perform skin care at the catheter insertion sites every 48 hours, using sterile technique. Cover the sites with an occlusive dressing.

PATIENT TEACHING

GENERAL
◆ Remind the patient to keep his extremity still; procure an order for soft restraints if needed to prevent injury to the patient.

RESOURCES
Organizations
American Medical Association: *www.ama-assn.org*
Continuous Renal Replacement Therapies: *www.crrtonline.com*

Selected references
American Nephrology Nurses Association. Standards and Guidelines of Practice for Continuous Renal Replacement Therapy (Revised 2005 edition). Pitman, N.J.
Niu, S.F., and Li, I.C. "Quality of Life of Patients Having Renal Replacement Therapy," *Journal of Advanced Nursing* 51(1):15-21, July 2005.
Schatell, D. "Home Dialysis, Home Dialysis Central, and What You Can Do Today," *Nephrology Nursing Journal* 32(2):235-38, March-April 2005.

Coronary artery bypass grafting

OVERVIEW

- Grafting of a blood vessel segment from another part of the body to create an alternate circulatory route that bypasses an occluded area of a coronary artery, thus restoring normal blood flow to the myocardium
- Saphenous vein or internal mammary artery commonly used
- Can relieve anginal pain and improve cardiac function, enhancing quality of life
- Sometimes involves a minimally invasive surgical procedure
- Commonly called *CABG*

INDICATIONS

- Medically uncontrolled angina that adversely affects quality of life
- Left main coronary artery disease (CAD)
- Severe proximal left anterior descending coronary artery stenosis
- Three-vessel CAD with proximal stenoses or left ventricular dysfunction
- Three-vessel CAD with normal left ventricular function at rest, but with inducible ischemia and poor exercise capacity

PROCEDURE

- The patient receives general anesthesia, and the surgeon makes a series of incisions in the patient's thigh or calf and removes a saphenous vein segment for grafting; internal mammarian artery segments also may be removed.
- A medial sternotomy is done and the heart is exposed.
- Cardiopulmonary bypass is initiated; cardiac hypothermia and standstill are induced.
- The surgeon sutures one end of the venous graft to the ascending aorta and the other end to a patent coronary artery distal to the occlusion; this procedure is repeated for each artery that will be bypassed.
- After the grafts are in place, the surgeon flushes the cardioplegic solution from the heart, and cardiopulmonary bypass is discontinued.
- Epicardial pacing electrodes are implanted and a chest tube is inserted.
- The incision is closed and a sterile dressing is applied.

COMPLICATIONS

- Cardiac arrhythmias
- Hypertension or hypotension
- Cardiac tamponade
- Thromboembolism
- Hemorrhage
- Postpericardiotomy syndrome
- Myocardial infarction
- Stroke
- Postoperative depression or emotional instability
- Pulmonary embolism
- Decreased renal function
- Infection

NURSING DIAGNOSES

- Decreased cardiac output
- Hypothermia
- Ineffective tissue perfusion: Cardiopulmonary

EXPECTED OUTCOMES
The patient will:
- maintain adequate cardiac output
- maintain a normal body temperature
- maintain hemodynamic stability.

PRETREATMENT CARE

- Explain the treatment and preparation and verify that an appropriate consent form has been signed.
- Explain what to expect during the immediate postoperative period, including endotracheal tube and mechanical ventilator, cardiac monitor, nasogastric tube, chest tube, indwelling urinary catheter, arterial line, epicardial pacing wires, and pulmonary artery catheter.
- Institute cardiac monitoring.
- The evening before surgery, have the patient shower with antiseptic soap as ordered, and restrict food and fluids after midnight as ordered.
- Provide sedation as ordered and assist with pulmonary artery catheterization and insertion of arterial lines.

POSTTREATMENT CARE

- Keep emergency resuscitative equipment immediately available.
- Maintain arterial pressure within the limits set by the practitioner.
- Adjust ordered I.V. medications according to your facility's protocol.
- Maintain chest tube patency.
- Assist with weaning the patient from the ventilator as appropriate.
- Promote chest physiotherapy; encourage coughing, deep breathing, and incentive spirometry use.
- Assist the patient with range-of-motion (ROM) exercises.
- Monitor the patient's vital signs and intake and output.
- Assess heart rate and rhythm, heart sounds, peripheral vascular status, electrocardiogram and hemodynamic values, and cardiovascular status.
- Monitor the patient for complications.
- Assess nutritional status.
- Monitor arterial blood gas levels, and assess respiratory status and breath sounds.
- Monitor the patient's neurologic status.
- Monitor the patient renal function.
- Assess surgical wounds and dressings.
- Monitor for electrolyte imbalances.

PATIENT TEACHING

GENERAL

- Review medications and possible adverse reactions with the patient.
- Review incentive spirometry therapy with the patient.
- Review ROM exercises with the patient.
- Instruct the patient about how to care for the incision site.
- Tell the patient about the signs and symptoms of infection, arterial reocclusion, and postpericardiotomy syndrome.
- Inform the patient about how to identify and cope with postoperative depression.
- Review complications of the procedure with the patient.
- Review dietary restrictions with the patient.
- Inform the patient about activity restrictions, adequate rest periods, and prescribed exercise program.
- If the patient smokes, advise him to stop.
- Refer the patient to the Mended Hearts Club and American Heart Association for information and support.

RESOURCES
Organizations
American College of Cardiology: *www.acc.org*
American Medical Association: *www.ama-assn.org*
HealthCenterOnline: *www.heartcenteronline.com*

Selected references

Akowuah, E., et al. "Above-Knee Vein Harvest for Coronary Revascularization Increases ASEPSIS Score," *Asian Cardiovascular & Thoracic Annals* 14(1):57-59, February 2006.

Egerod, I., and Hansen, G.M. "Evidence-Based Practice among Danish Cardiac Nurses: A National Survey," *Journal of Advanced Nursing* 51(5):465-73, September 2005.

Hartford, K. "Telenursing and Patients' Recovery from Bypass Surgery," *Journal of Advanced Nursing* 50(5):459-68, June 2005.

Kikura, M., et al. "A Double-Blind, Placebo-Controlled Trial of Epsilon-aminocaproic Acid for Reducing Blood Loss in Coronary Artery Bypass Grafting Surgery," *Journal of the American College of Surgeons* 202(2):216-22, February 2006.

Reid, T., et al. "Psychosocial Interventions for Panic Disorder After Coronary Artery Bypass Graft: A Case Study," *Dimensions of Critical Care Nursing* 24(4):165-70, July-August 2005.

Shimamura, Y., et al. "New Anastomosis Assist Devices for Coronary Artery Bypass Grafting," *Asian Cardiovascular & Thoracic Annals* 14(1):72-74, February 2006.

Corpus callosotomy

OVERVIEW

- Surgical technique that divides the corpus callosum, disconnecting the cerebral hemispheres
- Most effective in reducing atonic and tonic-clonic seizures
- Seizure frequency reduced 70% to 80% after partial callosotomy and 80% to 90% after complete callosotomy

INDICATIONS
- Atonic seizures
- Tonic-clonic seizures
- Tonic seizures

PROCEDURE

- After the patient is given general anesthesia, the surgeon makes an incision in the scalp, removes a piece of bone, and pulls back a section of the dura. This creates a window where he inserts instruments for disconnecting the corpus callosum.
- The surgeon gently separates the hemispheres to access the corpus callosum and uses surgical microscopes to magnify the brain structures.
- He then dissects the corpus callosum. The front two-thirds are cut in a partial callosotomy; this allows the hemispheres to share visual information. The other third is cut in a complete callosotomy, which may be done initially or in another procedure.
- After the corpus callosum is cut, the dura and bone are fixed back into place, and the scalp is closed using stitches or staples.

COMPLICATIONS
- Infection
- Bleeding
- Allergic reaction to anesthesia
- Increased intracranial pressure (ICP)
- Neurologic complications (such as lack of awareness of one side of the body, loss of coordination, problems with speech, memory, or words)
- Increase in partial seizures
- Stroke
- Scalp numbness
- Fatigue or depression
- Headache

NURSING DIAGNOSES

- Disturbed thought processes
- Ineffective tissue perfusion: Cerebral
- Risk for infection

EXPECTED OUTCOMES
The patient will:
- exhibit normal thought processes
- demonstrate normal neurologic functioning
- exhibit no signs of infection.

PRETREATMENT CARE

- Review the surgical procedure with the patient and his family, and verify that a consent form has been signed.
- Review laboratory study results and the patient's history and medications.
- Have the patient take a bath and wash his hair the evening before or the morning of the procedure.
- Perform a neurologic examination to obtain a baseline status.
- Tell the patient and his family that the face may be bruised and swollen after the surgery, but this will gradually reduce.
- Candidates for corpus callosotomy undergo an extensive presurgical evaluation—including seizure monitoring, electroencephalography, magnetic resonance imaging, and positron emission tomography.

POSTTREATMENT CARE

- Monitor the patient's vital signs, intake and output, and daily weight.
- Monitor the patient's level of consciousness and respiratory status and for signs of increased ICP.
- Monitor the patient's neurologic status and immediately report any changes to the surgeon.
- Monitor hemodynamic values and heart rate and rhythm.
- Monitor fluid and electrolyte balance.
- Monitor urine specific gravity.
- Maintain patency of any drains present, monitor surgical wound and dressings, and note drainage and monitor for signs of complications.
- Administer and assess effectiveness of analgesic.
- Maintain seizure precautions.
- Maintain oxygenation; encourage the patient to take deep breaths and cough; suction as indicated.

PATIENT TEACHING

GENERAL

- Tell the patient that activities will return gradually to normal within 2 or 3 months.

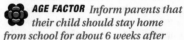 **AGE FACTOR** *Inform parents that their child should stay home from school for about 6 weeks after the surgery.*

- Review follow-up care and the need for continuing care.
- Tell the family it's unlikely that the patient's medications would be changed for at least 6 months.
- Inform the patient that hair will grow back over the incision site and cover the surgical scar.
- Review medications, dosage, and adverse effects with the patient. Tell the patient to continue taking antiseizure medication as ordered.

RESOURCES
Organizations
American Academy of Neurology: *www.aan.com*
American Medical Association: *www.ama-assn.org*
Epilepsy.com: *www.epilepsy.com*

Selected references
Dunn, D. "Preventing Perioperative Complications in Special Populations," *Nursing2005* 35(11):36-43, November 2005.
Schwartz, T.H., and Spencer, D.D. "Strategies for Reoperation after Comprehensive Epilepsy Surgery," *Journal of Neurosurgery* 95(4):615-23, October 2001.

Cortisone injection

- Cortisone injected directly into an affected joint to reduce severe, persistent inflammation
- Usually done because other treatment methods haven't worked effectively or quickly; designed to act longer and more potently

INDICATIONS
- Shoulder bursitis
- Arthritis
- Trigger finger
- Tennis elbow
- Carpal tunnel syndrome
- Any joint pain unresponsive to previous therapies

- The area to be injected is cleaned with povidone-iodine.
- Topical anesthetics are used to numb the area around the injection site.
- If there's a large amount of fluid in the joint, the practitioner will remove excess amounts.
- The practitioner then injects the cortisone into the joint. Lidocaine (or Marcaine) may also be injected with the cortisone.

COMPLICATIONS
- Crystallization of the cortisone at the injection site
- Whitening of the skin at the injection site
- Infection of the injection site

WARNING *More than three to four injections in 1 year in the same area of the body aren't recommended due to adverse effects of glucocorticoids. Research indicates that as few as six injections per year can permanently damage a joint or cause an increased risk of tendon rupture.*

- Weight gain
- High blood pressure
- Cataracts
- Diabetes
- Puffiness around the face
- Osteoporosis
- Reduced immunity and increased risk of infection
- Long-term joint and tendon damage
- Ulcers

- Acute pain
- Impaired physical mobility
- Risk for infection

EXPECTED OUTCOMES
The patient will:
- express feelings of increased comfort
- attain the highest degree of mobility possible within the confines of injury
- remain free from infection.

PRETREATMENT CARE

◆ Review the procedure with the patient, and verify that an informed consent form has been signed.

POSTTREATMENT CARE

◆ Place ice over the affected area if the patient experiences cortisone flare—the injected cortisone crystallizes and causes pain lasting for 1 or 2 days that's worse than before the shot.
◆ Observe for complications.
◆ Promote rest of the extremity; elevate the joint and position for comfort.

PATIENT TEACHING

GENERAL

◆ Advise the dark-skinned patient that whitening of the skin around the injection site is a common, but an unharmful, adverse effect.
◆ Review activity restrictions with the patient depending on the injection site: 3 days for knees, ankles, and hips, and 2 days for wrists, elbows, and shoulders. Tell the patient that complete rest helps keep cortisone in the joint, allowing the medication to work effectively.
◆ Tell the patient that the injected joint usually recovers within 1 to 4 days, whereas cortisone takes 2 to 3 weeks to be eliminated.
◆ Instruct the patient to report signs of complications, such as infection or sensitivity (increased pain and discomfort within the first 24 to 48 hours).
◆ Teach the patient the possible adverse effects of glucocorticoids.
◆ Inform the patient that there's a limit on the number of cortisone injections.

RESOURCES
Organizations
American Academy of Orthopedic Surgeons: *www.aaos.org*
American Medical Association: *www.ama-assn.org*
MedicineNet: *www.medicinenet.com*

Selected references
Buccilli, T.A. Jr., et al. "Sterile Abscess Formation Following a Corticosteroid Injection for the Treatment of Plantar Fasciitis," *Journal of Foot and Ankle Surgery* 44(6):466-68, November-December 2005.
Hanypsiak, B.T., and Shaffer, B.S. "Non-operative Treatment of Unicompartmental Arthritis of the Knee," *Orthopedic Clinics of North America* 36(4): 401-11, October 2005.
Nichols, A.W. "Complications Associated with the Use of Corticosteroids in the Treatment of Athletic Injuries," *Clinical Journal of Sports Medicine* 15(5):370-75, September 2005.

Craniotomy

OVERVIEW

- Surgical opening into the skull, exposing the brain for treatment
- Supratentorial craniotomy: involves such surgical approaches as frontal, parietal, temporal, occipital, or a combination
- Infratentorial craniotomy: involves surgical approach in which the surgeon makes an incision above the neck in the back of the skull

INDICATIONS

- Placement of ventricular shunt
- Tumor excision
- Abscess drainage
- Hematoma aspiration
- Aneurysm clipping

PROCEDURE

- The anesthetist starts a peripheral I.V. line, a central venous pressure line, and an arterial line; the patient receives a general or local anesthetic.
- The surgeon marks an incision line and cuts through the scalp to the cranium, forming a scalp flap that's folded to one side.
- The surgeon then bores four or five holes through the skull in the corners of the cranial incision and cuts out a bone flap.
- After pulling aside or removing the bone flap, the surgeon incises and retracts the dura, exposing the brain; the surgeon then proceeds with the required surgery.
- The dura mater is closed, and a drain may be used.
- The bone flap may not be replaced. If swelling is anticipated, it usually isn't replaced.
- Periosteum and muscle are approximated. Skin closure is performed and dressings are applied. (See *Craniotomy: A window to the brain.*)

COMPLICATIONS

- Infection
- Vasospasm
- Hemorrhage
- Increased intracranial pressure (ICP)
- Diabetes insipidus
- Syndrome of inappropriate antidiuretic hormone
- Seizures
- Cranial nerve damage

Craniotomy: A window to the brain

To perform a craniotomy, the surgeon incises the skin, clamps the aponeurotic layer, and retracts the skin flap. He then incises and retracts the muscle layer and scrapes the periosteum off the skull.

Next, using an air-driven or electric drill, he drills a series of burr holes in the corners of the skull incision. During drilling, warm saline solution is dripped into the burr holes, and the holes are suctioned to remove bone dust. When drilling is complete, the surgeon uses a dural elevator to separate the dura from the bone around the margin of each burr hole. He then saws between the burr holes to create a bone flap. He either leaves this flap attached to the muscle and retracts it or detaches the flap completely and removes it. In either case, the flap is wrapped to keep it moist and protected.

Finally, the surgeon incises and retracts the dura, exposing the brain.

INITIAL INCISION

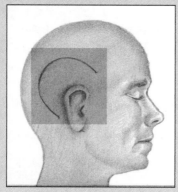

RETRACTION OF SKIN FLAP

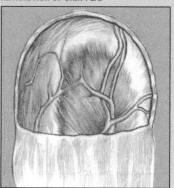

BURR HOLES DRILLED

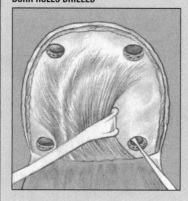

BRAIN EXPOSED

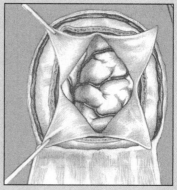

NURSING DIAGNOSES

- Disturbed sensory perception (all)
- Ineffective tissue perfusion: Cerebral
- Risk for injury

EXPECTED OUTCOMES
The patient will:
- exhibit improved or normal neurologic status
- maintain ICP within normal limits
- remain free from injury.

PRETREATMENT CARE

- Explain the treatment and preparation and verify that an appropriate consent form has been signed.
- Tell the patient that his head will be shaved in the operating room.
- Explain the intensive care unit and equipment the patient will see postoperatively.
- Perform a complete neurologic assessment.

POSTTREATMENT CARE

- Maintain a patent airway.
- Administer prescribed oxygen.
- Take steps to protect the patient's safety.
- Administer medications as ordered.
- Provide support to the patient's family members.
- Position the patient on his side with the head of the bed elevated 15 to 30 degrees; turn the patient carefully every 2 hours.
- Encourage careful deep breathing and coughing; suction gently as needed.
- Ensure a quiet, calm environment.
- Maintain seizure precautions.
- Monitor the patient's vital signs, intake and output, level of consciousness, respiratory status, ICP, heart rate and rhythm, and hemodynamic values.

⚡ **WARNING** *Notify the surgeon immediately if you detect a worsening mental status, pupillary changes, or focal signs such as increasing weakness in an arm or leg. These findings may indicate increased ICP.*

- Assess fluid and electrolyte balance, urine specific gravity, and daily weight.
- Monitor drain patency, surgical wound and dressings, and drainage.
- Apply antiembolism stockings to prevent deep vein thrombosis.
- Monitor the patient for complications.

PATIENT TEACHING

GENERAL
- Review medications and possible adverse reactions with the patient.
- Review care of the surgical wound with the patient.
- Tell the patient that headache and facial swelling will probably occur for 2 to 3 days after surgery.
- Instruct the patient on the importance of taking antiseizure medication postoperatively.
- Review postoperative leg exercises and deep breathing with the patient.
- Instruct the patient on the use of antiembolism stockings or a pneumatic compression device.
- Review signs and symptoms of infection and complications, and when to notify the practitioner.
- Discuss the use of a wig, hat, or scarf until hair grows back, as appropriate.
- Advise the patient to avoid alcohol and smoking.
- Emphasize follow-up care.

RESOURCES
Organizations
American Academy of Neurology: *www.aan.com*
American Medical Association: *www.ama-assn.org*
Epilepsy.com: *www.epilepsy.com*

Selected references
Dunn, D. "Preventing Perioperative Complications in Special Populations," *Nursing2005* 35(11):36-43, November 2005.

Horn, E.M., et al. "Bedside Twist Drill Craniotomy for Chronic Subdural Hematoma: A Comparative Study," *Surgical Neurology* 65(2):150-53, February 2006.

Movassaghi, K., et al. "Cranioplasty with Subcutaneously Preserved Autologous Bone Grafts," *Plastic and Reconstructive Surgery* 117(1):202-206, January 2006.

Nolan, S. "Traumatic Brain Injury: A Review," *Critical Care Nursing Quarterly* 28(2):188-94, April-June 2005.

Tazbir, J., et al. "Decompressive Hemicraniectomy with Duraplasty: A Treatment for Large-Volume Ischemic Stroke," *Journal of Neuroscience Nursing* 37(4):194-99, August 2005.

Tuncali, B., et al. "Intraoperative Fetal Heart Rate Monitoring During Emergency Neurosurgery in a Parturient," *Journal of Anesthesia* 20(1):40-43, January 2006.

Cryosurgery

OVERVIEW

- Destruction of tissue through application of extreme cold
- Success dependent on the type of lesion, extent and depth of the freeze, and duration between freezing and thawing; slow thaw destroys lesions more effectively
- Liquid nitrogen and nitrous oxide most commonly used; carbon dioxide and Freon less commonly used

INDICATIONS

- Actinic and seborrheic keratoses
- Leukoplakia
- Molluscum contagiosum
- Condyloma acuminatum
- Verrucae
- Basal cell epitheliomas
- Squamous cell carcinomas
- Cervicitis
- Chronic cervical erosion
- Cervical polyps
- Condyloma acuminate
- Cataracts
- Retinal tears or holes

PROCEDURE

- The procedure varies with the area being treated.

DERMATOLOGIC CRYOSURGERY

- A local anesthetic may be given based on the type and extent of the lesion.
- The correct temperature and depth are determined for freezing. For superficial lesions, this may be done by palpating the lesion. For skin cancers, a thermocouple needle and pyrometer are used to make sure that tissue at the deepest part of the lesion has been adequately frozen.
- The thermocoupler needles are inserted and secured to the base of the tumor. (See *Positioning thermocouple needles.*)
- The operative site is cleaned with povidone-iodine solution.
- The surgeon then uses a cotton-tipped applicator that has been dipped into liquid nitrogen or the complex cryosurgical unit to freeze the lesion. He may refreeze a tumor several times to ensure its destruction; for each cycle, monitor and record the number of seconds that elapse until the tissue reaches -4° F (20° C) and the number of seconds that it takes the tissue to thaw.
- After the surgery, the area is left uncovered.

GYNECOLOGIC CRYOSURGERY

- Anesthesia isn't usually given. The patient is placed in the lithotomy position and a speculum is inserted into the vagina.
- After locating and inspecting the cervix, the cryoprobe is inserted though the speculum and placed against the cervix. The tissue is frozen and later becomes necrotic and sloughs off.

OPHTHALMIC CRYOSURGERY

- After the eye dilates and becomes numb, the cryoprobe is positioned. Typically it's placed on the conjunctiva, directly over the anterior retinal break. However, if treating the posterior retinal area, an opening is first cut in the conjunctiva and the eye rotated to expose a large portion of the sclera.
- After the procedure, a patch is applied to the affected eye.

Positioning thermocouple needles

During cryosurgery, you may be responsible for positioning thermocouple needles and then operating them according to the surgeon's direction. These needles measure the temperature of the tissue at its tip and help the surgeon gauge the depth of freezing — a vitally important factor when destroying cancerous lesions. The needle may be placed in any of several positions.

Precise temperature measurement can be difficult because a variation of only 1 mm in the needle's position can translate into a difference of 50° to 59° F (10° to 15° C). For that reason, you'll usually place two or more needles in different areas to increase the accuracy of the reading.

In this illustration, the needle is shown inserted at an angle so that its tip rests about 5 mm below the base of the tumor to give a direct reading of tissue temperature. In this position, the temperature reading may be affected by chilling of the shaft within the frozen tissue, but the error isn't likely to be significant.

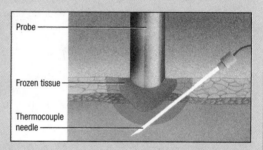

Here the probe is placed about 5 mm to one side of the frozen tissue at a depth of about 3 mm. In this position, it registers the same temperature as the probe above because both probe tips are about the same distance from the frozen tissue.

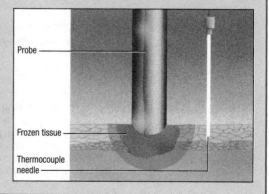

COMPLICATIONS

◆ Hypopigmentation (from destruction of melanocytes)
◆ Secondary infection
◆ Blood vessel, nerve, or tear duct damage
◆ Cervical stenosis (if too large an area of the cervix is frozen at one time)

NURSING DIAGNOSES

◆ Acute pain
◆ Disturbed body image
◆ Risk for infection

EXPECTED OUTCOMES

The patient will:
◆ state relief from pain
◆ express positive feelings about his body
◆ remain free from infection.

PRETREATMENT CARE

◆ Ask the patient if he has allergies or hypersensitivities, especially to lidocaine, iodine, or cold.
◆ Briefly explain the procedure to the patient and outline the basic steps. Tell him he will initially feel cold, followed by burning, during the procedure.
◆ Caution the patient to remain as still as possible to prevent inadvertent freezing of unaffected tissue.
◆ Gather equipment and make sure that it's working. Some surgeons use gentian violet or a surgical marker to delineate the margins of the lesion. If necessary, obtain the appropriate marker.
◆ Verify that the patient has signed an appropriate consent form.
◆ Position the patient comfortably.
◆ The gynecologic cryosurgery patient comes to the practitioner's office 1 week after her menstrual cycle.
◆ Tell the patient undergoing gynecologic cryosurgery that she may experience headache, dizziness, flushing, or cramping during the procedure. Reassure her that these adverse reactions are transient.

◆ For ophthalmic cryosurgery, mydriatic and anesthetic eyedrops are inserted into the affected eye.

POSTTREATMENT CARE

◆ After gynecologic cryosurgery, tell the patient to expect a heavy, watery discharge for the next several weeks. Warn her that the discharge will be heavy enough to require a peripad. Monitor the amount and type of drainage.
◆ After dermatologic cryosurgery, clean the area gently with a cotton-tipped applicator soaked in hydrogen peroxide. Don't apply a bandage.
◆ After ophthalmic cryosurgery, remove the eye patch when the anesthesia has worn off.
◆ Apply an ice bag to relieve swelling, and give analgesics as ordered.

PATIENT TEACHING

GENERAL
◆ Tell the patient to expect pain but he may take the prescribed analgesic as needed.
◆ Tell the dermatologic patient to expect pain, redness, and swelling. Also tell him that a blister will form within 6 hours of treatment, which will flatten within a few days and slough off in 2 to 3 weeks. Serous exudate may follow during the first week, accompanied by the development of a crust. Advise the patient to avoid breaking the blister.
◆ Warn the dermatologic patient that the blister may be large and may bleed. Warn him not to touch it to promote healing and prevent infection. Tell him that if the blister becomes uncomfortable or interferes with daily activities, he should call the practitioner, who will decompress it with a sterile blade or pin.
◆ Tell the dermatologic patient to clean the area gently with soap and water, alcohol, or a cotton-tipped applicator soaked in hydrogen peroxide, as instructed by the practitioner. To prevent hypopigmentation, instruct him

to cover the wound with a loose dressing when he's outdoors. After the wound heals, he should apply a sunscreen over the area.
◆ Tell the gynecologic patient that she'll have a watery vaginal discharge for several weeks. Advise her not to use tampons and to avoid sexual intercourse while the discharge is present because the cervix is fragile during this time.
◆ Emphasize the importance of notifying the practitioner promptly if the dermatologic patient experiences extreme pain, a widening area of erythema, oozing (of other than serous material), or fever; if the gynecologic patient experiences a vaginal discharge other than a watery appearance and fever; or if the ophthalmic patient experiences sudden changes in vision or an increase in eye pain.
◆ If the patient had a cancerous lesion destroyed, urge him to have regular checkups because cancers may recur.

RESOURCES
Organizations
American College of Emergency Physicians: *www.acep.org*
American Medical Association: *www.ama-assn.org*

Selected references
"Cryoablation Proves Effective, Safe, Durable Treatment for Prostate Cancer," *Oncology* 19(9):1142, August 2005.
Fikrle, T., and Pizinger, K. "Cryosurgery in the Treatment of Earlobe Keloids: Report of Seven Cases," *Dermatologic Surgery* 31(12):1728-31, December 2005.
Sinha, A., et al. "An Update on Second-Generation Devices for Endometrial Ablation," *Expert Review of Medical Devices* 2(5):635-41, September 2005.

Cystectomy

- Partial or total removal of the urinary bladder and surrounding structures (see *Types of cystectomy*)
- Total cystectomy: necessitates permanent urinary diversion into an ileal or colonic conduit

INDICATIONS

- Advanced bladder cancer
- Bladder disorders such as interstitial cystitis
- Frequent recurrence of widespread papillary tumors not responding to endoscopic or chemotherapeutic management

---

Types of cystectomy

In cystectomy, surgery may be partial, simple, or radical.
- *Partial cystectomy* involves resection of a portion of the bladder wall. Commonly preserving bladder function, this surgery is typically indicated for a single, easily accessible bladder tumor.
- *Simple or total cystectomy* involves resection of the entire bladder. It's indicated for benign conditions limited to the bladder. It may also be performed as a palliative measure, such as to stop bleeding, when cancer isn't curable.
- *Radical cystectomy* is generally indicated for muscle-invasive primary bladder carcinoma. Besides removing the bladder, this procedure removes several surrounding structures. This extensive surgery typically causes impotence in men and sterility in women.
    After removal of the entire bladder, the patient requires a permanent urinary diversion, such as an ileal conduit or a continent urinary pouch.

PARTIAL CYSTECTOMY

- The surgeon makes a midline low or transverse incision from the umbilicus to the symphysis pubis.
- The bladder is opened and the tumor removed, along with a small portion of healthy tissue.
- The wound is closed, leaving a Penrose drain and suprapubic catheter in place.

SIMPLE CYSTECTOMY

- The surgeon makes a midline abdominal incision.
- The entire bladder is removed, leaving only a portion of the urethra.

RADICAL CYSTECTOMY

- In addition to the bladder, the seminal vesicles and prostate in male patients and the uterus, ovaries, fallopian tubes, and anterior vagina in female patients are removed.
- Depending on the extent of the cancer, the urethra and surrounding lymph nodes may also be removed.

TO COMPLETE A SIMPLE OR RADICAL CYSTECTOMY

- Urinary diversion is done by attaching the ureters to an external collection device, such as a cutaneous ureterostomy, conduit of the large or small bowel, or continent urinary neobladder.

COMPLICATIONS

- Bleeding
- Hypotension
- Nerve injury such as to the genitofemoral or peroneal nerve
- Anuria
- Stoma stenosis
- Urinary tract infection
- Pouch leakage
- Electrolyte imbalances
- Ureteroileal junction stenosis
- Vascular compromise
- Loss of sexual or reproductive function
- Psychological problems relating to changes in body image

- Deficient fluid volume
- Impaired urinary elimination
- Risk for infection

EXPECTED OUTCOMES

The patient will:
- maintain adequate fluid volume
- maintain hemodynamic stability
- remain free from infection.

PRETREATMENT CARE

- Explain the treatment and preparation to the patient and his family.
- Verify that the patient has signed an appropriate consent form.
- Arrange for a visit by an enterostomal therapist.
- Address the patient's concerns about inevitable loss of sexual or reproductive function.
- Explain the equipment the patient will see immediately after surgery.
- If possible, arrange for the patient to visit the intensive care unit.
- Perform standard bowel preparation as ordered.
- Administer enemas or oral polyethylene glycol-electrolyte solution as ordered.
- Administer antibiotics as ordered.

POSTTREATMENT CARE

- Administer medications as ordered.
- Report urine output of less than 30 ml/hour.
- Maintain patency of the indwelling urinary catheter or stoma, as appropriate, and irrigate as ordered.
- Test all drainage from the nasogastric tube, abdominal drains, indwelling urinary catheter, and urine collection appliance for blood; notify the practitioner of positive findings.
- Change abdominal dressings, maintaining sterile technique.
- Encourage frequent position changes, coughing, deep breathing, and early ambulation.
- Offer emotional support.
- Monitor the patient's vital signs, intake and output, and drainage.
- Observe surgical wound and dressings.
- Assess the patient for hypovolemic shock, frank hematuria, and clots.
- Provide stoma care.
- Assess the patient's respiratory status.
- Monitor the patient for signs of infection.

PATIENT TEACHING

GENERAL

- Review the signs and symptoms of infection.
- Warn the patient about abnormal bleeding, including persistent hematuria, and that he should report it to the practitioner immediately.
- Review complications with the patient.
- Instruct the patient about urinary diversion care.
- Tell the patient about the possibility of cancer recurrence.
- Emphasize follow-up care.
- Refer the patient for home care nursing visits if appropriate.
- Refer the patient for psychological and sexual counseling as appropriate.
- Refer the patient to a support group, such as the United Ostomy Association, if appropriate.

RESOURCES
Organizations
American Association of Clinical Urologists: *www.aacuweb.org*
American Medical Association: *www.ama-assn.org*
eMedicine: *www.emedicine.com*

Selected references
Dunn, D. "Preventing Perioperative Complications in Special Populations," *Nursing2005* 35(11):36-43, November 2005.

Montie, J.E. "Lymph Node Metastases in Non-muscle Invasive Bladder Cancer Are Correlated with the Number of Transurethral Resections and Tumour Upstaging at Radical Cystectomy," *Journal of Urology* 175(1):95-96, January 2006.

Perimenis, P., and Koliopanou, E. "Postoperative Management and Rehabilitation of Patients Receiving an Ileal Orthotopic Bladder Substitution," *Urologic Nursing* 24(5):383-86, October 2004.

Ruggeri, E.M., et al. "Adjuvant Chemotherapy in Muscle-Invasive Bladder Carcinoma," *Cancer* 106(4):783-88, February 2006.

Zaghloul, M.S., et al. "Long-Term Results of Primary Adenocarcinoma of the Urinary Bladder: A Report on 192 Patients," *Urologic Oncology* 24(1): 13-20, January-February 2006.

Cystostomy

- Urinary diversion techniques: ensure adequate drainage from kidneys or bladder and help prevent urinary tract infection or kidney failure
- Tube usually placed percutaneously (sometimes surgically inserted); drains urine from bladder, diverting it from the urethra
- Tube inserted above the symphysis pubis; may be used alone or with an indwelling urinary catheter

INDICATIONS
- After certain gynecologic procedures
- Bladder surgery
- Prostatectomy
- Severe urethral strictures
- Traumatic injury

- After the patient is anesthetized, the surgeon makes a midline or para-medical abdominal incision.
- An opening is made through the abdomen into the urinary bladder and a drainage tube inserted.
- Percutaneous large-bore suprapubic cystostomy catheters can be placed under fluoroscopic guidance as an alternative to surgical cystostomy.

COMPLICATIONS
- Infection
- Discomfort
- Pressure when urinating
- Bleeding

- Acute pain
- Anxiety
- Risk for infection

EXPECTED OUTCOMES
The patient will:
- demonstrate or express feelings of increased comfort
- demonstrate or express decreased anxiety
- remain free from infection.

PRETREATMENT CARE

◆ Explain the procedure, reinforcing the practitioner's explanations as necessary.
◆ Have an enterostomal therapist visit with the patient and review information.
◆ Provide preoperative preparation as ordered; the patient may receive a liquid or low-residue diet a few days before surgery and be kept on nothing-by-mouth status after midnight the night before surgery.
◆ Verify that the patient has signed an appropriate consent form.

POSTTREATMENT CARE

◆ Irrigate a cystostomy tube as you would an indwelling urinary catheter.
◆ Perform irrigation to avoid damaging suture lines.
◆ Curve a cystostomy tube to prevent kinks; kinks are likely if the patient lies on the insertion site.
◆ Suspect an obstruction when the amount of urine in the drainage bag decreases or when the amount of urine around the insertion site increases.
◆ If a blood clot or mucus plug obstructs a cystostomy tube, try milking the tube to restore patency.
◆ Check cystostomy hourly for postoperative urologic patients.
◆ To check tube patency, note the amount of urine in the drainage bag and check the patient's bladder for distention.
◆ Keep the drainage bag below the level of the kidney at all times.
◆ Notify the practitioner immediately if the tube becomes dislodged.
◆ Cover the site with a sterile dressing; provide wound care as ordered.
◆ Monitor the patient's vital signs, intake and output, and urine quality.
◆ Monitor the patient for complications.

PATIENT TEACHING

GENERAL
◆ Explain how to clean the site with soap and water, check for skin breakdown, and change the dressing daily.
◆ Teach the patient how to change the leg bag or drainage bag.
◆ Explain how and when to wash the drainage bag.
◆ Encourage the patient to increase fluid intake to 3 qt (3 L) daily, if no contraindications.
◆ Discuss the signs of infection and tell the patient to notify the practitioner if they occur.
◆ Review activity restrictions.

RESOURCES
Organizations
American Association of Clinical Urologists: *www.aacuweb.org*
American College of Obstetrics and Gynecology: *www.acog.org*

Selected references
Burch, J. "The Pre- and Postoperative Nursing Care for Patients with a Stoma," *British Journal of Nursing* 14(6):310-18, March-April 2005.
Faenza, A., et al. "Urological Complications in Kidney Transplantation: Ureterocystostomy Versus Ureteroureterostomy," *Transplantation Proceedings* 37(6):2518-20, July-August 2005.
Gomez, M. "Promising New Suprapubic Catheter," *Urologic Nursing* 25(4):288, 291-92, August 2005.
Modi, P., et al. "Laparoscopic Ureteroneocystostomy for Distal Ureteral Injuries," *Urology* 66(4):751-53, October 2005.

Debridement

OVERVIEW

- Removes necrotic tissue by mechanical, chemical, or surgical means
- Includes wet-to-dry dressings, irrigation, hydrotherapy, and excision of dead tissue with forceps and scissors
- May be performed at the bedside or a specially prepared area such as a hydrotherapy tub
- Conservative sharp debridement: removes necrotic tissue by using a scalpel, scissors, or a laser
- Wet-to-dry dressings: used for wounds with extensive necrotic tissue and minimal drainage
- Irrigation of a wound with a pressurized antiseptic solution: cleans tissue and removes wound debris and excess tissue
- Hydrotherapy: involves immersing the patient in a tank of warm water, with intermittent agitation of the water
- Other debridement techniques: chemical debridement (with wound-cleaning beads or topical agents that remove exudate and debris) or surgical excision and skin grafting (usually reserved for deep burns or ulcers)
- Daily debridement: prevents hemorrhage and the need for surgical interventions
- May involve combination of debridement techniques
- Local or general anesthesia: commonly used for surgical debridement

INDICATIONS

- Remove eschar
- Manage or prevent infection
- Promote healing
- Prepare the wound surface to receive a graft

⚡ **WARNING** *Debridement is contraindicated with closed blisters over partial-thickness burns.*

PROCEDURE

CONSERVATIVE SHARP DEBRIDEMENT

- Expose only the area to be debrided to prevent chilling and fluid and electrolyte loss.
- Wash your hands and put on a cap, mask, gown or apron, and clean gloves.
- Remove the dressings and clean the wound.
- Remove your dirty gloves, and put on sterile gloves.
- Lift loosened edges of eschar with forceps.
- Use the blunt edge of scissors or forceps to probe the eschar.
- Cut the dead tissue from the wound with scissors.
- Leave a ¼" (0.6-cm) edge on remaining eschar to avoid cutting into viable tissue.
- Irrigate the wound to remove debris.
- Because debridement removes only dead tissue, bleeding should be minimal. If bleeding occurs, apply gentle pressure on the wound with sterile gauze pads and apply a hemostatic drug.
- If bleeding persists, notify the practitioner; maintain pressure on the wound until he arrives.
- Excessive bleeding or spurting vessels may require ligation.
- Perform additional procedures, such as an applying topical drugs and replacing dressings as ordered.

WET-TO-DRY DRESSING

- Put on clean gloves.
- Slowly remove the old dressings, using saline solution to moisten parts of the dressing that don't easily pull away. Discard old dressing and gloves in a waterproof trash bag.
- Put on sterile gloves.
- Using sterile technique, moisten a gauze pad with saline solution and loosely pack it into the wound. Make sure that the entire wound surface is lightly covered.
- Apply an outer dressing and secure it with tape or an adhesive bandage.

- Remove the dressing after it completely dries and becomes adherent to the necrotic tissue (4 to 6 hours).

IRRIGATION

- Using sterile technique, instill a slow, steady stream of solution into the wound with an irrigating syringe or catheter.

HYDROTHERAPY

- Prepare the tub and check the patient's vital signs.
- Assist the patient into the tub.
- After the affected area has been in the water for the prescribed time, put on clean gloves, remove old dressings, and discard items in a waterproof trash bag.
- Spray rinse and pat dry the patient before reapplying sterile dressings.

⚡ **WARNING** *Debride no more than 4" (10 cm) square at one time with debridement procedures.*

COMPLICATIONS

- Infection
- Bleeding or hemorrhage
- Fluid and electrolyte imbalance

NURSING DIAGNOSES

◆ Acute pain
◆ Impaired skin integrity
◆ Risk for infection

EXPECTED OUTCOMES
The patient will:
◆ express relief from pain
◆ maintain or improve skin integrity
◆ remain free from infection.

PRETREATMENT CARE

◆ Explain the procedure to the patient to lessen anxiety and promote cooperation.
◆ Tell the patient that the procedure is painful but that he'll be given pain medication.
◆ Provide privacy.
◆ Give an analgesic 20 minutes before debridement begins, or give an I.V. analgesic immediately before the procedure.
◆ Make sure that the room is warm.

POSTTREATMENT CARE

◆ Monitor the patient's vital signs, peripheral pulses, and pulse oximetry.
◆ Monitor the patient for signs of bleeding.
◆ Assess the patient for complications.
◆ Assess the patient's pain level and response to analgesics.
◆ Assess the patient for signs and symptoms of infection.
◆ Monitor laboratory test results.

PATIENT TEACHING

GENERAL
◆ Teach the patient distraction and relaxation techniques to ease his pain.

RESOURCES
Organizations
American Medical Association: *www.ama-assn.org*
Trauma Organization: *www.trauma.org*

Selected references
Beitz, J.M. "Wound Debridement: Therapeutic Options and Care Considerations," *Nursing Clinics of North America* 40(2):233-49, June 2005.
Davies, C.E., et al. "Exploring Debridement Options for Chronic Venous Leg Ulcers," *British Journal of Nursing* 14(7):393-97, April 2005.
Ichioka, S., et al. "Benefits of Surgical Reconstruction in Pressure Ulcers with a Non-advancing Edge and Scar Formation," *Journal of Wound Care* 14(7):301-305, July 2005.

Deep brain stimulation

OVERVIEW

- Suppresses tremors by delivering mild electrical stimulation to block signals from the thalamus, subthalamic nucleus, or globus pallidus that cause tremors without destroying brain tissue
- Target areas identified by a computed tomography scan or magnetic resonance imaging of the brain; many practitioners use microelectrode recording technique to map the brain
- Components of a deep brain stimulator: implantable lead with four electrodes at the end; neurostimulator with an external programming system to change stimulation settings; extension wire to connect the lead to the neurostimulator
- Can be performed on one or both sides of the brain (Majority of patients with Parkinson's disease require stimulators placed on both sides of the brain.)
- Procedure usually staged with each side of the brain done on separate days
- Stimulation adjustable and can be changed as symptoms change

INDICATIONS

- Essential tremor
- Parkinson's disease

PROCEDURE

LEAD PLACEMENT

- The patient's scalp is anesthetized with local anesthetic. Occasional I.V. sedation is also used for patient comfort but generally the patient is awake during the lead placement.
- An incision is made on the top of the head behind the hairline and a small opening (burr hole) is made.
- The neurologist and neurosurgeon identify the target sites using microelectrode mapping.
- Once the target site has been confirmed a permanent DBS lead is inserted through the burr hole.
- The patient is asked to answer questions and perform some tasks during the procedure to test the stimulation and maximize symptom control.
- I.V. sedation is administered and the lead is anchored to the skull with a plastic cap and the scalp incision is sutured shut.

NEUROSTIMULATOR PLACEMENT

- The neurostimulator is generally placed at a later time.
- This surgery is performed under general anesthesia.
- A small incision is made in the upper chest near the collar bone. A subcutaneous pocket is formed and the neurostimulator is implanted under the skin.
- The lead is attached to an extension cable which is passed under the skin of the scalp, neck, and shoulder and connected to the neurostimulator. (See *Deep brain stimulation.*)
- Programming of the neurostimulator usually takes place 3 to 4 weeks after implantation.

COMPLICATIONS

- Infection
- Paresthesia
- Paralysis
- Ataxia
- Intracerebral hemorrhage
- Seizures
- Stroke
- Confusion

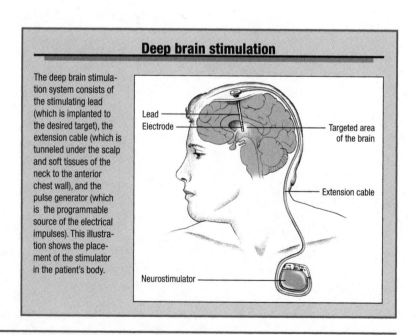

Deep brain stimulation

The deep brain stimulation system consists of the stimulating lead (which is implanted to the desired target), the extension cable (which is tunneled under the scalp and soft tissues of the neck to the anterior chest wall), and the pulse generator (which is the programmable source of the electrical impulses). This illustration shows the placement of the stimulator in the patient's body.

Lead
Electrode
Targeted area of the brain
Extension cable
Neurostimulator

NURSING DIAGNOSES

- Deficient knowledge (deep brain stimulation)
- Impaired physical mobility
- Risk for infection

EXPECTED OUTCOMES
The patient will:
- express an understanding of the procedure
- show improved mobility
- remain free from infection.

PRETREATMENT CARE

- Perform a complete neurologic assessment.
- Explain the treatment and preparation to the patient and his family.
- Verify that the patient has signed an appropriate consent form.
- Tell the patient that his head may be shaved in the operating room.

POSTTREATMENT CARE

- Monitor vital signs and closely observe neurologic status.
- Ensure a quiet, calm environment.
- Monitor fluid and electrolyte balance.
- Make sure dressings stay clean, dry and intact

  ⚡ **WARNING** *Notify the surgeon immediately if you detect a worsening of mental status, pupillary changes, or focal signs, such as increasing weakness in an arm or leg.*
- Assist with activities of daily living as appropriate.
- Administer medications as ordered.
- Observe for signs of infection.

PATIENT TEACHING

GENERAL
- Review medications and possible adverse effects with the patient.
- Review care of the surgical wound with the patient.
- Tell the patient that headache and facial swelling may occur for 2 or 3 days after surgery.
- Review postoperative leg and deep-breathing exercises and the use of antiembolism stockings or a pneumatic compression device.
- Discuss the signs and symptoms of infection, complications, and when to notify the practitioner.
- Explain the importance of follow-up care.
- Tell the patient not to engage in light activities for 2 weeks after surgery and heavy activities for 4 to 6 weeks after surgery.
- Explain to the patient that he will be provided with a magnet to activate and deactivate the neurostimulator.

RESOURCES
Organizations
American Academy of Neurology: *www.aan.com*
National Institute of Neurological Disorders and Stroke : *www.nids.nih.gov*
National Parkinson Foundation: *www.parkinson.org*

Selected references
Dunn, D. "Preventing Perioperative Complications in Special Populations," *Nursing2005* 35(11):36-43, November 2005.

Miller, J.L. "Parkinson's Disease Primer," *Geriatric Nursing* 23(2):69-75, March-April 2002.

Plaha, P., and Gill, S. "Bilateral Deep Brain Stimulation of the Pedunculopontine Nucleus for Parkinson's Disease," *Neuroreport* 16(17):1883-87, November 2005.

Dilatation and curettage or evacuation

OVERVIEW

- Involves cervical expansion or dilatation to allow access to the endocervix and uterus
- Dilatation and curettage (D&C): curette used to scrape endometrial tissue
- Dilatation and evacuation (D&E): suction applied to extract uterine contents

INDICATIONS

- Incomplete abortion
- Abnormal uterine bleeding
- Obtaining an endometrial or endocervical tissue sample for cytologic study
- D&E for incomplete or a therapeutic abortion (usually up to 12 weeks' gestation but occasionally as late as 16 weeks)

PROCEDURE

- After receiving a local or general anesthetic, the patient is placed in the lithotomy position.
- A preliminary bimanual pelvic examination is done.
- The cervix is exposed and the depth and direction of the uterine cavity is checked; in a D&E, this confirms gestational size.
- The cervical canal is dilated.

D&C

- Metal dilators of increasing size are used to dilate the cervix.
- The uterine cavity is explored and polyps are removed. If cervical or uterine cancer is suspected, specimens are obtained for biopsy from the endocervical canal.
- Standard curettage is done to remove the superficial layer of the endometrium, taking tissue specimens from the four quadrants of the cervix.
- If done to treat an incomplete abortion, the remaining products of conception are also removed.

D&E

- A suction curette is used to extract the contents of the uterus. The uterine cavity is explored to ensure complete removal of the products of conception.

COMPLICATIONS

- Uterine perforation
- Hemorrhage
- Infection

> **WARNING** *If cervical trauma occurs during these procedures, subsequent pregnancies may be affected. In fact, such trauma can lead to spontaneous abortion, cervical incompetence, or premature birth.*

NURSING DIAGNOSES

- Acute pain
- Anticipatory grieving
- Risk for trauma

EXPECTED OUTCOMES

The patient will:
- express relief from pain
- use support systems to help with coping
- remain free from trauma during the procedure.

PRETREATMENT CARE

- Review the procedure with the patient and answer her questions. Tell her that she may have some uterine cramping during the procedure and that she'll have some vaginal drainage and a perineal pad in place afterward. Explain that temporary abdominal cramping and pelvic and lower back pain normally occur after the procedure.
- Make sure that preliminary studies have been completed, including a history, physical examination, urinalysis, Papanicolaou test, and hematocrit and hemoglobin measurements. Alert the practitioner of abnormalities.
- Make sure that the patient has followed preoperative directions for fasting and used an enema to empty her colon before admission. Remind her that she won't be alert after the procedure and won't be able to drive. Make sure that she has arranged transportation.
- Ask the patient to void before administering preoperative medications, such as meperidine (Demerol) or diazepam (Valium). Start I.V. fluids as ordered to facilitate administration of the anesthetic. For the procedure, tell the patient that she may receive a general anesthetic, a regional paracervical block, or a local anesthetic.
- Offer emotional support and allow the patient to verbalize her feelings.
- Make sure that the patient has signed an informed consent form for the procedure.

POSTTREATMENT CARE

- Administer analgesics as ordered. Expect the patient to have moderate cramping and pelvic and lower back pain, but report any continuous, sharp abdominal pain that doesn't respond to analgesics. This may indicate perforation of the uterus.
- Monitor the patient for hemorrhage and signs of infection (such as purulent, foul-smelling vaginal discharge). Also check the color and volume of urine; hematuria indicates infection. Report these signs immediately.
- Administer fluids as tolerated, and allow food if the patient requests it. Keep the bed rails raised and help the patient to walk to the bathroom, if appropriate.

PATIENT TEACHING

GENERAL

- Instruct the patient to report signs of infection. Tell her to use analgesics to control pain but to report unrelenting sharp pain. (See *What to expect with a D&C.*)
- Inform the patient that spotting and discharge may last for 1 week or more. Tell her to notify the practitioner if bright red blood is observed.

- Instruct the patient to schedule an appointment with the practitioner for a routine checkup.
- Tell the patient to resume activity as tolerated but to follow her practitioner's instructions for vigorous exercise and sexual intercourse, which are usually discouraged until after the follow-up visit.
- Advise the patient to seek birth control counseling, if needed, and refer her to an appropriate center. Also advise her to seek psychological counseling, if indicated.

RESOURCES
Organizations
American College of Obstetrics and Gynecology: *www.acog.org*

Selected references
Greenhouse, L. "Justices Reaffirm Abortion Access for Emergencies," *The New York Times,* January 19, 2006, p. A1, A18.

Kirby, T.O., et al. "Surgical Staging in Endometrial Cancer," *Oncology* 20(1):45-50, January 2006.

Takeda, A., et al. "Management of Patients with Ectopic Pregnancy with Massive Hemoperitoneum by Laparoscopic Surgery with Intraoperative Autologous Blood Transfusion," *Journal of Minimally Invasive Gynecology* 13(1):43-48, January 2006.

PATIENT-TEACHING AID

What to expect with a D&C

Dear Patient,

Dilatation and curettage (D&C) is a surgical procedure designed to control abnormal uterine bleeding and to determine its cause.

BEFORE THE PROCEDURE

Before you enter the hospital, you'll describe your health history, and your health care provider will give you a physical and gynecological examination. You'll have a Papanicolaou test and blood and urine tests to make sure that you're ready for surgery.

You may be asked to shower with an antibacterial soap the night before the procedure; you may also be given an enema to clean your bowel — a precaution against infection. You'll probably be told not to eat or drink anything after midnight.

In the hospital, you'll be given a mild tranquilizer before surgery, and an I.V. line will be started to give you fluids or medicine that you may need during the procedure.

DURING THE PROCEDURE

If you have a general anesthetic to let you sleep through the procedure, you'll wake up in about 1 hour in the post-anesthesia care unit, where a nurse will check your progress. If you have a local anesthetic, you'll be awake during the procedure. Here's what to expect:

The surgical team will help you lie on your back on the operating table. You'll see stirrups for your legs.

The health care provider will examine you internally. Then he'll do the D&C using surgical instruments to stretch (dilate) your cervix and to gently scrape the surface lining of the uterus (endometrium). He may remove polyps (growths that can cause bleeding) and take tissue samples from your cervix and uterus. (The tissue will be studied to find out the reason for your bleeding.)

If you feel temporary cramping, nausea, or light-headedness, breathe deeply and try to relax. It's unlikely you'll feel discomfort. However, if you do, tell your health care provider. He can give you medicine.

AFTER THE PROCEDURE

When your anesthetic wears off, you'll feel mild to severe cramping, similar to a menstrual period. You may also have lower back pain for 1 or 2 days. Here are tips for your recovery:

- Ask your health care provider or nurse to recommend a pain medicine.
- Use a sanitary napkin, *not a tampon,* for mild spotting or staining that may last a few days or more.
- Resume your normal activities, but ask your health care provider about vigorous exercise.
- Don't have sexual intercourse until healing is complete (about 2 weeks).
- Report the following to your health care provider: vaginal bleeding that resembles a menstrual period; fever; sharp, constant pelvic pain; increased pulse rate; or foul-smelling vaginal drainage.
- Be sure to make and keep your appointment for a checkup.

Electroconvulsive therapy

OVERVIEW

- Electric current delivered to the patient's brain by electrodes placed (bilaterally or unilaterally) on his temples
- Produces seizure lasting from 30 seconds to 1 minute
- Requires a multidisciplinary approach—physician: obtains consent, titrates drug dosages, and administers the treatment; nurse: provides care during the assessment, preparation, treatment, and recovery; certified registered nurse anesthetist (CRNA): responsible for ensuring a patent airway, administering positive pressure oxygen during the treatment and until the patient is breathing well on his own, and administering specific drugs during the procedure

INDICATIONS
- Affective disorders
- Selective schizophrenias
- Severe depression when other therapies are ineffective

PROCEDURE

- Attach the patient to an electronic blood pressure monitor and check his baseline vital signs. Attach a pulse oximeter, insert an I.V. catheter, and attach him to the electrocardiogram (ECG) monitor.
- Attach the EEG electrodes and stimulus electrodes to the rubber headband. Coat the electrodes with conduction gel and place the band around the patient's head. Place the large, silver-colored stimulus electrodes on each temple at about eye level. Space the small, brown EEG electrodes across the forehead.
- Connect the stimulus electrodes to the stimulus output receptacle on the machine.
- Run the EEG/ECG machine in the self-test mode. When the machine is ready, it displays the message "Self Test Passed" and prints the date,

time, treatment parameters, a brief ECG strip, and EEG monitors.
- The CRNA or physician administers glycopyrrolate (Robinul) or atropine, followed by methohexital (Brevital). Methohexital acts very rapidly. Expect an abrupt loss of consciousness when the appropriate dose is infused.
- After the patient is unconscious, succinylcholine (Anectine) is administered. A tremor or fasciculation of various muscle groups occurs due to the depolarizing effect of this drug. Because succinylcholine also causes complete facial paralysis, mechanical ventilation is started at this time. A rubber mouthpiece is inserted and positive-pressure oxygen is given.
- The physician initiates the stimulus, and mild seizurelike activity occurs for about 30 seconds. The patient's jaw and extremities must be supported while avoiding contact with metal.
- Monitor the patient's vital signs as well as ECG and EEG rhythm strips. Assess the skin for burns.

COMPLICATIONS
- Respiratory distress
- Malignant hyperthermia
- Persistent memory loss

NURSING DIAGNOSES

- Disturbed sensory perception (all)
- Ineffective breathing pattern
- Ineffective tissue perfusion: Cerebral

EXPECTED OUTCOMES
The patient will:
- return to baseline or improved neurologic status
- maintain adequate ventilation
- exhibit improved or normal neurologic status.

PRETREATMENT CARE

- Review the procedure with the patient and what to expect before, during, and after the procedure.
- Verify that the patient has signed an appropriate consent form.

- If the patient is taking benzodiazepines before the procedure, obtain an order to begin tapering and discontinue the drugs 3 to 4 days preprocedure. Benzodiazepines and anticonvulsant drugs (such as lorazepam [Ativan] and phenytoin [Dilantin]) negatively affect the patient's response to treatment.
- Make sure that all equipment, drugs, and emergency equipment are available.
- Attach the ECG and EEG monitors.
- Complete a preprocedure assessment.
- The treatment parameters are set as ordered for pulse width (ms), frequency (Hz), duration (sec), and current (amp).

AGE FACTOR *These parameters represent the total volume of electrical stimulus applied, which differs depending on the patient's age, medication use, seizure threshold, and other factors.*

- Plug in the electronic blood pressure monitor. Make sure that the crash cart, with emergency drug kit, defibrillator, suction equipment, an endotracheal intubation tray, and oxygen is readily available and that needed medications are properly prepared. (See *Preparing medications for ECT*.)
- Verify the orders and gather the appropriate equipment.
- After arrival in the electroconvulsive therapy (ECT) room, identify the patient and check his nothing-by-mouth status.
- Make sure that the patient's history (including allergies to medications or latex), physical examination, and dental evaluation are documented in his chart.

WARNING *Contraindications to ECT include brain tumors, space-occupying lesions, and other brain diseases that cause increased intracranial pressure. The seriousness of any physical illness, such as heart, liver, or kidney disease as well as the psychiatric disorder, should be weighed against each other before ECT is initiated.*

- Make sure that the following diagnostic tests have been completed and assessed: complete blood count,

thyroid profile, urinalysis, ECG, pseudocholinesterase activity determination (especially in patients with severe liver disease, malnutrition, or a history of sensitivity to muscle relaxants or similar substances), chest X-ray, spine radiographs, EEG, and cranial computed tomography scan.
◆ Help the patient remove dentures, partial plates, or other foreign objects from his mouth to prevent choking. Make sure that the patient removes all jewelry, metal objects, and prosthetic devices before the procedure to prevent injury.
◆ Have the patient wear a hospital gown and ask him to void to prevent incontinence during the procedure. Assist the patient onto the stretcher.

POSTTREATMENT CARE

◆ When spontaneous ventilation returns, usually in 3 to 5 minutes, discontinue mechanical ventilation. Continue to monitor the patient's vital signs.
◆ As the patient becomes more alert, speak quietly and explain what's happening. Remove the rubber mouthpiece.
◆ Place the patient on his side to maintain a patent airway. Measure and document his vital signs every 15 minutes until they stabilize.
◆ Discharge the patient from the recovery area when he's able to move all four extremities voluntarily, can breathe and cough adequately, is roused and oriented when called, has an Aldrete score of 7 or greater, has stable vital signs and temperature within 1° F (0.6° C) of the pretreatment value, and has a normal swallowing reflex. A physician's order is required to release the patient from the recovery area.
◆ Obtain and record the patient's vital signs 1 hour after treatment. Check the patient's temperature to assess for malignant hyperthermia. Then continue to check his vital signs every hour as necessary until stable.

PATIENT TEACHING

GENERAL
◆ Review signs and symptoms to report to the practitioner.

RESOURCES
Organizations
American Academy of Neurology: *www.aan.com*
American Psychiatric Association: *www.healthyminds.org*
National Mental Health Association: *www.nmha.org*

Selected references
Gitlin, M. "Treatment-Resistant Bipolar Disorder," *Molecular Psychiatry* 11(3):227-40, March 2006.
Hanss, R., et al. "Bispectral Index-controlled Anaesthesia for Electroconvulsive Therapy," *European Journal of Anaesthesiology* 23(3):202-207, March 2006.
Howland, R.H. "Therapeutic Brain Stimulation for Mental Disorders," *Journal of Psychosocial Nursing Mental Health Services* 43(2):16-19, February 2005.
Sharma, A., et al. "Electroconvulsive Therapy after Repair of Cerebral Aneurysm," *The Journal of ECT* 21(3):180-81, September 2005.

Preparing medications for ECT

Even though the physician or certified registered nurse anesthetist administers medications during electroconvulsive therapy (ECT), you should become familiar with the medications that can be used so you can assess the patient for adverse effects. Brief descriptions of the most commonly used drugs appear below.

DRUG	ACTIONS	ADVERSE EFFECTS
Dantrolene (Dantrium)	Dantrolene is a direct-acting skeletal muscle relaxant that's effective against malignant hyperthermia.	◆ Seizures ◆ Muscle weakness ◆ Drowsiness ◆ Fatigue ◆ Headache ◆ Hepatitis ◆ Nervousness ◆ Insomnia
Glycopyrrolate (Robinul)	Glycopyrrolate has desirable cholinergic blocking effects because it reduces secretions in the respiratory system as well as oral and gastric secretions. It also prevents a drop in heart rate caused by vagal nerve stimulation during anesthesia.	◆ Dilated pupils ◆ Tachycardia ◆ Urine retention ◆ Anaphylaxis ◆ Confusion (in elderly patients) ◆ Dry mouth
Methohexital (Brevital)	Methohexital is a rapid, ultra-short-acting barbiturate anesthetic agent.	◆ Hypotension ◆ Tachycardia ◆ Respiratory arrest ◆ Bronchospasm ◆ Anxiety ◆ Hypersensitivity reaction ◆ Emergent delirium
Succinylcholine (Anectine)	Succinylcholine is an ultra-short-acting depolarizing skeletal muscle relaxant. Given I.V., it causes rapid, flaccid paralysis.	◆ Bradycardia ◆ Arrhythmias ◆ Cardiac arrest ◆ Prolonged respiratory depression ◆ Malignant hyperthermia ◆ Anaphylaxis

Endarterectomy, carotid

- Surgical removal of atheromatous plaque from inner lining of carotid artery
- Improves intracranial perfusion by increasing blood flow through the carotid artery
- Often considered a prophylactic treatment for stroke

INDICATIONS

- Reversible ischemic neurologic deficit
- Completed stroke
- Transient ischemic attack
- High-grade asymptomatic or ulcerative lesions

- Cervical block anesthesia, sedatives, or light general anesthesia may be given to the patient.
- A longitudinal incision is made over the area of the carotid bifurcation and the soft tissue is dissected for exposure of the carotid artery and its bifurcation.
- The patient is systemically heparinized.
- The external, common, and internal carotid arteries are clamped.
- An arteriotomy is made over the stenotic area. The incision is lengthened to expose the full extent of the occluding plaque.
- The plaque or plaques are dissected free from the arterial wall. The intima is cleaned with heparin solution.
- The arteriotomy is closed, and a synthetic or autogenous patch may be used to restore the arterial lumen if it's small.
- The occluding clamps are removed from the external and common carotid arteries. The internal carotid artery clamp is removed last to make sure that minor debris missed is flushed harmlessly into the external rather than the internal carotid artery.
- A drain is inserted through a separate stab incision, the wound is closed, and a dressing is applied.

COMPLICATIONS

- Blood pressure lability
- Perioperative stroke
- Temporary or permanent loss of carotid body function
- Recurrent thrombosis
- Respiratory distress
- Wound infection
- Ipsilateral vascular headache
- Seizures
- Intracerebral hemorrhage
- Vocal cord paralysis
- Transient or permanent neurologic deficit

- Ineffective tissue perfusion: Cerebral
- Risk for impaired gas exchange
- Risk for injury

EXPECTED OUTCOMES

The patient will:
- maintain baseline neurologic status
- remain free from respiratory distress
- remain free from injury.

PRETREATMENT CARE

- Explain the treatment and preparation to the patient, and verify that the patient has signed an appropriate consent form.
- Explain postoperative care and equipment.
- Perform a complete neurologic assessment.
- Assist with any invasive procedures as appropriate.
- Obtain a baseline EEG before the patient is anesthetized as ordered.
- Tell the patient that he'll have some postoperative discomfort or pain, but that pain medication will be available.

POSTTREATMENT CARE

- Perform a neurologic assessment every hour for the first 24 hours; check extremity strength, fine hand movements, speech, orientation, and level of consciousness.
- Obtain an electrocardiogram if the patient experiences chest pain or arrhythmias.
- Monitor the patient's vital signs, intake and output, heart rate and rhythm, neurologic status, respiratory status, surgical wound and dressings, drainage, cervical edema, infection, seizures, and complications.
- Asses for pain and administer medications as ordered.

PATIENT TEACHING

GENERAL
- Discuss care of the surgical wound.
- Review the signs and symptoms of infection.
- Review potential complications of the procedure.
- Discuss risk factor modification.
- Discuss the management of neurologic, sensory, or motor deficits.
- Review medication administration, dosing, and potential adverse effects with the patient and his family.

RESOURCES
Organizations
American Heart Association: *www.americanheart.org*
American Medical Association: *www.ama-assn.org*

Selected references
Hacke, W., et al. "Carotid Endarterectomy Versus Stenting: An International Perspective Response," *Stroke* 37(2): 344, February 2006.

Madycki, G., et al., "Carotid Plaque Texture Analysis Can Predict the Incidence of Silent Brain Infarcts among Patients Undergoing Carotid Endarterectomy," *European Journal of Vascular and Endovascular Surgery* 31(4):373-80, April 2006.

Middleton, S., et al. "Nursing Intervention after Carotid Endarterectomy: A Randomized Trial of Co-ordinated Care Post-Discharge (CCPD)," *Journal of Advanced Nursing* 52(3):250-61, November 2005.

Mitka, M. "Carotid Artery Surgery Guidelines Updated: New Data Also Support Stents in High-Risk Cases," *JAMA* 294(23):2955-56, December 2005.

Endometrial ablation

OVERVIEW

- Involves removal of the lining of the uterus; considered an outpatient surgical procedure
- Offers an effective alternative to hysterectomy
- Commonly chosen when other medical treatments have failed or are otherwise undesirable

  AGE FACTOR *Most women can't have children after this procedure. Because there's still a slight possibility of pregnancy, however, the patient should continue to use contraception until menopause.*

- Laparoscopy: may be performed at the same time to rule out other conditions that could require further therapy

INDICATIONS

- Heavy or prolonged bleeding during menses

PROCEDURE

ELECTROCAUTERY

- After the patient is under anesthesia in the operating room, a "roller-ball" or wire loop is used through a hysteroscope and the lining of the uterus is cauterized. Alternately, freezing may be done to destroy the uterine lining.
- The lining of the uterus is then vaporized, using a heat-generating tool inserted through the hysteroscope. About 90% of women experience relief of their symptoms within the first few months, with many having brief or no menstrual periods after the procedure.

BALLOON ENDOMETRIAL ABLATION

- This technique is performed in an outpatient surgical center or in a physician's office.
- The patient receives either a local or general anesthetic.
- A hysteroscope is inserted through the vagina and cervix into the uterus. A tiny camera is attached to allow the uterine cavity to be shown on a TV monitor during surgery. A triangular balloon is placed into the uterus and filled with fluid. The fluid is heated for several minutes and most of the uterine lining is destroyed.

COMPLICATIONS

- Cardiac arrest
- Respiratory arrest
- Uterine perforation with resultant bowel injury
- Fluid overload
- Infection

NURSING DIAGNOSES

- Acute pain
- Anxiety
- Risk for infection

EXPECTED OUTCOMES

The patient will:
- verbalize relief from pain
- demonstrate decreased anxiety and increased comfort
- exhibit no signs of infection.

PRETREATMENT CARE

- Make sure that a medical history and physical examination have been completed.
- Verify that the patient has signed an appropriate consent form.
- Make sure pretreatment testing has been completed, including complete blood count, uterine lining sampling (biopsy), and hysteroscopy and ultrasonography. These procedures are usually done in the practitioner's office before the treatment.

   ⚡ **WARNING** *A biopsy of the uterine lining may be needed to exclude cancer because endometrial ablation isn't appropriate if cancer is suspected.*

- For 1 or 2 months before the procedure, the patient may be prescribed a gonadotropin-releasing hormone analog medication or receive injections to decrease the thickness of the endometrium. Thinning the uterine lining exposes the basal layer of endometrial cells, which are removed by electrosurgery.
- The day before surgery, the practitioner may choose to insert medication to gradually dilate the cervix before surgery.

POSTTREATMENT CARE

- Monitor the patient's vital signs and cardiovascular and respiratory status
- Monitor for complications.
- Monitor drainage and the patient's comfort level; perform perineal care and apply peripads as indicated.
- If specimens are obtained, make sure that they're labeled appropriately and sent to the laboratory.
- Assess the effect of the analgesic.
- Women who have undergone endometrial ablation may be treated with progestogens to reduce the risk of developing uterine cancer when postmenopausal estrogen replacement therapy is prescribed. Women who have undergone hysterectomy, in contrast, generally don't require progestogens.

PATIENT TEACHING

GENERAL

- Review activity restrictions with the patient: strenuous activity may be avoided for a period, usually for 24 hours after the procedure.
- Tell the patient to refrain from sexual intercourse, usually 2 weeks or until the discharge stops.
- Tell the patient to schedule a postoperative appointment about 1 week after the procedure for follow-up.
- Tell the patient that she may experience frequent urination during the first 24 hours and that this is normal.
- Tell the patient that she may experience a small amount of bloody, watery discharge for up to 6 weeks postoperatively.
- Warn the patient that it's impossible to evaluate the effectiveness of surgery until at least 3 months postoperatively.
- Tell the patient that heavy bleeding may recur several years after the ablation, requring additional surgery.
- Review prescribed medications and their potential adverse effects with the patient.

RESOURCES
Organizations
American College of Obstetrics and Gynecology: *www.acog.org*
American Medical Association: *www.ama-assn.org*

Selected references
Bachmann, G. "Expanding Treatment Options for Women with Symptomatic Uterine Leiomyomas: Timely Medical Breakthroughs," *Fertility and Sterility* 85(1):46-67, January 2006.
League, D.D. "Endometrial Ablation as an Alternative to Hysterectomy," *AORN Journal* 77(2):322-24, 327-38, February 2003.
Paddison, K. "Menorrhagia: Endometrial Ablation or Hysterectomy?" *Nursing Standards* 18(1):33-37, September 2003.

Episiotomy

- Procedure in which skin between the vagina and anus (perineum) is cut
- Enlarges the vaginal opening so that the neonate can be easily delivered
- Usually heals without problems and may heal more quickly than a tear; also thought to help prevent vaginal stretching and to tighten the vagina after delivery

INDICATIONS
- Infant's head is too big for the mother's vaginal opening
- Infant in a breech or shoulder position
- To prevent vaginal tearing
- Preterm birth
- Fetal distress necessitating rapid delivery

- Just before birth, the obstetrician numbs the vaginal area.
- The episiotomy is usually performed when the fetal head has stretched the vaginal opening to several centimeters during a contraction.
- One of two types of episiotomies may be done. A mediolateral cut is angled down away from the vagina and into the muscle. This type of episiotomy doesn't tend to tear or extend, but is associated with greater blood loss and may not heal as well.
- A midline cut is made straight down between the vagina and anus. This type of episiotomy usually heals well but may be more likely to tear and extend into the rectal area (a third- or fourth-degree laceration).
- The area is sutured closed after the infant and placenta are delivered.

COMPLICATIONS
- Infection
- Bleeding
- Bruising
- Intercourse-related pain after pregnancy
- Incontinence
- Formation of hematoma

- Acute pain
- Anxiety
- Deficient knowledge (condition and treatment)

EXPECTED OUTCOMES
The patient will:
- demonstrate or express feelings of increased comfort
- verbalize feelings of reduced anxiety
- verbalize understanding of labor and delivery process.

PRETREATMENT CARE

◆ Check for allergies (especially latex) to iodine or medications before the procedure.
◆ Verify that the patient has signed an appropriate consent form.
◆ Explain the purpose of and intended effect of the procedure.
◆ Place the patient in the lithotomy position just before childbirth.

⚡ **WARNING** *Notify the practitioner if there's a history of bleeding disorders or if the patient is taking anticoagulants, aspirin, or other medications that affect blood clotting. It may be necessary to stop these medications before the procedure.*

POSTTREATMENT CARE

◆ Monitor the patient's vital signs and intake and output.
◆ Monitor for vaginal discharge.
◆ Apply ice to the area.
◆ Perform perineal care.
◆ Inspect the sutures and surgical site for complications.
◆ Perform routine postpartum care and care of the neonate.
◆ Monitor the incision site for infection.

PATIENT TEACHING

GENERAL

◆ Inform the patient that the stitches are absorbed by the body and don't need to be removed.
◆ Review pain-relief measures with the patient: warm sitz baths and analgesics and creams or local anesthetic sprays may be used on the perineum as directed by the practitioner.
◆ Review perineal care and how to prevent infection.
◆ If stool softeners are ordered, instruct the patient about their use.
◆ Tell the patient not to douche, use tampons, or have intercourse until approved by the practitioner.
◆ Tell the patient to avoid strenuous lifting until seen by the practitioner.
◆ Tell the patient to notify the practitioner if bleeding from the episiotomy site occurs, there are signs of infection (such as foul-smelling drainage from the vagina, fever, or chills), or if she's experiencing severe perineal pain.

RESOURCES
Organizations
American College of Obstetrics and Gynecology: *www.acog.org*
American Medical Association: *www.ama-assn.org*

Selected references
Dencker, A., et al. "Suturing after Childbirth — A Randomised Controlled Study Testing a New Monofilament Material," *BJOG: An International Journal of Obstetrics and Gynaecology* 113(1):114-16, January 2006.
Eogan, M., et al. "Does the Angle of Episiotomy Affect the Incidence of Anal Sphincter Injury?" *BJOG: An International Journal of Obstetrics and Gynaecology* 113(2):190-94, February 2006.

Jensen, K. "Preventing Episiotomies," *Midwifery Today International Midwife* (75):49, Autumn 2005.
Kearney, R., et al. "Obstetric Factors Associated with Levator Ani Muscle Injury after Vaginal Birth," *Obstetrics and Gynecology* 107(1):144-49, January 2006.
Premkumar, G. "Perineal Trauma: Reducing Associated Postnatal Maternal Morbidity," *RCM Midwives* 8(1):30-32, January 2005.

Esophagectomy

- Surgical removal of the esophagus
- Minimally invasive esophagectomy: not performed as frequently as traditional esophagectomy because it isn't suitable for all patients; advantages: less trauma to the body, less blood loss, smaller surgical scars, less need for pain medication, shorter hospital stay, and faster return to normal activities
- Minimally invasive (laparoscopic) surgery: done through small incisions (requiring only 1 or 2 stitches to close), using specialized techniques, miniature cameras with microscopes, tiny fiber-optic flashlights and high-definition monitors; method not appropriate for all patients

AGE FACTOR *The type of surgery performed depends on many factors, such as the patient's age; size and location of the cancer; whether the cancer has grown into other structures in the chest, such as the lungs or large blood vessels; overall health of the patient; and experience of the surgeon in performing the surgical technique.*

INDICATIONS

- Esophageal cancer
- Achalasia (abnormal esophageal nerve function, making swallowing difficult)

PROCEDURE

- The patient receives general anesthesia and is positioned appropriately.
- The transhiatal or transthoracic esophagectomy (Ivor-Lewis procedure) is performed. Transhiatal esophagectomy is performed without an incision in the chest cavity and results in reduced pain and faster recovery for appropriate patients. The other approach involves a thoracic approach.
- After the incision is made, the surgeon will examine the peritoneal cavity for metastatic disease. If metastases are found, the operation isn't continued.
- During an esophagectomy, the surgeon removes a portion of the esophagus and the top part of the stomach. The esophagus is reconstructed using one of several other organs, most commonly the stomach or large intestine.
- A portion of the stomach is then pulled up into the chest and connected to the remaining normal portion of the esophagus. The patient then has a "new" esophagus made up of the normal portion of the esophagus not removed at surgery, connected to a portion of the stomach pulled up into the chest.

MINIMALLY INVASIVE ESOPHAGEAL SURGERY

- The surgeon makes four to five small incisions and inserts tubelike instruments through them.
- The abdomen is filled with gas to help the surgeon view the abdominal cavity.
- A camera inserted through one tube displays images on a monitor located in the operating room. Other instruments are placed through additional tubes, allowing the surgeon to work inside the abdomen without using a larger incision.
- After the stomach is exposed, the fundus is stapled off and cut from the rest of the stomach.

- The second part of the procedure is the thorascopic stage. Instruments are inserted into the chest to remove the damaged parts of the esophagus. After the fundus and lower esophagus are free, both are removed. To reestablish continuity of the digestive tract, the stomach is pulled upward to join with the remaining portion of the esophagus.

COMPLICATIONS

- Infection
- Bleeding
- Leakage from the area where the remaining esophagus is reattached
- Myocardial infarction
- Arrhythmias

- Acute pain
- Imbalanced nutrition: Less than body requirements
- Risk for infection

EXPECTED OUTCOMES

The patient will:
- demonstrate or express feelings of increased comfort
- maintain a normal weight
- remain free from infection.

PRETREATMENT CARE

- Required, presurgical diagnostic tests include blood tests, computed tomography scanning of the chest, endoscopy, and a chest X-ray.
- An electrocardiogram and echocardiogram may also be done to check for cardiovascular disease that could complicate surgery.
- Make sure that the patient has nothing to eat or drink from midnight before surgery.
- Tell the patient that he may also have to undergo preparatory therapies, such as bowel cleaning and antibiotic therapy to help sterilize the bowel.
- Explain the treatment and preparation to the patient and his family.
- Verify that the patient has signed an appropriate consent form.
- Tell the patient that a nasogastric (NG) tube will be in place after surgery and will be removed in a few days.
- Prepare the patient for early postoperative ambulation.
- Tell the patient to expect to have an I.V. line and abdominal drains after surgery.

POSTTREATMENT CARE

- Maintain I.V. replacement therapy as ordered.
- Keep the NG tube patent, but don't reposition it.
- Provide wound care as indicated.
- Encourage regular coughing and deep-breathing exercises.
- Encourage splinting of the incision site as necessary.
- Monitor the patient's vital signs, intake and output, and daily weight.
- Report signs of dehydration, peritonitis, sepsis, and infection.
- Monitor drainage from the wound.

⚡ **WARNING** *Monitor for and immediately report signs and symptoms of anastomotic leakage, including low-grade fever, malaise, slight leukocytosis, abdominal distention, tenderness, hemorrhage, hypovolemic shock, and bloody stool or wound drainage.*

- Administer medications as ordered.
- Assess for abdominal pain, abdominal cramps, or shoulder pain. Explain that bloating or abdominal fullness from laparoscopy will subside as gas is absorbed, as appropriate.
- Provide comfort measures.

PATIENT TEACHING

GENERAL

- Review with the patient coughing and deep-breathing exercises and splinting of the incision site.
- Tell the patient to avoid abdominal straining and heavy lifting until the sutures are completely healed and the practitioner approves.
- Tell the patient to return to activities as directed. Because a laparoscopic procedure is less traumatic, he can usually resume normal activities soon after leaving the health care facility.
- Tell the patient that after 1 month, he can resume his normal diet, but needs to eat smaller quantities. The reduced size of the stomach limits its capacity to hold food. Instead of eating three large meals, he may choose to eat several small meals each day. He can expect to lose about 20 lb (9 kg) after surgery.
- Tell the patient to keep follow-up appointments.
- Be sure to review medications and their possible adverse reactions, care for the incision site, signs and symptoms of infection and complications, and prescribed activity restrictions.

RESOURCES
Organizations
American College of Gastroenterology: *www.acg.gi.org*
American Gastroenterological Association: *www.gastro.org*
American Medical Association: *www.ama-assn.org*

Selected references
DeMeester, S.R. "Endoscopic Mucosal Resection and Vagal-Sparing Esophagectomy for High-Grade Dysplasia and Adenocarcinoma of the Esophagus," *Seminars in Thoracic and Cardiovascular Surgery* 17(4):320-25, Winter 2005.

Mackenzie, D.J., et al. "Care of Patients after Esophagectomy," *Critical Care Nurse* 24(1):16-29, February 2004.

Pennathur, A., et al. "Surgical Aspects of the Patient with High-Grade Dysplasia," *Seminars in Thoracic and Cardiovascular Surgery* 17(4):326-32, Winter 2005.

External enhanced coronary perfusion

OVERVIEW

◆ Noninvasive procedure that can reduce the symptoms of angina pectoris by increasing coronary blood flow in ischemic areas of the heart
◆ Involves the use of the external enhanced coronary perfusion (EECP) device to inflate and deflate a series of compressive cuffs wrapped around the patient's calves, lower thighs, and upper thighs; inflation and deflation of cuffs modulated by events in the cardiac cycle via computer-interpreted electrocardiogram (ECG) signals
◆ Concept of counterpulsation: based on a favorable response of the left ventricle to reduce arterial pressure during the systolic period; heart can be rested and its demand for oxygen reduced, if left ventricular pressure can be reduced; increases stroke volume per unit work and efficiency of the left ventricle; coronary flow and collateral flow to ischemic regions of myocardium increased

INDICATIONS

◆ Stable or unstable angina pectoris
◆ Patients considered at high risk for revascularization procedures or in whom revascularization isn't technically possible
◆ Heart failure
◆ Cardiogenic shock

PROCEDURE

◆ The EECP device is placed on the patient's legs and set to inflate and deflate a series of compression cuffs wrapped around the patient's calves, lower thighs, and upper thighs. (See *External enhanced coronary perfusion device.*)
◆ At the start of treatment, external compression is progressively increased, as needed, to raise diastolic pressures gradually. Finger plethysmography is used to monitor correct timings.
◆ Inflation and deflation of the cuffs are modulated by events in the cardiac cycle via computer-interpreted ECG signals.
◆ During diastole, the cuffs inflate sequentially from the calves proximally, resulting in augmented diastolic central aortic pressure and increased coronary perfusion pressure. Rapid and simultaneous decompression of the cuffs at the onset of systole permits systolic unloading and decreased cardiac workload.

◆ Patients are treated with EECP 1 or 2 hours per day for a total of 35 hours. The first week of treatment is limited to 1 hour daily to facilitate familiarization and monitor patient tolerance before increasing the daily treatment time. Two hours of treatment on the same day is usually separated by a rest period.

COMPLICATIONS

◆ Discomfort from the pulsatile movement and pressure on legs and buttocks

NURSING DIAGNOSES

◆ Activity intolerance
◆ Decreased cardiac output
◆ Ineffective tissue perfusion: Cardiopulmonary

EXPECTED OUTCOMES

The patient will:
◆ carry out activities of daily living without excess fatigue or decreased energy
◆ maintain adequate cardiac output
◆ be free from signs of decreased cardiopulmonary tissue perfusion.

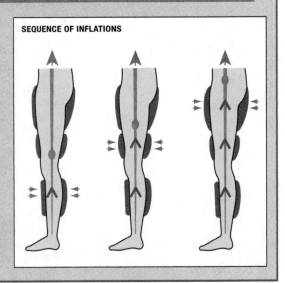

External enhanced coronary perfusion device

The external enhanced coronary perfusion device is a series of compression cuffs that are placed on the patient's legs and set to inflate and deflate. This illustration shows the sequence of inflations: the calves are inflated first, then the thighs, then the buttocks.

SEQUENCE OF INFLATIONS

PRETREATMENT CARE

◆ At each visit and before treatment begins, take and record the patient's resting blood pressure readings. Also measure and record the sitting pulse and respiratory rates.

⚡ **WARNING** *Patients with blood pressure over 180/110 mm Hg or a heart rate of more than 120 beats/ minute should have these conditions treated before beginning EECP.*

◆ The patient's legs are examined for areas of redness, ecchymosis, and signs of other vascular problems.

◆ Advise the patient to urinate immediately before treatment.

◆ Ask the patient about symptoms of angina and review the patient's record.

⚡ **WARNING** *EECP shouldn't be used to treat patients with uncontrolled heart failure, severe valvular disease, uncontrolled arrhythmias, hemorrhage, coagulopathy, thrombophlebitis, and peripheral vascular diseases involving iliofemoral arterial obstruction.*

POSTTREATMENT CARE

◆ Place the patient in a comfortable position and give supplemental oxygen as indicated.

◆ Provide continuous cardiac monitoring as indicated.

◆ Administer medications and monitor for effect as ordered.

◆ Provide support for the patient's family.

◆ Monitor the patient's vital signs and intake and output as ordered.

PATIENT TEACHING

GENERAL

◆ Review the signs and symptoms of heart failure.

◆ Tell the patient that discomfort from the pulsatile movement and pressure on legs and buttocks may be eliminated or minimized by using suitable protective clothing during treatment, such as tights or bicycle pants.

◆ Advise the patient that if the pulsating sensation becomes uncomfortable, he should notify the treatment supervisor immediately to stop the treatment.

◆ Instruct the patient to record each anginal attack, its time of occurrence, duration, severity, its relationship to precipitating factors, and the number of nitroglycerin tablets used to ease the attack. Check the patient's diaries for accuracy and completeness at each treatment visit.

◆ Emphasize the importance of follow-up care.

RESOURCES
Organizations
American College of Cardiology: *www.acc.org*
American Medical Association: *www.ama-assn.org*

Selected references
Michaels, A.D., et al. "The Effects of Enhanced External Counterpulsation on Myocardial Perfusion in Patients with Stable Angina: A Multicenter Radionuclide Study," *American Heart Journal* 150(5):1066-73, November 2005.

Shea, M.L., et al. "An Update on Enhanced External Counterpulsation," *Clinical Cardiology* 28(3):115-18, March 2005.

Soran, O., et al. "Two-Year Clinical Outcomes after Enhanced External Counterpulsation (EECP) Therapy in Patients with Refractory Angina Pectoris and Left Ventricular Dysfunction (report from the International EECP Patient Registry)," *American Journal of Cardiology* 97(1):17-20, January 2006.

Extracorporeal membrane oxygenation

OVERVIEW

- Group of supportive therapies that oxygenizes blood outside the body
- Exposes a patient's lungs to low pressures, allowing them to rest and providing a means for oxygen delivery and carbon dioxide removal
- Lowers fraction of inspired oxygen (FIO_2) concentrations and volumes via mechanical ventilation, thereby reducing the risk of oxygen toxicity and barotrauma
- Also called *ECMO* or *extracorporeal life support*

INDICATIONS

- Severe acute respiratory failure in patients of all ages
- Acute respiratory distress syndrome
- Perioperative cardiac failure
- Primary myocardial failure
- Bridge to transplantation

PROCEDURE

- The physician uses strict aseptic technique to insert a cannula (adult size ranging from 16 French to 23 French) percutaneously into the appropriate vessel.
- The patient receives a loading dose of heparin I.V.
- The catheter is connected to the ECMO circuit and therapy is initiated; a continuous heparin infusion is maintained throughout therapy. An ECMO specialist remains at the patient's bedside. (See *ECMO setup.*)
- As blood leaves the patient's body, it's pumped through a membrane oxygenator, which acts as an artificial lung, supplying oxygen to the blood.
- A roller pump regulates the blood flow to the oxygenator, turning off whenever the pump flow is greater than blood return to the patient; excessive pressure on the right atrium or major vessels is averted. The pump automatically restarts when the flow rate balances.

    AGE FACTOR *Typical blood flow rates for adults range from 70 to 90 ml/kg/minute; for children, 80 to 100 ml/kg/minute; and for neonates, 120 to 170 ml/kg/minute.*
- An in-line fiber-optic catheter is used to monitor venous oxygen levels.
- Before returning to the patient, the blood passes through a heat exchanger where it's warmed to prevent hypothermia.

COMPLICATIONS
- Numerous complications (see *Complications of ECMO*)

NURSING DIAGNOSES
- Impaired gas exchange
- Ineffective tissue perfusion: Cardiopulmonary
- Risk for infection

EXPECTED OUTCOMES
The patient will:
- maintain adequate ventilation
- maintain tissue perfusion
- remain free from infection.

PRETREATMENT CARE
- Instruct the patient and his family about the procedure and the rationale for treatment. Reinforce the practitioner's explanation of the procedure, equipment, and follow-up care,

---

ECMO setup

Extracorporeal membrane oxygenation (ECMO) is managed by either a critical care nurse or respiratory therapist with special training in its operation. Illustrated and described here is a typical ECMO setup:

- *arterial filter* — removes air bubbles and clots from the blood as it travels through the ECMO circuit
- *cannula* — catheter through which blood travels to and from the patient
- *control desk module* — continuously monitors pressure throughout the circuit and regulates blood flow rate as needed in response to changing pressures in the system

- *heater* — generates heat needed to keep blood at a constant temperature
- *heat exchanger* — uses heat generated by a heater to maintain the temperature of the blood as it's oxygenated
- *hemochron* — monitors blood clotting
- *I.V. pump* — allows injection of medications, such as antibiotics, into the cannula of the ECMO circuit
- *membrane oxygenator* — serves as the artificial lung supplying oxygen to the blood
- *transonic blood flowmeter* — measures the amount of blood flowing through the cannula at various places along the ECMO circuit.

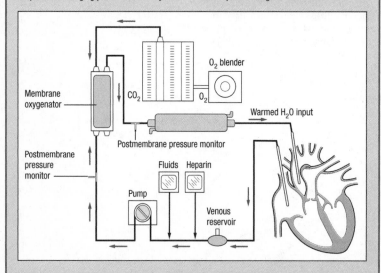

---

and verify that an appropriate consent form is signed.

- As appropriate, inform the patient that he'll have an endotracheal (ET) tube in place and will be connected to a mechanical ventilator. Review other equipment that may be used and provide emotional support.
- Administer sedation as ordered to reduce pain and restrict movement during catheter insertion and treatment initiation.

POSTTREATMENT CARE

- Assess cardiopulmonary and hemodynamic status closely, including central venous pressure, pulmonary artery pressure, and cardiac output, as indicated by the patient's condition or your facility's policy.
- If the patient becomes hemodynamically unstable, expect to administer dopamine (Intropin) to raise blood pressure and dobutamine (Dobutrex) to improve cardiac output; titrate dosages to desired response.

- Assess ET tube patency, position, and function, and mechanical ventilation. Monitor oxygen saturation levels and arterial blood gas levels as ordered. Administer supplemental oxygen and suction as necessary.
- After ECMO is initiated and the patient's gas exchange shows signs of improvement, expect to lower ventilator settings. Stay alert for changes in tidal volumes, which should increase as the lungs improve.
- Perform chest physiotherapy and change the patient's position frequently. Make sure that the ECMO circuit is unimpaired.
- Administer sedatives and analgesia and apply soft restraints as ordered.
- Monitor intake and output, daily weight, blood urea nitrogen, and serum creatinine levels closely for renal dysfunction. Administer diuretics as ordered to maintain fluid balance.
- Assess for signs and symptoms of acute renal failure; anticipate the need for hemofiltration, which can be added to the ECMO circuit.
- Monitor activated clotting times as indicated and assist with adjustments to heparin infusion.

- Expect to administer blood transfusions, including packed red blood cells to increase the oxygen carrying capacity of the blood and help stabilize the patient's intravascular volume. Anticipate platelet transfusion if the patient's platelet count drops below $100,000/mm^3$.
- Inspect catheter insertion sites for oozing or hematoma; change dressings as needed to keep the site clean and dry. If necessary, weigh saturated dressings to determine fluid volume loss.
- If a hematoma develops, palpate and mark the borders to monitor for an increase in size.
- Assess the affected extremity distal to the ECMO catheter insertion site for pulses, color, and temperature at least every 2 hours.

WARNING *A thready or absent pulse; a pale, cyanotic, or cool extremity; and a decrease in sensation indicate that the extremity isn't receiving adequate blood flow. This is an emergency that must be reported to the practitioner immediately.*

PATIENT TEACHING

GENERAL
- Offer emotional support to the patient's family; encourage them to visit and interact with the patient.

RESOURCES
Organizations
American Medical Association: *www.ama-assn.org*
The Society of Thoracic Surgeons: *www.sts.org*

Selected references
Gay, S.E., et al. "Critical Care Challenges in the Adult ECMO Patient," *Dimensions of Critical Care Nursing* 24(4): 157-62, July-August 2005.
Vlasselaers, D., et al. "Ventricular Unloading with a Miniature Axial Flow Pump in Combination with Extracorporeal Membrane Oxygenation," *Intensive Care Medicine* 32(2):329-33, February 2006.

Complications of ECMO

Extracorporeal membrane oxygenation (ECMO) is associated with numerous complications.

MECHANICAL COMPLICATIONS
- Clots in the circuit (most common mechanical complication) leading to oxygenator failure, consumption coagulopathy, and pulmonary and systemic emboli
- Cannula placement leading to damage of internal jugular vein or dissection of the carotid arterial intima
- Air in the circuit
- Oxygenator failure
- Cracks in connectors and tube rupture
- Pump malfunction
- Heat exchanger malfunction
- Failure of entire circuit
- Failure of circuit monitoring equipment

PATIENT COMPLICATIONS
- Seizures
- Intracranial bleeding
- Hemorrhage at catheter site, surgical site, or site of previous invasive procedures; intrathoracic, intra-abdominal, or retroperitoneal hemorrhage
- Thrombocytopenia
- Myocardial stun (decrease in left ventricular shortening fraction on initiation with return to normal after 48 hours of ECMO)
- Hypertension
- Pericardial tamponade
- Pneumothorax
- Pulmonary hemorrhage
- Oliguria
- Acute tubular necrosis
- Hemorrhage from stress, ischemia, or bleeding tendencies
- Hyperbilirubinemia
- Biliary calculi
- Infection; sepsis
- Metabolic acidosis or alkalosis
- Electrolyte imbalances (either high or low) involving potassium, sodium, and calcium
- Hyperglycemia or hypoglycemia

Extratemporal cortical resection

OVERVIEW

- Surgery to resect brain tissue that contains a seizure focus
- May involve tissue removal from more than one area or lobe of the brain
- Successful in eliminating or reducing seizures in 45% to 65% of cases; generally more effective if only one area of the brain is involved

INDICATIONS

- Disabling seizures uncontrolled by medication
- For patients who can't tolerate anti-seizure medication due to severe effects on quality of life

PROCEDURE

- After the patient receives general anesthesia, the surgeon creates a window to insert special instruments to remove brain tissue by making an incision in the scalp, and performs a craniotomy by removing a piece of bone and pulling back a section of the dura. Surgical microscopes are used to give the surgeon a magnified view of the area of the brain involved.
- In some cases, a portion of the surgery is performed while the patient is awake, using medication to keep the person relaxed and pain-free. This is done so that the patient can help the surgeon find and avoid areas in the brain responsible for vital functions, such as brain regions of language and motor control.
- After the brain tissue is removed, the dura and bone are fixed back into place, and the scalp is closed using stitches or staples.

COMPLICATIONS

- Infection
- Bleeding
- Allergic reaction to anesthesia
- Swelling of the brain
- Failure to relieve seizures
- Changes in personality or behavior
- Partial loss of vision, memory, or speech
- Stroke

NURSING DIAGNOSES

- Acute pain
- Disturbed sensory perception (all)
- Risk for infection

EXPECTED OUTCOMES

The patient will:
- verbalize relief from pain
- exhibit improved or normal neurologic status
- exhibit no signs of infection.

- An extensive presurgery evaluation is usually done and includes such testing as video electroencephalographic seizure monitoring, magnetic resonance imaging, and positron emission tomography. Other tests include neuropsychological memory testing, Wada test (to lateralize the side of language), ictal single-photon emission computed tomography, and magnetic resonance spectroscopy. These tests help pinpoint the seizure focus and determine if surgery is possible.
- Explain the treatment and preparation to the patient and his family.
- Verify that the patient has signed an appropriate consent form.
- Tell the patient that his head may be shaved in the operating room.
- Perform a complete neurologic assessment.

POSTTREATMENT CARE

- Position the patient on his side with the head of the bed elevated 15 to 30 degrees.
- Encourage careful deep breathing and coughing; suction gently as needed.
- Provide a quiet, calm environment.
- Maintain seizure precautions.
- Monitor the patient's vital signs, intake and output, level of consciousness, respiratory status, intracranial pressure (ICP), heart rate and rhythm, hemodynamic values, fluid and electrolyte balance, urine specific gravity, daily weight, drain patency, surgical wound and dressings, drainage, and complications.

 WARNING *Notify the practitioner immediately if you detect a worsening mental status, pupillary changes, or focal signs, such as increasing weakness in an arm or leg. These findings may indicate increased ICP.*

- Seizure medications are continued and unchanged to evaluate the initial effects of surgery. Afterward, medications should be adjusted to maximal effect.

PATIENT TEACHING

GENERAL

- Review care of the surgical wound with the patient.
- Inform the patient that headache and facial swelling will likely occur for 2 or 3 days after surgery.
- Review postoperative leg exercises and deep breathing and the use of antiembolism stockings or a pneumatic compression device.
- Review signs and symptoms of infection, complications, and when to notify the practitioner.
- Explain the importance of follow-up care.
- Tell the patient that most people who undergo this procedure can return to their normal activities, including work or school 4 to 6 weeks after surgery.
- Inform the patient that hair will grow over the incision site and hide the surgical scar.
- Inform the patient that although he may need to continue taking antiseizure medication for 2 or more years after surgery, when seizure control is established, the medications may be reduced or eliminated.

RESOURCES
Organizations
American Academy of Neurology:
   www.aan.com
American Medical Association:
   www.ama-assn.org
Epilepsy Therapy Development Project:
   www.epilepsy.com

Selected references
Cascino, G.D. "Surgical Treatment for Extratemporal Epilepsy," *Current Treatment Options in Neurology* 6(3):257-62, May 2004.

Cascino, G.D., et al. "Ictal SPECT in Nonlesional Extratemporal Epilepsy," *Epilepsia* 45(Suppl 4):32-34, 2004.

Cho, D.Y., et al. "Application of Neuronavigator Coupled with an Operative Microscope and Electrocorticography in Epilepsy Surgery," *Surgical Neurology* 64(5):411-17, discussion 417-18, November 2005.

Femoral popliteal bypass

OVERVIEW

- Used to restore blood flow to the leg with a femoral artery occlusion
- Also called *femoral-popliteal or fem-pop bypass*

INDICATIONS

- Vessel damaged by an arteriosclerotic or thromboembolic disorder
- Arterial occlusive disease
- Limb-threatening acute arterial occlusion unresponsive to thrombolytic drug therapy
- Vessel trauma, infection, or congenital defect
- Vascular disease unresponsive to drug therapy or nonsurgical revascularization

PROCEDURE

- The procedure may be done under local or general anesthesia. (See *Femoropopliteal bypass.*)
- I.V. antibiotics may be administered prophylactically during or just after the procedure; blood pressure drugs may be titrated to maintain the desired range.
- The surgical area is thoroughly cleaned with an antiseptic solution.
- Immediately before starting the procedure, the surgical team takes a "time out" to verify the correct patient, procedure, and site.
- If the saphenous vein will be used, an incision is made in the thigh and the other tissues are retracted until the vein can be seen. An appropriate length of the vein is excised for grafting and prepared (the vein is reversed so that the end that was originally located in the groin is now connected to the popliteal artery to eliminate hindrance of the valves).
- If the saphenous vein is inadequate, a synthetic vein graft is used.
- The saphenous access incision is closed and smaller incisions are made in the groin area to access the femoral artery, and behind the knee for the popliteal artery.
- One end of the vein graft is attached above the blockage femorally, and the free end of the graft is tunneled next to the artery to the popliteal site, where it's sutured in place.
- Blood flow is initiated through the graft and the connections are assessed for leakage.
- A repeat arteriogram is performed to confirm that blood flow has been restored.
- The incisions are closed and dressings are applied.

COMPLICATIONS

- Vessel or nerve injury
- Thrombus or emboli formation
- Myocardial infarction
- Cardiac arrhythmias
- Hemorrhage
- Infection
- Edema
- Pulmonary edema
- Graft occlusion, narrowing, dilation, or rupture

NURSING DIAGNOSES

- Acute pain
- Impaired tissue integrity
- Risk for infection

EXPECTED OUTCOMES

The patient will:

- verbalize and demonstrate feelings of increased comfort
- demonstrate improvement in peripheral pulsations and circulation in the affected extremity
- not show signs of incisional or deep leg infection.

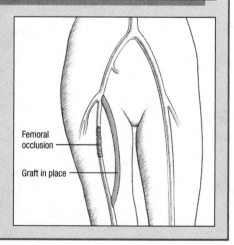

Femoropopliteal bypass

A femoropopliteal bypass graft is used to restore blood flow to the leg with a femoral occlusion. The surgeon bypasses the occluded part of the artery with an autogenous graft from the patient's saphenous vein. If this vein can't be used, a synthetic graft is placed.

Femoral occlusion

Graft in place

PRETREATMENT CARE

- ◆ Explain the treatment and preparation to the patient and his family.
- ◆ Verify that the patient has signed an appropriate consent form.
- ◆ Explain postoperative care.
- ◆ Perform a complete neurovascular assessment; mark the location of distal peripheral pulses bilaterally (if present) for ease of monitoring during and after the procedure (may require Doppler ultrasound localization in affected extremity).
- ◆ Obtain baseline vital signs and blood pressure.
- ◆ Obtain or verify the completion of the baseline 12-lead electrocardiogram and laboratory studies.
- ◆ Restrict food and fluids as ordered.
- ◆ Give the patient an aspirin before the procedure, if ordered by the surgeon.
- ◆ Notify the surgeon if the patient is sensitive to or is allergic to any medications, latex, iodine, tape, contrast dyes, or anesthetic agents (local or general).
- ◆ Notify the surgeon if there's a history of bleeding disorders or if the patient is taking anticoagulants, aspirin, or other medications that affect blood clotting. It may be necessary to stop these medications before the procedure.
- ◆ Make sure the surgeon marks the site where the procedure is to be performed.
- ◆ Complete the preoperative verification process.
- ◆ Shave the areas around the surgical sites as ordered.
- ◆ Initiate peripheral I.V. access; inform the patient that his heart rhythm will be monitored during the procedure.
- ◆ Insert a urinary catheter after preparing the patient for the procedure.
- ◆ Administer sedation as ordered.

POSTTREATMENT CARE

- ◆ Monitor the patient's vital signs, heart rate and rhythm, and neurovascular status per facility policy. (Use Doppler ultrasonography if peripheral pulses aren't palpable.)
- ◆ Administer medications as ordered.
- ◆ Position the patient, as ordered, and encourage frequent turning, keeping pressure off the graft site.
- ◆ Provide comfort measures and analgesics as needed.
- ◆ Assist with initial transfers and ambulation when cleared by the practitioner, and explain recommended activity levels to the patient.
- ◆ Encourage frequent incentive spirometer use, coughing, and deep breathing.
- ◆ Assist with and teach the patient range-of-motion exercises.
- ◆ Assess incisions frequently for bleeding and infection, and provide care and dressing changes as ordered.
- ◆ Record intake and output; remove urinary catheter as ordered.
- ◆ Assess for complications, including abnormal bleeding, graft occlusion, signs of infection, chest pain, and breathing difficulty with embolism or pulmonary edema.

PATIENT TEACHING

GENERAL

- ◆ Review medications and possible adverse reactions with the patient, including possible new antiplatelet drugs.
- ◆ Teach the patient to monitor his lower extremities for changes in temperature, color, and sensation, and any return of preoperative symptoms, and to notify the surgeon of changes noted.
- ◆ Teach the patient how to care for the incision sites.
- ◆ Review the signs and symptoms of infection with the patient.
- ◆ Tell the patient about signs and symptoms of possible complications, and to call the practitioner promptly.
- ◆ Advise the patient to stop smoking, if appropriate, and encourage him to follow a low-cholesterol diet, exercise regularly per the practitioner's instructions, and have regular monitoring of his blood pressure and cholesterol levels.

RESOURCES
Organizations
American College of Surgeons:
www.facs.org
American Heart Association:
www.americanheart.org
Vascular Disease Foundation:
www.vdf.org

Selected references
D'Addio, V., et al. "Femorofemoral Bypass with Femoral Popliteal Vein," *Journal of Vascular Surgery* 42(1):35-39, July 2005.

Galaria, I.I., et al. "Popliteal-to-Distal Bypass: Identifying Risk Factors Associated with Limb Loss and Graft Failure," *Vascular and Endovascular Surgery* 39(5):393-400, September-October 2005.

Lee, T.L., and Bokovoy, J. "Understanding Discharge Instructions After Vascular Surgery: An Observational Study," *Journal of Vascular Nursing* 23(1):25-29, March 2005.

Gastric bypass

- Malabsorption and restriction procedure in which a small stomach pouch is created using sutures and is attached to a portion of the jejunum; reduces the body's intake of calories, thus achieving potentially significant weight loss
- Postoperatively, because stomach is smaller, allows patient to feel fuller faster
- Also referred to as a *Roux-en Y bypass*

INDICATIONS

- Body mass index (BMI) of 40 or more; a patient with a BMI of 40 or more is at least 100 lb (45 kg) over his recommended weight (normal BMI, 18.5 to 25)
- BMI of 35 or more plus a life-threatening illness that can be improved with weight loss, such as sleep apnea, type 2 diabetes, and heart disease

PROCEDURE

- Immediately before starting the procedure, the surgical team takes a "time out" to verify the correct patient, procedure, and site.
- The surgery is performed under general anesthesia.
- The surgeon divides the stomach into a small upper section and a larger bottom section using staples similar to stitches.
- After the stomach has been divided, the surgeon connects a section of the small intestine (commonly the jejunum) to the pouch.
- The surgeon then reconnects the base of the Roux limb with the remaining portion of the small intestines from the bottom of the stomach, forming a Y-shape. (See *Understanding gastric bypass.*)
- Gastric bypass can be performed using a laparoscope.

  WARNING *If the patient weighs more than 350 lb (159 kg) or if he has had previous abdominal surgery, he isn't a good candidate for laparoscopy.*

- With laparoscopy, small incisions are made in the abdomen. Carbon dioxide is insufflated to separate the organs from one another. The surgeon passes slender surgical instruments through these incisions with a laparoscope to perform the procedure and video monitoring during the surgery.

COMPLICATIONS

- Bleeding
- Infections
- Gallstones
- Gastritis
- Vomiting
- Iron or vitamin B_{12} deficiencies leading to anemia
- Calcium deficiency leading to osteoporosis
- Dumping syndrome (nausea, vomiting, diarrhea, dizziness, and sweating)

NURSING DIAGNOSES

- Activity intolerance
- Chronic low self-esteem
- Imbalanced nutrition: More than body requirements

EXPECTED OUTCOMES

The patient will:
- perform activities of daily living
- express positive feelings about self
- exhibit weight loss.

PRETREATMENT CARE

- A complete medical examination is done to evaluate the patient's overall health. A psychological evaluation is also performed to determine if he'll be adhering to the new lifestyle.
- Extensive nutritional counseling is done with the patient.
- Explain the treatment and preparation to the patient and his family.
- Verify that the patient has signed an appropriate consent form.
- Obtain blood samples for hematologic and chemistry studies as ordered.
- Withhold food and fluids as ordered.
- Begin I.V. fluid replacement and total parenteral nutrition (TPN) as ordered.
- Prepare the patient for abdominal X-rays as ordered.
- Explain postoperative care and equipment.
- Monitor the patient's vital signs, intake and output, nutritional status, and laboratory test results.
- Complete the preoperative verification process.

Understanding gastric bypass

In gastric bypass surgery, most of the stomach is bypassed as shown.

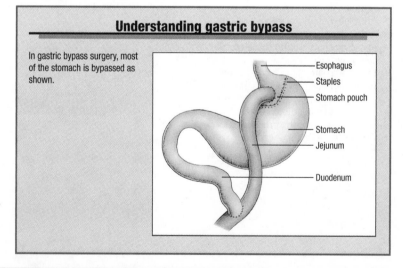

Labels: Esophagus, Staples, Stomach pouch, Stomach, Jejunum, Duodenum

---

POSTTREATMENT CARE

- Maintain I.V. replacement therapy as ordered.
- Keep the nasogastric tube patent, but don't reposition it.
- Encourage regular turning, coughing and deep-breathing exercises, and use of incentive spirometry.
- Encourage splinting of the incision site with coughing and movement.
- Monitor vital signs, intake and output, and daily weight.
- Report signs of dehydration, peritonitis, sepsis, infection, or postresection obstruction.

⚡ **WARNING** *Monitor for and immediately report signs and symptoms of anastomotic leakage, including low-grade fever, malaise, slight leukocytosis, abdominal distension, tenderness, hemorrhage, hypovolemic shock, and bloody stool or wound drainage.*

- Administer medications as ordered.
- Assess for abdominal pain, cramping, or shoulder pain. Explain that bloating or abdominal fullness from laparoscopy will subside as carbon dioxide is absorbed.
- Provide comfort measures.
- Administer medications as ordered.
- Place the patient in low or semi-Fowler's position.
- Monitor bowel sounds. After bowel sounds return, begin oral intake, providing six small feedings per day.
- Monitor laboratory test results.
- Provide wound care, and assess the type and amount of drainage.
- Assess for signs of dehydration; encourage fluids to prevent dehydration.
- Monitor for complications of morbid obesity, such as pneumonia, thromboembolism, skin breakdown, and delayed wound healing.

PATIENT TEACHING

GENERAL

- Review medications and possible adverse reactions with the patient.
- Instruct the patient to report excessive bleeding from surgical sites.
- Review the signs and symptoms of infection with the patient.
- Teach the patient about the signs and symptoms of obstruction or perforation.
- Advise the patient to continue coughing and performing deep-breathing exercises.
- Teach the patient how to care for the surgical wound.
- Inform the patient about dumping syndrome (weakness, nausea, flatulence, and palpitations occurring within 30 minutes after a meal) and how to prevent it.
- Inform the patient that he'll receive extensive nutritional counseling.
- Tell the patient that about 10 lb (4.5 kg) per month is usually lost and that a stable weight occurs between 18 and 24 months after surgery. Inform him that most weight loss occurs at the beginning.
- Inform the patient that during his follow-up visits in the first year after surgery, physical and mental health status, change in weight, and nutritional needs will be addressed.
- Instruct the patient that to achieve weight loss and avoid complications, he must exercise and eat as directed.
- Tell the patient he'll remain on liquid or pureed food for several weeks after the surgery. Even then, he'll feel full quickly because the new stomach pouch initially holds only 1 tablespoonful of food. Tell him that the pouch eventually expands.
- Advise the patient that he may need replacement of iron, calcium, vitamin B_{12}, or other nutrients and that supplements, such as a multivitamin with minerals, may be prescribed.

- Instruct that patient that after his diet includes solid food, he'll need to chew slowly and thoroughly. He'll be instructed on eating small meals frequently during the day, rather than large meals.
- Advise the patient that he may need to separate fluid and food intake by at least 30 minutes and to sip fluids only.
- Tell the patient he won't be able to tolerate large amounts of fat, alcohol, or sugar. Advise him to reduce his intake of fat (especially fast-food meals, deep-fried foods, and high-fat foods) and sugar (such as cakes, cookies, and candy).

RESOURCES
Organizations
American College of Gastroenterology: *www.acg.gi.org*
American Gastroenterological Association: *www.gastro.org*
American Society of Bariatric Surgery: *www.asbs.org*

Selected references
Blackwood, H.S. "Help Your Patient Downsize with Bariatric Surgery," *Nursing* (Suppl):4-9, Fall 2005.
Cottam, D.R., et al. "A Case-Controlled Matched-Pair Cohort Study of Laparoscopic Roux-En-Y Gastric Bypass and Lap-Band Patients in a Single U.S. Center With Three-Year Follow-Up," *Obesity Surgery* 16(5):534-40, May 2006.
Smith, B.L. "Bariatric Surgery. It's No Easy Fix," *RN* 68(6):58-63, June 2005.

Gastric lavage

◆ Irrigation of the stomach and aspiration of stomach contents through a large-bore gastric tube

INDICATIONS
◆ Preparation for endoscopic examination
◆ Life-threatening poisoning
◆ Life-threatening drug overdose
◆ Upper GI bleeding

⚡ **WARNING** *Gastric lavage is contraindicated after ingestion of corrosive substances (such as lye, petroleum distillates, ammonia, alkalis, or mineral acids); the lavage tube may perforate the already compromised esophagus.*

◆ If the patient has a decreased level of consciousness (LOC), he may require endotracheal intubation before the procedure.
◆ After positioning the patient in a left lateral position with his head in a dependent position, the practitioner inserts the gastric tube nasally or orally and advances it slowly; forceful insertion may injure tissues. Tube placement is verified by aspiration of stomach contents. (See *Using wide-bore gastric tubes.*)

⚡ **WARNING** *The patient may vomit when the gastric tube reaches the posterior pharynx; be prepared to suction the airway immediately.*

◆ After securing the tube with tape and making sure the irrigant inflow tube on the lavage setup is clamped, connect the unattached end of the irrigant inflow tube to the lavage tube.
◆ Allow stomach contents to empty into the drainage container before instilling the irrigant. This decreases the risk of overfilling the stomach with irrigant and inducing vomiting.
◆ Save a sample of the aspirated stomach contents in a labeled container and send it for laboratory analysis to identify the ingested substance.

◆ If using a syringe irrigation set, aspirate stomach contents with a 50-ml bulb or catheter-tip syringe before instilling the irrigant.
◆ If using a syringe, after confirming proper tube placement, instill about 50 ml of solution at a time until 250 to 500 ml has been instilled. Clamp the inflow tube and unclamp the outflow tube to allow the irrigant to flow out.

⚡ **WARNING** *Correct tube placement is essential; accidental misplacement in the lungs followed by lavage can be fatal.*

◆ If using the syringe irrigation kit, aspirate the irrigant with the syringe and empty it into a calibrated container. Measure inflow and outflow to make sure that outflow equals at least the amount of irrigant instilled; this prevents stomach distention and vomiting.
◆ If the drainage amount is significantly less than the instilled amount, reposition the tube until sufficient solution flows out. Gently massage the abdomen over the stomach to promote outflow.
◆ Repeat the inflow-outflow cycle until returned fluids appear clear, signaling that the stomach no longer contains harmful substances or that bleeding has stopped.
◆ After the practitioner completes the lavage, an absorbent may be instilled through the tube. After instillation, the tube is clamped so that the absorbent can remain in the stomach and inactivate the toxic substance.

COMPLICATIONS
◆ Vomiting
◆ Aspiration
◆ Bradyarrhythmias
◆ After iced lavage, body temperature may fall, triggering cardiac arrhythmias

◆ Disturbed sensory perception (all)
◆ Impaired gas exchange
◆ Ineffective tissue perfusion: Renal, cerebral, cardiopulmonary, peripheral

EXPECTED OUTCOMES
The patient will:
◆ exhibit improved neurologic status
◆ maintain patent airway and adequate oxygenation
◆ demonstrate hemodynamic stability.

◆ Explain the procedure to the patient and his family.
◆ Remove the patient's dentures if appropriate.
◆ Maintain a patent airway.
◆ Gather equipment and set up per facility protocol. A prepackaged, syringe-type irrigation kit may be used for intermittent lavage. For poisoning or drug overdose, the continuous lavage setup is faster and more effective for diluting and removing the harmful substance.
◆ Make sure suction equipment is readily available.
◆ Monitor the patient's vital signs.
◆ Assess the patient's LOC as well as respiratory, cardiac, and GI status.

Using wide-bore gastric tubes

To deliver a large volume of fluid rapidly through a gastric tube (for such conditions as profuse gastric bleeding or poisoning), a wide-bore gastric tube works best. Typically inserted orally, the tube remains in place long enough to complete the lavage and evacuate stomach contents.

EWALD TUBE

In an emergency, using the Ewald tube—a single-lumen tube with several openings at the distal end—allows you to aspirate large amounts of gastric contents quickly.

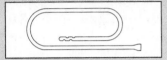

LEVACUATOR TUBE

The Levacuator tube has two lumens. Use the larger lumen for evacuating gastric contents; the smaller, for instilling an irrigant.

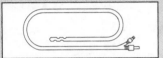

EDLICH TUBE

The Edlich tube is a single-lumen tube that has four openings near the closed distal tip. A funnel or syringe may be connected at the proximal end. Like the Ewald tube, the Edlich tube lets you withdraw large quantities of gastric contents quickly.

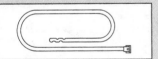

POSTTREATMENT CARE

- Assess the patient's vital signs, urine output, and LOC every 15 minutes. Notify the practitioner of changes.
- If ordered, remove the gastric tube.
- To control GI bleeding, the practitioner may order continuous stomach irrigation before withdrawing the gastric tube.
- Never leave the patient alone during gastric lavage.
- Keep tracheal suctioning equipment nearby; watch closely for airway obstruction caused by vomiting or excess oral secretions.
- Suction the oral cavity often to ensure an open airway and prevent aspiration.
- Obtain blood samples to check levels of the ingested substance, electrolytes, blood urea nitrogen, and creatinine (if the substance was toxic).
- If gastric lavage was performed to control bleeding, obtain blood for hematology studies, and monitor for signs of increased bleeding.
- When lavage is done to stop bleeding, keep precise intake and output records to determine the amount of bleeding. When large volumes of fluid are instilled and withdrawn, serum electrolyte and arterial blood gas levels may be measured during or after lavage.
- Monitor intake and output and record volume and type of irrigant and amount of drained gastric contents.
- Note color and consistency of drainage.

PATIENT TEACHING

GENERAL

- Provide follow up for the patient; admit to facility as indicated, and inform authorities as appropriate.
- Teach the patient how to prevent recurrent overdose, and instruct him about poison prevention.
- Refer the patient for resource and support services.
- Refer the patient for psychiatric treatment if poisoning was intentional.

RESOURCES
Organizations
American Academy of Neurology: *www.aan.com*
American Association of Poison Control Centers: *www.aapcc.org*
American College of Emergency Physicians: *www.acep.org*

Selected references

Bartlett, D. "Acetaminophen Toxicity," *Journal of Emergency Nursing* 30(3): 281-83, June 2004.
Heard, K. "Gastrointestinal Decontamination," *Medical Clinics of North America* 89(6):1067-78, November 2005.
Littlejohn, C. "Management of Intentional Overdose in A&E Departments," *Nursing Times* 100(33):38-43, August 2005.

Gastrostomy

- Creation of a channel that extends from the gastric lumen to the skin for insertion of a gastrostomy feeding tube or button
- Gastrostomy feeding tube: may be inserted through a midline abdominal incision or through percutaneous endoscopy
- Gastrostomy feeding button: may be inserted laparoscopically

INDICATIONS

- Extensive oral or esophageal cancer, obstruction, or trauma
- Prevention of starvation or malnutrition

⚡ **WARNING** *Contraindications include intestinal obstruction that prohibits the use of the bowel, diffuse peritonitis, intractable vomiting, paralytic ileus, and severe diarrhea that makes metabolic management difficult. Cautions include severe pancreatitis, enterocutaneous fistulae, and GI ischemia.*

STANDARD FEEDING TUBE INSERTION

- Immediately before starting the procedure, the surgical team takes a "time out" to verify the correct patient, procedure, and site and to make sure that the gastrostomy feeding tube is readily available.
- After the patient receives a general anesthetic or moderate sedation, the surgeon makes a vertical abdominal incision directly over the stomach.
- He then inserts a gastrostomy tube into the anterior gastric wall, inflates the balloon or tests the mushroom disk to hold it in place, and aspirates the gastric contents.
- The tube is clamped and several purse-string sutures are inserted to hold it in place.
- A sterile dressing is applied around the tube.

PERCUTANEOUS ENDOSCOPIC GASTROSTOMY TUBE INSERTION

- Immediately before starting the procedure, the surgical team takes a "time out" to verify the correct patient, procedure, and site and to make sure that the gastrostomy feeding tube is readily available.
- After the patient receives moderate sedation, the patient receives a local anesthetic to the throat and the abdomen over the stomach.
- The endoscopic tube is passed into the stomach and the area for tube insertion is visualized.
- A small incision is made and the tube is pushed through the stomach and abdominal walls, and the balloon inflated to hold it in position.

GASTROSTOMY FEEDING BUTTON INSERTION

- Immediately before starting the procedure, the surgical team takes a "time out" to verify the correct patient, procedure, and site and to make sure that the gastrostomy feeding button is readily available.
- After the patient receives general anesthesia, a small incision is made and a laparoscope is inserted to visualize the stomach and the area for insertion.
- A small incision is made in the abdominal wall into the stomach and the feeding button is placed and then tested.

COMPLICATIONS

- Nausea and vomiting
- Abdominal distention
- Exit-site infection
- Exit-site leakage
- Peritonitis

- Acute pain
- Imbalanced nutrition: Less than body requirements
- Risk for infection

EXPECTED OUTCOMES

The patient will:

- verbalize and demonstrate increased feelings of comfort
- have stable weight and laboratory values that return to within normal parameters
- experience no signs and symptoms of skin or peritoneal cavity infection.

- Tell the patient that the surgeon will perform the initial insertion.
- Make sure that a consent form has been signed.
- Explain to the patient (if appropriate) and his family the purpose of a gastrostomy tube, how and where it's inserted, and what it looks like. Answer questions, and address concerns to allay their anxiety.
- Tell the patient (if appropriate) and his family if the gastrostomy is expected to be permanent. Provide emotional support.
- If the patient is receiving nasogastric (NG) feedings, withhold them after midnight on the day of surgery. Don't remove the NG tube unless the surgeon orders its removal—he may want it to remain in place to decompress the stomach during surgery or until gastrostomy tube feedings are started.
- Initiate I.V. therapy as indicated.
- Complete the preoperative verification process.

- Take the patient's vital signs as ordered postoperatively until he's fully recovered from the anesthesia.
- Prepare the patient for the first fluid administration through the gastrostomy tube soon after surgery. Assess for tube patency and leakage around the tube. Ensure the patient's privacy, and place him in semi-Fowler's position before the instillation.
- Prepare the patient for further gastrostomy instillations in the same manner. Check tube patency by aspirating gastric fluids with a syringe and administering 30 to 60 ml of water at room temperature through the tube. Expect to gradually increase the amount given as the patient tolerates it and if no leaking occurs. After instillation, clamp the tube, and follow the facility's protocol for covering and securing the tube and dressing the site.
- Administer intermittent (bolus) tube feedings as ordered. Check for residual stomach contents before each feeding. Keep the patient in semi-Fowler's position for at least 30 minutes after each feeding to facilitate digestion and prevent aspiration. Record the amount and contents of each feeding as well as the patient's tolerance.
- If continuous feedings are ordered, periodically check for residual stomach contents and give feedings according to the surgeon's guidelines. To maintain patency, flush the gastrostomy tube with water at least once every 8 hours.
- Monitor the gastrostomy site for signs of skin irritation and infection.
- Wash the area around the tube daily with soap and water or normal saline solution. A barrier ointment, such as zinc oxide or petroleum jelly, may be ordered to protect the skin from irritation. Keep the gastrostomy site clean and dry.
- If the button pops out while feeding, reinsert it, estimate the formula already delivered, and resume feeding. (See *How to reinsert a gastrostomy feeding button.*)

(continued)

How to reinsert a gastrostomy feeding button

If a gastrostomy feeding button pops out, follow these procedures to reinsert the device.

PREPARE THE EQUIPMENT

- Collect the feeding button (shown below); wash it with soap and water; rinse thoroughly and dry. Also obtain an obturator and water-soluble lubricant.

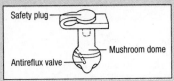

Safety plug

Mushroom dome

Antireflux valve

INSERT THE BUTTON

- Check the depth of the patient's stoma to make sure you have a feeding button of the correct size; clean around the stoma.
- Lubricate the obturator with water-soluble lubricant and distend the button several times to ensure the patency of the antireflux valve within the button.
- Lubricate the mushroom dome and stoma. Push the button through the stoma into the stomach (as shown).

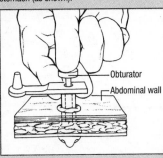

Obturator

Abdominal wall

- Remove the obturator by rotating it as you withdraw it, to keep the antireflux valve from adhering to it. If the valve sticks, push the obturator back into the button until the valve closes.
- After removing the obturator, make sure the valve is closed.
- Close the flexible safety plug, which should be relatively flush with the skin surface (as shown).

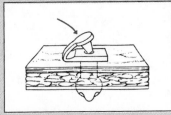

- If you need to give a feeding right away, open the safety plug and attach the feeding adapter and feeding tube (as shown). Deliver feeding as ordered.

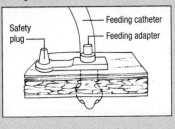

Safety plug

Feeding catheter

Feeding adapter

- Once daily, clean the peristomal skin with mild soap and water or povidone-iodine, and let the skin air-dry for 20 minutes, to avoid skin irritation.
- Clean the peristomal site whenever spillage from the feeding bag occurs.

PATIENT TEACHING

GENERAL
- Explain how the gastrostomy feeding button is inserted and cared for. Tell the patient how to use the button for feedings.
- Advise the patient how to clean the equipment.
- Teach the patient about peristomal skin care.
- Tell the patient when and whom to call with questions.
- Tell the patient or caregiver to notify the practitioner if signs of infection (such as redness, swelling, and purulent drainage), problems with administering feedings, or leakage occurs around the tube.
- Teach the patient or caregiver how to care for the gastrostomy tube. If the gastrostomy is permanent, show the patient or caregiver how to change the tube every 2 to 3 days. Explain that the tube may be removed after several weeks and reinserted only for feedings and that, between feedings, the gastrostomy opening may be protected by a small gauze pad held in place by adhesive. (See *Caring for your gastrostomy tube.*)

- Provide skin care instructions, stressing the importance of keeping the skin around the tube clean and dry to prevent skin breakdown.
- Explain that the patient should be positioned with his head elevated at least 30 degrees during the feeding and for 30 minutes afterward.
- Teach the patient or caregiver how to prepare and administer the type of gastrostomy tube feedings ordered. Tell them to flush the tube or button with 30 ml of water after feedings. If continuous feedings are to be administered, make sure the patient or caregiver understands how to operate the pump used for this procedure.
- Explain the importance of keeping open cans of tube feeding formula refrigerated and to use them within 2 days of opening. However, explain that the formula should be administered at room temperature.
- Provide instructions for clearing a clogged tube.
- Teach the patient or caregiver what they should do if the tube or button become dislodged.
- Help arrange for visiting nurse follow-up after discharge.

RESOURCES
Organizations
American College of Gastroenterology: *www.acg.gi.org*
American Gastroenterological Association: *www.gastro.org*
The Society of American Gastrointestinal and Endoscopic Surgeons: *www.sages.org*

Selected references
Borkowski, S. "G Tube Care: Managing Hypergranulation Tissue," *Nursing* 35(8):24, August 2005.
Ditchburn, L., and Chapman, W. "Joint Primary-Secondary Care Design of PEG Care Pathways," *Nursing Times* 101(18):34-36, May 2005.
Owada, K. "Use of a Hydrofiber Dressing to Manage PEG Sites," *Advanced Skin and Wound Care* 18(4):183-89, May 2005.
Rimon, E., et al. "Percutaneous Endoscopic Gastrostomy: Evidence of Different Prognosis in Various Patient Subgroups," *Age and Ageing* 34(4):353-57, July 2005.

Caring for your gastrostomy tube

Dear Patient:

Use these guidelines to review what the nurse taught you about caring for your gastrostomy tube.

CHECKING TUBE POSITION

◆ Make sure the tube is in place. Look for a mark in indelible ink on the tube where it should exit from your body.

◆ If you can't see the mark, the tube is slipping too far into your body. If you see more tube below the mark than usual, the tube is pulling out of your body.

◆ Either way, contact the home care nurse or health care provider immediately before trying to administer feedings or medicine through the tube.

◆ When you're sure the tube is positioned correctly, remove the cap or plug and, if necessary, unclamp the tube.

CLEARING THE TUBE

◆ Pour 2 tablespoons (30 ml) of water into the funnel or syringe used for feeding or giving medicine. Let the water flow into the stomach by gravity.

◆ Before the water has flowed out completely, reclamp or pinch the tube and remove the funnel or syringe.

◆ Cap the tube or insert the plug and, if necessary, clamp the tubing.

◆ Wash the funnel or syringe thoroughly in hot, soapy water and store it in a clean, covered container.

CHANGING THE DRESSING

Change your dressing daily or whenever it's wet or soiled, as follows. Don't use scissors to remove the old dressing; you might cut the tube accidentally.

1. Carefully clean the skin around the tube with mild soap and warm water. Then rinse and dry the skin thoroughly.

2. Position two 4″ × 4″ gauze pads around the tube so that the slit sides overlap, to protect the skin from gastric leakage.

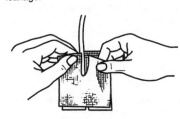

3. Then cover the slit pads with uncut gauze pads. Secure them with hypoallergenic tape. If your skin is tender, use a skin preparation before taping.

CARING FOR YOUR SKIN

◆ Keep the skin around your stomach opening clean and dry to avoid skin irritation and infection. Check it several times per day.

◆ If you see leakage of food or medicine around the tube, immediately apply a warm, moistened towel to soften encrusted fluid, and wash, rinse, and dry the skin. Then call your health care provider.

◆ If the skin becomes irritated, dust it with karaya gum powder.

◆ Notify your home care nurse or health care provider if the skin around the tube feels sore, looks red, or seems puffy or if you feel any discomfort in your stomach.

Heart valve annuloplasty

OVERVIEW

- Surgery performed on the valve's annulus (the connection between the valve leaflets and the heart wall) to improve functioning of the heart's valves

INDICATIONS
- Severe aortic valvular stenosis or insufficiency
- Severe mitral valvular stenosis or insufficiency

PROCEDURE

- Immediately before the procedure, the surgical team takes a "time out" to verify the correct patient, procedure, and site and to make sure that the annuloplasty ring is readily available (if being used for the procedure).
- After the patient is anesthetized, a medial sternotomy is performed.
- Cardiopulmonary bypass is initiated by cannulating the great vessels and perfusing them with a cold cardioplegic solution.
- An esophageal echocardiogram may be done to help determine the functioning of the valve before and after surgery.
- The surgeon reshapes or tightens the valve using purse-string sutures or by sewing an annuloplasty ring to the annulus which may be made of tissue or of synthetic material. The opening is made smaller which allows the leaflets to meet again at valve closure. (See *Annuloplasty ring insertion.*)
- The patient is removed from the bypass machine.
- Epicardial pacemaker leads and a chest tube are inserted.
- The incision is closed, and a sterile dressing is applied.

COMPLICATIONS
- Postpericardiotomy syndrome
- Cardiac arrhythmias
- Hemorrhage
- Coagulopathy
- Stroke
- Valve dysfunction or failure
- Renal failure
- Pulmonary embolism
- Thromboembolism
- Infection

NURSING DIAGNOSES

- Decreased cardiac output
- Ineffective tissue perfusion: Cardiopulmonary
- Risk for infection

EXPECTED OUTCOMES
The patient will:
- maintain adequate cardiac output
- maintain hemodynamic stability as evidenced by adequate blood pressure and cardiac rhythm
- be free from signs and symptoms of infection

PRETREATMENT CARE

- Explain the procedure and preparation to the patient and his family.
- Verify that the patient has signed an appropriate consent form.
- Explain postoperative care and equipment.
- Obtain results of laboratory studies, including blood typing and cross-matching.
- Obtain a 12-lead electrocardiogram (ECG) as ordered.
- Make sure that a chest X-ray has been obtained.
- Perform a preoperative assessment and complete the preoperative verification process.
- Withhold food and fluids as ordered.
- Initiate I.V. therapy as prescribed.

Annuloplasty ring insertion

(A) Mitral valve insufficiency, leaflets don't close. (B) Insertion of an annuloplasty ring. (C) Completed valvuloplasty, leaflets close.

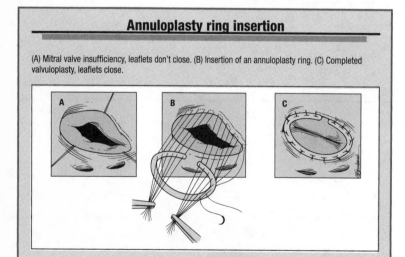

POSTTREATMENT CARE

- Administer medications as ordered.
- Assist with temporary epicardial pacing as indicated.
- Monitor the ECG for development of arrhythmias and ischemia.
- Maintain mean arterial pressure within prescribed guidelines (usually between 70 and 100 mm Hg in an adult).
- Maintain the chest tube system as ordered. Report a sudden change in the amount of drainage or an output of 200 ml/hour.
- Administer I.V. fluids and blood products as ordered.
- Assist with weaning from the mechanical ventilator as indicated.
- Encourage coughing, turning, and deep breathing.
- Encourage use of incentive spirometry.
- Assist with early ambulation.
- Monitor vital signs, heart rate and rhythm, cardiovascular status, heart sounds, and hemodynamic values.
- Record and evaluate daily weight, sternal stability and drainage, and intake and output.
- Monitor for complications such as abnormal bleeding.
- Assess respiratory status, including pulse oximetry and arterial blood gas analysis.
- Monitor laboratory test results.
- Perform surgical wound care and dressing changes, as prescribed, and monitor the wound for signs of infection.

PATIENT TEACHING

GENERAL

- Review medications and possible adverse reactions with the patient.
- Teach the patient how to care for the surgical wound.
- Tell the patient about the signs and symptoms of infection.
- Tell the patient about the signs and symptoms of postpericardiotomy syndrome.
- Inform the patient about possible complications.
- Teach the patient about anticoagulant therapy precautions such as monitoring for bleeding and prevention of trauma (such as by using a soft toothbrush and electric razors).
- Tell the patient to notify the practitioner if bleeding occurs.
- Advise the patient to follow the prescribed activity restrictions and to balance activity with rest periods.
- Advise the patient to follow dietary restrictions directed by the practitioner.
- Tell the patient to follow the prescribed exercise program.
- Stress the need for follow-up care.
- Emphasize the importance of informing all health care providers of his valve surgery.
- Stress the importance of wearing medical identification at all times.

RESOURCES
Organizations
American College of Chest Surgeons: *www.chestnet.org*
American College of Surgeons: *www.facs.org*
American Heart Association: *www.americanheart.org*

Selected references
Babaliaros, V., et al. "Surgery Insight: Current Advances in Percutaneous Heart Valve Replacement and Repair," *Nature Clinical Practice, Cardiovascular Medicine* 3(5):256-64, May 2006.
Eastwood, G.M. "Evaluating the Reliability of Recorded Fluid Balance to Approximate Body Weight Change in Patients Undergoing Cardiac Surgery," *Heart and Lung* 35(1):27-33, January-February 2006.
Goskin, I., et al. "Modified Semicircular Constricting Annuloplasty (Sagban's Annuloplasty) in Severe Functional Tricuspid Regurgitation: Alternative Surgical Technique and Its Mid-Term Results," *Journal of Cardiac Surgery* 21(2):172-75, March-April 2006.

Heart valve chordoplasty

OVERVIEW

- Surgery performed to replace or shorten the chordae tendineae to promote cardiac output and heart valve functioning
- Missing chordae replaced by moving a few chordae from one side of the valve to the other, or by reconstructing from durable Gore-Tex sutures
- Leakage eliminated when cords and muscles are the right length and valve leaflet edges meet

INDICATIONS

- Severe mitral valvular insufficiency
- Severe tricuspid valvular insufficiency (rare)

PROCEDURE

- After the patient is anesthetized, a medial sternotomy is performed.
- Cardiopulmonary bypass is initiated by cannulating the great vessels and perfusing them with a cold cardioplegic solution.
- An esophageal echocardiogram is done to help determine the functioning of the valve before, during, and after surgery.
- When there's prolapse of the anterior mitral valve leaflet, repair is more complex. Posterior leaflet chordae may be transferred to the anterior leaflet. (See *Chordae tendineae repair*.)
- Alternatively, a premeasured loop of Gore-Tex suture may be attached to the head of the papillary muscle with a special suture, then attached to the damaged area of the anterior leaflet.
- The repair is tested by saline infusion and transesophageal echocardiogram imaging.
- The patient is removed from the bypass machine.
- Epicardial pacemaker leads and a chest tube are inserted.
- The incision is closed, and a sterile dressing is applied.

COMPLICATIONS

- Postpericardiotomy syndrome
- Cardiac arrhythmias
- Hemorrhage
- Coagulopathy
- Stroke
- Valve dysfunction or failure
- Renal failure
- Pulmonary or thromboembolism
- Infection

NURSING DIAGNOSES

- Decreased cardiac output
- Ineffective tissue perfusion: Cardiopulmonary
- Risk for infection

EXPECTED OUTCOMES

The patient will:

- maintain adequate cardiac output
- maintain blood pressure and cardiac rate within normal limits, and have clear lung sounds
- be free from signs and symptoms of infection.

PRETREATMENT CARE

- Explain the procedure and preparation to the patient and his family.
- Verify that the patient has signed an appropriate consent form.
- Explain postoperative care and equipment.
- Obtain results of laboratory studies, including blood typing and cross-matching.
- Obtain a 12-lead electrocardiogram (ECG) as ordered.
- Perform a preoperative assessment and complete the preoperative verification process.
- Withhold food and fluids as ordered.
- Initiate I.V. therapy as prescribed.

Chordae tendineae repair

When sufficient intact chordae remain after a tear or rupture, functional ones may be moved to the opposite leaflet to replace the damaged ones.

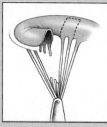

A rectangle of posterior leaflet tissue with intact chordae is dissected free.

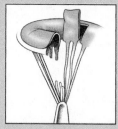

The intact chordae and leaflet tissue is sutured into place on the anterior leaflet, replacing the damaged chordae.

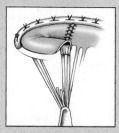

The posterior leaflet surgical edges are anastomosed and sutured together. An annuloplasty ring is then molded and sutured in place to support the repair.

POSTTREATMENT CARE

- ◆ Administer medications as ordered.
- ◆ Assist with temporary epicardial pacing as indicated.
- ◆ Monitor the ECG for the development of arrhythmias and ischemia.
- ◆ Maintain mean arterial pressure within prescribed guidelines (usually between 70 and 100 mm Hg in an adult).
- ◆ Maintain the chest tube system as ordered. Report a sudden change in the amount of drainage or an output of 200 ml/hour.
- ◆ Administer I.V. fluids and blood products as ordered.
- ◆ Assist with weaning from the mechanical ventilator as indicated.
- ◆ Encourage coughing, turning, and deep breathing.
- ◆ Encourage use of incentive spirometry.
- ◆ Assist with early ambulation.
- ◆ Monitor vital signs, heart rate and rhythm, cardiovascular status, heart sounds, and hemodynamic values.
- ◆ Record and evaluate daily weight, sternal stability and drainage, and intake and output.
- ◆ Monitor for complications such as abnormal bleeding.
- ◆ Assess respiratory status, including arterial blood gas analysis.
- ◆ Monitor laboratory test results.
- ◆ Perform surgical wound care and dressing changes, as prescribed, and monitor the wound for signs of infection.

PATIENT TEACHING

GENERAL

- ◆ Review medications and possible adverse reactions with the patient.
- ◆ Teach the patient how to care for the surgical wound.
- ◆ Tell the patient about the signs and symptoms of infection.
- ◆ Tell the patient about the signs and symptoms of postpericardiotomy syndrome.
- ◆ Inform the patient about possible complications.
- ◆ Teach the patient about anticoagulant therapy precautions such as monitoring for bleeding and prevention of trauma (such as by using a soft toothbrush and electric razors).
- ◆ Tell the patient to notify the practitioner if bleeding occurs.
- ◆ Advise the patient to follow prescribed activity restrictions and to balance activity with rest periods.
- ◆ Advise the patient to follow dietary restrictions directed by the practitioner.
- ◆ Instruct the patient to follow the prescribed exercise program.
- ◆ Stress the need for follow-up care.
- ◆ Emphasize the importance of informing all health care providers of his valve surgery.
- ◆ Stress the importance of wearing medical identification at all times.

RESOURCES

Organizations

American College of Chest Surgeons: *www.chestnet.org*
American College of Surgeons: *www.facs.org*
American Heart Association: *www.americanheart.org*

Selected references

Dang, N.C., et al. "Simplified Placement of Multiple Artificial Mitral Valve Chords," *The Heart Surgery Forum* 8(3):E129-31, 2005.

Fox, E., et al. "Cardiac Papillary Fibroelastoma Presents as an Acute Embolic Stroke in a 35-year-old African American Male," *American Journal of the Medical Sciences* 331(2):91-94, February 2006.

Urbanski, P.P. "Modified Technique of Chordal Replacement for Mitral Valve Repair," *The Thoracic and Cardiovascular Surgeon* 53(5):315-17, October 2005.

Heart valve commissurotomy

OVERVIEW

- Surgically increases the opening of a stenotic valve caused by fusion of the commissures, thereby promoting more normal valve functioning and promoting improved cardiac output and circulation
- May be performed on any heart valve, but most commonly done on the mitral valve
- May also be accomplished by percutaneous balloon valvuloplasty

INDICATIONS

- Symptomatic mitral valve stenosis
- Valvular stenosis in patients who are poor surgical risks

PROCEDURE

- The patient is given general anesthesia, intubated, and mechanically ventilated. A hemodynamic monitoring catheter is inserted.
- Open commissurotomy with complete visualization of the valve requires the circulatory bypass.
- A medial sternotomy or left thoracic incision is made.
- Cardiopulmonary bypass is initiated.
- The area of the heart affected is incised so that the valve can be fully seen.
- The fused leaflets are separated, and other accompanying problems, such as a thrombus or chord or papillary muscle tear, is fixed.
- When proper valve function has been tested, cardiopulmonary bypass is removed and the heart restarted. Epicardial pacing wires may be left in place.
- A chest tube is inserted.
- Incisions are closed, and a sterile dressing is applied.

COMPLICATIONS

- Valvular insufficiency
- Embolism
- Valve leaflet damage
- Arrhythmias
- Myocardial ischemia and infarction
- Restenosis
- Cardiac arrhythmias
- Infection
- Stroke

NURSING DIAGNOSES

- Decreased cardiac output
- Ineffective tissue perfusion: Cardiopulmonary
- Risk for infection

EXPECTED OUTCOMES

The patient will:

- maintain adequate cardiac output
- maintain hemodynamic stability as evidenced by blood pressure and cardiac rate within normal limits
- be free from signs and symptoms of infection.

PRETREATMENT CARE

◆ Review with the patient the purpose of the surgery and what nursing care to expect after its completion.
◆ Verify that an appropriate consent form has been signed.
◆ Provide emotional support.
◆ Monitor electrocardiogram (ECG), pulmonary artery and hemodynamic status, and intake and output.
◆ Restrict food and fluid intake as ordered.
◆ Obtain routine laboratory studies; report abnormal results; and make sure blood typing and crossmatching are completed.
◆ Initiate I.V. therapy as prescribed.
◆ Perform a preoperative assessment and complete the preoperative verification process.
◆ Administer a sedative as ordered.

POSTTREATMENT CARE

◆ Administer I.V. medications and fluids as ordered.

⚡ WARNING *Be sure to assess for signs of fluid overload and hypoxemia especially in the compromised patient; report symptoms immediately.*

◆ Assist with temporary epicardial pacing as indicated.
◆ Monitor the ECG for development of arrhythmias and ischemia.
◆ Maintain mean arterial pressure within prescribed guidelines (usually between 70 and 100 mm Hg in an adult).
◆ Maintain the chest tube system as ordered. Report a sudden change in the amount of drainage or an output of 200 ml/hour.
◆ Administer I.V. fluids and blood products as ordered.
◆ Assist with weaning from the mechanical ventilator as indicated.
◆ Encourage coughing, turning, and deep breathing.
◆ Encourage use of incentive spirometry.
◆ Assist with early ambulation.
◆ Monitor vital signs, heart rate and rhythm, cardiovascular status, heart sounds, and hemodynamic values.
◆ Record and evaluate daily weight, sternal stability and drainage, and intake and output.
◆ Monitor for complications such as abnormal bleeding.
◆ Assess respiratory status, including pulse oximetry and arterial blood gas analysis.
◆ Monitor laboratory test results.
◆ Perform surgical wound care and dressing changes, as prescribed, and monitor the wound for signs of infection.

PATIENT TEACHING

GENERAL

◆ Review medications and possible adverse reactions with the patient.
◆ Teach the patient how to care for the surgical wound.
◆ Tell the patient about the signs and symptoms of infection.
◆ Inform the patient about possible complications.
◆ Advise the patient to follow the prescribed activity restrictions and to balance activity with rest periods.
◆ Advise the patient to follow dietary restrictions directed by the practitioner.
◆ Stress the need for follow-up care.
◆ Emphasize the importance of informing all health care providers of his valve surgery.

RESOURCES
Organizations
American College of Chest Surgeons: *www.chestnet.org*
American College of Surgeons: *www.facs.org*
American Heart Association: *www.americanheart.org*

Selected references

Bauer, F., et al. "Left Atrial Appendage Function Analyzed by Tissue Doppler Imaging in Mitral Stenosis: Effect of Afterload Reduction After Mitral Valve Commissurotomy," *Journal of the American Society of Echocardiography* 18(9):934-39, September 2005.

Harikrishnan, S., et al. "Percutaneous Transmitral Commissurotomy in Juvenile Mitral Stenosis—Comparison of Long Term Results of Inoue Balloon Technique and Metallic Commissurotomy," *Catheter and Cardiovascular Interventions* 67(3):453-59, March 2006.

Trehan, V.K., et al. "Bedside Percutaneous Transseptal Mitral Commissurotomy under Sole Transthoracic Echocardiographic Guidance in a Critically Ill Patient," *Echocardiography* 23(4): 312-14, April 2006.

Heart valve minimally invasive surgery

OVERVIEW

- Surgical technique for valve replacement or repair, which avoids full sternotomy and chest opening, but usually takes longer because of its complexity
- Requires heart-lung bypass machine use, but this may be applied through "ports" or small incisions accessing the femoral artery or thoracic aorta
- Benefits: reduction of blood loss, chest wall trauma, scarring, and length of hospital stay
- Percutaneous replacement and repairs to the valve leaflets and robotic techniques: now being experimentally evaluated in some large medical centers

INDICATIONS

- Stenotic or insufficient valves

  WARNING *The procedure is generally contraindicated in patients with severe valve damage, more than one valve requiring repair or replacement, atherosclerosis, and a body mass index over 30.*

PROCEDURE

- After the patient is anesthetized, endotracheal intubation and mechanical ventilation are started.
- A pulmonary artery catheter is inserted for hemodynamic monitoring and a transesophageal echocardiogram is done to confirm abnormalities.
- A partial sternotomy, removal of the second and third rib cartilage, or an incision between two ribs will be made according to the treatment being given.
- Cardiopulmonary bypass is initiated.
- The damaged valve is repaired or replaced.
- The incisions in the heart are closed and the heart is defibrillated to restart pumping.
- When the heart is beating well, cardiac bypass is discontinued.
- Epicardial pacemaker leads and a chest tube are inserted.
- The incision is closed, and a sterile dressing is applied.

COMPLICATIONS

- Postpericardiotomy syndrome
- Cardiac arrhythmias
- Hemorrhage
- Coagulopathy
- Stroke
- Prosthetic valve endocarditis
- Valve dysfunction or failure
- Renal failure
- Pulmonary or thromboembolism
- Postanesthesia memory loss
- Infection

NURSING DIAGNOSES

- Decreased cardiac output
- Ineffective tissue perfusion: Cardiopulmonary
- Risk for infection

EXPECTED OUTCOMES

The patient will:
- maintain adequate cardiac output
- maintain blood pressure and cardiac rate within normal limits, and have clear lung sounds
- be free from signs and symptoms of infection.

PRETREATMENT CARE

- Explain the treatment and preparation to the patient and his family.
- Make sure the patient has signed an appropriate consent form.
- Explain postoperative care and equipment.
- Obtain results of laboratory studies, including blood typing and cross-matching. Make sure a chest X-ray has been obtained.
- Obtain a 12-lead electrocardiogram (ECG) as ordered.
- Perform a preoperative assessment and complete the preoperative verification process.
- Withhold food and fluids as ordered.
- Initiate I.V. therapy as prescribed.

POSTTREATMENT CARE

◆ Administer medications as ordered.
◆ Assist with temporary epicardial pacing as indicated.
◆ Monitor the ECG for development of arrhythmias.
◆ Maintain mean arterial pressure within prescribed guidelines (usually between 70 and 100 mm Hg in an adult).
◆ Maintain the chest tube system as ordered.
◆ Administer I.V. fluids and blood products as ordered.
◆ Assist with weaning from the mechanical ventilator as indicated.
◆ Encourage coughing, turning, and deep breathing.
◆ Encourage use of incentive spirometry.
◆ Assist with early ambulation.
◆ Monitor vital signs, heart rate and rhythm, cardiovascular status, heart sounds, and hemodynamic values.
◆ Record and evaluate daily weight, sternal stability and drainage, and intake and output.
◆ Monitor for complications such as abnormal bleeding.
◆ Assess respiratory status, including arterial blood gas analysis.
◆ Monitor laboratory test results.
◆ Perform surgical wound care and dressing changes, as prescribed, and monitor the wound for signs of infection.

PATIENT TEACHING

GENERAL

◆ Review medications and possible adverse reactions with the patient.
◆ Teach the patient how to care for the surgical wound.
◆ Tell the patient about the signs and symptoms of infection.
◆ Tell the patient about the signs and symptoms of postpericardiotomy syndrome.
◆ Inform the patient about possible complications.
◆ Teach the patient about anticoagulant therapy precautions such as monitoring for bleeding and prevention of trauma (such as by using a soft toothbrush and electric razors).
◆ Tell the patient to notify the practitioner if bleeding occurs.
◆ Advise the patient to follow prescribed activity restrictions and to balance activity with rest periods.
◆ Advise the patient to follow dietary restrictions directed by the practitioner.
◆ Tell the patient to follow the prescribed exercise program.
◆ Stress the need for follow-up care.
◆ Emphasize the importance of informing all health care providers of his valve surgery.
◆ Stress the importance of wearing medical identification at all times.

RESOURCES
Organizations
American College of Chest Surgeons: *www.chestnet.org*
American College of Surgeons: *www.facs.org*
American Heart Association: *www.americanheart.org*

Selected references
Aybek, T., et al. "Two Hundred Forty Minimally Invasive Mitral Operations Through Right Minithoracotomy," *The Annals of Thoracic Surgery* 81(5):1618-24, May 2006.
Feldman, T., et al. "Percutaneous Mitral Valve Repair Using the Edge-To-Edge Technique: Six-Month Results of the EVEREST Phase I Clinical Trial," *Journal of the American College of Cardiology* 46(11):2134-40, December 2005.
Lee, S., et al. "Clinical Results of Minimally Invasive Open-Heart Surgery in Patients With Mitral Valve Disease: Comparison of Parasternal and Low-Sternal Approach," *Yonsei Medical Journal* 47(2):230-36, April 2006.

Heart valve percutaneous balloon valvuloplasty

OVERVIEW

- Insertion of a balloon-tipped catheter through the femoral vein or artery and into the heart, followed by repeated balloon inflation against the leaflets of a diseased heart valve
- Helps expand the constricted valve, promoting more adequate cardiac output and heart functioning

INDICATIONS

- Congenital valve defects
- Valve calcifications
- Valvular stenosis
- Poor candidate for invasive valve surgery

PROCEDURE

- After the patient is sedated, the catheter site is cleaned and draped. A local anesthetic is then injected into the tissue surrounding the catheter insertion site.
- The physician inserts a catheter into the femoral artery (for left heart valve) or the femoral vein (for a right heart valve).
- The balloon-tipped catheter is passed through this catheter and guided by fluoroscopy into the heart.
- The deflated balloon is inserted in the valve opening and repeatedly inflated with a solution containing normal saline solution and a contrast media.
- As the balloon inflates, the valve leaflets split free from one another, permitting them to open and close properly and increase the valvular orifice. (See *Percutaneous balloon valvuloplasty.*)
- The physician removes the balloon-tipped catheter.
- The femoral catheter may be left in place in case the patient needs to return to the laboratory for a repeat procedure.

COMPLICATIONS

- Valvular insufficiency
- Embolism
- Valve leaflet damage
- Infection
- Bleeding and hematoma at the arterial or venous puncture site
- Arrhythmias
- Myocardial ischemia and infarction
- Circulatory insufficiency distal to the catheter entry site
- Restenosis
- Guidewire perforation of the ventricle, leading to tamponade

 AGE FACTOR *Elderly patients with aortic valve disease commonly experience restenosis 1 or 2 years after undergoing valvuloplasty.*

NURSING DIAGNOSES

- Decreased cardiac output
- Ineffective tissue perfusion: Cardiopulmonary
- Risk for infection

EXPECTED OUTCOMES

The patient will:
- maintain adequate cardiac output
- maintain hemodynamic stability as evidenced by blood pressure and cardiac rate within normal limits
- be free from signs and symptoms of infection.

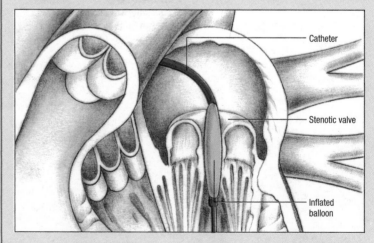

Percutaneous balloon valvuloplasty

In balloon valvuloplasty, the physician inserts a balloon-tipped catheter through the femoral vein or artery and threads it into the heart. After locating the stenotic valve, he inflates the balloon, increasing the size of the valve opening.

Catheter

Stenotic valve

Inflated balloon

◆ Review the purpose of the procedure and what nursing measures to expect after insertion of the device.
◆ Initiate I.V. therapy as prescribed.
◆ Prepare the patient's groin area.
◆ Verify that an appropriate consent form has been signed.
◆ Provide emotional support.
◆ Monitor electrocardiogram (ECG), pulmonary artery and hemodynamic status; if central catheter already in place, monitor vital signs and intake and output.
◆ Restrict food and fluid intake as ordered.
◆ Obtain routine laboratory studies; report abnormal results; and verify that blood typing and crossmatching are complete.
◆ Palpate bilateral distal pulses and complete a vascular assessment of the extremities, mark the pulse points with a skin marker, and record the assessment findings. Use Doppler ultrasonography, if needed, to locate all pulses.
◆ Administer a sedative and withhold other medications as ordered.
◆ Complete the preoperative verification process.

◆ Monitor I.V. medications; administer I.V. fluids.

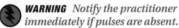 **WARNING** *Be sure to assess for signs and symptoms of fluid overload and hypoxemia; report them immediately.*

◆ Maintain sandbag or other compression device over cannulation site to minimize bleeding as ordered.
◆ Prevent excessive hip flexion by keeping affected leg straight and elevating the head of the bed no more than 15 degrees.
◆ If needed, prepare for catheter removal in 6 to 12 hours after valvuloplasty. Afterward, apply a pressure dressing and assess vital signs.
◆ Monitor vital signs, intake and output, ECG, hemodynamic status if central catheter in place, peripheral pulses distal to insertion site, and color, temperature, and capillary refill of extremities.

WARNING *Notify the practitioner immediately if pulses are absent.*

◆ Observe catheter insertion site for hematoma formation, ecchymosis, or hemorrhage. If an expanding ecchymotic area appears, mark the area to help determine the pace of expansion. If bleeding occurs, apply direct pressure and notify the practitioner.
◆ Auscultate for murmurs, which may indicate worsening valvular insufficiency. Report changes to the practitioner immediately.

GENERAL

◆ Review with the patient signs to report to the practitioner, including bleeding or increased bruising at the puncture site or recurrence of symptoms of valvular insufficiency, such as breathlessness or decreased exercise tolerance.
◆ Review diet and activity restrictions.
◆ Teach the patient about his medication regimen and adverse effects of the medications.
◆ Stress the need for prophylactic antibiotics during dental surgery or other invasive procedures.
◆ Stress the importance of regular follow-up care.

RESOURCES
Organizations
American College of Chest Surgeons: *www.chestnet.org*
American College of Surgeons: *www.facs.org*
American Heart Association: *www.americanheart.org*

Selected references

Chlan, L.L., et al. "Effects of Three Groin Compression Methods on Patient Discomfort, Distress, and Vascular Complications Following a Percutaneous Coronary Intervention Procedure," *Nursing Research* 54(6):391-98, November-December, 2005.

Krittayaphong, R., et al. "One-year Outcome of Cardioversion of Atrial Fibrillation in Patients With Mitral Stenosis After Percutaneous Balloon Mitral Valvuloplasty," *American Journal of Cardiology* 97(7): 1045-50, April 2006.

Tagney, J., and Lackie, D. "Bed-rest Post-Femoral Arterial Sheath Removal— What Is Safe Practice? A Clinical Audit," *Nursing in Critical Care* 10(4):167-73, July-August 2005.

Heart valve replacement

OVERVIEW

- Excision of a diseased heart valve and replacement with a mechanical or biological valve prosthesis
- May be done using a medial sternotomy approach or minimally invasive approach
- Heart valve replaced with mechanical valves, tissue valves, or homografts (valves from a human donor) to promote improved cardiac output (see *Replacement heart valves*)

INDICATIONS

- Severe aortic valvular stenosis or insufficiency
- Severe mitral valvular stenosis or insufficiency
- Damage or disease from bacterial endocarditis, rheumatic fever, calcific degeneration, or congenital abnormalities

PROCEDURE

- After the patient is anesthetized, a medial sternotomy is performed, and cardiopulmonary bypass is initiated.
- For aortic valve replacement, the aorta is clamped above the right coronary artery; for mitral valve replacement, the left atrium is incised to expose the mitral valve.
- The diseased valve is excised.
- The surgeon sutures around the margin of the valve annulus.
- The suture is threaded through the sewing ring of the prosthetic valve.
- Using a valve holder, the prosthesis is positioned, and the sutures are secured.
- The patient is removed from the bypass machine.
- As the heart fills with blood, the surgeon vents the aorta and ventricle for air.
- Epicardial pacemaker leads and a chest tube are inserted.
- The incision is closed, and a sterile dressing is applied.

COMPLICATIONS

- Postpericardiotomy syndrome
- Cardiac arrhythmias
- Hemorrhage
- Coagulopathy
- Stroke
- Prosthetic valve endocarditis
- Valve dysfunction or failure
- Renal failure
- Pulmonary or thromboembolism
- Infection

NURSING DIAGNOSES

- Decreased cardiac output
- Ineffective tissue perfusion: Cardiopulmonary
- Risk for infection

EXPECTED OUTCOMES
The patient will:
- maintain adequate cardiac output
- maintain hemodynamic stability as evidenced by blood pressure and cardiac rate within normal limits
- be free from signs and symptoms of infection.

PRETREATMENT CARE

- Explain the procedure and preparation to the patient and his family.
- Verify that the patient has signed an appropriate consent form.
- Explain postoperative care and equipment.
- Obtain results of chest X-ray, 12-lead electrocardiogram (ECG), and laboratory tests, including blood typing and crossmatching.
- Perform a preoperative assessment, and complete the preoperative verification process.

POSTTREATMENT CARE

- Administer medications as ordered.
- Assist with temporary epicardial pacing as indicated.
- Monitor the ECG for development of arrhythmias and ischemia.
- Maintain mean arterial pressure within prescribed guidelines.
- Maintain the chest tube system as ordered. Report a sudden change in the amount of drainage or an output of 200 ml/hour.
- Administer I.V. fluids and blood products as ordered.
- Assist with weaning from the mechanical ventilator as indicated.
- Encourage coughing, turning, and deep breathing.
- Encourage use of incentive spirometry.
- Assist with early ambulation.
- Monitor vital signs, respiratory status, heart rate and rhythm, cardiovascular status, heart sounds, and hemodynamic values.
- Record and evaluate daily weight, sternal stability and drainage, and intake and output.
- Monitor for complications such as abnormal bleeding.
- Monitor laboratory test results.
- Perform surgical wound care and dressing changes, as prescribed, and monitor for signs of infection.

PATIENT TEACHING

GENERAL
- Review medications and possible adverse reactions with the patient.
- Teach the patient how to care for the surgical wound.
- Tell the patient about the signs and symptoms of infection.
- Tell the patient about the signs and symptoms of postpericardiotomy syndrome.
- Teach the patient about anticoagulant therapy precautions such as monitoring for bleeding and prevention of trauma (such as by using a soft toothbrush and electric razors).

- Tell the patient to notify the practitioner if bleeding occurs.
- Advise the patient to follow prescribed activity restrictions and to balance activity with rest periods.
- Advise the patient to follow dietary restrictions directed by the practitioner.
- Stress the need for follow-up care.
- Emphasize the importance of informing all health care providers of his valve surgery.
- Stress the importance of wearing medical identification at all times.

RESOURCES
Organizations
American College of Chest Surgeons: *www.chestnet.org*
American College of Surgeons: *www.facs.org*
American Heart Association: *www.americanheart.org*

Selected references
Edmundson, S., et al. "Upsetting the Apple Cart: A Community Anticoagulation Clinic Survey of Life Event Factors That Undermine Safe Therapy," *Journal of Vascular Nursing* 23(3):105-11, September 2005.

Falcoz, P.E., et al. "Blood Warm Reperfusion: A Necessary Adjunct to Heart-Valve Surgery in Low-Risk Patients?" *Journal of Cardiovascular Surgery (Torino)* 46(6):577-81, December 2005.

Fink, A.M. "Endocarditis After Valve Replacement Surgery. Early Recognition and Treatment are Essential to Averting Deadly Complications," *AJN* 106(2): 40-51, February 2006.

Replacement heart valves

When the patient's heart valve malfunctions, he may undergo surgery to replace the malfunctioning valve with a prosthetic one. Here are the most commonly used valves.

TILTING-DISK VALVE

The tilting-disk valve was developed as an alternative to the ball-in-cage valve. It has a hingeless design and contains open-ended, elliptical struts. These features reduce the risk of thrombus formation and offer improved blood flow. It also causes minimal damage to blood cells. The most common tilting-disk valve is the Medtronic Hall prosthesis. (Photo courtesy of Medtronic, Inc.)

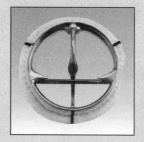

BILEAFLET VALVE

The most commonly used prosthetic valve, a bileaflet valve consists of two semicircular leaflets that pivot on hinges. The leaflets swing partially open and are designed to close so that an acceptable amount of regurgitant blood flow is permitted. In the United States, the St. Jude Medical Valve is the most commonly inserted bileaflet valve. (Photo courtesy of St. Jude Medical.)

PORCINE VALVES

A porcine valve is made using the aortic valve of a pig that's sewn to a frame called a stent. The stent is commonly made from a plastic composite that's covered with a polyester cloth. Porcine valves include the Carpentier-Edwards Duraflex Low-Pressure Bioprosthesis Valve and the Medtronic Hancock II Valve. (Photos courtesy of Edwards Lifesciences [top] and Medtronic, Inc. [middle].)

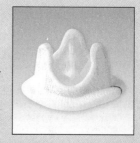

BOVINE VALVE

A bovine valve is made from the pericardial tissue of a cow. Ionescu-Shiley constructed the first bovine valve; however, it's been discontinued. The Carpentier-Edwards PERIMOUNT Pericardial Bioprosthesis Valve is now widely used. (Photo courtesy of Edwards Lifesciences.)

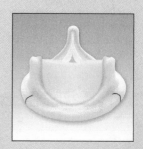

Hemapheresis

OVERVIEW

- Involves separation and removal of specific blood components that are being overproduced or causing disease or an autoimmune reaction; also called *pheresis* or *apheresis*
- Procedure named according to component of blood that's removed from the patient; type of procedure varies with different diseases
- Typical components removed: plasma (plasmapheresis), all types of white blood cells ([WBCs], leukopheresis), lymphocyte WBCs (lymphapheresis), red blood cells, (erythropheresis), platelets (plateletcytapheresis), and total plasma exchange (removal of plasma and replacement with fresh frozen plasma)

INDICATIONS

- Myasthenia gravis
- Waldenström's macroglobulinemia
- Goodpasture's syndrome
- Cryoglobulinemia
- Refsum's disease
- Leukostasis caused by severely elevated WBC count in leukemia
- Severely elevated platelet counts in leukemia or myeloproliferative disorders
- Systemic lupus with life-threatening complications
- Severe vasculitis
- Polymyositis or dermatomyositis
- Severe rheumatoid arthritis
- Rapidly progressive glomerulonephritis
- Chronic autoimmune polyneuropathy
- Familial hyperlipoproteinemia
- Thrombocytopenic purpura
- Autoimmune hemolytic anemia
- Pemphigus
- Aplastic anemia
- Hairy cell leukemia

PROCEDURE

- The hemapheresis technician sets up the machine according to the practitioner's orders and patient's disorder.
- All hemapheresis procedures involve connecting the blood in the patient's veins through tubing to a machine that separates the blood components. The separation is done by either a centrifuge process or a filtration process on the blood in the machine specified depending on the condition of the patient and results desired.
- After the separation, the component of the blood that's believed to contain the disease-provoking elements is discarded, whereas the remainder of the blood components are reinfused back into the patient; the procedure typically takes about 2 hours.

COMPLICATIONS

- Bleeding
- Infection
- Immunosuppression
- Hypotension
- Electrolyte imbalance
- Muscle cramping

NURSING DIAGNOSES

- Activity intolerance
- Deficient fluid volume
- Risk for infection

EXPECTED OUTCOMES

The patient will:
- demonstrate increased ability to perform activities of daily living
- maintain adequate fluid volume
- be free from signs and symptoms of infection.

PRETREATMENT CARE

- Explain all procedures and their purpose to the patient.
- Review the patient's history for presence of blood disorders or allergies.
- Complete a physical and mental health nursing assessment.
- Verify that an appropriate consent form has been signed.
- **WARNING** *Hemapheresis is generally avoided if a patient has an active infection, an unstable heart or a lung disorder, a severely low WBC or platelet count, a bleeding tendency, or a significantly low blood pressure.*
- Assist with setting up of the equipment as necessary.
- Perform a baseline electrocardiogram if indicated, and record vital signs.
- Institute dietary restrictions before the procedure as ordered.

POSTTREATMENT CARE

- Provide adequate hydration.
- Administer blood or plasma transfusions or other components as ordered.
- Administer medications as ordered.
- Provide emotional support.
- Monitor vital signs, blood pressure, heart and lung sounds, peripheral pulses, and intake and output.
- Monitor for signs of bleeding.
- Monitor patient for signs and symptoms of infection.

Learning about hemapheresis

Dear Patient:

Your health care provider has ordered hemapheresis to help improve your symptoms of muscle weakness and fatigue. This procedure filters your blood to clean it of harmful substances that cause disease symptoms.

BEFORE THE PROCEDURE

Eat lightly before the procedure. Drink at least one glass of milk 30 to 60 minutes before the procedure and another one during the procedure. This will prevent calcium levels in your body from falling too low.

Also, be sure to empty your bladder to prevent your blood pressure from dropping too low.

DURING THE PROCEDURE

A specially trained nurse or technician will insert a needle into one or both of your arms. This is about the most discomfort you'll feel.

Then you'll see your blood travel through the needle into an attached tube that leads into a filtering machine called a cell separator. Here the blood is filtered and cleaned. Then it's returned to your body.

The entire procedure may take up to 5 hours to complete, so take a book or a radio with earphones to help you pass the time.

During the treatment, a specially trained nurse or technician will take blood samples from you to make sure your calcium and potassium levels are all right. She'll also check your blood pressure and heart rate frequently.

If you feel a tingling or "pins and needles" sensation in your body, tell the nurse or technician. She'll allow you to move around in your chair to relieve the sensation and prevent stiffness.

AFTER THE PROCEDURE

When hemapheresis ends, the nurse or technician will turn off the cell separator. Then she'll remove the needles from your arms. Next, she'll apply pressure to the puncture sites and then secure a bandage to make sure that you don't bleed more than usual. She'll check your bandage periodically for drainage.

WHEN YOU GO HOME

You may feel tired for 1 or 2 days after hemapheresis. Here are some tips for handling your daily activities after hemapheresis:
◆ Avoid strenuous activities, such as aerobic exercise or housecleaning (including vacuuming and furniture moving).
◆ Rest frequently.
◆ Eat a high-protein diet, and take a multivitamin with iron daily.
◆ Avoid contact with people who have colds, and stay out of crowds because you're more susceptible now to an infection.
◆ If your skin or the whites of your eyes turn yellowish, contact your practitioner.

PATIENT TEACHING

GENERAL
◆ Refer the patient to appropriate resources and support services.
◆ Refer the patient for appropriate follow-up care as his diagnosis indicates. (See *Learning about hemapheresis.*)

RESOURCES
Organizations
American Medical Association: *www.ama-assn.org*

The Leukemia & Lymphoma Society: *www.leukemia.org*
Myasthenia Gravis Foundation of America: *www.myasthenia.org*

Selected references
Basic-Jukic, N., et al. "Complications of Therapeutic Plasma Exchange: Experience with 4,857 Treatments," *Therapeutic Apheresis and Dialysis* 9(5):391, October 2005.
Chen, W., et al. "Clearance Studies During Subsequent Sessions of Double Filtration Plasmapheresis," *Artificial Organs* (30)2:111, February 2006.
Henry, J.B., et al. "Mean Arterial Pressure and Systolic Blood Pressure for Detection of Hypotension During Hemapheresis: Implications for Patients with Baseline Hypertension," *Journal of Clinical Apheresis* 20(3):154-165, October 2005.

Hemispherectomy, functional

- Surgical disconnection of one side of the brain from the other (with some tissue removal) to treat intractable seizures
- Leads to partial or complete seizure control in about 80% of patients; in those with partial control, medication can be significantly decreased
- Originally involved removal of whole hemisphere with several attendant risks postoperatively; now involves just partial resection and complete separation

INDICATIONS
- Medically intractable epilepsy
- Hemimeganencephaly
- Sturge-Weber Syndrome
- Rasmussen's encephalitis

- The anesthetist starts a peripheral I.V. line, a central venous pressure line, and an arterial line; the patient receives general anesthesia.
- The surgeon marks an incision line and cuts through the scalp to the cranium, forming a scalp flap that's folded to one side.
- After pulling aside or removing the bone section, the surgeon incises and retracts the dura, exposing the brain.
- The surgeon removes the affected temporal lobe, and a corpus callosotomy is performed, which disconnects the frontal and occipital lobes completely from the intact hemisphere. The blood supply to the remaining brain is left intact.

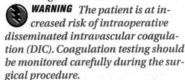 **WARNING** *The patient is at increased risk of intraoperative disseminated intravascular coagulation (DIC). Coagulation testing should be monitored carefully during the surgical procedure.*
- The dura mater is closed, and a drain may be used.
- The bone flap may not be replaced if swelling is anticipated. Intracranial pressure monitor may be placed.
- Periosteum and muscle are approximated. Skin closure is performed and dressings are applied.

COMPLICATIONS
- Infection
- Hemorrhage or DIC
- Increased intracranial pressure (ICP)
- Loss of peripheral vision
- Loss of movement or sensation on the opposite side of the body
- Continued seizures
- Cranial nerve damage or damage to the functional hemisphere

- Disturbed sensory perception (all)
- Risk for imbalanced fluid volume
- Risk for infection

EXPECTED OUTCOMES
The patient will:
- exhibit stable or improved neurosensory assessment findings
- maintain stable level of consciousness (LOC), pupil size and reactivity, sensorimotor skills, and ICP
- exhibit no signs of infection as evidenced by laboratory studies within normal limits, normal white blood count and differential, vital signs, and wound findings.

PRETREATMENT CARE

- Reinforce the practitioner's explanation of the treatment and review the nursing care to be provided.
- Verify that an appropriate consent form has been signed.
- Tell the patient that his head will be shaved in the operating room.
- Explain the intensive care unit and equipment the patient will see postoperatively.
- Explain to the patient that he'll be on a mechanical ventilator (initially) after surgery; therefore, he won't be able to speak. Reassure him that he'll be provided with a means to communicate with hospital staff and his family.
- Tell the patient that he may experience scalp numbness, headache, facial swelling or puffy eyes, nausea, fatigue or depression, difficulty speaking or remembering or finding words, and a transient decrease in contralateral muscle strength after surgery.
- Perform and document a complete neurologic assessment.
- Make sure that ordered examinations and testing have been completed, including magnetic resonance imaging of the brain, EEG, and video seizure monitoring.

WARNING *Extensive testing is required to confirm true seizures and their source due to the severity and complexity of the treatment.*

POSTTREATMENT CARE

- Position the patient on his side with the head of the bed elevated 15 to 30 degrees; turn him carefully every 2 hours.
- Monitor respiratory status and maintain appropriate ventilator settings.
- Encourage careful deep breathing and coughing; suction gently as needed.
- Ensure a quiet, calm environment.
- Maintain seizure precautions.
- Monitor vital signs, intake and output, LOC, ICP, heart rate and rhythm, and hemodynamic values.
- Assess fluid and electrolyte balance, intake and output, and daily weight.
- Monitor drain patency, the surgical wound and dressings, and drainage.
- Monitor for complications.

WARNING *Notify the practitioner immediately if there's a worsening of mental status, pupillary changes, or focal signs, such as increasing weakness in an arm or leg; these findings may indicate increased ICP.*

- Maintain a patent airway after ventilator weaning, and administer prescribed oxygen if ordered.
- Administer medications as ordered.
- Provide support to the patient and his family.

PATIENT TEACHING

GENERAL

- Review medication dosages and possible adverse reactions with the patient and his family.
- Teach the patient and his family how to monitor the surgical wound for signs of infection, and how to clean and dress it daily.
- Tell the patient that headaches and facial or eye swelling will likely last for 2 or 3 days after surgery.
- Tell the patient that the decrease in contralateral muscle strength, fatigue, nausea, and difficulties with speech or memory may last for 2 to 4 weeks.
- Review the signs and symptoms complications; instruct the patient to notify the practitioner when these occur.
- Discuss the use of a wig, hat, or scarf until the patient's hair grows back as appropriate.
- Advise the patient to avoid alcohol and smoking.
- Stress the need for regular follow-up care.

RESOURCES

Organizations
American Academy of Neurology: *www.aan.com*
American Medical Association: *www.ama-assn.org*
Epilepsy Therapy Development Project: *www.epilepsy.com*

Selected references
Dunn, D. "Preventing Perioperative Complications in Special Populations," *Nursing* 35(11):36-45, November 2005.
González-Martínez, J.A., et al. "Hemispherectomy for Catastrophic Epilepsy in Infants," *Epilepsia* 46(9): 1518-25, September 2005.
Mani, J., et al. "Postoperative Seizures After Extratemporal Cortical Resection and Hemispherectomy in Pediatric Epilepsy," *Neurology* 66(7):1038-43, April 2006.

Hemodialysis

- Extracts toxic wastes from the blood by removing the blood from the body, circulating it through a purifying dialyzer, then returning it to the body
- Restores or maintains balance of the body's buffer system and electrolyte level, promoting rapid return to normal serum values and preventing uremia-associated complications
- For long-term treatment: various access sites, including arteriovenous (AV) fistula or shunt may be used (see *Hemodialysis access sites*)

INDICATIONS

- Chronic end-stage renal disease
- Acute renal failure
- Acute poisoning
- Drug overdose

PROCEDURE

- Support the access site and rest it on a clean drape.

BEGINNING HEMODIALYSIS WITH A DOUBLE-LUMEN CATHETER

- If extension tubing isn't already clamped, clamp it to prevent air from entering the catheter.
- Clean each catheter extension tube, clamp, and Luer-lock injection cap with povidone-iodine pads to remove contaminants.
- Place a sterile gauze pad under the extension tubing, and place two 5-ml syringes and two sterile gauze pads on the drape.
- Prepare the anticoagulant regimen as ordered.
- Identify arterial and venous blood lines, and place them near the drape.

- To remove clots and ensure catheter patency, remove catheter caps, attach syringes to each catheter port, open the clamp, aspirate 1.5 to 3 ml of blood, close the clamp, and flush each port with 5 ml of heparin flush solution.

- To gain patient access, remove the syringe from the arterial port and attach the line to it; administer the heparin according to protocol to prevent clotting in the extracorporeal circuit.

Hemodialysis access sites

Hemodialysis requires vascular access. The site and type of access depends on expected duration of dialysis, surgeon's preference, and patient's condition.

SUBCLAVIAN VEIN CATHETERIZATION

Using the Seldinger technique, the surgeon inserts an introducer needle into the subclavian vein. He then inserts a guide wire through the introducer needle and removes the needle. Using the guide wire, he threads a 5″ to 12″ (12.5- to 30.5-cm) plastic or Teflon catheter (with a Y-hub) into the patient's vein.

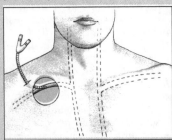

FEMORAL VEIN CATHETERIZATION

Using the Seldinger technique, the surgeon inserts an introducer needle into the left or right femoral vein. He then inserts a guide wire through the introducer needle and removes the needle. Using the guide wire, he threads a 5″ to 12″ plastic or Teflon catheter with a Y-hub or two catheters, one for inflow and the other placed about ½″ (1.3 cm) distal to the first for outflow.

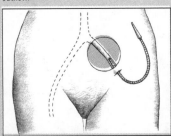

ARTERIOVENOUS FISTULA

To create a fistula, the surgeon makes an incision in the patient's lower forearm, then a small incision in the side of an artery, and another in the side of a vein. He sutures the edges of the incisions together to make a common opening ⅛″ to ¼″ (3 to 6 mm) long.

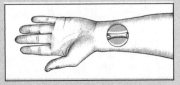

ARTERIOVENOUS SHUNT

To create a shunt, the surgeon makes an incision in the patient's lower forearm or (rarely) ankle. He inserts a 6″ to 10″ (15- to 25-cm) transparent Silastic cannula into an artery and another into a vein. Finally, he tunnels the cannulas out through stab wounds and joins them with a piece of Teflon tubing.

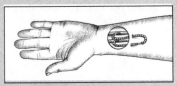

ARTERIOVENOUS GRAFT

To create a graft, the surgeon makes an incision in the patient's forearm, upper arm, or thigh. He then tunnels a natural or synthetic graft under the skin and sutures the distal end to an artery and the proximal end to a vein.

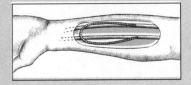

- Grasp the venous blood line and attach it to the venous port; open the clamps on the extension tubing and secure the tubing to the patient's extremity with tape to reduce tension on the tube and minimize trauma at insertion site.
- Begin hemodialysis according to facility protocol.

BEGINNING HEMODIALYSIS WITH AN AV FISTULA OR SHUNT

- Flush the fistula needles, using attached syringes containing heparinized saline solution, and set them aside.
- Place a linen-saver pad under the patient's arm.
- Using sterile technique, clean a 3″ × 10″ (8 × 25 cm) area of skin over the fistula with povidone-iodine pads. If the patient is sensitive to iodine, use chlorhexidine gluconate or alcohol instead. Discard each pad after one wipe.
- Apply a tourniquet above the fistula to distend the veins and facilitate venipuncture; avoid occluding the fistula.
- Put on clean gloves and remove the fistula needle guard and squeeze the wing tips firmly together. Insert the arterial needle at least 1″ (2.5 cm) above the anastomosis, being careful not to puncture the fistula.
- Release the tourniquet and flush the needle with heparin flush solution to prevent clotting.
- Clamp the arterial needle tubing with a hemostat, and secure the wing tips of the needle to the skin with adhesive tape.
- Perform another venipuncture with the venous needle a few inches above the arterial needle.
- Flush the venous needle with heparin flush solution.
- Clamp the venous needle tubing, and secure the wing tips of the venous needle with tape.
- Remove the syringe from the end of the arterial tubing, uncap the arterial line from the hemodialysis machine, and connect the two lines.

- Tape the connection securely to prevent separation during the procedure.
- Remove the syringe from the end of the venous tubing, uncap the venous line from the hemodialysis machine, and connect the two lines.
- Tape the connection securely.
- Release the hemostat and start hemodialysis.
- Monitor vital signs throughout hemodialysis at least hourly or as often as every 15 minutes.
- Perform periodic tests for clotting time on patient's blood samples and samples from the dialyzer.
- Give necessary drugs during dialysis unless the drug would be removed in the dialysate.

DISCONTINUING HEMODIALYSIS WITH A DOUBLE-LUMEN CATHETER

- Clamp the extension tubing to prevent air from entering the catheter.
- Clean all connection points on all lines and clamps to reduce risk of infections.
- Place a clean drape under the catheter, and place two sterile povidone-iodine soaked gauze pads on the drape beneath the catheter lines.
- Prepare the catheter flush solution with normal saline or heparin flush solution, as ordered.
- Put on clean gloves and grasp each blood line with a gauze pad and disconnect each line from the catheter.
- Flush each port with saline solution to clear extension tubing and catheter of blood.
- Administer additional heparin flush solution as ordered to ensure catheter patency. Attach Luer-lock injection caps to prevent air entry or loss of blood.
- Clamp the extension tubing.
- Re-dress catheter site per facility policy.

DISCONTINUING HEMODIALYSIS WITH AN AV FISTULA

- Turn the blood pump on the hemodialysis machine to 50 to 100 ml/ minute.
- Put on clean gloves and remove the tape from the connection site of arterial lines.
- Clamp the needle tubing with a hemostat and disconnect the lines. The blood in the machine's arterial line will continue to flow toward the dialyzer, followed by a column of air. Just before the blood reaches the point where the normal saline solution enters the line, clamp the blood line with another hemostat.
- Unclamp the normal saline solution to allow a small amount to flow through the line.
- Unclamp the hemostat on the machine line to allow all blood to flow into the dialyzer where it passes through the filter and back to the patient through the venous line.
- After the blood is retransfused, clamp the venous needle tubing and the machine's venous line with hemostats and turn off the blood pump.
- Remove the tape from connection site of the venous lines and disconnect the lines.
- Remove the venipuncture needle and apply pressure to the site with a folded gauze pad until all bleeding stops, usually within 10 minutes.
- Apply an adhesive bandage.
- Repeat the procedure on the arterial line.
- Disinfect and rinse the delivery system according to manufacturer's instructions.
- If bleeding continues after you remove an AV fistula needle, apply pressure with a sterile, absorbable gelatin sponge or topical thrombin solution.

(continued)

Learning about hemodialysis

Dear Patient:

Your health care provider has ordered hemodialysis for you. This procedure uses a dialyzer (pictured below) to do your kidneys' job. By filtering your blood through its internal membranes, it removes extra fluids and impurities and returns purified blood to your body.

BEFORE DIALYSIS

The nurse or dialysis technician will weigh you. Your blood pressure will also be taken—once while you're standing and once while you're lying down.

Before your first treatment, the physician will create an opening in your collarbone, groin area, wrist, or lower forearm. He'll make the area numb first so that you aren't uncomfortable.

For an opening in the collarbone or groin area, your physician will insert a thin, hollow tube called a *catheter*. In the wrist or forearm, the physician will create a passage (fistula) and insert a different kind of tube called a *shunt* or *graft*. Stitches will keep the tube in place. The tube will be used to transfer some of your blood to the machine.

DURING DIALYSIS

Next, the nurse will connect you to the machine and turn it on to begin the treatment. She'll check the dialyzer and the connections frequently.

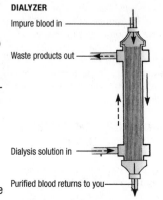

DIALYZER

Impure blood in

Waste products out

Dialysis solution in

Purified blood returns to you

During hemodialysis, the nurse will check your blood pressure every 10 to 30 minutes. She'll also collect blood samples occasionally during hemodialysis and when it ends. The blood samples will be tested to see how well hemodialysis is working for you.

Be sure to tell the nurse how you feel, especially if you experience a headache, dizziness, backache, nausea, vomiting, muscle twitching, difficulty breathing, or pain.

When hemodialysis is over, the nurse will disconnect the tube from the dialyzer.

AFTER DIALYSIS

When you go home, remember to keep the skin around the tube clean and dry. If the nurse has taught you how, you may clean the incision daily until healing is complete and the stitches are removed.

Call your health care provider if you have pain, swelling, redness, or drainage in the tube area.

COMPLICATIONS
- Dialysis disequilibrium syndrome
- Hypotension
- Cardiac arrhythmias
- Cardiovascular disease
- Air embolism
- Thrombosis of AV fistula
- Stenosis of AV fistula
- Bleeding
- Infection
- Electrolyte imbalance
- Fluid imbalance
- Anemia

NURSING DIAGNOSES

- Risk for deficient fluid volume
- Risk for infection
- Risk for injury

EXPECTED OUTCOMES
The patient will:
- maintain vital signs within normal limits and avoid signs and symptoms of hypovolemic shock
- remain free from infection
- remain free from injury during and after the procedure.

PRETREATMENT CARE

- Prepare hemodialysis equipment following manufacturer's instructions and facility protocol.

WARNING *To avoid pyrogenic reactions and bacteremia with septicemia, use strict sterile technique while preparing machine.*

- Test the dialyzer and dialysis machine for residual disinfectant after rinsing, and test all alarms.
- Maintain strict sterile technique to prevent introducing pathogens into the patient's bloodstream.
- If the patient is undergoing hemodialysis for the first time, explain the procedure. (See *Learning about hemodialysis.*)
- Wear appropriate personal protective equipment throughout all procedures.
- Weigh the patient and record his weight.
- Record baseline vital signs, taking blood pressure while he's sitting and standing; auscultate the heart for rate, rhythm, and abnormalities; assess for edema; observe respiratory rate, rhythm, and quality; and check his mental status.
- Assess the condition and patency of the access site.
- Auscultate for bruits and palpate for a thrill to confirm patency of the AV fistula or shunt before beginning and periodically throughout the procedure; notify the practitioner if bruits or a thrill is absent.
- Help the patient into a comfortable position (supine or sitting in recliner chair with feet elevated).
- Obtain blood samples from the patient, as ordered, before beginning hemodialysis; evaluate the results.
- Immediately report machine malfunction or equipment defect.

WARNING *Complete each step of dialysis correctly to avoid unnecessary blood loss or inefficient treatment from poor clearances or inadequate fluid removal. Failure to perform hemodialysis properly can lead to injury to the patient and death.*

POSTTREATMENT CARE

- Monitor the patient's vital signs.
- Evaluate postreatment laboratory values.
- Weigh the patient and record his weight; compare to his pretreatment weight.
- Observe the patient for adverse effects of treatment.
- Assess the catheter insertion site for signs of infection, such as purulent drainage, inflammation, and tenderness.
- Provide emotional support.

PATIENT TEACHING

GENERAL
- Tell the patient to notify the practitioner if pain, swelling, redness, or drainage occurs in the accessed arm.
- Provide the telephone number of the dialysis center.
- Remind the patient not to allow any treatments or procedures on the accessed arm, including blood pressure monitoring or needle punctures. Tell him to avoid putting excessive pressure on the arm. He shouldn't sleep on it, wear constricting clothing over it, or lift heavy objects or strain with it. He should also avoid getting it wet for several hours after dialysis.
- Review the dialysis schedule with the patient and his family. Make sure that they're aware of the next scheduled treatment.
- Review fluid and diet restrictions as needed.

RESOURCES
Organizations
American Nephrology Nurses' Association: *www.anna.inurse.com*
National Kidney and Urologic Diseases Information Clearinghouse: *www.kidney.niddk.nih.gov*
National Kidney Foundation: *www.kidney.org*

Selected references
American Nephrology Nurses' Association, "ANNA Position Statements (revised or reaffirmed April 2005)," *Nephrology Nursing Journal* 32(3): 313-27, May-June 2005.
Holley, J.L., et al. "Managing Homeless Dialysis Patients," *Nephrology News Issues* 20(1):49-50, 52-53, January 2006.
Kanagasundaram, N.S., and Paganini, P. "Acute Renal Failure on the Intensive Care Unit," *Clinical Medicine* 5(5): 435-40, September-October 2005.

Hemorrhoidectomy

- Removal of hemorrhoidal varicosities
- May involve rubber band ligation, use of surgical staples, radiofrequency ablation, cryotherapy, infrared coagulation, sclerotherapy, laser excision, or harmonic scalpel surgery
- Hemorrhoids classified from Grade I to IV based on degree and tractability of prolapse outside the anal canal; treatments based on the grade

INDICATIONS

- Intolerable and prolonged hemorrhoidal pain
- Excessive bleeding of hemorrhoids
- Grade III to IV prolapse
- Infection

PROCEDURE

- A local or general anesthetic is administered, depending on the procedure.
- The surgeon dilates the rectal sphincter digitally or with an anoscope.
- Grade I or II symptomatic hemorrhoidal varicosities are usually removed by banding (ligating), injecting a sclerosing agent, freezing (cryosurgery), or coagulating with an infrared beam. A combination of these methods may also be used. (See *Ligating hemorrhoidal tissue*.)
- In conventional hemorrhoidectomy for Grade III or IV disease, the practitioner excises the hemorrhoidal tissues with a scalpel and sutures, coagulates, or cauterizes, the wound. The harmonic scalpel is an ultrasound driven cutting tool used for excising and coagulating the tissue. Radiofrequency ablation can also be used to excise the tissues.
- In stapled hemorrhoidectomy, the hemorrhoid tissue isn't necessarily resected, but the relapsing tissues are drawn into a circular stapling device, which attaches them to the lower rectal vault, thus retracting and flattening out the prolapsed areas.

- A small, lubricated tube may be placed in the anus to drain fluid, blood, and flatus, or the area may be packed with petroleum gauze.

COMPLICATIONS

- Hemorrhage
- Anal stenosis
- Infection locally or into the peritoneum
- Recurrence
- Fecal incontinence or constipation
- Urine retention
- Fistula

- Acute pain
- Risk for infection
- Risk for injury

EXPECTED OUTCOMES

The patient will:
- demonstrate or express feelings of increased comfort
- show no signs of infection as evidenced by laboratory test results within normal limits
- experience minimal site bleeding postoperatively and regain normal bowel function.

Ligating hemorrhoidal tissue

Removal of large internal hemorrhoids commonly requires ligation. In this surgical technique, the practitioner inserts an anoscope to dilate the rectal sphincter, then uses grasping forceps to pull the hemorrhoid into position. He then inserts a ligator through the anoscope and slips a small rubber band over the pedicle of the hemorrhoid to bind it and cut off blood flow. Next, he excises the hemorrhoid or allows it to slough off naturally, which usually occurs within 5 to 7 days.

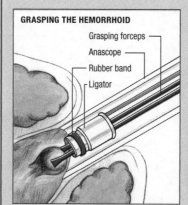

GRASPING THE HEMORRHOID

- Grasping forceps
- Anascope
- Rubber band
- Ligator

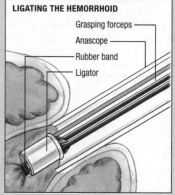

LIGATING THE HEMORRHOID

- Grasping forceps
- Anascope
- Rubber band
- Ligator

PRETREATMENT CARE

◆ Review the treatment and preparation to the patient and family.
◆ Verify that the patient has signed an appropriate consent form.
◆ Explain postoperative care.
◆ Administer an enema as ordered.
◆ Shave and clean the perianal area as ordered.
◆ Administer a sedative as ordered

POSTTREATMENT CARE

◆ Administer medications as ordered.
◆ Position the patient comfortably in bed; support the buttocks with pillows if necessary.
◆ Help the patient change positions regularly and to assume a prone position for 15 minutes every few hours.
◆ Check the dressing regularly, and immediately report excessive bleeding or drainage. If bleeding is excessive, insert a balloon-tipped catheter into the rectum and inflate it to exert pressure on the hemorrhagic area and reduce blood loss as ordered.

⚡ **WARNING** *Watch for acute hemorrhage and hypovolemic shock. Monitor vital signs every 2 to 4 hours, monitor intake and output, and assess for signs of fluid volume deficit, such as poor skin turgor, dry mucous membranes, and feelings of faintness, weakness, and confusion.*

◆ Verify that the patient voids within the 6 to 8 hours after surgery. If necessary, help stimulate voiding with such measures as massages and warm sitz baths; catheterize him only if other measures fail.
◆ Using warm water and a mild soap, clean the perianal area to prevent infection and irritation. Gently pat the area dry. Apply a wet dressing (a 1:1 solution of cold water and witch hazel) or a commercially available product to the perianal area.

◆ Provide analgesics and sitz baths or warm compresses to reduce local pain, swelling, and inflammation and to prevent rectoanal spasms.
◆ As soon as bowel sounds return and oral feeding is initiated, administer a stool-softener, as ordered, to ease defecation.

PATIENT TEACHING

GENERAL

◆ Review medications and possible adverse reactions with the patient.
◆ Tell the patient to notify the practitioner if excessive bleeding occurs.
◆ Stress the need for follow-up surgical evaluation.
◆ Tell the patient how to prevent the recurrence of hemorrhoids by exercising daily; increasing his intake of dietary fiber, and drinking about 2 gallons of fluid daily.
◆ Before discharge, teach the patient proper perianal hygiene, such as wiping gently with soft, white toilet paper (the dyes used in colored paper may cause irritation); cleaning with mild soap and warm water; and applying a sanitary pad until drainage stops.
◆ Teach the patient to take sitz baths three or four times daily and after each bowel movement to reduce swelling and discomfort.
◆ Instruct the patient to report increased rectal bleeding, purulent drainage, fever, constipation, or rectal spasm to the surgeon.
◆ Stress the importance of regular soft, formed bowel movements to prevent recurrence of hemorrhoids.
◆ Warn against overusing stool-softening laxatives. Explain that a firm stool is necessary to dilate the anal canal and prevent stricture formation.

RESOURCES
Organizations
American College of Emergency Practitioners: *www.acep.org*
American Society of Colon and Rectal Surgeons: *www.ascrs.affiniscape.com*

Selected references
Felicie, G., et al. "Doppler-Guided Hemorrhoidal Artery Ligation: An Alternative to Hemorrhoidectomy," *Diseases of the Colon and Rectum* 48(11):2090-93, November 2005.
Gupta, P.J. "Hemorrhoidal Ablation and Fixation: An Alternative Procedure for Relapsing Hemorrhoids." *Digestion* 72(2-3):181-88, September 2005.
Gupta, P.J., et al., "Radiofrequency Ablation and Plication—A New Technique for Relapsing Hemorrhoidal Disease," *Current Surgery* 63(1):44-50, January-February 2006.
Oughriss, M., et al., "Complications of Stapled Hemorrhoidectomy: A French Multicentric Study," *Gastroenterology Clinique et Biologique* 29(4):429-33, April 2005.

Hernia repair, diaphragmatic

- Surgical repair of abnormal hole in the muscle separating the abdomen and chest (diaphragm), which may interfere with digestion and normal respiration
- Frequently congenital, left-sided, and causing compression of the left lung in the neonate; if severe, requiring emergency surgery (Congenital form is also called *Bochdalek hernia.*)
- Laparoscopic repair performed for small hernias; however, herniation generally requires open procedure
- Fetal surgery being researched for large congenital defects

INDICATIONS

- Hernias of the diaphragm, congenital or traumatic

- General anesthesia is used and mechanical ventilation is initiated.
- The surgeon makes an incision between the ribs over the herniated area or into the upper abdomen.
- The herniated intestinal organs are manipulated back to their proper positions.
- The defect in the muscle or fascia is tightly sutured.
- If necessary, the defect is reinforced with wire, mesh, or another material.
- A chest tube is inserted and connected to the drainage system.
- The incision is closed and a dressing is applied.

COMPLICATIONS

- Infection
- Bleeding
- Pulmonary hypertension
- Recurrence (rare)
- Respiratory impairment

> **AGE FACTOR** *Neonates with large congenital diaphragmatic hernias may have permanent lung impairment from failure of the affected lung to develop fully in utero.*

- Failure to thrive
- Gastroesophageal reflux
- Breast bone abnormalities

- Acute pain
- Ineffective tissue perfusion: GI, pulmonary
- Risk for infection

EXPECTED OUTCOMES

The patient will:

- demonstrate or express feelings of increased comfort
- regain normal bowel function, exhibit respiratory rate and pattern within normal limits for age, and demonstrate clear bilateral breath sounds
- remain free from infection.

PRETREATMENT CARE

- Review the treatment and preparation with the patient and his family.
- Verify that the patient or a family member has signed an appropriate consent form.
- Explain postoperative care.
- Assess vital signs, blood pressure, heart and lung sounds, and bowel sounds.
- Obtain laboratory tests, electrocardiogram, and X-rays as ordered.
- Administer I.V. therapy as ordered.
- Withhold food and oral fluids as ordered.
- Place a nasogastric tube to low suction as ordered.
- Monitor mechanical ventilation and pulse oximetry and arterial blood gas analysis results.

POSTTREATMENT CARE

- Administer medications as ordered.
- Monitor chest tube drainage and insertion site frequently for bleeding, infection, and excessive drainage.
- Help wean the patient from mechanical ventilation as ordered.
- Assess heart, lung, and abdominal sounds frequently.
- Take measures to prevent constipation when bowel sounds return.
- Teach coughing and deep-breathing exercises as appropriate.
- Provide comfort measures.
- Monitor vital signs and intake and output.
- Monitor the surgical wound, dressings and drainage, and provide care as ordered.
- Provide nutritional support as ordered.
- Provide emotional support to the patient and his family.

PATIENT TEACHING

GENERAL

- Review medications and possible adverse reactions with the patient and his family.
- Tell the patient about resuming activity per practitioner instructions.
- Teach the patient and his family how to care for the incision.
- Tell the patient about the signs and symptoms of lung or incisional infection.
- Instruct the patient and his family to report abdominal pain or abnormal patterns of bowel function to the practitioner.
- Stress the need for follow-up care.
- Teach parents of neonates who required large patch grafts that the grafts don't grow with the child so monitoring for recurrence of herniation is essential.
- Refer the parents of an affected neonate to sources of information and emotional support.

RESOURCES

Organizations

American Academy of Pediatrics: *www.aap.org*
American College of Surgeons: *www.facs.org*
CHERUBS—The Association of Congenital Diaphragmatic Hernia Research, Advocacy, and Support: *www.cherubs-cdh.org*

Selected references

Chiu, P.P., et al. "The Price of Success in the Management of Congenital Diaphragmatic Hernia: Is Improved Survival Accompanied by an Increase in Long-Term Morbidity?" *Journal of Pediatric Surgery* 41(5):888-92, May 2006.

Conforti, A., and Losty, P. "Perinatal Management of Congenital Diaphragmatic Hernia," *Early Human Development* 82(5):283-87, April 2006.

Mousa, A., et al. "Hand-assisted Thoracoscopic Repair of a Bochdalek Hernia in an Adult," *Journal of Laparoendoscopic & Advanced Surgical Techniques, Part A* 16(1):54-58, February 2006.

Hernia repair, hiatal

- Surgical repair of bulging of stomach tissue through the opening (hiatus) in the diaphragm through which the esophagus passes into the abdominal cavity
- Laparoscopic repair typical for uncomplicated hernias
- Often accompanied by fundoplication of the stomach to prevent acid and gastric contents from refluxing into the esophagus
- Paraesophageal hernias more likely to cause twisting or incarceration of the stomach and receive similar treatment

INDICATIONS

- Hiatal hernia with potential for or that which presents with strangulation or constriction
- Esophageal stricture

- General or spinal anesthesia is used.
- In open procedures, an upper abdominal incision is made.
- In laparoscopic procedures, three or four small incisions are made to allow for the fiber-optic scope and surgical instruments.
- The stomach and lower esophageal sphincter are manipulated back into the abdomen and lightly sutured in place.
- The hiatus is tightened with a drawstring technique.
- Other nearby defects in the muscle are repaired.
- Increasingly, the repair is reinforced with wire or mesh.
- Nissen (full, or 360 degree) or partial fundoplication is commonly done with the repair. The fundus of the stomach is wrapped around the back of the stomach and sewed to itself creating a collar around the end of the esophagus.
- When the surgery is completed, the incision is closed and a dressing is applied.

COMPLICATIONS

- Infection
- Bleeding
- Injury to the liver, spleen, esophagus, or stomach
- Gastroesophageal reflux disease

- Acute pain
- Ineffective tissue perfusion: GI
- Risk for infection

EXPECTED OUTCOMES

The patient will:

- demonstrate or express feelings of increased comfort
- regain normal esophageal and stomach function
- be free from signs and symptoms of infection of the lungs, abdomen, or incision sites.

PRETREATMENT CARE

◆ Review the treatment and preparation with the patient and his family.
◆ Verify that the patient has signed an appropriate consent form.
◆ Explain postoperative care.
◆ Shave the surgical site as ordered.
◆ Start an I.V. line as ordered.
◆ Assess vital signs, blood pressure, heart and lung sounds, and bowel sounds.
◆ Obtain laboratory tests, electrocardiogram, X-rays as ordered.
◆ Withhold food and oral fluids as ordered.
◆ Administer a sedative as ordered.
◆ Review proper coughing and deep-breathing techniques and use of an incentive spirometer.

POSTTREATMENT CARE

◆ Administer medications as ordered.
◆ Encourage early ambulation.
◆ Provide comfort measures.
◆ Monitor vital signs and intake and output.
◆ Assess for complications, such as infection, bleeding, and abnormal abdominal pain or sounds.
◆ Monitor the surgical wound, dressings, and drainage.
◆ Encourage proper coughing and deep-breathing techniques and use of an incentive spirometer.

PATIENT TEACHING

GENERAL

◆ Review medications and possible adverse reactions with the patient.
◆ Tell the patient about resuming his activity gradually per practitioner orders.

WARNING *Adults should avoid heavy lifting or straining for 6 to 8 weeks after surgery; such activity can disrupt the hernia repair. Any lifting may increase intra-abdominal pressure and rupture the sutures that have been placed to wrap the stomach around the esophagus.*

◆ Teach the patient how to care for the incision and to notify the practitioner of reddening, warmth, drainage, or pain at the site.
◆ Tell the patient about the signs and symptoms of abdominal infection.
◆ Stress the need for follow-up care.
◆ Inform the patient about the signs and symptoms of the recurrence of hernia.
◆ Refer the patient to a weight-reduction program if indicated.
◆ Refer the patient to a smoking-cessation program if indicated.
◆ Review dietary restrictions as ordered.
◆ Tell the patient to expect significant gas, bloating, and diarrhea for some time after surgery, as appropriate.
◆ Tell the patient to continue antacid medications for 10 to 14 days before being gradually tapered off, as instructed by the practitioner.
◆ Tell the patient to avoid bathing in a tub for at least 5 days after the surgery. Soaking may separate the skin tapes and the wound could break open. Sponge bathing and showering are permitted the day after surgery. Instruct the patient to carefully pat the wound tapes dry after showering.

RESOURCES
Organizations
American College of Surgeons: *www.facs.org*
American Gastroenterological Association: *www.gastro.org*
The Society of American Gastrointestinal and Endoscopic Surgeons: *www.sages.org*

Selected references
Benassai, G., et al. "Laparoscopic Antireflux Surgery: Indications, Preoperative Evaluation, Techniques, and Outcomes," *Hepatogastroenterology* 53(67):77-81, January-February 2006.
Haider, M., et al. "Surgical Repair of Recurrent Hiatal Hernia," *Hernia* 10(1): 13-19, March 2006.
Muller-Stich, B.P., et al. "Laparoscopic Hiatal Hernia Repair: Long-Term Outcome With the Focus on the Influence of Mesh Reinforcement," *Surgical Endoscopy* 29(3):380-84, March 2006.

Hernia repair, inguinal

OVERVIEW

- Surgical repair of opening or weakness in the groin muscle that allows protrusion of the bowel
- Most common type of hernia; more common in males than females
- Classified as direct (acquired) or indirect (congenital)

   AGE FACTOR *Inguinal hernias in children are rarely caused by an injury or tearing of tissue and are usually the result of incomplete closure in the groin.*

- Femoral hernias found nearby, with bowel protrusion through the opening for the femoral vessels; more common in females than males
- Laparoscopic repair typical for uncomplicated hernias; hernia repair using mesh called *hernioplasty*
- Most hernias treated surgically after reduction by use of a truss; only a temporary measure to prevent restricted blood flow or blocked intestine

INDICATIONS
- Hernias of the inguinal area

   WARNING *Tissue, such as intestine and peritoneum, can become trapped in the hernia (incarcerated hernia). When blood flow is restricted, it's called a strangulated hernia. If blood flow is restricted or the intestine is blocked, emergency surgery may be needed to prevent necrosis of the bowel loop.*

PROCEDURE

- General, spinal, regional, or local anesthesia may be used, depending on the extent of herniation and the type of procedure.
- For open techniques, the surgeon makes an incision over the herniated area.
- The herniated tissue is manipulated back to its proper position. The area is also inspected carefully for other potential herniations which are also reduced.
- The defect in the muscle or fascia is closed with sutures or staples.
- A small or preshaped piece of surgical mesh may be used to repair the defect or hole. (See *Mesh plug for hernia repair.*)
- A larger piece of surgical mesh may be placed under the spermatic cord and over and around the deep inguinal ring to provide added support to the structures.
- The same basic procedure can be accomplished in a laparoscopic approach for uncomplicated repairs.
- When surgery is complete, the incision is closed and a dressing is applied.

COMPLICATIONS
- Infection
- Bleeding
- Hernia recurrence
- Chronic neuralgia from damage to nearby nerves
- Injury to abdominal structures or the intestines
- Spermatic cord injury
- Bowel or bladder injury

NURSING DIAGNOSES

- Acute pain
- Risk for impaired urinary elimination
- Risk for infection

EXPECTED OUTCOMES
The patient will:
- demonstrate or express feelings of increased comfort
- maintain normal urinary function
- be free from signs or symptoms of infection.

Mesh plug for hernia repair

The mesh plug technique is preferred for repairing initial and recurrent inguinal hernias.

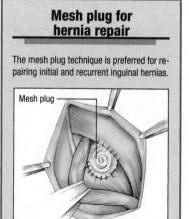

Mesh plug

PRETREATMENT CARE

◆ Review the basic procedure and preparation with the patient and his family.
◆ Verify that the patient or a family member has signed an appropriate consent form.
◆ Verify that ordered blood work, medical evaluation, chest X-ray, and electrocardiography are completed if required.
◆ Instruct the patient to temporarily stop drugs, such as aspirin, blood thinners, anti-inflammatory medications, and vitamin E, for several days to 1 week before surgery; also, tell him to stop taking diet medications or St. John's wort for 2 weeks before surgery.
◆ Tell the patient to stop smoking, and make arrangements for help he may need at home after the surgery.
◆ Explain postoperative care.
◆ Perform a complete overall assessment; obtain baseline vital signs.
◆ Insert an I.V. access device and administer prophylactic antibiotics or fluids as ordered.
◆ Shave the surgical site as ordered.
◆ Administer an enema as ordered.
◆ Administer a sedative as ordered.

POSTTREATMENT CARE

◆ Administer medications as ordered.
◆ Take measures to prevent constipation, such as increasing liquids and fiber in the diet as ordered.
◆ Encourage early ambulation.
◆ Make sure the patient voids within 8 hours after surgery; insert a urinary catheter, if necessary.
◆ Provide comfort measures.
◆ Apply an ice bag to the scrotum if appropriate.
◆ Monitor vital signs; heart, lung, and abdominal sounds; and intake and output.
◆ Assess for complications, such as infection and bleeding.
◆ Monitor the surgical wound, dressings, and drainage.

PATIENT TEACHING

GENERAL

◆ Review medications and possible adverse reactions with the patient.
◆ Tell the patient about resuming his usual activities per practitioner instructions.

AGE FACTOR *Small children have no restrictions after routine hernia repair. Older children should avoid contact sports for at least 3 weeks—a blow to the incision could burst the skin closure or disrupt the repair (less common). Adults should avoid heavy lifting or straining for about 4 to 8 weeks after surgery because such activity can disrupt the hernia repair.*

◆ Teach the patient and his family measures to reduce pressure on the incision site.
◆ Teach the patient how to care for the incision and to report redness, pain, warmth, or drainage to the practitioner promptly.
◆ Stress the need for follow-up care.
◆ Inform the patient about the signs and symptoms of the recurrence of hernia.
◆ Tell the patient how to prevent hernia recurrence.
◆ Instruct the patient to follow a high-fiber diet.
◆ Instruct the patient to have an adequate oral fluid intake.
◆ Refer the patient to a weight-reduction program if indicated.
◆ Refer the patient to a smoking-cessation program if indicated.
◆ Tell the patient to avoid tub bathing for at least 5 days after surgery. Soaking may separate the skin tapes and the wound could break open. Sponge bathing for infants and showering for older children are permitted the day after surgery. Instruct the patient to carefully pat the wound tapes dry after showering.

RESOURCES
Organizations
American College of Surgeons: *www.facs.org*
American Gastroenterological Association: *www.gastro.org*
The Society of American Gastrointestinal and Endoscopic Surgeons: *www.sages.org*

Selected references
Demirer, S., et al. "The Effect of Polypropylene Mesh on Ilioinguinal Nerve in Open Mesh Repair of Groin Hernia," *Journal of Surgical Research* 131(2): 175-81, April 2006.
Di Vita, G., et al. "Systemic Inflammatory Response in Elderly Patients Following Hernioplastical Operation," *Immunity & Ageing* 3(1):3, March 2006.
Rozen, D., and Parvez, U. "Pulsed Radiofrequency of Lumbar Nerve Roots for Treatment of Chronic Inguinal Herniorrhaphy Pain," *Pain Physician* 9(2):153-56, April 2006.

Hernia repair, umbilical and ventral

OVERVIEW

- Surgical repair of opening or weakness in the abdominal wall around the naval (umbilical) or where a previous surgical incision was made (ventral)

AGE FACTOR *Umbilical hernias that develop in infants usually heal naturally by age 3. Surgery is only indicated when bowel loops are irreversibly trapped in the herniated sac.*

- Ventral hernias: occur in about 11% of abdominal surgeries due to weakening of the muscles from incision and use of sutures alone to reapproximate the tissues; large midline sites most at risk
- Herniation usually discovered when bulging from a loop of intestines or other abdominal contents into a sac of tissue under the skin appears; pain is rarely the first indicator
- Abdominal contents stuck within the sac, becoming incarcerated, causing tissue death unless emergency surgery is performed
- Laparoscopic repair under local anesthesia typical for uncomplicated hernias in adults
- Most hernias repaired to prevent restricted blood flow or blocked intestine

WARNING *Complicated hernias occur in those patients with many prior abdominal surgeries, those in unusual or difficult to access sites, those with previous hernia repairs, and in those patients significantly over their ideal body weight or with other significant medical conditions.*

INDICATIONS
- Umbilical hernia
- Ventral hernia

PROCEDURE

- General anesthesia is used for children, or adults with complicated hernias.
- The surgeon makes an incision over the herniated area for ventral her-

nias, just below the naval for umbilical hernias.
- Generally, the protruding organs are returned to the abdominal cavity, then a mesh sheet is threaded between the muscle layers and sutured in place, allowing the muscle fibers to approximate and regrow together incorporating the strengthening mesh barrier.
- When surgery is complete, the incision is closed and a dressing applied.
- In laparoscopic repair, a laparoscope is inserted through a small incision near the hernia to visualize the area. Gas is insufflated into the abdomen to separate the structures from one another. Several smaller incisions are required for entrance of the special surgical tools to remove any scar tissue and to insert a surgical mesh into the abdomen. The mesh is held in place with special surgical tacks and sutures. When complete, incisions are sutured closed and dressings applied.

COMPLICATIONS
- Infection
- Bleeding
- Recurrence of hernia
- Injury to abdominal structures or the intestines

NURSING DIAGNOSES

- Acute pain
- Ineffective tissue perfusion: GI
- Risk for infection

EXPECTED OUTCOMES
The patient will:
- demonstrate or express feelings of increased comfort
- maintain normal bowel function
- be free from infection.

PRETREATMENT CARE

- Review the treatment and preparation with the patient and his family.
- Verify that the patient or a family member has signed an appropriate consent form.

- Obtain ordered blood work, chest X-ray, and electrocardiogram depending on the patient's age and medical condition.
- Ask the patient to shower the night before or morning of the surgery.
- Instruct the patient to temporarily stop drugs, such as aspirin, blood thinners, anti-inflammatory medications, and vitamin E, for several days to 1 week before surgery as ordered; also, tell him to stop taking diet medications or St. John's wort for 2 weeks before surgery.
- Explain postoperative nursing care.
- Shave the surgical site as ordered.
- Administer an enema as ordered.
- Administer a sedative as ordered.

POSTTREATMENT CARE

- Administer medications as ordered.
- Avoid placing pressure on the incision site.
- Make sure the patient voids within 8 hours after surgery; insert a urinary catheter, if needed.
- Encourage early ambulation.
- Take measures to prevent constipation.
- Provide comfort measures, including teaching the patient to splint the abdomen when coughing.
- Monitor vital signs, abdominal sounds, and intake and output.
- Assess for complications, such as infection or excessive bleeding.
- Assess the surgical wound and drainage, provide wound care as ordered.
- Teach patients with laparoscopic procedures that upper abdominal and shoulder pain is expected from the gas infused into the abdomen, and will resolve within 24 hours.

PATIENT TEACHING

GENERAL
- Review medications and possible adverse reactions with the patient and his family.
- Review the practitioner's instructions about activity resumption and lifting restrictions with the patient.

Recovering from hernia surgery

Dear Patient:

IIn most cases, hernias can be repaired on an outpatient basis. This means you'll probably leave the hospital on the same day that you have surgery.

After you're home, follow these guidelines to minimize discomfort and speed your recovery.

THE FIRST FEW DAYS

For the first 2 or 3 days, you may have a fever. Your temperature may be as high as 100° F (37.8° C). Use over-the-counter medications, such as acetominophen to reduce fever. It the fever persists or goes higher than 101° F, call your health care provider.

You may notice swelling, bruising, tenderness, or the feeling that there's a rope under the incision. Your health care provider may prescribe medication to relieve pain.

While the incision is still tender, you'll be most comfortable wearing soft, loose-fitting clothes.

Notify your health care provider immediately if you experience chest pain, nausea, trouble breathing, or if you have difficulty urinating.

PREVENT AND RECOGNIZE INFECTION

Keep the incision clean and covered to prevent infection.

Contact your health care provider if fever, pain, swelling, and tenderness last longer than 3 days. Also contact him if you notice bleeding, redness, or drainage at the incision site or if you have chills or other flu-like symptoms. These symptoms may signal infection.

Remember to make an appointment with your health care provider within 1 week after hernia surgery to check the wound and remove sutures.

TAKE IT EASY

Your health care provider will let you know when it's safe to resume your usual activities. You can probably return to work or school within 2 or 3 days. He may advise you to avoid bathing for a couple of days and to refrain from driving for about 2 weeks. You may resume sexual activity as soon as you feel comfortable. Try to use positions that don't strain your incision.

Avoid foods that might make you constipated and strain against you incision. Don't perform strenuous activities, such as bending, heavy lifting, or playing contact sports, until your health care provider says it's okay.

If you're a parent, you may have to restrict some of your usual activities with your children. Avoid picking them up or carrying them. Explain to them why you need to take it easy and reassure them that things will soon return to normal.

This patient-teaching aid may be reproduced by office copier for distribution to patients. © 2007 Lippincott Williams & Wilkins.

- ◆ Inform the patient about possible complications such as recurrence.
- ◆ Stress the need for follow-up care with the surgeon.
- ◆ Instruct the patient to decrease strain on the abdominal muscles when healed such as by using proper body mechanics for lifting.
- ◆ Tell the patient to follow a high-fiber diet with adequate fluid intake to prevent constipation.
- ◆ Refer the patient to a weight-reduction program if indicated.
- ◆ Tell the patient to avoid tub bathing for at least 5 days after regular surgery. Soaking may separate the skin tapes and the wound could break open. Sponge bathing for infants and showering for older children are permitted the day after surgery. Instruct the patient to carefully pat the wound tapes dry after showering. (See *Recovering from hernia surgery.*)

RESOURCES
Organizations
American Academy of Pediatrics: *www.aap.org*
American College of Surgeons: *www.facs.org*
Society of American Gastrointestinal Endoscopic Surgeons: *www.sages.org*

Selected references
Burger, J.W.A., et al. "Long-term Follow-up of a Randomized Controlled Trial of Suture Versus Mesh Repair of Incisional Hernia," *Annals of Surgery* 240(4): 578-85, April 2004.

Mussack, T., et al. "Cine Magnetic Resonance Imaging vs. High-Resolution Ultrasonography for Detection of Adhesions After Laparoscopic and Open Incisional Hernia Repair: A Matched Pair Pilot Analysis," *Surgical Endoscopy* 19(12):1538-43, December 2005.

Sorensen, L.T., et al. "Smoking Is a Risk Factor for Incisional Hernia," *Archives of Surgery* 140(2):119-23, February 2005.

AGE FACTOR *Small children have no restrictions after routine hernia repair. Older children should avoid contact sports for at least 3 weeks—a blow to the incision could burst the skin closure or disrupt the repair (less common). Adults should avoid heavy lifting or straining for 6 to 8 weeks after surgery; such activity can disrupt the hernia repair.*

- ◆ Teach the patient and his family how to care for the incision, including reporting new redness, warmth, drainage, or pain to the practitioner.

Hyperbaric oxygenation

OVERVIEW

- Medical treatment that delivers 100% oxygen while in special pressurized chamber
- Increases oxygen in the plasma and its availability to hypoxic cells and tissues
- Increases white blood cells and stimulates the formation of new capillaries and nerve endings around wound sites, pushes other dissolved harmful gases out of the circulatory system, and causes vasoconstriction without accompanying decrease in oxygenation
- Involves specialized chambers that deliver oxygen at atmospheric pressures 1½ to 3 times that at sea level and may house one or several patients at a time
  - Monoplace chambers: house one individual in a clear acrylic-shelled chamber; communication devices allow direct conversation between the patient and technician or practitioner
  - Multiplace chambers: can hold 2 to 16 patients with an attendant if needed
  - Portable chamber: nylon or fabric and vinyl tube-like lightweight and collapsible bag that can be pressurized with a manual pump to treat one patient in an out-of-hospital emergency
- Oxygen delivered in special masks or acrylic hoods that provide for a continuous flow of air across the face and venting of carbon dioxide outside the chamber
- Regular air pressurized within most chambers, although monoplace chambers are pressurized with 100% oxygen, thereby avoiding a mask
- Chambers humidified, heated, and cooled for comfort
- Treatment protocols varied in length, frequency, and inpatient or outpatient location by type of disorder

INDICATIONS

- Carbon monoxide or cyanide poisoning
- Gas or air embolism
- Decompression sickness
- Osteoradionecrosis
- Drug overdose
- Clostridial gas gangrene
- In combination with other treatments for:
  - Anemia from severe blood loss
  - Crush injuries or wounds with severe tissue ischemia
  - Compartment syndrome
  - Graft and flap salvage
  - Injury from radiation, thermal burns
  - Necrotizing soft tissue infections
- Neurologic disease

PROCEDURE

- The patient enters the hyperbaric chamber on a stretcher (monoplace) or may be treated while in a chair, recliner, or stretcher (multiplace).
- Oxygen delivery devices are applied to the patient, often with a transcutaneous oxygen monitor on the arm.
- The chamber is sealed and pressurized to the ordered air pressure, for the prescribed amount of time.
- Patients are monitored visually through the acrylic chamber or by video camera, and staff speak directly to the patient to assess adjustment and difficulties via special communication lines. An attendant monitors the chamber at all times during treatment.
- The pressure is gradually decompressed at the end of the treatment phase, and the oxygen delivery device is removed.

COMPLICATIONS

- Oxygen toxicity syndrome
- Pain, bloody discharge from sinuses
- Edema, rupture, or retraction of tympanic membrane
- Temporary deterioration of visual acuity; accelerated maturation of cataracts
- Ataxia
- Vertigo
- Tinnitus; hearing loss
- Hypoglycemia in patients with type 1 diabetes
- Nausea or vomiting
- Flatulence; colicky abdominal pain
- Tooth pain; tooth implosion or explosion
- Sudden decreased level of consciousness
- Hemiplegia

- Anxiety
- Disturbed sensory perception (visual, auditory)
- Ineffective tissue perfusion: Cardiopulmonary, peripheral

EXPECTED OUTCOMES
The patient will:
- remain calm during the course of treatment
- exhibit no new visual or auditory losses
- maintain tissue perfusion as evidenced by adequate blood pressure, heart rate, color, and respiratory rate.

PRETREATMENT CARE

- Baseline vital signs are obtained, and heart and lung sounds assessed. If wounds are involved, a pretreatment assessment is completed.
- Explain how therapy is delivered, safety measures in place, and communication devices used.
- Verify that an informed consent has been signed as appropriate.
- Determine if the patient has a history of claustrophobia, notify practitioner then administer mild sedation as ordered.
- Explain to the patient and family that an electrocardiogram, arterial line, hemodynamic monitoring lines, I.V. lines, or mechanical ventilation may be used within the chambers as needed.
- Teach the patient that cigarettes and fire risk materials; hand warmers; watches, jewelry, metal objects; hair spray, make-up, perfume, deodorant, shaving lotion, skin lotions, and any other alcohol or petroleum-based hair or skin product; newspapers (books are acceptable); battery-operated equipment; and personal aids, such as hearing aids, hard contact lenses, and dental plates, aren't permitted in the chamber for safety reasons.

- Instruct the patient that he may participate in diversional activities while in the chamber.
- Teach the patient methods to clear pressure in the eustachian tubes, and to notify the attendant promptly if the discomfort doesn't improve.
- Inform the patient that some ear discomfort or popping, an increase in temperature of the chamber, and motorlike noise are to be expected as the chamber is pressurized. The ambient temperature will be reduced to comfortable levels and the noise will stop once the chamber is pressurized fully.
- Inform the patient that he may experience light-headedness, fatigue, headache, or vomiting after the treatment, but the symptoms resolve quickly.
- Assist the patient, as needed, into all cotton clothes and shoe covers (required to reduce static electricity).

POSTTREATMENT CARE

- Monitor vital signs, hemodynamic values, heart rate and rhythm, intake and output, and pulse oximetry as appropriate.
- Monitor neurologic, pulmonary, skin, sensory, and mental status for complications.

PATIENT TEACHING

GENERAL
- Teach the patient and family the signs of oxygen toxicity and other complications to report to the practitioner promptly.
- Review follow-up appointments with the patient and his family.
- Explain medication administered and potential adverse reactions.
- Stress the need to follow safety guidelines for each treatment.

RESOURCES
Organizations
American Medical Association: *www.ama-assn.org*
National Heart, Lung and Blood Institute: *www.nhlbi.nih.gov*
Undersea & Hyperbaric Medicine Society: *www.uhms.org*

Selected references
Bailey, D.L., et al. "HBO Therapy: Beyond the Bends," *RN* 67(9):30-35, September 2004.
Gray, M., and Ratliff, C.R. "Is Hyperbaric Oxygen Therapy Effective for the Management of Chronic Wounds?" *The Journal of Wound, Ostomy, and Continence Nursing* 33(1):21-25, January-February 2006.
Harvey, C. "Wound Healing," *Orthopedic Nursing* 24(2):143-57, March-April 2005.

Hypophysectomy

OVERVIEW

- Surgical excision of all or part of the pituitary gland
- Three major approaches:
- Transfrontal entry approach: into the sella turcica through the skull (surgical flap or stereotaxic using 3-dimensional imaging and several small holes in the skull for instruments)
- Transsphenoidal entry approach: into the sella turcica from the inner aspect of the upper lip through the sphenoid sinus
- Endoscopic transnasal approach: entry into the sella turcica through a nostril and small opening into the sphenoid sinus
- Endoscopic approach most common in major medical centers today; transfrontal approach used when involvement of nearby structures and poorly defined tumors present

INDICATIONS
- Pituitary tumor
- Palliative measure for metastatic breast or prostate cancer (rare)

PROCEDURE

TRANSSPHENOIDAL HYPOPHYSECTOMY
- The patient receives general anesthesia.
- The surgeon makes an incision in the superior gingival tissue of the maxilla and membranes and tissues are dissected, and the nasal septum is removed.
- A speculum blade is placed slightly anterior to the sphenoid sinus. (See *Adenectomy: Alternative to hypophysectomy.*)
- The deeper anatomy is evaluated using an operating microscope with binocular vision and high-power lighting.
- Using a microdrill, the surgeon penetrates the sphenoid bone to view the anterior sella floor and the tumor is resected and aspirated.

- Hemostatic agents, subcutaneous fat plug (from the abdomen or outer thigh), or a muscle plug (from the thigh as graft tissue) may be placed to control bleeding or leakage of cerebrospinal fluid (CSF) and the sella floor may be sealed off with a small piece of bone or cartilage.
- The nasal septum is replaced.
- Nasal catheters are inserted, and petroleum gauze is packed around them.
- The initial incision is closed with stitches inside the inner lip.

ENDOSCOPIC TRANSNASAL HYPOPHYSECTOMY
- The patient receives general anesthesia.
- An endoscope in inserted into one nostril until the ostium (opening passageway) of the sphenoid sinus is visualized.
- The ostium is enlarged to allow passage of the endoscope into the sinus cavity.
- Using a microdrill, the surgeon penetrates the sphenoid bone to view the anterior sella floor and the tumor is resected and aspirated.
- Hemostatic agents or a fat plug may be used as needed.
- The endoscope is removed and a small mustache dressing applied.

COMPLICATIONS
- Diabetes insipidus
- Transient syndrome of inappropriate antidiuretic hormone (SIADH)
- Infection with possible brain abscess or meningitis
- Cerebrospinal fluid leakage
- Hemorrhage
- Vision defects
- Loss of smell and taste
- Nasal septum injury

NURSING DIAGNOSES

- Deficient fluid volume
- Disturbed sensory perception (olfactory, gustatory, visual)
- Risk for infection

EXPECTED OUTCOMES
The patient will:
- maintain adequate fluid volume as evidenced by adequate intake and output
- exhibit no reduction of smell or taste when the dressings are removed, and no decrease in visual acuity or fields
- remain free from infection.

Adenectomy: Alternative to hypophysectomy

Both adenectomy and hypophysectomy can be used to remove pituitary tumors. In hypophysectomy, the surgeon removes the tumor and all or part of the pituitary gland. However, for a tumor confined to the sella turcica, the surgeon may be able to perform an adenectomy, in which he removes the lesion while leaving the pituitary gland intact. Both surgeries involve the transsphenoidal approach shown here.

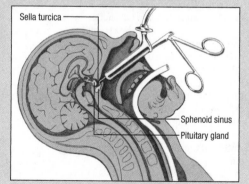

Sella turcica

Sphenoid sinus

Pituitary gland

- Review the treatment and preparation with the patient and his family.
- Verify that the patient has signed an appropriate consent form.
- Instruct the patient to begin taking hydrocortisone (Cortef) tablets the day before surgery as ordered, and explain what the drug is for, its adverse effects, and that it will be continued for a few days postoperatively.
- Instruct the patient to fast after midnight before surgery.
- Explain postoperative care, including the presence of a nasal catheter and packing for 2 to 4 days after surgery following transsphenoidal approach.
- Explain to the patient that he will have four or five special stick-on buttons applied to his skull and marked just before having a magnetic resonance imaging scan done of the brain before surgery. These marker buttons should be left in place as the scan results are used to guide the surgery.
- Arrange for a baseline visual field test and other appropriate tests and examinations as ordered.
- Administer antibiotics before the procedure as ordered.

- Administer medications, including antibiotics and hydrocortisone, as ordered.
- Maintain bed rest for 24 hours if ordered, then encourage ambulation (endoscopic transnasal approach may be done as same day surgery).
- Elevate the head of the bed to facilitate drainage and reduce swelling.
- For patients with diabetes insipidus, administer fluids, aqueous vasopressin, or sublingual desmopressin (DDAVP) as ordered.
- Arrange for visual field testing as ordered.
- Obtain laboratory tests as ordered.
- Monitor vital signs, neurologic status, and intake and output.
- Assess for complications, such as diabetes insipidus, SIADH, and CSF leakage (requires follow-up surgery).
- Monitor the drainage for signs of infection.

GENERAL

- Review medications and possible adverse reactions with the patient.
- Explain the signs and symptoms of diabetes insipidus and to notify the practitioner promptly if these occur.
- Tell the patient of fluid restrictions as indicated.
- Advise the patient to avoid sneezing, coughing, blowing his nose, or bending over for several days after surgery.
- Advise the patient to avoid brushing his teeth for 2 weeks, if directed by the practitioner (transsphenoidal approach); suggest he use a mouthwash instead.

- Inform the patient about the signs and symptoms of excessive or insufficient cortisol or thyroid hormone and to notify the practitioner of problems.
- Review other possible complications with the patient and clarify to notify the practitioner of new symptoms promptly.
- Emphasize the importance of wearing medical identification if hormone replacements are required.
- Stress the need for follow-up care.

RESOURCES
Organizations
American Association of Clinical Endocrinologists: *www.aace.com*
American Association of Endoscopic Surgeons: *www.endocrinesurgeons.org*
American Medical Association: *www.ama-assn.org*

Selected references
Colao, A., et al. "Partial Surgical Removal of Growth Hormone-Secreting Pituitary Tumors Enhances the Response to Somatostatin Analogs in Acromegaly," *Journal of Clinical Endocrinology and Metabolism* 91(1):85-92, January 2006.
Schneider, M., et al. "Anterior Pituitary Hormone Abnormalities Following Traumatic Brain Injury," *Journal of Neurotrauma* 22(9):937-46, September 2005.
Schubert, A., et al. "Anesthesia for Minimally Invasive Cranial and Spinal Surgery," *Journal of Neurosurgical Anesthesiology* 18(1):47-56, January 2006.

Hysterectomy

OVERVIEW

- Surgical removal of the uterus
- May be performed abdominally, vaginally, or laparoscopically
- Subtotal hysterectomy: removal of the entire uterus except the cervix
- Total hysterectomy (most common): removal of the uterus and cervix
- Panhysterectomy: removal of the entire uterus, ovaries, and fallopian tubes
- Radical hysterectomy: removal of the uterus, ovaries, fallopian tubes, adjoining ligaments and lymph nodes, upper one-third of the vagina, and surrounding tissues

INDICATIONS

- Malignant or benign tumor of the uterus, cervix, or adnexa
- Uterine bleeding and hemorrhage
- Uterine rupture or perforation
- Life-threatening pelvic infection
- Endometriosis unresponsive to conservative treatment
- Pelvic floor relaxation or prolapse

PROCEDURE

- The patient receives general anesthesia.

ABDOMINAL APPROACH

- The surgeon makes a midline vertical incision from the umbilicus to the symphysis pubis, or makes a horizontal incision in the lower abdomen.
- The uterus and accompanying structures are excised and removed.
- The incision is closed, and a dressing and perineal pad are applied.

VAGINAL APPROACH

- An incision is made above the vagina near the cervix.
- The uterus is excised and removed through the vaginal canal.
- The opening is closed to the peritoneal cavity with sutures.
- A perineal pad is applied.

LAPAROSCOPIC APPROACH

- An incision is made in the umbilicus.
- Nitrous oxide or carbon dioxide is infused into the abdominal cavity.
- The patient is placed in Trendelenburg's position.
- The laparoscope is inserted. (If an operative laparoscope is used, no other incision is required.)
- Several other small abdominal incisions are made to pass instruments.
- The uterus is excised vaginally after preparation through the laparotomy incisions.
- The incisions are closed, and dressings and perineal pad are applied.

COMPLICATIONS

- Urine retention
- Abdominal distention
- Pulmonary or thromboembolism
- Hemorrhage
- Ureteral or bowel injury
- Wound dehiscence
- Paralytic ileus
- Psychological problems
- Infection

NURSING DIAGNOSES

- Acute pain
- Impaired adjustment
- Impaired urinary elimination

EXPECTED OUTCOMES

The patient will:

- demonstrate and express feelings of increased comfort
- verbalize how the hysterectomy has affected her emotionally and measures to take to regain her emotional stability
- void normally after surgery and have no signs or symptoms of urine retention.

PRETREATMENT CARE

- Review the treatment and preparation to the patient and her family.
- Verify that the patient has signed an appropriate consent form.
- Administer an enema the evening before surgery.
- Administer prophylactic antibiotics as ordered.
- Make sure laboratory tests have been performed, including a pregnancy test if indicated; report abnormal results.
- Explain postoperative care, including expected abdominal cramping and moderate amounts of drainage. If the patient will have an abdominal hysterectomy, explain that an indwelling urinary catheter or suprapubic tube as well as a nasogastric tube, may be inserted.
- Institute prophylaxis for deep vein thrombosis as ordered.
- Provide information about estrogen replacement therapy, if appropriate.

POSTTREATMENT CARE

- Administer medications as ordered.
- Provide indwelling urinary catheter or suprapubic catheter care if appropriate.
- Provide regular perineal care.
- Encourage the patient to cough, breathe deeply, and turn at least every 2 hours.
- Administer I.V. fluids as ordered.
- Assess bowel sounds and withhold oral intake until peristalsis returns; then increase diet as ordered.
- Assist with early ambulation.
- Encourage the patient to perform prescribed leg and ankle exercises to prevent venous stasis and to apply sequential compression stockings as ordered.
- Monitor vital signs, intake and output, and heart and lung sounds.
- Assess for complications, such as abnormal bleeding and infection.
- Monitor the surgical wound and dressings and provide care as ordered.
- Assess vaginal drainage color, odor, and amount frequently.

  ⚡ **WARNING** *Notify the practitioner if the patient saturates more than one perineal pad every 4 hours.*

- Administer pain medication as needed and assess for effect.
- Assist with suture or staple removal (usually by the fifth postoperative day) in the patient who underwent an abdominal or laparoscopic hysterectomy.

PATIENT TEACHING

GENERAL

- Review medications, including appropriate use of pain medications, and possible adverse reactions with the patient.
- Instruct the patient to cough, to perform deep-breathing exercises, and to use an incentive spirometer frequently, especially after the abdominal procedure.
- Review the signs and symptoms of infection with the patient and instruct her to notify the practitioner immediately.
- Review the need to notify the practitioner promptly if the patient develops new onset of shortness of breath or chest pain, or warmth, redness, swelling, and tenderness in an extremity.
- If the patient had a vaginal or laparoscopic hysterectomy, instruct her to notify the practitioner immediately if severe cramping, heavy bleeding, or hot flashes occur.
- If the patient had an abdominal hysterectomy, tell her to avoid heavy lifting, rapid walking, or dancing, which can cause pelvic congestion. Encourage her to walk a little more each day and to avoid sitting for prolonged periods. Tell her that she can swim but she should avoid taking tub baths, douching, and sexual activity until after her 6-week follow-up visit.
- Encourage the patient to eat a high-protein, high-residue diet with plenty of fluids, to avoid constipation, which may increase abdominal pressure.
- Explain to the patient and her family that she may feel depressed or irritable temporarily because of abrupt hormonal fluctuations. Encourage the patient to express her feelings with significant others, and instruct family members that calm and understanding responses are most helpful.
- Teach the patient that a period of adjustment to loss of the ability to reproduce and any body image concerns is normal, but that if she experiences significant symptoms of ongoing depression, to talk with the practitioner for treatment options.
- If the patient had a panhysterectomy or radical hysterectomy, instruct her to discuss the potential for exogenous hormonal and calcium supplementation with her practitioner.
- Stress the importance of follow-up care.
- Teach the patient how to care for her incisions as appropriate and reassure her that vaginal sutures are usually absorbed.
- If the patient had an abdominal hysterectomy, explain that urine retention may occur, and to notify the practitioner if she hasn't voided for 8 to 12 hours.

RESOURCES
Organizations
American College of Obstetricians and Gynecologists: *www.acog.org*
American College of Surgeons: *www.facs.org*
American Medical Association: *www.ama-assn.org*

Selected references
Bojahr, B., et al. "Perioperative Complication Rate in 1706 Patients After a Standardized Laparoscopic Supracervical Hysterectomy Technique," *Journal of Minimally Invasive Gynecology* 13(3):183-89, May-June 2006.
Flory, N., et al. "The Psychosocial Outcomes of Total and Subtotal Hysterectomy: A Randomized Controlled Trial," *Journal of Sexual Medicine* 3(3):483-91, May 2006.
Rodriguez, J.F., et al. "The Effect of Performance Feedback on Wound Infection Rate in Abdominal Hysterectomy," *American Journal of Infection Control* 34(4):182-87, May 2006.

Ileoanal reservoir

OVERVIEW

- Forms a rectal pouch from the distal ileum and connects it directly to the anus when total colon removal (colectomy) and rectal lining removal (mucosal proctectomy) is required
- Requires that the rectal muscles and anal sphincter be unimpaired by previous surgery or illness
- Generally a two-stage procedure, may be done via open abdominal incision or laparoscopic incisions
- Ileostomy and pouch created in first stage
- Reanastomosis: occurs in second stage; at this stage ileostomy is reversed
- Performed so that patient can pass stool normally through the anus
- Also known as *ileal pouch-anal anastomosis* or *J-pouch, S-pouch,* or *W-pouch*

INDICATIONS

- Ulcerative colitis
- Familial adenomatous polyposis
- Extensive colorectal carcinoma
- Inflammatory bowel disease

PROCEDURE

STAGE 1

- After the patient receives general anesthesia, the surgeon makes a large midline incision in the abdominal wall, or several smaller incisions for laparoscopic instruments.
- The colon and most of the rectum are removed, leaving all of the small intestine and about 2″ (5 cm) of the rectum intact.
- A J, S, or W pouch is formed with a stapling instrument, using a portion of the distal ileum.
- The rectal mucosa may be removed by ultrasound or by hand before anastomosis of the ileal pouch, but the muscles of the rectum and the underlying anal sphincter muscles are left intact. The end of the pouch is then stapled to the anal tissue.
- A loop of the ileum about 12″ (30 cm) proximal to the pouch is used to

form a stoma after a small incision is made in the abdominal wall, thus diverting the ileal contents to the outside. (See *Ileoanal reservoir.*)

STAGE 2

- Generally performed 3 months after stage 1
- The patient is placed under general anesthesia. The ileum is reanastomosis to form a continuous tract to the pouch and anus either by an open or laparoscopic technique.
- The stoma is allowed to close naturally.

COMPLICATIONS

- Ileus or small-bowel obstruction
- Fluid and electrolyte imbalance
- Skin excoriation
- Pelvic abscess
- Bleeding or leakage from the anastomosis site
- Damage to the anal sphincter, which causes leakage of stool or gas

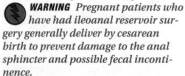 **WARNING** *Pregnant patients who have had ileoanal reservoir surgery generally deliver by cesarean birth to prevent damage to the anal sphincter and possible fecal incontinence.*

- Peritonitis
- Wound infection
- Psychological problems
- Inflammation of pouch
- Erectile dysfunction
- Urinary dysfunction
- Fistula

NURSING DIAGNOSES

- Acute pain
- Disturbed body image
- Ineffective tissue perfusion: GI
- Risk for infection

EXPECTED OUTCOMES

The patient will:
- demonstrate or express feelings of increased comfort
- express feelings about changes in body image
- be free from ileus or bowel obstruction
- show no signs or symptoms of incisional, pelvic, peritoneal, or blood infection.

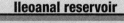

Ileoanal reservoir

A mucosal proctectomy precedes anastomosis of the ileal reservoir. A temporary loop ileostomy diverts effluent for several months.

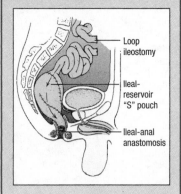

PRETREATMENT CARE

- Explain preoperative and postoperative procedures and equipment to the patient and his family.
- Discuss postoperative analgesia.
- Verify that the patient has signed an appropriate consent form.
- Tell the patient what to expect for fecal drainage and bowel movement control after ileostomy and after reversal of the ileostomy.
- Provide total parenteral nutrition as ordered.
- Administer antibiotics and other medications as ordered.
- Perform bowel preparation as ordered.
- Monitor vital signs, nutritional status, fluid and electrolyte status, intake and output, and daily weight.
- Arrange for the patient to meet with an enterostomal nurse to help explain the care of the temporary ileostomy and mark the abdomen with the best location for the stoma.
- Make sure that the patient doesn't eat or drink anything after midnight before the surgery.

POSTTREATMENT CARE

- Provide meticulous wound care.
- Administer analgesics as ordered.
- Maintain I.V. replacement therapy as ordered
- Keep the nasogastric tube patent but don't reposition it.
- Encourage the patient to express feelings and concerns about either procedure.
- Arrange for a consultation with an enterostomal therapist as appropriate.
- Arrange for the patient to meet with a well-adjusted ostomy patient if possible.
- Monitor vital signs and intake and output.
- Assess for dehydration (poor skin turgor, dry mucous membranes, tachycardia) and electrolyte imbalance.

- Assess appearance of stoma and drainage; assess for skin irritation and excoriation, as appropriate.
- Monitor for signs of infection, peritonitis, or sepsis.
- Encourage coughing and deep-breathing exercises. Encourage splinting of the incision site with a pillow during these exercises as necessary.
- If anastomosis is complete, encourage oral fluid intake and give stool softeners and laxatives as ordered.

⚡ **WARNING** *Monitor for and immediately report signs and symptoms of anastomotic leakage, including low-grade fever, malaise, slight leukocytosis, abdominal distention, tenderness, hemorrhage, hypovolemic shock, and bloody stool or wound drainage.*

PATIENT TEACHING

GENERAL

- Review medications and possible adverse reactions, including reduction or elimination of steroids, with the patient.
- Inform the patient about the ileostomy function, ostomy appliances, and stoma and skin care.
- Instruct the patient how to care for the surgical incision site and the signs and symptoms of infection.
- Reinforce the surgeon's instructions about resuming sexual activities, and provide teaching materials as needed while the ileostomy is in place.
- Stress the importance of adequate fluid intake.
- Advise the patient to avoid use of alcohol, laxatives, or diuretics unless approved by the practitioner.
- Inform the patient about bowel function after the patient has ileostomy closure, including to expect 8 to 10 watery bowel movements day or night initially, and that the pouch and the rectal musculature will develop better control with time, with decreased water in the stool and less frequency of movements (about five during the day, one at night).

- Tell the patient about the signs and symptoms of pouch inflammation (increased numbers of bowel movements, diarrhea, spoilage [especially at night], bleeding, and fatigue) and pelvic abscess or infection (increased temperature, increased abdominal discomfort or distension, abnormal or foul-smelling drainage).
- Tell the patient about other possible complications and when to notify the practitioner.
- Stress the need for regular follow-up care.
- Advise the patient to avoid spicy foods, raw vegetables, caffeine, and foods that causes cause gas after surgery is completed. Tell him that bread, bananas, rice, and bulk-forming supplements, such as Citrucel, may help form firmer stools.
- Refer the patient for nutritional counseling as needed.

RESOURCES
Organizations
American College of Gastroenterology: *www.acg.gi.org*
American Gastroenterological Association: *www.gastro.org*
International Foundation for Functional Gastrointestinal Disorders: *www.iffgd.org*
The Wound, Ostomy and Continence Nurses Society: *www.wocn.org*

Selected references
Beitz, J.M. "Continent Diversions: The New Gold Standards of Ileoanal Reservoir and Neobladder," *Ostomy Wound Management* 50(9):26-35, September 2004.
Hassan, I., et al. "Quality of Life After Ileal Pouch-Anal Anastomosis and Ileorectal Anastomosis in Patients with Familial Adenomatous Polyposis," *Diseases of the Colon and Rectum* 48(11):2032-37, November 2005.
Shen, B., et al. "Clinical Approach to Diseases of Ileal Pouch-Anal Anastomosis," *American Journal of Gastroenterology* 100(12):2796-807, December 2005.

Ileostomy, continent

- Removal of the colon and rectum with creation of an internal reservoir from the terminal ileum
- Contains a one-way valve to prevent fecal material from advancing through the stoma opening
- Fecal drainage achieved by insertion of small tube through the stoma opening into the reservoir
- Alternative to conventional ileostomy
- Also called a *Kock ileostomy* or an *ileal pouch*

INDICATIONS
- Ulcerative colitis
- Familial adenomatous polyposis
- Extensive colorectal cancer
- Crohn's disease (selected patients)

- After the patient receives general anesthesia, the surgeon makes an incision in the abdominal wall.
- The surgeon removes the colon, rectum, and anus, and closes the anus.
- A reservoir is constructed from a loop of the terminal ileum.
- A portion of the ileal reservoir is stapled back onto itself to form a one-way nipple valve.
- The nipple valve is used to create a stoma by pulling it through the abdominal wall and suturing it flush with the skin. (See *Anatomy of a Kock pouch.*)

COMPLICATIONS
- Fistula formation
- Pouch perforation
- Nipple valve dysfunction or slippage
- Abscess
- Bacterial overgrowth in the pouch (pouchitis)
- Hemorrhage
- Sepsis
- Ileus or bowel obstruction
- Fluid and electrolyte imbalance
- Wound infection
- Psychological problems

- Acute pain
- Disturbed body image
- Ineffective tissue perfusion: GI
- Risk for infection

EXPECTED OUTCOMES
The patient will:
- demonstrate or express feelings of increased comfort
- express feelings about change in body image
- be free from ileus or bowel obstruction
- show no signs or symptoms of incisional, pelvic, peritoneal, or blood infection.

Anatomy of a Kock pouch

A Kock pouch is formed by surgically looping part of the distal ileum, stapling the loops together, and opening the inner canals to form a reservoir for the soft, watery stool to be held until catheterized for removal. The nipple valve is formed as shown, by pulling part of the pouch tissue back over the terminal end of the ileum and stapling it closed to reduce the size of the opening and form a canal for the catheter. The length and smaller diameter of the nipple valve prevents waste products from escaping, although some mucus drainage may be expected.

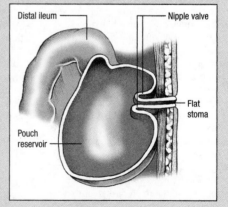

Distal ileum · Nipple valve · Flat stoma · Pouch reservoir

- Explain preoperative and postoperative procedures and equipment to the patient and his family.
- Reinforce and supplement the practitioner's explanation of the procedure and implications for the patient.
- Assess the attitudes of the patient and his family about the surgery and forthcoming changes in the patient's body image.
- Provide encouragement and support.
- Discuss postoperative analgesia.
- Verify that the patient has signed an appropriate consent form.
- Tell the patient what to expect for fecal drainage and bowel movement control for the type of ostomy performed.
- Provide I.V. fluids and total parenteral nutrition as ordered.
- Administer antibiotics and other medications as ordered.
- Monitor vital signs, nutritional status, fluid and electrolyte status, intake and output, and daily weight.

- Provide meticulous wound care.
- Administer analgesics as ordered.
- Administer antibiotics as ordered.
- Maintain I.V. replacement therapy as ordered.
- Keep nasogastric tube patent but don't reposition it.
- Attach the drainage catheter emerging from the ileostomy to continuous gravity drainage.
- Clamp and unclamp the pouch catheter to increase its capacity as ordered.
- Irrigate the catheter, as ordered, to prevent obstruction and allow fluid return by gravity.
- Monitor fluid intake and output.
- Assess the patient for signs and symptoms of bowel obstruction.
- Check the stoma frequently for color, edema, and bleeding.

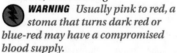 **WARNING** *Usually pink to red, a stoma that turns dark red or blue-red may have a compromised blood supply.*

- Encourage the patient to express his feelings and concerns.
- Arrange for a consultation with an enterostomal therapist to explain care of stoma and associated equipment.
- Arrange for the patient to meet with a well-adjusted ostomy patient if possible.
- Monitor vital signs.
- Assess for dehydration and electrolyte imbalance.
- Assess skin for irritation and excoriation.
- Monitor for signs of infection, peritonitis, or sepsis.

WARNING *Immediately report excessive blood or mucus draining from the stoma, which may indicate hemorrhage or infection.*

- Encourage coughing and deep-breathing exercises. Encourage splinting of the incision as necessary.

GENERAL

- Review medications and possible adverse reactions with the patient.
- Teach the patient about stoma and catheter care and arrange for a consultation; reassure him that follow-up visits with a home care nurse or enterostomal therapist will be arranged to assist with care.
- Reinforce the surgeon's instructions about resuming sexual activities.
- Advise the patient about dietary restrictions to avoid excess gas or other irritation as indicated.
- Stress the importance of a high-fluid intake.
- Advise the patient to avoid use of alcohol, laxatives, and diuretics unless approved by the practitioner.
- Teach the patient about bowel training as indicated during the first 2 to 6 weeks postoperatively.
- Tell the patient about the signs and symptoms of inflammation and infection of the abdominal incision or the bowel itself, and when to call the practitioner.
- Stress the need for regular follow-up care.
- Make sure the patient feels comfortable calling the practitioner, nurse, or other caregivers to ask questions or discuss problems. (See *Care of the continent ileostomy,* page 180.)
- Refer the patient to a local ostomy group.

(continued)

Care of the continent ileostomy

Dear Patient:

These are some instructions to help you care for your continent ileostomy.

PROVIDING STOMA CARE (WITH CATHETER IN PLACE)

◆ Make sure your hands are clean.
◆ Remove the dressing, gently clean the peristomal area with water, and pat dry.
◆ Use skin sealant around the stoma to prevent skin irritation.
◆ Apply a stoma dressing by slipping a precut drain dressing around the catheter.
◆ Cut a hole slightly larger than the lumen of the catheter in the center of a piece of foam.
◆ Disconnect the catheter from the drainage bag and insert the distal end of the catheter through the hole in the foam and slide it onto the dressing. Secure it with Montgomery straps.
◆ Secure the catheter by wrapping the strap ties around it or use a commercial catheter-securing device.
◆ Reconnect the catheter to the drainage bag.
◆ The drainage catheter will be removed by the surgeon when he determines that the suture line has healed.
◆ Assess the peristomal skin for irritation from moisture.

DRAINING THE POUCH

◆ Wash your hands.
◆ Sit on the toilet to be at ease during the procedure.
◆ Remove the stoma dressing.
◆ Relax the abdominal muscles to allow the catheter to slide easily into the pouch.
◆ Lubricate the tip of the drainage catheter tip with the water-soluble lubricant and insert it in the stoma.
◆ Gently push the catheter downward; note the direction of insertion may vary.
◆ When the catheter reaches the nipple valve of the internal pouch or reservoir (after 2″ [5 cm]), you'll feel resistance.
◆ Take a deep breath as you exert gentle pressure on the catheter to insert it through the valve.
◆ If this fails, lie in a supine position and rest for a few minutes, then try again.
◆ Advance the catheter to the suture mark made by the surgeon.
◆ Let the pouch drain completely. It usually takes 5 to 10 minutes, but with thick drainage or a clogged catheter, it may take 30 minutes.
◆ If the tube clogs, irrigate it with 30 ml of water or normal saline solution using the 50-ml catheter-tip syringe.
◆ Rotate and milk the tube, as needed, to continue flow of fecal matter.

◆ If these steps fail, remove, rinse, and reinsert the catheter.
◆ Remove the catheter after completing drainage.
◆ Measure output, subtracting the amount of irrigant used.
◆ Rinse the catheter thoroughly with warm water.
◆ Clean the peristomal area and apply a fresh stoma dressing.

WHAT TO REMEMBER

◆ Never aspirate fluid from the catheter because resulting negative pressure may damage inflamed tissue.
◆ To shorten drainage time, cough, then press gently on the abdomen over the pouch, or suddenly tighten and relax the abdominal muscles.
◆ Keep a record of intake and output to check fluid and electrolyte balance.
◆ Average daily output should be 1,000 ml.
◆ Report low or high output (more than 1,400 ml daily).
◆ Minimize gas pains by chewing food well, limiting talking while eating, and not drinking from a straw.
◆ Walk frequently to reduce gas pain.

RESOURCES

Organizations

American College of Gastroenterology: *www.acg.gi.org*

American Gastroenterological Association: *www.gastro.org*

The Wound, Ostomy and Continence Nurses Society: *www.wocn.org*

Selected references

Burch, J. "The Pre- and Postoperative Nursing Care for Patients with a Stoma," *British Journal of Nursing* 14(6):310-18, March-April 2005.

Delaini, G.G., et al. "Is the Ileal Pouch an Alternative for Patients Requiring Surgery for Crohn's Proctocolitis," *Techniques in Coloproctology* 9(3):222-24, December 2005.

Nessar, G., et al. "Long-term Outcome and Quality of Life After Continent Ileostomy," *Diseases of the Colon and Rectum* 49(3):336-44, March 2006.

Ileostomy, conventional

OVERVIEW

- Removal of colon and rectum
- Forms stoma for external bowel drainage by bringing out the ileum through the abdominal wall

INDICATIONS

- Ulcerative colitis
- Crohn's disease
- Familial adenomatous polyposis
- Extensive colorectal cancer

PROCEDURE

- After the patient receives a general anesthetic, the surgeon makes an incision in the abdominal wall.
- All or part of the colon and rectum (proctocolectomy) is removed.
- A stoma ileostomy is created by bringing the end of the ileum out through a small abdominal incision in the right lower quadrant.

COMPLICATIONS

- Hemorrhage
- Sepsis
- Ileus or bowel obstruction
- Fluid and electrolyte imbalance
- Skin excoriation
- Psychological problems
- Infection

NURSING DIAGNOSES

- Acute pain
- Disturbed body image
- Ineffective tissue perfusion: GI
- Risk for infection

EXPECTED OUTCOMES

The patient will:
- demonstrate or express feelings of increased comfort
- express feelings about changes in body image
- be free from ileus or bowel obstruction
- show no signs or symptoms of incisional, pelvic, peritoneal, or blood infection.

PRETREATMENT CARE

- Explain preoperative and postoperative procedures and equipment to the patient and his family.
- Discuss postoperative analgesia.
- Verify that the patient has signed an appropriate consent form.
- Tell the patient what the stoma will look like and what type of fecal drainage to expect.
- Provide I.V. fluids and total parenteral nutrition as ordered.
- Administer antibiotics and other medications as ordered.
- Monitor vital signs, nutritional status, fluid and electrolyte status, intake and output, and daily weight.

POSTTREATMENT CARE

- Provide meticulous wound care.
- Administer analgesics as ordered.
- Maintain I.V. replacement therapy as ordered
- Keep nasogastric tube patent but don't reposition it.
- Administer antibiotics as ordered.
- Assess the appearance of the stoma and drainage; also assess for skin irritation and excoriation.

    ⚡ **WARNING** *Usually pink to red, a stoma that turns dark red or blue-red may have a compromised blood supply.*

- Encourage the patient to express his feelings and concerns.
- Arrange for a consultation with an enterostomal therapist to further explain care of ileostomy and associated equipment.
- Arrange for the patient to meet with a well-adjusted ostomy patient if possible.
- Monitor vital signs and intake and output.
- Assess for dehydration and electrolyte imbalance.
- Monitor for signs of infection, peritonitis, or sepsis.

    ⚡ **WARNING** *Immediately report if excessive blood or mucus drains from the stoma, which could indicate hemorrhage or infection.*

- Encourage coughing and deep-breathing exercises. Encourage splinting of the incision during coughing or movement as necessary.

PATIENT TEACHING

GENERAL

- Review medications and possible adverse reactions with the patient.
- Teach the patient about the function of the ileostomy.
- Show the patient how to use the ostomy appliances.
- Reinforce the surgeon's instructions about resuming sexual activities.
- Instruct the patient how to care for the stoma and skin.
- Advise the patient about dietary restrictions.
- Stress the importance of a high-fluid intake.
- Advise the patient to avoid use of alcohol, laxatives, and diuretics unless approved by the practitioner.
- Tell the patient about the signs and symptoms of infection and when to notify the practitioner.
- Tell the patient about possible complications.
- Stress the need for regular follow-up care.

RESOURCES

Organizations

American College of Gastroenterology: *www.acg.gi.org*
American Gastroenterological Association: *www.gastro.org*
The Wound, Ostomy and Continence Nurses Society: *www.wocn.org*

Selected references

Burch, J. "The Pre- and Postoperative Nursing Care for Patients with a Stoma," *British Journal of Nursing* 14(6):310-18, March-April 2005.

Sica, J., and Burch, J. "Ileostomy Products: An Overview of Recent Developments," *British Journal of Community Nursing* 9(10):420-24, October 2004.

Turnbull, G.B. "The Issue of Oral Medications and a Fecal Ostomy," *Ostomy Wound Management* 51(3):14, 16, March 2005.

Implantable cardioverter-defibrillator

- Electronic device inserted into the body with electrodes connected to the heart
- Monitors the heart for bradycardia, ventricular tachycardia, and fibrillation; delivers shocks or paced beats when indicated
- Stores information and electrocardiograms (ECGs) and tracks treatments and their outcomes
- Allows information retrieval to evaluate the device's function and battery status and to adjust the settings
- Depending on the model, may deliver bradycardia pacing (both single- and dual-chamber), antitachycardia pacing, cardioversion, and defibrillation (see *Types of ICD therapies*)
- Also called an *ICD*

INDICATIONS

- Cardiac arrhythmias refractory to drug therapy, surgery, or catheter ablation

PROCEDURE

- The transvenous route with fluoroscopy is the most commonly used procedure for ICD placement. The thoracotomy approach may be used for patients who have mediastinal adhesions from previous sternal surgery. The subxiphoid approach may also be used. A median sternotomy may be used if the patient requires other cardiac surgery such as revascularization.
- One or more leadwires are attached to the epicardium.
- A programmable pulse generator is inserted into a pocket made under the right or left clavicle. (See *Location of an ICD*.)
- The device is programmed and checked for proper functioning.

COMPLICATIONS

- Infection
- Venous thrombosis and embolism
- Pneumothorax
- Pectoral or diaphragmatic muscle stimulation
- Arrhythmias
- Cardiac tamponade
- Cardiac arrest
- Myocardial infarction
- Lead dislodgment
- ICD malfunction

NURSING DIAGNOSES

- Activity intolerance
- Decreased cardiac output
- Ineffective tissue perfusion: Cardiopulmonary

EXPECTED OUTCOMES
The patient will:
- carry out activities of daily living without excess fatigue or decreased energy
- maintain adequate cardiac output
- maintain blood pressure and heart rate within normal limits.

Types of ICD therapies

Implantable cardioverter-defibrillators (ICDs) can deliver a range of therapies, depending on the arrhythmia detected and how the device is programmed. Therapies include antitachycardia pacing, cardioversion, defibrillation, and bradycardia pacing. Some newer ICDs can also provide biventricular pacing.

THERAPY	DESCRIPTION
Antitachycardia pacing	A series of small, rapid electrical pacing pulses used to interrupt atrial arrhythmias or ventricular tachycardia and return the heart to its normal rhythm. Antitachycardia pacing isn't appropriate for all patients; it's initiated by the practitioner after appropriate evaluation of electrophysiology studies.
Cardioversion	A low- or high-energy shock (up to 34 joules) that's timed to the R wave to terminate atrial fibrillation or ventricular tachycardia and return the heart to its normal rhythm.
Defibrillation	A high-energy shock (up to 34 joules) to the heart to terminate atrial fibrillation or ventricular fibrillation and return the heart to its normal rhythm.
Bradycardia pacing	Electrical pacing pulses used when the natural electrical signals are too slow. ICD systems can pace one chamber (VVI pacing) of the heart at a preset rate or sense and pace both chambers (DDD pacing).

PRETREATMENT CARE

- Explain the treatment and preparation
- Verify that an appropriate consent form has been signed.
- Obtain baseline vital signs and a 12-lead ECG.
- Evaluate the patient's radial and pedal pulses.
- Assess his mental status.
- Restrict food and fluids before the procedure as ordered.
- Explain postoperative care.
- If the patient is monitored, document and report arrhythmias.
- Administer medications as ordered, and prepare to assist with medical procedures, such as defibrillation, if indicated.

Location of an ICD

To insert an implantable cardioverter-defibrillator (ICD), the cardiologist makes a small incision near the collarbone and accesses the subclavian vein. The leadwires are inserted through the subclavian vein, threaded into the heart, and placed in contact with the endocardium.

The leads are connected to the pulse generator, which is placed under the skin in a specially prepared pocket in the right or left upper chest. (Placement is similar to that used for a pacemaker.) The cardiologist then closes the incision and programs the device.

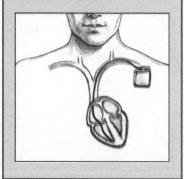

POSTTREATMENT CARE

- Obtain a printed status report verifying the ICD type and model, status (on or off), detection rates, and therapies to be delivered (such as pacing, antitachycardia pacing, cardioversion, and defibrillation).
- Maintain the occlusive dressing for the first 24 hours.
- After the first 24 hours, begin passive range-of-motion exercises if ordered, and progress as tolerated.
- If the patient experiences cardiac arrest, initiate cardiopulmonary resuscitation (CPR) and advanced cardiac life support (wearing latex gloves to avoid experiencing an ICD shock).

> **WARNING** *For external defibrillation, use anteroposterior paddle placement; don't place paddles directly over the pulse generator.*

- Monitor the patient's vital signs, intake and output, heart rate and rhythm, complications, surgical incision and dressings, drainage, and infection.

> **WARNING** *Monitor for signs and symptoms of a perforated ventricle with resultant cardiac tamponade, distant heart sounds, pulsus paradoxus, hypotension accompanied by narrow pulse pressure, increased venous pressure, bulging neck veins, cyanosis, decreased urine output, restlessness, and complaints of fullness in the chest. Notify the practitioner immediately, and prepare the patient for emergency surgery.*

PATIENT TEACHING

GENERAL

- Review medications and possible adverse reactions with the patient.
- Tell the patient about possible complications.
- Tell the patient about the signs and symptoms of infection.
- Instruct the patient to wear a medical identification that indicates placement of an ICD and to always carry information about the ICD.

- Advise the patient to avoid placing excessive pressure over the insertion site.
- Instruct the patient to follow activity restrictions, as directed by the practitioner.
- Inform the patient about what to expect when the ICD discharges and to notify the practitioner after the ICD discharges.
- Tell the patient to inform airline personnel and health care workers who perform diagnostic tests (such as computed tomography scans and magnetic resonance imaging) of the presence of an ICD and possible disruption of the ICD by electrical or electronic devices.
- Stress the need for follow-up care
- Advise the patient about what to do in an emergency, such as calling 911 and having a family member perform CPR if the ICD fails.

RESOURCES
Organizations
American Academy of Family Physicians: *www.aafp.org*
American College of Cardiology: *www.acc.org*
American Heart Association: *www.americanheart.org*

Selected references
Gura, M.T. "Implantable Cardioverter Defibrillator Therapy," *Journal of Cardiovascular Nursing* 20(4):276-87, July-August 2005.
O'Brien, M.C., et al. "Implantable Cardioverter Defibrillator Storm: Nursing Care Issues for Patients and Families," *Critical Care Nursing Clinics of North America* 17(1):9-16, March 2005.
Prystowsky, E.N. "Prevention of Sudden Cardiac Death," *Clinical Cardiology* 28(11 Suppl 1):I12-18, November 2005.

Incision and drainage

◆ Drainage of accumulated pus from an infected area through a surgically created incision
◆ Also called *I & D*

INDICATIONS
◆ Infection that fails to respond to antibiotics
◆ Localized infection

◆ The surgeon anesthetizes the affected area.
◆ If the infection is superficial and ready to rupture, pus may be aspirated with a needle and syringe.
◆ If the area is large, an incision is made directly over the suppurative area, spreading its edges to allow pus to drain.
◆ The area may be irrigated with normal saline solution.
◆ The pus is cultured and allowed to drain.
◆ The cavity is left open to promote healing, or a drainage tube may be placed to continue drainage for 1 to 2 days.
◆ If the cavity is large, it may be packed with gauze.
◆ A sterile dressing is applied.

COMPLICATIONS
◆ Persistent infection

◆ Acute pain
◆ Impaired tissue integrity
◆ Risk for infection

EXPECTED OUTCOMES
The patient will:
◆ verbalize and demonstrate feelings of comfort
◆ demonstrate healing of wound
◆ not show recurrent signs or symptoms of infection.

PRETREATMENT CARE

- Explain the treatment and preparation to the patient.
- Verify that the patient has signed an appropriate consent form.
- Assemble required sterile equipment.
- Label all medications, medication containers, and solutions on and off the sterile field.
- Obtain appropriate specimen tubes for culture samples.
- Prepare the skin with antiseptic solution as ordered.
- Cover the operative area with sterile drapes.
- Provide emotional support.

POSTTREATMENT CARE

- Administer medications as ordered.
- Change the wound dressings as ordered.
- Clean or irrigate the wound as ordered.
- Report complaints of excessive pain.
- Monitor vital signs.
- Assess for systemic infection and localized infection.
- Monitor results of wound culture.
- Assess the appearance and amount of drainage.
- Maintain drainage tube, if present.

PATIENT TEACHING

GENERAL

- Review medications and possible adverse reactions with the patient.
- Inform the patient about the signs and symptoms of infection and when to notify the practitioner.
- Teach the patient how to care for the incision site.
- Teach the patient proper hand-washing techniques.
- Stress the importance of maintaining asepsis.
- Teach the patient how to dispose of soiled dressings properly.
- Stress the need for follow-up care.

RESOURCES

Organizations

American Academy of Pediatrics: *www.aap.org*
American College of Surgeons: *www.facs.org*
American Medical Association: *www.ama-assn.org*

Selected references

Al-Sehly, A.A., et al. "Pediatric Poststernotomy Mediastinitis," *Annals of Thoracic Surgery* 80(6):2314-20, December 2005.

Bona, S., et al. "Minimally Invasive Echoguided Treatment of Gluteal and Deep Muscular Abscesses: An Effective Option for an Old Problem," *Academic Emergency Medicine* 13(3):359-360, March 2006.

Puccio, F., et al. "Primary Retroperitoneal Abscess Extending to the Calf," *Archives of Surgery* 140(12):1230-31, December 2005.

Insulin pump

- External device that delivers insulin continuously under the surface of the skin
- Keeps blood glucose levels as close to normal as possible
- Has a reservoir that contains only fast-acting insulin
- Provides lifestyle flexibility—for traveling, exercising, working, or eating—without worry of injections and when insulin will take effect
- Also called *continuous subcutaneous insulin infusion*

INDICATIONS
- Diabetes mellitus

- A small soft cannula (called an *infusion set*) is inserted under the skin of the patient's abdomen, thigh, or leg. (Usually the patient requires 12 insertions per month.)
- The infusion set is connected to the insulin pump.
- The pump is programmed according to the patient's needs. The basal rate (a continuous preprogrammed rate) is usually 40% to 50% of the total daily dose of insulin. There may be several different basal rates throughout a 24-hour period based on activity patterns, hormonal changes, and other factors that affect the insulin needs.
- Bolus rates are programmed by the user to compensate for eating. This is usually a pre-meal bolus dose given around the time of a meal or snack.
- The pump is clipped to the patient's clothing for easy access.

COMPLICATIONS
- Pump malfunction resulting in hypoglycemia or hyperglycemia
- Skin site infection

- Deficient fluid volume
- Imbalanced nutrition: Less than body requirements
- Risk for infection

EXPECTED OUTCOMES
The patient will:
- maintain adequate fluid volume as evidenced by adequate intake and output
- maintain optimum body weight
- show no signs or symptoms of skin site infection.

PRETREATMENT CARE

◆ Review the information about the procedure and the functioning of the pump.
◆ Verify that an appropriate consent form has been signed.

POSTTREATMENT CARE

◆ Monitor vital signs.
◆ Monitor blood glucose levels.
◆ Make sure the pump is functioning properly and assess the patency of the infusion set.
◆ Watch for complications.

PATIENT TEACHING

GENERAL

◆ Review the operation of the pump with the patient and supply him with manuals and available resources.
◆ Give the patient the vendor information for contact information.
◆ Tell the patient that the pump gives a precise dose of insulin based on his current needs, as established by his practitioner. Reinforce the need to follow set guidelines for safety purposes.
◆ Tell the patient to follow good nutrition and exercise habits, test blood glucose levels frequently, and how to make decisions about how much insulin to take for the food.
◆ Review diabetes education with the patient as indicated.
◆ Teach the patient and his family about signs and symptoms of hypoglycemia and hyperglycemia. Review emergency measures if such complications should occur.
◆ Teach the patient and his family about signs and symptoms of infection at the infusion insertion sites. Encourage him to change infusion sites as instructed.
◆ Teach the patient about insulin needs during illness or stress.
◆ Reinforce appropriate follow-up care. Arrange for the patient to consult with a diabetes educator, if available.

RESOURCES
Organizations
The American Diabetes Association: *www.diabetes.org*
American Medical Association: *www.ama-assn.org*
Diabetes Services, Inc., Diabetes Mall: *www.diabetesnet.com*

Selected references
Fisher, L.K., and Halvorson, M. "Future Developments in Insulin Pump Therapy: Progression from Continuous Subcutaneous Insulin Infusion to a Sensor-Pump System," *Diabetes Educator* 32(1):47S-52S, January-February 2006.
Low, K.G., et al. "Insulin Pump Use in Young Adolescents with Type 1 Diabetes: A Descriptive Study," *Pediatric Diabetes* 6(1):22-31, March 2005.
Wittlin, S.D. "Treating the Spectrum of Type 2 Diabetes: Emphasis on Insulin Pump Therapy," *Diabetes Educator* 32(1):39S-46S, January-February 2006.

Intra-aortic balloon counterpulsation

- Temporarily supports the heart's left ventricle by mechanically displacing blood by an intra-aortic balloon attached to an external pump console
- Increases the supply of oxygen-rich blood to the myocardium and decreases myocardial oxygen demand
- Also used to monitor myocardial perfusion and the effects of drugs on myocardial function and perfusion
- Usually inserted through the common femoral artery and positioned with its tip just distal to the left subclavian artery
- Also called *IABC*

INDICATIONS

- Low cardiac output disorders
- Refractory angina
- Ventricular arrhythmias
- Cardiogenic shock
- Cardiac instability
- Myocardial infarction
- High-grade lesions
- Support measures
- Bypass surgery
- Angioplasty
- Cardiac catheterization

- Before the physician inserts the balloon, he puts on sterile gloves, a gown, and a mask, cleans the site with povidone-iodine solution, and covers the area with a sterile drape.

INSERTING THE INTRA-AORTIC BALLOON PERCUTANEOUSLY

- The physician may insert the balloon percutaneously through the femoral artery into the descending thoracic aorta, using a modified Seldinger technique.
- He accesses the vessel with an 18G angiography needle, removes the inner stylet, passes the guide wire through the needle, and then removes the needle.
- An introducer (dilator and sheath assembly) is passed over the guide wire into the vessel until 1″ (2.5 cm) remains above the insertion site.
- The inner dilator is removed, leaving the introducer sheath and guide wire in place.
- After passing the balloon over the guide wire into the introducer sheath, the physician advances the catheter into position, ⅜″ to ¾″ (1 to 2 cm) distal to the left subclavian artery under fluoroscopic guidance.
- The balloon is then attached to the control system to start counterpulsation.

INSERTING THE INTRA-AORTIC BALLOON SURGICALLY

- The surgeon may decide to insert the catheter through a femoral arteriotomy.
- After making an incision and isolating the femoral artery, the surgeon attaches a Dacron graft to a small opening in the arterial wall and passes the catheter through this graft.
- Using fluoroscopic guidance, he advances the catheter up the descending thoracic aorta and positions the catheter tip between the left subclavian and renal arteries.

- The Dacron graft is sewn around the catheter at the insertion point and the other end is connected to the pump console.
- If the balloon can't be inserted through the femoral artery, the surgeon may use the transthoracic method and insert it in an antegrade direction through the anterior wall of the ascending aorta.
- He positions it ⅜″ to ¾″ beyond the left subclavian artery and brings the catheter out through the chest wall.

COMPLICATIONS

- Arterial embolism
- Extension or rupture of an aortic aneurysm
- Femoral or iliac artery perforation
- Femoral artery occlusion
- Sepsis
- Bleeding at the insertion site

- Decreased cardiac output
- Ineffective breathing pattern
- Ineffective tissue perfusion: Cardiopulmonary

EXPECTED OUTCOMES

The patient will:

- maintain adequate cardiac output
- maintain adequate breathing pattern as evidenced by oxygen saturation and respiratory rate within normal limits
- maintain hemodynamic stability as evidenced by blood pressure and heart rate within normal limits.

PRETREATMENT CARE

- Depending on facility policy, you or a perfusionist must balance the pressure transducer in the external pump console and calibrate the oscilloscope monitor to ensure accuracy.
- Tell the patient that the physician will place a special balloon catheter in his aorta to help his heart pump more easily.
- Let the patient know that the balloon will be removed after his heart can resume an adequate workload.
- Explain the insertion procedure; mention that the catheter will be connected to a large console next to the patient's bed.
- Verify that the patient has signed an appropriate consent form.
- Record the patient's baseline vital signs and hemodynamic results, if available.
- Monitor the electrocardiogram (ECG) continuously in lead II.
- Obtain a baseline 12-lead ECG.
- Provide oxygen, as needed.
- Maintain and monitor arterial line and pulmonary artery catheter.
- Insert an indwelling urinary catheter; monitor intake and output.
- Assess the patient's left arm and peripheral leg pulses and document sensation, movement, color, and temperature of the arm and legs.
- Give the patient a sedative as ordered.

WARNING Have a defibrillator, suction, temporary pacemaker, and emergency drugs readily available in case the patient develops complications, such as an arrhythmia, during insertion.

POSTTREATMENT CARE

WARNING If the control system malfunctions or becomes inoperable, don't let the balloon catheter remain dormant for more than 30 minutes. Inflate the balloon manually until another control system is available.

- Verify correct balloon placement with chest X-ray.
- Assess and record pedal and posterior tibial pulses as well as color, sensation, and temperature in the affected limb every 15 minutes for 1 hour and then hourly.

WARNING Notify the practitioner immediately if circulatory changes occur; the balloon may need to be removed.

- Monitor the patient's arm pulses, arm sensation and movement, and arm color and temperature every 15 minutes for 1 hour after balloon insertion; repeat every 2 hours while the balloon is in place. (See *Interpreting intra-aortic balloon waveforms,* page 192.)

WARNING Loss of left arm pulses may indicate upward balloon displacement. Notify the practitioner of changes in left-arm pulse.

- Monitor intake and output.
- Monitor laboratory test results.
- Monitor vital signs every 15 minutes to 1 hour, according to facility policy and patient condition.
- Watch for signs of bleeding, especially at the insertion site.
- Adjust heparin drip according to protocol to maintain partial thromboplastin time (PTT) at 1½ to 2 times the normal value; monitor PTT according to facility policy.
- Measure pulmonary artery pressure and pulmonary artery wedge pressure (PAWP) every 1 or 2 hours.

WARNING A rising PAWP reflects preload, signaling increased ventricular pressure and workload; notify the practitioner if this occurs. Some patients require I.V. nitroprusside (Nipride) during intra-aortic balloon counterpulsation to reduce preload and afterload.

WEANING THE PATIENT FROM INTRA-AORTIC BALLOON COUNTERPULSATION

- Assess hemodynamic status.
- To begin weaning, gradually decrease the frequency of balloon augmentation to 1:2 and 1:4, as ordered.
- Assist frequency is usually maintained for 1 hour or longer, depending on facility policy. If the patient's hemodynamic status remain stable during this time, weaning may continue.

WARNING Don't leave the patient on a low augmentation setting for more than 2 hours to prevent embolus formation.

- Assess the patient's tolerance of weaning.

WARNING Notify the practitioner immediately if the patient shows signs of hemodynamic instability.

REMOVING THE INTRA-AORTIC BALLOON

- If the balloon was inserted surgically, the surgeon closes the Dacron graft and sutures the insertion site. If the balloon was inserted percutaneously, the cardiologist usually removes the catheter.
- Make sure PTT is within normal limits before the balloon is removed to prevent hemorrhage at insertion site.
- Turn off the control system and disconnect the connective tubing from the catheter to ensure balloon deflation.
- The practitioner withdraws the balloon until the proximal end of the catheter contacts the distal end of the introducer sheath.
- The practitioner then applies pressure below the puncture site and removes the balloon and introducer sheath as a unit, allowing a few seconds of free bleeding to prevent thrombus formation.
- To promote distal bleed-back, apply pressure above the puncture site for 30 minutes or until bleeding stops, if facility policy permits. (Sometimes this is the practitioner's responsibility.)

(continued)

Interpreting intra-aortic balloon waveforms

During intra-aortic balloon counterpulsation, you can use electrocardiogram and arterial pressure waveforms to determine whether the balloon pump is functioning properly.

NORMAL INFLATION-DEFLATION TIMING

Balloon inflation occurs after aortic valve closure; deflation, during isovolumetric contraction, occurs just before the aortic valve opens. In a properly timed waveform such as the one shown at right, the inflation point lies at or slightly above the dicrotic notch. Both inflation and deflation cause a sharp V. Peak diastolic pressure exceeds peak systolic pressure; peak systolic pressure exceeds assisted peak systolic pressure.

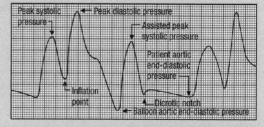

EARLY INFLATION

With early inflation, the inflation point lies before the dicrotic notch. Early inflation dangerously increases myocardial stress and decreases cardiac output.

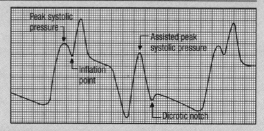

EARLY DEFLATION

With early deflation, a U shape appears and peak systolic pressure is less than or equal to assisted peak systolic pressure. This won't decrease afterload or myocardial oxygen consumption.

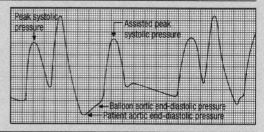

LATE INFLATION

With late inflation, the dicrotic notch precedes the inflation point, and the notch and the inflation point create a W shape. This can lead to a reduction in peak diastolic pressure, coronary and systemic perfusion augmentation time, and augmented coronary perfusion pressure.

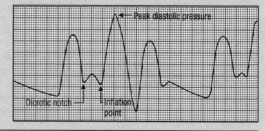

LATE DEFLATION

With late deflation, peak systolic pressure exceeds assisted peak systolic pressure. This threatens the patient by increasing afterload, myocardial oxygen consumption, cardiac workload, and preload. It occurs when the balloon has been inflated for too long.

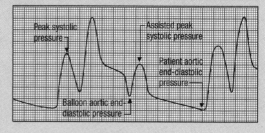

- After balloon removal, provide wound care according to facility policy.
- Monitor and record the patient's pedal and posterior tibial pulses and the color, temperature, and sensation of the affected limb.
- Enforce bed rest, with the head of the bed elevated no more than 30 degrees, usually for 24 hours.
- Change the dressing at the balloon insertion site every 24 hours or as needed, using strict sterile technique.

PATIENT TEACHING

GENERAL
- Reinforce the practitioner's explanation of the procedure, the reason for the pump, and potential complications as needed; and tell the patient and his family about the nursing care provided.
- Inform the patient about positioning and movement restrictions.
- Teach the patient and his family to report changes in alertness or thinking; unexplained sweating; chest, back, or abdominal pain; shortness of breath; feeling or becoming faint; new mass in the abdomen; change in color, sensation, or temperature of an extremity; bleeding anywhere; or feverishness to the nurse or practitioner immediately.

RESOURCES
Organizations
American College of Cardiology:
  www.acc.org
American Heart Association:
  www.americanheart.org

Selected references
Ellis, T.C., et al. "Therapeutic Strategies for Cardiogenic Shock, 2006," *Current Treatment Options in Cardiovascular Medicine* 8(1):79-94, February 2006.
Vohra, H.A., and Dimitri, W.R. "Elective Intraaortic Balloon Counterpulsation in High-Risk Off-Pump Coronary Artery Bypass Grafting," *Journal of Cardiac Surgery* 21(1):1-5, January-February 2006.

In vitro fertilization and embryo transfer

- Procedure in which one or more mature oocytes are laparoscopically removed from the woman's ovary, fertilized with sperm, and transferred into the woman's uterus
- Performed about 40 hours after fertilization
- Ideally, one or more of the zygotes implant in the uterus
- Also called *IVF-ET*

INDICATIONS

- Infertility as the result of damaged or blocked fallopian tubes
- Oligospermia
- Cervical mucus that's unable to allow sperm to travel from the vagina into the uterus
- Endometriosis
- Pelvic adhesions
- Male infertility
- Ovulatory dysfunction

- Before the procedure, the patient is given fertility medication to stimulate the production of mature ova.
- During ovulation, the patient receives local or general anesthesia, depending on the technique used.
- After the ovaries have been determined to be ready for IVF-ET, laparoscopy is used to visualize and aspirate fluid containing the eggs from the ovarian follicles. Alternatively, guided ultrasound may be used to visualize the ovarian follicles and guide a needle through the back of the vagina to retrieve fluid and eggs from the ovarian follicles.
- The collected eggs are placed in a test tube or laboratory dish containing a culture medium for 3 to 6 hours and monitored by an embryologist.
- Sperm from the patient's partner or donor is added to the dish.
- Two days after fertilization, the embryo is transferred into the patient's uterus through a fine plastic catheter, where it may implant and establish a pregnancy.
- A maximum of four pre-embryos are transferred to the uterus for possible implantation. The patient has an option to freeze unused pre-embryos for later use; other options include donation or disposal.

COMPLICATIONS

- Unsuccessful implantation
- Bleeding, perforation of organs, or gas pains with laparoscopy
- Medication reaction
- Multiple pregnancy
- Emotional stress

- Acute pain
- Anxiety
- Decisional conflict (fertilization)

EXPECTED OUTCOMES

The patient will:

- express relief of pain
- verbalize feelings of decreased anxiety
- demonstrate positive feelings related to procedure.

PRETREATMENT CARE

- Obtain a history and make sure a physical examination has been completed.
- The patient should have undergone thorough infertility testing; make sure results of testing are obtained.
- Explain the procedure to the patient and answer any questions she may have.
- Verify that a consent form has been signed.
- Explain that an ovulation drug, such as clomiphene (Clomid) or menotropin (Pergonal), is given before the procedure. About the tenth day of the menstrual cycle, the ovaries are examined, and when the size of the follicles appears to be mature, the patient is given an injection of human chorionic gonadotropin. This hormone causes ovulation to occur within 38 to 42 hours. The IVG-ET procedure is then performed.

POSTTREATMENT CARE

- Monitor vital signs.
- Provide assurance and support.
- Pregnancy can be confirmed using blood tests about 13 days after egg aspiration. Pregnancy can be confirmed by ultrasound 30 to 40 days after aspiration.

PATIENT TEACHING

GENERAL

- Review all procedures and their purpose with the patient.
- Review medication administration, dosage, and possible adverse effects, with the patient.
- Tell the patient what to expect during and after the procedure.
- Advise the patient to be sedentary for 24 hours following pre-embryo placement in the uterus. Tell her to avoid strenuous exercises, such as jogging, horseback riding, or swimming, until pregnancy is confirmed.

RESOURCES
Organizations
American Board of Obstetrics and Gynecology: *www.abog.org*
American Medical Association: *www.ama-assn.org*
Georgia Reproductive Specialists: *www.ivf.com*

Selected references
Blennborn, M., et al. "The Couple's Decision-Making in IVF: One or Two Embryos at Transfer?" *Human Reproduction* 20(5):1292-97, May 2005.
Fisher-Jeffes, L.J., et al. "Parents' Concerns Regarding Their ART Children," *Reproduction* 131(2):389-94, February 2006.
Mitchell, A., et al. "A Survey of Nurses who Practice in Infertility Settings," *Journal of Obstetric, Gynecologic, and Neonatal Nursing* 34(5):561-68, September-October 2005.

Iridectomy and iridotomy

- Iridectomy: removal of a small full-thickness piece of the iris either surgically or by laser
- Iridotomy: formation of a small hole in the iris by a laser
- Both procedures performed to reduce the level of fluid pressure in the affected eye by opening normal channels of perfusion
- Iridectomy: also known as *corectomy*
- Iridotomy: also known as *laser peripheral iridotomy*

INDICATIONS
Iridectomy
- Angle-closure glaucoma
- Melanoma of the iris
- Pre-cataract surgery

Iridotomy
- Angle-closure or narrow-angle glaucoma
- Nanophthalmos (small eyes)
- Malignant glaucoma

SURGICAL IRIDECTOMY
- The patient receives general anesthesia.
- An incision is made in the cornea just below the iris and a piece of the iris is removed. The incision in the cornea is self-sealing. (See *Surgical iridectomy.*)

LASER IRIDECTOMY AND IRIDOTOMY
- The patient is seated in a special chair that has a frame with a chin rest for his head.
- Anesthetic eye drops are instilled.
- When the eye is numb and the patient positioned correctly, a special magnification lens is placed on the eye. Then the ophthalmologist directs the laser beam to either make a hole in the iris or remove a small portion of the iris.
- Argon lasers have photocoagulation capabilities and are used initially when patients have many blood vessels in the area from other disease processes or have bleeding tendencies. The Nd:YAG laser, however, is more precise and is used for the actual procedure in most cases.

COMPLICATIONS
Surgical iridectomy
- Infection
- Bleeding
- Scarring
- Continued increased intraocular pressure (IOP)
- Formation of a cataract

Laser iridotomy or iridectomy
- Anterior uveitis
- Bleeding
- Scarring
- Failure of the iridotomy hole to remain open over time
- Increased IOP
- Retinal perforation (rare)
- Rupture of the lens capsule
- Opacification of anterior lens
- Swelling of or damage to the cornea
- Macular edema

- Glare or double vision if the area isn't fully covered by the eyelid

- Acute pain
- Disturbed sensory perception (visual)
- Risk for infection

EXPECTED OUTCOMES
The patient will:
- express and demonstrate feelings of increased comfort
- regain accurate visual function
- demonstrate intact postsurgical eye tissue without signs or symptoms of infection.

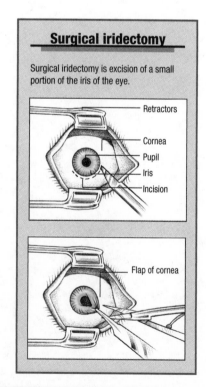

Surgical iridectomy

Surgical iridectomy is excision of a small portion of the iris of the eye.

Retractors
Cornea
Pupil
Iris
Incision

Flap of cornea

PRETREATMENT CARE

- Explain preprocedure and postprocedure nursing care to the patient and his family.
- Verify that an informed consent form has been signed.
- Instruct the patient having a laser procedure that fasting beforehand isn't required.
- Instruct the patient having a surgical iridectomy to avoid eating or drinking for 8 hours before the procedure.
- A sedative may be given to help the patient relax.
- Encourage the patient and his family to express concerns related to the procedure.
- Give corticosteroid eye drops, antibiotic eye drops, and pressure-reducing eye drops as ordered.

POSTTREATMENT CARE

- Monitor the patient's vital signs.
- Monitor the patient for pain.
- Assess and monitor vision changes, such as blurriness, double vision, or other complaints.
- Repeat administration of corticosteroid eye drops, antibiotic eye drops, and pressure-reducing eye drops as ordered.
- Maintain eye shield as ordered.
- Assist the practitioner in hourly IOP checks as ordered.

PATIENT TEACHING

GENERAL

- Review all procedures and treatments with the patient.
- Emphasize proper eye care and hand-washing.
- Tell the patient with a laser procedure that he can go to work the next day and resume other activities with no restrictions, but must continue corticosteroid drops for 1 week as ordered, and may experience some cloudy vision for 1 or 2 days.
- Tell the patient who had a surgical iridectomy that he must wear a patch over the affected eye for several days, must use drops to minimize the risk of infection and reduce inflammation or discomfort as ordered, and may have blurred or cloudy vision for a few weeks after the procedure with full healing in about 6 weeks.
- Inform the patient that he will need follow-up appointments with the ophthalmologist in 1 week and then as prescribed.
- Inform the patient who underwent an iridectomy for angle-closure glaucoma that for the long term, he must continue using eye drops to lower IOP, and have periodic reevaluations by the ophthalmologist.
- Inform the patient with melanoma of the iris that regular eye examinations for tumor recurrence and possible spread to the liver will be needed. Tell him that sunlight and other sources of ultraviolet light, if seen without protective lenses, may increase his risk of recurrence.
- Teach the patient signs and symptoms of possible complications, and when to contact the practitioner.

RESOURCES

Organizations

American Academy of Ophthalmology: *www.aao.org*
Glaucoma Research Foundation: *www.glaucoma.org*
National Eye Institute: *www.nei.nih.gov*

Selected references

Johnson, G.J., and Foster, P.J. "Can We Prevent Angle-Closure Glaucoma?" *Eye* 19(10):1119-24, October 2005.
Spaeth, G.L., et al. "The Effects of Iridotomy Size and Position on Symptoms Following Laser Peripheral Iridotomy," *Journal of Glaucoma* 14(5):364-67, October 2005.
Yamamoto, Y., et al. "Demonstration of Aqueous Streaming Through a Laser Iridotomy Window Against the Corneal Endothelium," *Archives of Ophthalmology* 124(3):387-93, March 2006.

Joint replacement, hand

OVERVIEW

- Total replacement of joint in the hand with a synthetic prosthesis; new joint commonly composed of silicone rubber or the patient's own tissues such as a portion of tendon
- Restores joint mobility and stability and relieves pain
- Also called *arthroplasty*

INDICATIONS

- Rheumatoid arthritis
- Degenerative joint disorders
- Extensive joint trauma
- Psoriatic arthritis
- Osteoarthritis

PROCEDURE

- The patient is placed in a lateral decubitus position and receives regional or general anesthesia.
- An incision is made to expose the joint.
- The capsule is incised or excised as indicated.
- The joint is dislocated to expose the surfaces, then it's reshaped to accept the prosthesis.
- The device is secured in place. Polymethylmethacrylate adhesive may be used to secure the device if the prosthesis is cemented.
- With hand and wrist joint replacement, the fusion of the joint closest to the fingertip may be done. This procedure relieves pain and only minimally compromises hand function due to lack of motion at this joint.
- Joint replacement is commonly performed in the second joint from the fingertip. Surgery of the index finger isn't recommended because it must endure sideway forces that accompany movements. Silicone rubber joints may be used to provide stability, which have a flexible hinge in the middle and stems at the ends.
- With thumb basal joint replacement, the natural material that's used in a ligament reconstruction procedure is used. The patient's own tendon stabilizes the thumb and resurfaces the joint; providing stability and pain relief. It's also called the *tendon roll* because the tendon used is curled to form the new joint cushion.

COMPLICATIONS

- Infection
- Nerve compromise
- Prosthesis slippage, breakage, or loosening
- Scar tissue formation
- Thrombophlebitis

NURSING DIAGNOSES

- Acute pain
- Dressing or grooming self-care deficit
- Impaired physical mobility
- Ineffective tissue perfusion: Peripheral

EXPECTED OUTCOMES

The patient will:
- express and demonstrate feelings of increased comfort
- demonstrate improved ability for self-care before discharge
- attain the highest degree of mobility possible within the confines of the disorder
- exhibit pink, warm fingers, and adequate radial pulse on the affected side.

PRETREATMENT CARE

- Explain the procedure and patient preparation.
- Verify that the patient has signed an appropriate consent form.
- Explain postoperative care and hand precautions.
- Reassure the patient that analgesics will be available postoperatively as needed.
- Provide emotional support.
- Make sure that a physical examination and a X-ray of the joints has been completed as well as any blood testing ordered.
- The surgeon or member of the surgical team must mark the affected extremity before surgery.

POSTTREATMENT CARE

- Administer medications as ordered.
- Help the patient get out of bed and ambulate without using the affected extremity.
- Assess the patient's pain level and provide analgesics as ordered.
- Reinforce exercises and precautions taught by the physical therapist as needed.
- Encourage coughing and deep-breathing exercises.
- Encourage adequate fluid intake.
- Monitor vital signs, lung sounds, and intake and output.
- Assess for signs and symptoms of infection.
- Monitor the neurovascular status of the affected extremity.
- Monitor wound dressing.
- Arrange rehabilitation requirements as appropriate.
- Provide assistance in self-care as appropriate.

PATIENT TEACHING

GENERAL

- Review medications and possible adverse reactions with the patient.
- Tell the patient about the signs and symptoms of infection, and to notify the practitioner promptly.
- Teach the patient the signs and symptoms of prosthesis slippage, loosening, or breakage, and to notify the practitioner promptly.
- Teach the patient that the dressing will be removed in the surgeon's office visit in about 3 days, and the sutures removed in about 10 days.
- Instruct the patient to follow the prescribed exercise regimen and hand safety precautions as ordered in order to maximize recovery of function.
- Show the patient how to care for the postoperative splint as appropriate.
- Educate the patient about rehabilitation expectations.

RESOURCES

Organizations

American Academy of Orthopaedic Surgeons: *www.orthoinfo.aaos.org/*
American College of Rheumatology: *www.rheumatology.org*
Arthritis Foundation: *www.arthritis.org*

Selected references

Minami, A., et al. "A Long-Term Follow-Up of Silicone-Rubber Interposition Arthroplasty for Osteoarthritis of the Thumb Carpometacarpal Joint," *Hand Surgery* 10(1):77-82, July 2005.

Parkkila, T., et al. "Comparison of Swanson and Sutter Metacarpophalangeal Arthroplasties in Patients with Rheumatoid Arthritis: A Prospective and Randomized Trial," *The Journal of Hand Surgery* 30(6):1276-81, November 2005.

Sharp, J.T., et al. "Measurement of Joint Space Width and Erosion Size," *Journal of Rheumatology* 32(12):2456-61, December 2005.

Joint replacement, hip

OVERVIEW

- Total or partial replacement of the hip joint with a synthetic prosthesis consisting of two major parts: the acetabular cup and femoral stem
- Newer techniques for minimally invasive surgery: two-incision or mini-incision
- Restores joint mobility and stability and relieves pain

INDICATIONS

- Osteoarthritis
- Rheumatoid arthritis
- Trauma
- Avascular necrosis
- Ankylosing spondylitis

PROCEDURE

- General or regional (spinal) anesthesia is administered.
- The surgeon removes the head of the femur, exposing the marrow cavity of the femur's shaft.
- The femoral component of the prosthesis is inserted into the cavity so that its head articulates with the acetabular cup.
- The acetabular cup is attached to the pelvic bones.
- A cemented or noncemented technique is used. (See *Total hip replacement*.)

CEMENTED TECHNIQUE

- The surgeon cements the head of the prosthesis into a position that allows articulation with a studded cup.
- The studded cup is then cemented into the deepened acetabulum.

NONCEMENTED TECHNIQUE

- In a porous-coated prosthesis, the smooth metal surface is studded with metal beads and sprayed with a bone-stimulating material.
- The coated beads are designed to stimulate bone growth between the beads to hold the prosthesis in place.

COMPLICATIONS

- Hip fracture or dislocation
- Stroke
- Myocardial infarction
- Fat embolism
- Infection
- Hypovolemic shock
- Pulmonary edema
- Arterial thrombosis
- Pseudoaneurysm
- Hematoma
- Fracture of the joint cement
- Displaced prosthetic head
- Heterotrophic ossification (mainly in men

NURSING DIAGNOSES

- Acute pain
- Impaired physical mobility
- Risk for infection

EXPECTED OUTCOMES

The patient will:

- express feelings of increased comfort
- attain the highest degree of mobility possible within the confines of the disorder
- be free from signs and symptoms of infection.

PRETREATMENT CARE

- Explain the treatment and preparation to the patient and his family.
- Make sure the patient has signed an appropriate consent form.
- Explain postoperative care.
- Make sure the patient's medical history and physical examination, laboratory studies, and diagnostic tests are completed; report abnormal results.
- Check for a history of allergies.
- Make sure blood typing and cross-matching is completed; verify if blood is to be kept on hold for the patient.
- The affected limb must be marked by someone from the surgical team before surgery.

POSTTREATMENT CARE

- Administer medications as ordered.
- Administer I.V. fluids as ordered.
- Transfuse blood products as ordered.
- Maintain bed rest for the prescribed period, then assist with exercises.
- Maintain hip in proper alignment, using a triangular abduction pillow.

⚡ **WARNING** *Stay alert for and report signs and symptoms of dislocation; these include sudden, severe pain; shortening of the involved leg; and external leg rotation.*

- Reposition the patient frequently.
- Encourage frequent coughing and deep-breathing exercises.
- Assess for complications, such as infection and abnormal bleeding.
- Monitor neurovascular status distal to the operative site.
- Monitor the surgical wound, dressings, and drainage.
- Monitor vital signs and pulse oximetry.

⚡ **WARNING** *Watch for and immediately report early clinical changes that may indicate fat embolism syndrome, including altered*

Total hip replacement

To form a totally artificial hip, the surgeon cements a femoral head prosthesis in place to articulate with a cup, which he then cements into the deepened acetabulum. He may avoid using cement by implanting a prosthesis with a porous coating that promotes bony ingrowth.

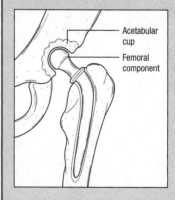

Acetabular cup

Femoral component

Adjusting to a total hip replacement

Dear Patient:

Your new artificial hip should eliminate hip pain and help you get around better. But go easy at first.

    To give your hip time to heal and to avoid too much stress on it, follow these "do's and don'ts" for the next 3 months or for as long as your health care provider orders.

DO'S

◆ Sit only in chairs with arms that can support you when you get up. When you want to stand up, first ease to the edge of your chair. Place your affected leg in front of the unaffected one, which should be well under your chair. Now, grip the chair's arms firmly, and push up with your arms—not with your legs. You should be supporting most of your weight with your arms and your unaffected leg.

◆ Wear your support stockings (except when you're in bed at night).

◆ Keep your affected leg facing forward, whether you're sitting, lying down, or walking.

◆ Exercise regularly as ordered. Stop exercising immediately, however, if you feel severe hip pain.

◆ Lie down and elevate your feet and legs if they swell after walking.

◆ Obtain a raised toilet seat for use at home, and use public toilets designated for the disabled.

◆ Turn in bed only as directed.

◆ Place a pillow between your legs when you lie on your side and when you go to bed at night. (This keeps your leg from twisting and dislodging your new hip.)

◆ Sit on a firm pillow when riding in a car, and keep your affected leg extended.

DON'TS

◆ Don't lean far forward to stand up.
◆ Don't sit on low chairs or couches.

◆ Don't reach far when picking up objects or tying your shoes.
◆ Don't cross your legs or turn your hip or knee inward or outward.
◆ Don't scrub your hip incision.
◆ Don't take tub baths.
◆ Don't lift heavy items.
◆ Don't have sexual intercourse until your health care provider says you can.
◆ Don't play tennis, run, jog, or do other strenuous activities.
◆ Don't drive a car until your health care provider gives you permission.
◆ Don't reach to the end of the bed to pull the blankets up.

WHAT TO REPORT

◆ Redness, swelling, or warmth around your incision
◆ Drainage from your incision
◆ Fever or chills
◆ Severe hip pain uncontrolled by prescribed pain medicine
◆ Sudden sharp pain and a clicking or popping sound in your joint
◆ Leg shortening, with your foot turning outward
◆ Loss of control over leg motion or complete loss of leg motion

AN IMPORTANT PRECAUTION

You'll need to take an antibiotic just before dental procedures (other than routine fillings), any surgery, and some diagnostic procedures.

---

level of consciousness, tachypnea, dyspnea, elevated temperature without other cause, and tachycardia.
◆ Consult with physical therapy.
◆ Arrange for rehabilitation as appropriate.

PATIENT TEACHING

GENERAL
◆ Reinforce physical therapy teaching.
◆ Teach the patient about the signs and symptoms of infection.
◆ Inform the patient about possible complications.
◆ Teach the patient how to care for the incision site.
◆ Teach the patient the signs and symptoms of joint dislodgment.
◆ Stress the need for follow-up care.
◆ Teach the patient the signs and symptoms of deep vein thrombosis and pulmonary embolism.
◆ Stress the importance of maintaining hip abduction.
◆ Instruct the patient to avoid flexing his hips more than 90 degrees when rising from a bed or chair.
◆ Teach the patient the proper use of crutches or a cane. (See *Adjusting to a total hip replacement.*)

RESOURCES
Organizations
American Academy of Orthopaedic Surgeons: *www.orthoinfo.aaos.org/*
American College of Rheumatology: *www.rheumatology.org*
Arthritis Foundation: *www.arthritis.org*

Selected references
Kalra, S., et al. "Intracapsular Hip Fractures in End-Stage Renal Failure," *Injury* 37(2):175-84, February 2006.
Ostergaard, M., et al. "Magnetic Resonance Imaging in Rheumatoid Arthritis Advances and Research Priorities," *Journal of Rheumatology* 32(12):2462-64, December 2005.
Persson, P.E., et al. "Do Non-Steroidal Anti-Inflammatory Drugs Cause Endoprosthetic Loosening? A 10-Year Follow-Up of a Randomized Trial on Ibuprofen for Prevention of Heterotopic Ossification After Hip Arthroplasty," *Acta Orthopaedica* 76(6):735-40, December 2005.

Joint replacement, knee

OVERVIEW

- Total or partial replacement of a knee joint with a synthetic prosthesis
- Restores joint mobility and stability and relieves pain

INDICATIONS

- Severe chronic arthritis
- Degenerative joint disorders
- Extensive joint trauma
- Joint contractures
- Conditions that prohibit full extension or flexion

PROCEDURE

- General anesthesia is administered.
- The orthopedic surgeon makes an incision over the affected knee.
- After the patella is moved, the prosthesis is placed, with adjustments made to the femur, tibia, and undersurface of the patella.
- Bone cement is used to secure the prosthesis, then the area is sutured closed with a surgical drain in place.

COMPLICATIONS

- Infection
- Hypovolemic shock
- Fat embolism
- Thromboembolism
- Pulmonary embolism
- Nerve compromise
- Prosthesis dislocation or loosening
- Heterotrophic ossification
- Avascular necrosis
- Atelectasis
- Pneumonia
- Deep vein thrombosis (DVT)

NURSING DIAGNOSES

- Acute pain
- Impaired physical mobility
- Risk for infection

EXPECTED OUTCOMES

The patient will:

- express feelings of increased comfort
- attain the highest degree of mobility possible within the confines of injury
- be free from signs and symptoms of infection.

PRETREATMENT CARE

- Explain the treatment and patient preparation.
- Verify that the patient has signed an appropriate consent form.
- Explain postoperative care.
- Reassure the patient that analgesics will be available as needed.
- Provide emotional support.
- The affected limb must be marked by someone from the surgical team before the procedure.

POSTTREATMENT CARE

- Administer medications as ordered.
- Maintain bed rest for the prescribed period.
- Maintain the affected joint in proper alignment.
- Assess the patient's pain level and provide analgesics as ordered.
- Change dressings as ordered.
- Reposition the patient frequently.
- Encourage frequent coughing and deep-breathing exercises.
- Encourage adequate fluid intake.
- Exercise the affected joint as ordered.
- If joint displacement occurs, notify the practitioner.
- If traction is used to correct joint displacement, periodically check the weights and other equipment.
- Monitor vital signs and intake and output.
- Assess for complications, such as infection and abnormal bleeding.
- Monitor the surgical wound, dressings, and drainage.
- Assess respiratory status.
- Monitor neurovascular status of the affected extremity.
- Use continuous passive motion (CPM) device as instructed.

PATIENT TEACHING

GENERAL

- Review medications and possible adverse reactions with the patient.
- Tell the patient about the signs and symptoms of infection.
- Teach the patient the signs and symptoms of joint dislodgment.
- Tell the patient about possible complications.
- Teach the patient how to care for the incision site.
- Stress the need for follow-up care.
- Teach the patient the signs and symptoms of DVT and pulmonary embolism.
- Instruct the patient to follow the exercise program prescribed by the practitioner and the physical therapist, including using a CPM device as ordered.
- Tell the patient to wear anti-embolism stockings or inflatable pneumatic compression stockings as ordered.
- Instruct the patient to use the incentive spirometry device hourly.
- Instruct the patient to follow the activity restrictions as directed by the practitioner. Tell him to avoid contact sports, but that he can perform low-impact activities, such as swimming and golf, after he has recovered from surgery.

RESOURCES

Organizations

American Academy of Orthopaedic Surgeons: *www.orthoinfo.aaos.org*
American College of Rheumatology: *www.rheumatology.org*
Arthritis Foundation: *www.arthritis.org*

Selected references

Campbell, D.G., et al. "Patellar resurfacing in total knee replacement: A Ten-Year Randomised Prospective Trial," *The Journal of Bone and Joint Surgery, British Volume* 88(6):734-39, June 2006.

Jeong, G.K., et al. "Floating Total Knee": Ipsilateral Periprosthetic Fractures of the Distal Femur and Proximal Tibia After Total Knee Arthroplasty," *Journal of Arthroplasty* 21(1):138-40, January 2006.

Quintana, J.M., et al. "Health-Related Quality of Life and Appropriateness of Knee or Hip Joint Replacement," *Archives of Internal Medicine* 23:166(2):220-26, January 2006.

Joint replacement, shoulder

OVERVIEW

- Total or partial replacement of shoulder joint with synthetic prosthesis
- Restores joint mobility and stability and relieves pain

INDICATIONS
- Degenerative joint disorders
- Extensive joint trauma
- Osteoarthritis
- Rheumatoid arthritis
- Charcot's arthropathy

PROCEDURE

- General or local anesthesia is administered.
- The surgeon makes an incision and the area is exposed.
- Total shoulder replacement involves replacing the arthritic joint surfaces with a highly polished metal ball that's attached to a stem and a plastic socket.
- If the bone is soft, bone cement may be used. In most patients, an all-plastic glenoid component is implanted with bone cement.
- In some cases, the surgeon may replace only the ball, for example when the shoulder is severely fractured and the socket is normal.
- Reverse total shoulder replacement (the socket and metal ball are switched) is used for patients who have completely torn rotator cuffs and severe arthritis (cuff tear arthropathy), or patients who previously had a shoulder replacement that failed.
- In reverse total shoulder replacement, the metal ball is attached to the shoulder bone and a plastic socket is attached to the humerus, thereby allowing the use of the deltoid muscle instead of the torn rotator cuff to lift the arm.
- After replacement, the surgeon sutures the area closed and may leave a surgical drain in place.

COMPLICATIONS
- Infection
- Fat embolism
- Thromboembolism
- Pulmonary embolism
- Nerve compromise
- Prosthesis dislocation or loosening
- Heterotrophic ossification
- Avascular necrosis
- Pneumonia
- Deep vein thrombosis (DVT)
- Fracture
- Biceps tendon rupture

NURSING DIAGNOSES

- Acute pain
- Dressing and grooming self-care deficit
- Impaired physical mobility
- Ineffective tissue perfusion: Peripheral

EXPECTED OUTCOMES
The patient will:
- express feelings of increased comfort
- demonstrate improved self-care before discharge
- attain the highest degree of mobility possible within the confines of injury
- exhibit adequate tissue perfusion and pulses distally.

PRETREATMENT CARE

◆ Explain the treatment and patient preparation.
◆ Verify that the patient has signed an appropriate consent form.
◆ Explain postoperative care.
◆ Reassure the patient that analgesics will be available as needed.
◆ Provide emotional support.
◆ The affected limb must be marked by someone from the surgical team before the procedure.

POSTTREATMENT CARE

◆ Administer medications as ordered.
◆ Maintain the affected joint in proper alignment.
◆ Assess the patient's pain level and provide analgesics as ordered.
◆ Change dressings as ordered.
◆ Reposition the patient frequently.
◆ Encourage frequent coughing and deep-breathing exercises.
◆ Encourage adequate fluid intake.
◆ Exercise the affected joint as ordered.
◆ If joint displacement occurs, notify the practitioner.
◆ Monitor vital signs and intake and output.
◆ Assess for complications such as infection.
◆ Monitor the surgical wound, dressings, and drainage.
◆ Monitor respiratory status.
◆ Assess neurovascular status of the affected extremity.
◆ Arrange for rehabilitation care as appropriate.

PATIENT TEACHING

GENERAL
◆ Review medications and possible adverse reactions with the patient.
◆ Tell the patient about the signs and symptoms of infection.
◆ Teach the patient the signs and symptoms of joint dislodgment.
◆ Tell the patient about possible complications.
◆ Teach the patient how to care for the incision site.
◆ Stress the need for follow-up care.
◆ Teach the patient the signs and symptoms of DVT and pulmonary embolism.
◆ Tell the patient to follow the exercise regimen and activity restrictions prescribed by the practitioner.
◆ Instruct the patient to perform range-of-motion exercises and to use a pulley device as instructed by physical therapy.
◆ Stress the importance of keeping the affected arm in a sling as ordered.
◆ Tell the patient not to use the affected arm to push up in bed or from a chair.
◆ Tell the patient not to place his arm in an extreme position, such as straight out to the side or behind his body for the first 6 weeks after surgery.

RESOURCES
Organizations
American Academy of Orthopaedic Surgeons: *www.orthoinfo.aaos.org*
American College of Rheumatology: *www.rheumatology.org*
Arthritis Foundation: *www.arthritis.org*

Selected references
Keller, J., et al. "Glenoid Replacement in Total Shoulder Arthroplasty," *Orthopedics* 29(3):221-26, March 2006.
Lin, J.S., et al. "Effectiveness of Replacement Arthroplasty With Calcar Grafting and Avoidance of Greater Tuberosity Osteotomy for the Treatment of Humeral Surgical Neck Nonunions," *Journal of Shoulder and Elbow Surgery* 15(1):12-18, January-February 2006.
Pfahler, M., et al. "Hemiarthroplasty Versus Total Shoulder Prosthesis: Results of Cemented Glenoid Components," *Journal of Shoulder and Elbow Surgery* 15(2):154-63, March-April 2006.

Laparoscopy

- Allows examination of the pelvic and abdominal cavity—via a laparoscope (endoscope) inserted through abdominal wall near umbilicus—and repair or removal of diseased or injured structures
- Also called *pelvic peritoneoscopy*

INDICATIONS

- Repair or removal of diseased or injured structures or organs
- Certain abdominal surgical procedures such as cholecystectomy
- Tubal ligation
- Ovarian cyst aspiration
- Graafian follicle aspiration
- Cauterization of endometrial implants (endometriosis)
- Lysis of adhesions
- Oophorectomy
- Salpingectomy
- Laparoscopic-assisted hysterectomy
- Pediatric biliary atresia

PROCEDURE

- The patient receives local or general anesthesia.
- The patient is placed in the lithotomy position.
- A needle is inserted below the umbilicus, and carbon dioxide is infused into the pelvic cavity.
- An infra-umbilical incision is made, and a trocar and cannula are inserted.
- The trocar is removed, and the laparoscope is inserted through the cannula.
- The pelvic cavity is visualized, and additional instruments are inserted through a second small incision close to the infraumbilical incision, or they may be passed through the laparoscope.
- The cannula is removed.
- The incisions are sutured, and dressings applied.

COMPLICATIONS

- Infection
- Hemorrhage
- Other complications associated with the specific procedure performed

NURSING DIAGNOSES

- Acute pain
- Ineffective tissue perfusion: GI
- Risk for infection

EXPECTED OUTCOMES

The patient will:

- demonstrate or express feelings of increased comfort
- regain normal bowel function
- be free from signs and symptoms of infection.

PRETREATMENT CARE

- Explain the treatment and preparation.
- Verify that an appropriate consent form has been signed.
- Explain postoperative care.
- Restrict food and fluids as ordered.
- Obtain and document laboratory test results and report abnormal findings to the practitioner.

POSTTREATMENT CARE

- Administer medications as ordered.
- Assess for abdominal pain, abdominal cramps, and shoulder pain.
- Provide comfort measures.
- Explain that bloating or abdominal fullness and shoulder pain from laparoscopy will subside as the carbon dioxide gas is absorbed.
- Monitor the patient's vital signs, intake and output, complications, abnormal bleeding, surgical wound and dressings, drainage, and for signs of possible infection.

PATIENT TEACHING

GENERAL

- Review medications and possible adverse reactions with the patient.
- Tell the patient to perform coughing and deep-breathing exercises.
- Instruct the patient to use an incentive spirometer.
- Teach the patient how to care for the incision site.
- Inform the patient about the signs and symptoms of infection.
- Tell the patient about possible complications.
- Instruct the patient to follow the activity restrictions as directed by the practitioner.
- Stress the need for follow-up care. (See *Learning about laparoscopy.*)

RESOURCES

Organizations

American Academy of Pediatrics: *www.aap.org*

American Board of Obstetrics and Gynecology: *www.abog.org*

American College of Surgeons: *www.facs.org*

American Society of Colon and Rectal Surgeons: *www.ascrs.affiniscape.com*

Selected references

Bax, N.M. "Laparoscopic Surgery in Infants and Children," *European Journal of Pediatric Surgery* 15(5):319-24, October 2005.

Cothren, C.C., et al. "Can We Afford to do Laparoscopic Appendectomy in an Academic Hospital?" *American Journal of Surgery* 190(6):950-54, December 2005.

Galli, B., et al. "Laparoscopic Radical Nephrectomy in Renal Cell Carcinoma," *Urological Nursing* 25(2):83-86, 133, April 2005.

Learning about laparoscopy

Dear Patient:

Your health care provider has scheduled you for a laparoscopy. This procedure lets him see your reproductive and abdominal organs through a slender, telescope-like instrument. Laparoscopy allows for diagnosis and, sometimes, treatment of your disorder during the same procedure.

Laparoscopy takes about 1 hour. It's performed in the operating room, and you'll probably receive a general anesthetic. Usually, you can go home the same day.

GETTING READY

Beforehand, a few routine laboratory tests will be done to assess your general health. These tests include a complete blood count, blood chemistry studies, and urinalysis.

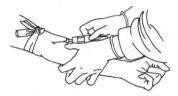

Because you'll be receiving an anesthetic, don't eat or drink anything after midnight on the night before the procedure. If you're a smoker, don't smoke for about 12 hours before surgery. Remove eye makeup and nail polish beforehand.

DURING THE PROCEDURE

When the anesthetic takes effect, the surgeon will make a small incision in the lower part of your navel. Then he'll insert a needle through the incision and inject carbon dioxide or nitrous oxide into your pelvic area. This inflates the area. It creates a viewing space by lifting the abdominal wall away from the organs below.

Next, the surgeon will insert a thin, flexible, optical instrument called a laparoscope through the incision. This instrument magnifies the view of your organs.

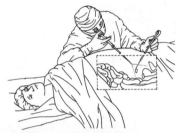

REMOVING IMPLANTS AND ADHESIONS DURING LAPAROSCOPY

If the laparoscopic findings confirm endometriosis, the surgeon may decide to remove the implants and adhesions.

To remove them, the surgeon will make a second, smaller incision just above your pubic hairline. Then he'll insert a special instrument for moving your internal organs aside. He may also insert a blunt instrument called a cannula through your vagina and into your uterus to move your uterus. The implants and adhesions will be removed by inserting instruments through the laparoscope.

Next, the surgeon will release the gas through the incision and remove the laparoscope. Then he'll close the incision and apply an adhesive bandage.

AFTER THE PROCEDURE

After laparoscopy, you'll go to the postanesthesia care unit, where nurses will monitor you until you're fully alert. If necessary, you'll receive an analgesic for minor discomfort in the incisional area when the anesthetic wears off. Expect vaginal bleeding similar to a menstrual period for a few days.

TIPS FOR RECOVERY

When you get home, keep these points in mind:

◆ Wait until the day after surgery to remove your bandage and to bathe or shower.

◆ Eat lightly because some gas will remain in your abdomen; you'll probably belch or feel bloated for 1 or 2 days.

◆ Take acetaminophen (Tylenol) or ibuprofen to relieve shoulder pain. Called *referred pain,* this results from the remaining gas in your abdomen, which can irritate your diaphragm and cause a pain in your shoulders.

◆ Expect to resume your normal activities after 1 or 2 days, but avoid strenuous work or sports for 1 week.

◆ Resume sexual activity when the bleeding stops or when your health care provider gives approval.

WHEN TO CALL YOUR HEALTH CARE PROVIDER

In rare instances, a laparoscopy may be complicated by infection, hemorrhage, or a burn or a small cut on an organ. Call your health care provider if you experience any of the following:

◆ a fever of 100.4° F (38° C) or higher
◆ persistent or excessive vaginal bleeding
◆ severe abdominal pain
◆ redness, puffiness, or drainage from your incision
◆ nausea, vomiting, or diarrhea.

Laparotomy

- Surgical incision made into the abdominal wall
- Called an *exploratory laparotomy* when extent of abdominal injury or disease unknown

INDICATIONS
- Examination of the pelvic cavity
- Repair or removal of diseased or injured structures
- Extensive surgical repair
- Pelvic conditions untreatable by laparoscopy
- Resection of ovarian cysts containing endometrial tissue
- Identification and removal of ectopic pregnancy

- The patient receives general anesthesia.
- An abdominal incision is made, and the abdominal cavity is explored.
- Necessary repairs or excisions are made.
- The incision is sutured, and a sterile dressing is applied.

COMPLICATIONS
- Infection
- Hemorrhage
- Other complications associated with the specific procedure performed

- Acute pain
- Ineffective tissue perfusion: GI
- Risk for infection

EXPECTED OUTCOMES
The patient will:
- demonstrate or express feelings of increased comfort
- regain normal bowel function as evidenced by normal bowel movements
- be free from signs and symptoms of infection.

PRETREATMENT CARE

- Explain the treatment and preparation.
- Verify that an appropriate consent form has been signed.
- Explain postoperative care.
- Restrict food and fluids as ordered.
- Obtain and document laboratory results and report abnormal findings to the practitioner.

POSTTREATMENT CARE

- Administer medications as ordered.
- Assess for abdominal pain.
- Provide comfort measures.
- Monitor the patient's vital signs, intake and output, complications, abnormal bleeding, surgical wound and dressings, drainage, and for signs of possible infection.

PATIENT TEACHING

GENERAL

- Review medications and possible adverse reactions with the patient.
- Tell the patient to perform coughing and deep-breathing exercises.
- Instruct the patient to use an incentive spirometer.
- Teach the patient how to care for the incision site.
- Inform the patient about the signs and symptoms of infection.
- Tell the patient about possible complications.
- Instruct the patient to follow the activity restrictions as directed by the practitioner.
- Stress the need for follow-up care.

RESOURCES

Organizations

American Society of Colon and Rectal Surgeons: *www.ascrs.affiniscape.com*
Gynecologic Surgery Society: *www.gynecologicsurgerysociety.org*

Selected references

Ertekin, C., et al. "Unnecessary Laparotomy by Using Physical Examination and Different Diagnostic Modalities for Penetrating Abdominal Stab Wounds," *Emergency Medical Journal* 22(11): 790-94, November 2005.

Shaver, S.M., and Shaver, D.C. "Perioperative Assessment of the Obstetric Patient Undergoing Abdominal Surgery," *Journal of Perianesthesia Nursing* 20(3):160-66, June 2005.

Laryngectomy

OVERVIEW

- Partial or complete surgical removal of the larynx
- May be performed with other treatments for cancer, such as radiation therapy or chemotherapy
- Total laryngectomy: entire larynx removed, along with any affected surrounding structures such as the lymph nodes
- Partial laryngectomy: performed if small tumor; usually, one vocal chord removed

INDICATIONS

- Cancer
- Relieve symptoms associated with cancer

PROCEDURE

- General anesthetic is administered.

ENDOSCOPIC RESECTION

- The surgeon places an endoscope into the patient's throat.
- He inserts surgical instruments through the endoscope to remove the cancer or laser the affected tissues away. The laser, similar to a scalpel, can cut through tissue, but causes less bleeding.

PARTIAL LARYNGECTOMY

- In this procedure, part of the larynx is removed and at least part of one vocal cord is kept so that the patient's retains the ability to speak, but his voice may be hoarse or weak.
- There are several different types of partial laryngectomy, depending on the location of the cancer:
- Cordectomy removes the vocal cords only
- Supraglottic laryngectomy removes the supraglottis only
- Hemilaryngectomy removes half of the larynx; retaining the patient's voice
- Partial laryngectomy removes portion of the larynx; helping retain the patient's ability to speak.

TOTAL LARYNGECTOMY

- This procedure involves the removal of the entire larynx with the formation of a permanent stoma.
- If the patient has nodes larger than 1 cm, a neck dissection may be done in which all the lymph nodes on the affected side are removed. The sternocleidomastoid, internal jugular vein, and accessory nerve may also be removed if the lymph nodes adjacent to them are cancerous. Because the accessory nerve controls shoulder movement, the shoulder may be stiff and difficult to move after surgery. If the muscle is removed, the patient's neck might appear thinner and sunken on the affected side over time.

COMPLICATIONS

- Infection
- Hemorrhage (ruptured carotid artery)
- Edema
- Aspiration
- Fistula
- Tracheostomy stenosis
- Neurovascular injury
- Complications from anesthesia

- Impaired gas exchange
- Ineffective breathing pattern
- Ineffective tissue perfusion: Cardio-pulmonary

EXPECTED OUTCOMES
The patient will:
- maintain adequate ventilation as evidenced by arterial blood gas levels within normal limits
- exhibit normal breathing pattern
- maintain tissue perfusion as evidenced by blood pressure and cardiac rhythm within normal limits.

- Make sure that diagnostic testing has been completed and documented and any abnormal findings reported to the practitioner; this may include physical examination of the throat and neck, laryngoscopy, endoscopy with tissue samples and lymph nodes taken for biopsy, computer tomography or magnetic resonance imaging scan, biopsy, or barium swallow.
- Tell the patient what to expect postoperatively, such as a feeding tube, neck edema, drains to help reduce the swelling, attachment to a ventilator, and the inability to speak.

- Arrange a visit with a patient who has undergone a laryngectomy.
- Arrange for the speech language pathologist to meet the patient and his family before surgery.
- Help the patient choose a temporary way to communicate, such as writing, alphabet board, or sign language.
- Verify that a consent form has been signed.

- Monitor vital signs and intake and output.
- Assess respiratory status; suction patient as indicated; assess breath sounds and pulse oximetry; monitor response to ventilator settings; and assist with weaning as indicated.
- Make sure there's a spare tracheotomy tube at the bedside that's the same size as the patient's tube.
- Monitor for bleeding and edema at wound site; assess for wound dehiscence; and monitor dressings and drainage.
- Keep the head of bed elevated as ordered.
- Provide tracheostomy care.
- Maintain patency of I.V. tubes; administer fluids as ordered.
- Help the patient turn and perform deep-breathing exercises to help mobilize secretions in the lungs. Suction the patient as indicated.
- Maintain patency of nasogastric (NG) tube; begin tube feedings or parenteral therapy as ordered.
- Provide mouth care.
- Assess for pain and effect of pain medication.
- Provide emotional support; keep call bell within reach and provide a means of communication for the patient. (See *Alternative speech methods.* See also *Learning to communicate without speech,* page 212.)
- Monitor laboratory test results and report any abnormal results to the practitioner.

Alternative speech methods

During convalescence, your patient may work with a speech pathologist, who can teach him new ways to speak using various communication techniques—some of which are outlined below.

ESOPHAGEAL SPEECH

By drawing air in through the mouth, trapping it in the upper esophagus, and releasing it slowly while forming words, the patient can again communicate by voice. With training and practice, a highly motivated patient can master esophageal speech in about 1 month. Recognize that speech will sound choppy at first, but with increasing skill, words will flow more smoothly and understandably.

Because esophageal speech requires strength, an elderly patient or one with asthma or emphysema may find it too physically demanding to learn. And because it also requires frequent sessions with a speech pathologist, a chronically ill patient may find learning esophageal speech overwhelming.

ARTIFICIAL LARYNGES

The throat vibrator and the Cooper-Rand device are basic artificial larynges. Both types vibrate to produce speech that's easy to understand, although it sounds monotonous and mechanical.

Tell the patient to operate a throat vibrator by holding it in place against his neck. A pulsating disk in the device vibrates the throat tissue as the patient forms words with his mouth. The throat vibrator may be difficult to use immediately after surgery, when the patient's neck wounds are still sore.

The Cooper-Rand device vibrates sounds piped into the patient's mouth through a thin tube, which the patient positions in the corner of his mouth. Easy to use, this device may be preferred soon after surgery.

SURGICALLY IMPLANTED PROSTHESES

Most surgical implants generate speech by vibrating when the patient manually closes the tracheostomy, forcing air upward. One such device is the Blom-Singer voice prosthesis. Only hours after it's inserted through an incision in the stoma, the patient can speak in a normal voice. The surgeon may implant the device when radiation therapy ends or within a few days (or even years) after laryngectomy.

To speak, the patient covers his stoma while exhaling. Exhaled air travels through the trachea, passes through an airflow port on the bottom of the prosthesis, and exits through a slit at the esophageal end of the prosthesis. This creates the vibrations needed to produce sound.

Not all patients are eligible for tracheoesophageal puncture, the procedure needed to insert the prosthesis. Considerations include the extent of the laryngectomy, pharyngoesophageal muscle status, stoma size and location, and the patient's mental and emotional status, visual and auditory acuity, hand-eye coordination, bimanual dexterity, and self-care skills.

(continued)

Learning to communicate without speech

Dear Caregiver:

As the person in your care weakens, his speech may become impaired. To prevent isolation, you'll need to find new ways for him to communicate, such as by lip-reading or using a communication board or a talking computer. Whichever method you choose, begin to practice it with the person before he must rely on it totally.

GENERAL POINTERS

◆ Ask simple questions that require a yes-or-no answer. For example, ask, "Would you like to sit outside now?" rather than, "What do you feel like doing this afternoon?"

◆ Try to anticipate the person's needs so you can communicate more efficiently. Pay attention to nonverbal cues. For instance, if he looks bored or depressed while watching television, suggest a game of cards or a visit with a neighbor to cheer him up.

◆ Don't put words in the person's mouth. Give him the opportunity to express himself in his own way, even if it takes more time.

LIP-READING

Lip-reading is one of the most effective ways to communicate without speech; however, it will take you time and effort to learn. Here are some tips to make lip-reading easier:

◆ Make sure that the person who is lip-speaking has his face in the light so you can see well.

◆ Tell the person in your care to pause after forming each word with his lips. Then repeat the word aloud to make sure that you understood him. If you can't make out the word, ask him to spell it by forming each letter with his lips.

◆ Watch the person's gestures and facial expressions to get clues.

◆ Keep a pen and paper handy.

COMMUNICATION BOARDS

With a communication board, a person can express his thoughts by pointing to words, letters, pictures, or phrases on the board. Communication boards come in various forms, including manual versions and ones that operate on a home computer.

When using a communication board:

◆ Make sure that the person can see it clearly.

◆ Decide how the person will identify the figure or character on the board. If he can't lift his arm to point, perhaps you can point for him. Alternatively, think about getting a special pointer that requires only slight hand or arm movement.

◆ Talk to a speech pathologist, who can help you decide which board best suits the person's needs and teach you both how to use it.

TALKING COMPUTERS

If you own or wish to purchase a home computer, you may want to investigate "talking software." These programs provide a mechanical voice for the person, who controls the program through a computer keyboard. Ask your speech specialist for information.

PATIENT TEACHING

GENERAL
♦ Tell the patient that he won't be able to smell aromas, blow his nose, whistle, gargle, or sip or suck on a straw.
♦ Arrange for home care nursing and speech therapy referrals.
♦ Teach the patient and caregiver how to care for the permanent tracheostomy as indicated, how to perform care and cleaning of the stoma, and how to provide humidification and oxygenation.

RESOURCES

Organizations
American Cancer Society:
  www.cancer.org
International Association of Laryngectomees: *www.larynxlink.com*
National Cancer Institute:
  www.cancer.gov

Selected references
Al-Fattah, H.A., et al. "Partial Laser Arytenoidectomy in the Management of Bilateral Vocal Fold Immobility: A Modification Based on Functional Anatomical Study of the Cricoarytenoid Joint," *Otolaryngology—Head and Neck Surgery* 134(2):294-301, February 2006.
Dobbins, M., et al. "Improving Patient Care and Quality of Life After Laryngectomy/Glossectomy," *British Journal of Nursing* 14(12):634-40, June-July 2005.
Rodriguez, C.S., et al. "Pain Measurement in Older Adults with Head and Neck Cancer and Communication Impairments," *Cancer Nursing* 27(6):425-33, November-December 2004.

Laser eye surgery: keratectomy

OVERVIEW

- Laser-assisted in-situ keratomileusis (LASIK): corrects vision by changing the curvature of the cornea
- Recovery normally quick with fewer adverse effects and complications than other methods of vision correction
- Significant improvement in vision common soon after surgery
- Newer technique: *wavefront-guided LASIK*, involving special mapping of small irregularities in the patient's cornea and customizing of the laser shaping procedure to correct these defects

INDICATIONS

- Low to high levels of nearsightedness, farsightedness, and astigmatism

PROCEDURE

- The area around the eyes is draped with a sterile towel and anesthetic eye drops are applied. When the eye is completely numb, an eyelid holder is placed between the eyelids to keep the patient from blinking.
- A special ring is applied to the eye and suction pressure is applied.
- A microkeratome is used to create a hinged flap of thin corneal tissue, which is suctioned open with the ring and then removed.
- The patient looks directly at a target light while the laser reshapes the cornea. The protective layer is folded back into place. (See *Laser keratectomy.*)
- For the patient who's nearsighted, the surgeon makes the steep cornea flatter by removing tissue from the cornea's center, thus moving the point of focus from in front of the retina to directly on the retina. Similarly, for the patient who's farsighted, the surgeon makes the flat cornea steeper by removing tissue outside of the central optical zone, thus moving the point of focus from behind the retina to directly on the retina.
- For the patient with astigmatism, the cornea is made more spherical, thus eliminating multiple focusing points within the eye.
- After the procedure, the patient's eyes are examined with a slit lamp microscope and an eye shield is applied.

COMPLICATIONS

- Infection
- Failure of treatment

NURSING DIAGNOSES

- Anxiety
- Disturbed sensory perception (visual)
- Risk for injury

EXPECTED OUTCOMES

The patient will:

- demonstrate decreased anxiety
- regain visual function
- experience no postsurgical injury to the eye.

Laser keratectomy

A microkeratome is used during laser-assisted in-situ keratomileusis surgery to create a hinged flap of corneal tissue. This tissue is folded out of the way until the procedure is completed. The tissue is then folded back into place where it adheres by itself without sutures.

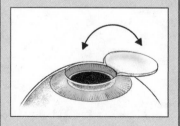

PRETREATMENT CARE

◆ Explain the treatment and preparation to the patient and his family.
◆ Verify that the patient had a baseline visual evaluation and refraction before the procedure and, if he's a contact lens wearer, hasn't worn his lenses for at least 2 weeks before the baseline examination for soft lenses, 3 weeks for rigid gas permeable or toric soft lenses, or 4 weeks for hard lenses; nor worn them since the examination.
◆ Make sure the patient has signed an appropriate consent form.
◆ Verify that the patient isn't wearing eye makeup, lotions, perfume, or creams, and the eyelids and lashes have been washed.
◆ Explain that a protective shield may be placed over the eye postoperatively.
◆ Explain that, immediately after surgery, his eye may feel itchy, burning, watery, or as if a foreign body is in it; however, he must avoid rubbing the eye because rubbing can result in dislodging the flap and injuring the surgical area.
◆ Inform the patient that his vision may be blurry and he may see halos or starbursts around lights and he may also be sensitive to glare for a few days.
◆ Make sure the patient has someone to drive him home after the procedure.
◆ Administer a sedative or an osmotic agent, as ordered, to reduce intraocular pressure.

POSTTREATMENT CARE

◆ Instill corticosteroid eyedrops or topical antibiotics as ordered.
◆ Assess for pain and administer analgesics as ordered.
◆ Help the patient lie on his back or the unaffected side.
◆ Keep the head of the bed flat or slightly elevated as ordered.
◆ Assist the patient with ambulation.
◆ Keep all personal items within the patient's field of vision.
◆ Monitor vital signs.
◆ Inform the patient about the postsurgical follow-up appointment in 24 to 48 hours.

⚡ **WARNING** *Immediately report sudden, sharp, or excessive pain; bloody, purulent, or clear viscous drainage; and fever.*

PATIENT TEACHING

GENERAL
◆ Review medications and possible adverse reactions with the patient.
◆ Emphasize the need for follow-up care.
◆ Instruct the patient to avoid eye makeup for 1 to 2 weeks after the procedure, not to engage in sports for about 3 days, to avoid strenuous or contact sports for about 1 month, and to avoid swimming, whirlpools, and hot tubs for about 8 weeks depending on his practitioner's follow-up instructions.
◆ Advise the patient to take precautions for photophobia, such as avoiding bright sunlight and wearing protective sunglasses.
◆ Emphasize the importance of using an eye shield when sleeping for about 1 month.
◆ Tell the patient to avoid driving until approved by the practitioner.
◆ Advise the patient to immediately report sudden, sharp, or excessive pain; bloody, purulent, or clear viscous drainage; and fever to his practitioner.

RESOURCES
Organizations
American Academy of Ophthalmology: *www.aao.org*
American Society of Ophthalmic Plastic and Reconstructive Surgery: *www.asoprs.org*
U.S. Food and Drug Administration, Centers for Devices and Radiological Health, LASIK Eye Surgery: *www.fda.gov/cdrh/LASIK/default.htm*

Selected references
Brilakis, H.S., and Holland, E.J. "Anterior Stromal Puncture in the Treatment of Loose Epithelium after LASIK," *Journal of Refractive Surgery* 22(1):103-105, January-February 2006.
Noda-Tsuruya, T., et al. "Autologous Serum Eye Drops for Dry Eye After LASIK," *Journal of Refractive Surgery* 22(1):61-66, January-February 2006.

Laser eye surgery: keratectomy, photorefractive

OVERVIEW

- Photorefractive keratectomy (PRK): uses the Excimer laser to correct vision by reshaping the cornea
- Difference between laser in-situ keratomileusis (LASIK) and PRK: in PRK, epithelium is removed and laser applied to the surface of the cornea, but no corneal flap is created as in LASIK surgery
- Performed on patients who have corneas too thin for LASIK or on those with large pupils

INDICATIONS

- Low to high levels of nearsightedness, farsightedness, and astigmatism

PROCEDURE

- The area around the eyes is draped with a sterile towel and anesthetic eye drops are applied. When the eye is completely numb, an eyelid holder is placed between the eyelids to keep the patient from blinking.
- The surgeon removes the epithelium of the cornea. The patient looks directly at a target light while the laser reshapes the cornea. The laser is programmed with the information gathered in the preoperative examination. The laser treatment is completed in less than 2 minutes, depending on the amount of correction needed.
- For the patient who's nearsighted, the surgeon makes the steep cornea flatter by removing tissue from the cornea's center. For the patient who's farsighted, he makes the flat cornea steeper by removing tissue outside of the central optical zone of the cornea. The point of focus is then redirected to the retina.
- For the patient with astigmatism, the cornea is made more spherical, eliminating multiple focusing points within the eye.
- After the procedure, the patient's eyes are examined with a slit lamp microscope and a bandage contact lens is applied as well as anti-inflammatory and antibiotic medications and an eye shield.

COMPLICATIONS

- Infection
- Failure of treatment
- Double vision (diplopia)
- Night vision problems
- New astigmatism
- Glare or hazy vision

NURSING DIAGNOSES

- Anxiety
- Disturbed sensory perception (visual)
- Risk for injury

EXPECTED OUTCOMES

The patient will:

- demonstrate decreased anxiety
- regain visual function
- experience no post-surgical injury to the eye.

PRETREATMENT CARE

- Explain the treatment and preparation to the patient and his family.
- Verify that the patient has signed an appropriate consent form.
- Explain that a bandage and protective shield may be placed over the eye postoperatively.
- Verify that the patient had a baseline visual evaluation and refraction before the procedure and, if he's a contact lens wearer, hasn't worn his lenses for at least 2 weeks before the baseline examination for soft lenses, 3 weeks for rigid gas permeable or toric soft lenses, or 4 weeks for hard lenses; nor worn them since the examination.
- Verify that the patient isn't wearing eye makeup, lotions, perfume, or creams, and the eyelids and lashes have been washed.
- Explain that, immediately after surgery, his eye may feel itchy, burning, watery, or as if a foreign body is in it; however, he must avoid rubbing the eye because rubbing can result in dislodging the flap and injuring the surgical area.
- Inform the patient that his vision may be blurry and he may see halos or starbursts around lights and may also be sensitive to glare for a few days.
- Make sure the patient has someone to drive him home after the procedure.
- Administer a sedative or an osmotic agent, as ordered, to reduce intraocular pressure.

POSTTREATMENT CARE

- Instill corticosteroid eyedrops or topical antibiotics as ordered.
- Assess for pain and administer analgesics as ordered.
- Help the patient lie on his back or the unaffected side.
- Keep the head of the bed flat or slightly elevated as ordered.
- Assist the patient with ambulation.
- Keep all personal items within the patient's field of vision.
- Monitor vital signs.
- Inform the patient about the postsurgical follow-up appointment in 24 to 48 hours.

⚡ **WARNING** *Immediately report sudden, sharp, or excessive pain; bloody, purulent, or clear viscous drainage; and fever.*

PATIENT TEACHING

GENERAL

- Review medications and possible adverse reactions with the patient.
- Review the signs and symptoms of possible complications.
- Explain that visual changes will be gradual and it may take up to 6 months for vision to fully stabilize.
- Emphasize the need for follow-up care.
- Explain that the bandage contact lens is usually worn for the first 2 to 3 days until the eye surface epithelium has healed and should be removed only by the practitioner.
- Instruct the patient to avoid eye makeup for 1 to 2 weeks after the procedure, not to engage in sports for about 3 days, to avoid strenuous or contact sports for about 1 month, and to avoid swimming, whirlpools, and hot tubs for about 8 weeks depending on his practitioners follow-up assessments.

- Advise the patient to take precautions for photophobia such as wearing protective sunglasses.
- Emphasize the importance of using an eye shield when sleeping.
- Tell the patient to avoid driving or participating in physical activities until approved by the practitioner.
- Tell the patient to inform the practitioner immediately if he experiences sudden, sharp, or excessive pain; bloody, purulent, or clear viscous drainage; or fever.

RESOURCES
Organizations
American Academy of Ophthalmology: *www.aao.org*
American Society of Ophthalmic Plastic and Reconstructive Surgery: *www.asoprs.org*
U.S. National Library of Medicine, National Institutes of Health, MedlinePlus: *www.nlm.nih.gov/medlineplus/lasereyesurgery.html*

Selected references
Aslanides, M., et al. "Phacoemulsification and Implantation of an Accommodating IOL after PRK," *Journal of Refractive Surgery* 22(1):106-108, January-February 2006.
Kymionis, G.D., et al. "Dry Eye After Photorefractive Keratectomy With Adjuvant Mitomycin C," *Journal of Refractive Surgery* 22(5):511-13, May 2006.

Laser eye surgery: keratectomy, phototherapeutic

OVERVIEW

- Phototherapeutic keratectomy (PTK): removes roughness or cloudiness from corneas, which doesn't allow rays of light to focus properly on the retina, resulting in blurry images
- May be used alone or with traditional corneal surgical techniques

INDICATIONS

- Corneal degenerations and dystrophies
- Corneal irregularities
- Superficial scars

PROCEDURE

- The area around the eyes is cleaned and draped with a sterile towel and aesthetic eye drops are applied. When the eye is completely numb, an eyelid holder is placed between the eyelids to keep the patient from blinking.
- PTK treatments vary depending on the corneal disorder, and goals vary based on the patient's symptoms. The laser allows corneas to be treated with a cool beam of light that evaporates tissue, producing a smoother surface.
- After PTK, the patient's eyes are examined with a slit lamp microscope and a bandage contact lens and an eye shield applied.

COMPLICATIONS

- Infection
- Poor wound healing
- Excessive corneal flattening resulting in farsightedness
- Irregular astigmatism or poor vision that can't be corrected completely with eyeglasses

NURSING DIAGNOSES

- Disturbed sensory perception (visual)
- Risk for infection
- Risk for injury

EXPECTED OUTCOMES

The patient will:
- regain visual function
- be free from signs and symptoms of infection
- experience no postsurgical injury to his eye.

PRETREATMENT CARE

◆ Explain the treatment and preparation to the patient and family.
◆ Verify that the patient has signed an appropriate consent form.
◆ Explain that a bandage and protective shield may be placed over the eye postoperatively.
◆ Administer a sedative or an osmotic agent, as ordered, to reduce intraocular pressure.

POSTTREATMENT CARE

◆ Instill corticosteroid eyedrops or topical antibiotics as ordered.
◆ Administer analgesics as ordered.
◆ Help the patient lie on his back or the unaffected side.
◆ Keep the head of the bed flat or slightly elevated as ordered.
◆ Assist the patient with ambulation.
◆ Keep all personal items within the patient's field of vision.
◆ Monitor the patient's vital signs.
◆ Assess the patient for pain.

⚡ **WARNING** *Immediately report sudden, sharp, or excessive pain; bloody, purulent, or clear viscous drainage; and fever.*

PATIENT TEACHING

GENERAL
◆ Review medications and possible adverse reactions with the patient.
◆ Review the signs and symptoms of possible complications.
◆ Emphasize the need for follow-up care.
◆ Review activity restrictions as ordered by the practitioner.
◆ Explain that the bandage contact lens is usually worn for the first 2 to 3 days until the eye surface epithelium has healed and should be removed only by the practitioner.
◆ Advise the patient to take precautions for photophobia such as wearing protective sunglasses.
◆ Emphasize the importance of using an eye shield when sleeping.
◆ Tell the patient to avoid driving or participating in physical activities until approved by the practitioner.
◆ Tell the patient to inform the practitioner immediately if he experiences sudden, sharp, or excessive pain; bloody, purulent, or clear viscous drainage; or fever.

RESOURCES
Organizations
American Academy of Ophthalmology: *www.aao.org*
American Society of Ophthalmic Plastic and Reconstructive Surgery: *www.aso-prs.org*

Selected references
Chow, A.M., et al. "Shallow Ablations in Phototherapeutic Keratectomy: Long-Term Follow-Up," *Journal of Cataract Refractive Surgery* 31(11):2133-36, November 2005.
Kim, T.I., et al. "Mitomycin C Inhibits Recurrent Avellino Dystrophy After Phototherapeutic Keratectomy," *Cornea* 25(2):220-23, February 2006.

Lesionectomy

- Removal of a lesion in the brain causing seizures in 20% to 30% of people with epilepsy who are unresponsive to medication (intractable or refractory epilepsy)
- Includes removal of a small rim of brain tissue around the lesion (lesionectomy plus corticectomy)
- Requirement for surgery: possibility of removing the lesion and surrounding brain tissue without causing damage to areas of the brain responsible for vital functions, such as movement, sensation, language, and memory

INDICATIONS

- Tumors
- Scars from a head injury or infection
- Abnormal blood vessels
- Hematoma

- The anesthetist starts a peripheral I.V. line, a central venous pressure line, and an arterial line; the patient receives local or general anesthesia.
- A lesionectomy requires exposing an area of the brain using a craniotomy. The surgeon makes an incision in the scalp, removes a piece of bone and pulls back a section of the dura. He will use the information gathered preoperatively to help identify abnormal brain tissue and to avoid areas of the brain responsible for vital functions.
- In some cases, part of the surgery is performed with the patient awake so that contact with vital areas of the brain are avoided. Probes are used to stimulate different areas of the brain while the patient counts, identifies pictures, or performs other tasks.
- After the brain tissue is removed, the dura and bone are fixed back into place, and the scalp is closed using stitches or staples.

COMPLICATIONS

- Infection
- Vasospasm
- Hemorrhage
- Air embolism
- Respiratory compromise
- Increased intracranial pressure (ICP)
- Diabetes insipidus
- Syndrome of inappropriate antidiuretic hormone
- Failure to relieve seizures
- Nerve damage

- Impaired gas exchange
- Ineffective breathing pattern
- Ineffective tissue perfusion: Cardiopulmonary; cerebral

EXPECTED OUTCOMES

The patient will:

- maintain adequate ventilation as evidenced by arterial blood gas levels within normal limits
- exhibit normal breathing pattern
- maintain tissue perfusion as evidenced by blood pressure and cardiac rhythm within normal limits and improved Glasgow Coma Scale score.

PRETREATMENT CARE

- Make sure that preoperative evaluation has been completed, including seizure monitoring, electroencephalography, and magnetic resonance imaging. These tests help to locate the lesion and confirm that it's the source of the seizures.
- Explain the treatment and preparation to the patient.
- Make sure that an appropriate consent form has been signed.
- Tell the patient that his head will be shaved in the operating room.
- Review the intensive care unit and equipment the patient will see postoperatively.
- Perform a complete neurologic assessment.

POSTTREATMENT CARE

- Position the patient on his side with the head of the bed elevated 15 to 30 degrees; turn the patient carefully every 2 hours.
- Encourage coughing and deep-breathing exercises; suction gently as needed.
- Ensure a quiet, calm environment.
- Maintain seizure precautions.
- Monitor vital signs, intake and output, level of consciousness, respiratory status, ICP, heart rate and rhythm, and hemodynamic values.
- Assess fluid and electrolyte balance and urine specific gravity.
- Monitor drain patency, surgical wound and dressings, and drainage.
- Maintain a patent airway.
- Administer prescribed oxygen.
- Take steps to protect the patient's safety.
- Administer medications as ordered.
- Monitor for complications.

WARNING *Notify the practitioner immediately if there's a worsening in mental status, pupillary changes, or focal signs such as increasing weakness in an arm or leg. These findings may indicate increased ICP.*

PATIENT TEACHING

GENERAL

- Review medications and possible adverse reactions with the patient.
- Review care of the surgical wound with the patient.
- Tell the patient that headache and facial swelling will likely occur for 2 or 3 days after surgery.
- Review postoperative deep-breathing exercises with the patient.
- Instruct the patient about the use of antiembolism stockings as ordered.
- Review the signs and symptoms of infection, possible complications, and when the patient should notify the practitioner.
- Advise the patient to avoid alcohol and smoking.

- Tell the patient that most people who have undergo a lesionectomy can return to their normal activities, including work or school, in 6 to 8 weeks after surgery.
- Inform the patient that he will likely need to continue taking antiseizure medication; once seizure control is established, his medications may be reduced or eliminated.
- Tell the patient that scalp numbness, nausea, feelings of tiredness or depression, headaches, difficulty speaking, or remembering or finding words are temporary adverse effects that should subside.
- Stress the importance of follow-up care.

RESOURCES
Organizations
American Academy of Neurology:
www.aan.com
American Medical Association:
www.ama-assn.org
Epilepsy Therapy Development Project:
www.epilepsy.com

Selected references
Ferroli, P., et al. "Cerebral Cavernomas and Seizures: A Retrospective Study on 163 Patients Who Underwent Pure Lesionectomy," *Neurological Science* 26(6):390-94, February 2006.
Giulioni, M., et al. "Lesionectomy in Epileptogenic Gangliogliomas. Seizure Outcome and Surgical Results," *Journal of Clinical Neuroscience* 13(5):529-35, June 2006.
Giulioni, M., et al. "Seizure Outcome of Lesionectomy in Glioneural Tumors Associated with Epilepsy in Children," *Journal of Neurosurgery* 102(3 Suppl): 280-87, April 2005.

Lithotripsy

- Procedures for removing obstructive renal calculi or gallstones
- May be repeated for large or multiple calculi
- Extracorporeal shock-wave lithotripsy (ESWL): non-invasive, high-energy shock wave treatment
- Percutaneous ultrasonic lithotripsy (PUL): invasive procedure using ultrasonic shock waves at close range
- Common replacements for surgical removal of renal calculi (except when kidney is nonfunctional and must be removed)
- Now commonly replaced by laparoscopic cholecystectomy for gallstones
- Contraindicated in patients with urinary or biliary tract obstruction distal to the calculi; in renal or gallbladder cancer; calculi that are fixed to the kidney, ureter, or gallbladder or located below the iliac crest level; pacemakers; and during pregnancy

INDICATIONS
- Potentially obstructive calculi
- Emergency treatment for acute renal obstruction

- The patient receives I.V. or oral sedation, or the use of a transcutaneous electrical nerve stimulator.

ESWL
- The patient is placed in a semi-reclining or supine position on the hydraulic stretcher of the ESWL machine on a water-filled cushion (or submerged in lukewarm water for gallstones) through which the shock waves are directed from the lithotriptor.
- The generator is focused on the calculi using biplane fluoroscopy confirmation.
- The generator is activated to direct high-energy shock waves through the cushion or water at the calculi.
- Shock waves are synchronized to the patient's R waves on the electrocardiogram (ECG) and fired during diastole.
- The number of waves fired depends on the size, number, and composition of the calculi (500 to 2,000 shocks delivered during a treatment).

PUL
- The patient receives local anesthesia or oral sedation.
- Gallstones can be broken up by several percutaneous fragmentation devices besides ultrasound, such as laser pulses and electrohydraulics, utilizing electric sparks.
- Overall procedures for gallstones and renal calculi are similar, except for placement of the percutaneous device into the gallbladder or common bile duct versus the renal pelvis. (See *Understanding percutaneous ultrasonic lithotripsy.*)

COMPLICATIONS
- Hemorrhage
- Hematomas
- Obstruction (biliary or ureteral)

- Acute pain
- Risk for imbalanced fluid volume
- Risk for infection

EXPECTED OUTCOMES
The patient will:
- demonstrate signs of comfort
- remain free from signs and symptoms of bleeding
- remain free from signs and symptoms of infection.

Understanding percutaneous ultrasonic lithotripsy

In this lithotripsy technique, an ultrasonic probe inserted through a nephrostomy tube into the renal pelvis generates ultrahigh-frequency sound waves to shatter calculi, while continuous suctioning removes the fragments. (See the illustration below.)

Percutaneous ultrasonic lithotripsy (PUL) may be used instead of extracorporeal shock-wave lithotripsy (ESWL), or it may be performed following ESWL to remove residual fragments. It's particularly useful for radiolucent calculi lodged in the kidney, which aren't treatable by ESWL.

TWO STAGES

Some practitioners prefer to perform PUL in two stages, with nephrostomy tube insertion on the first day followed by lithotripsy 1 or 2 days later, after intrarenal bleeding has subsided and the calculi can be better visualized. The day before scheduled treatment, the patient will have an excretory urography or lower abdominal radiographs to locate the calculi.

POTENTIAL COMPLICATIONS

Because PUL is an invasive procedure, it has many of the risks associated with surgical methods. In addition to possibly causing hemorrhage and infection, it may lead to renal damage from nephrostomy tube insertion and ureteral obstruction from incomplete passage of calculi fragments.

POSTPROCEDURE CARE

After PUL, care measures include increased fluid intake, frequent nephrostomy tube irrigations, and straining of urine to capture passed calculi fragments and allow laboratory analysis of their composition. One or 2 days after treatment, the patient will have kidneys, ureters, and bladder radiograph or a nephrostogram to check for retained fragments. If none are revealed, the practitioner usually will remove the nephrostomy tube. Occasionally, a patient will be discharged with the tube temporarily in place.

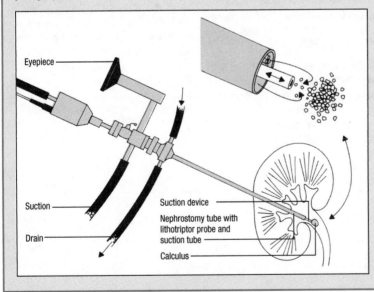

Eyepiece

Suction

Drain

Suction device

Nephrostomy tube with lithotriptor probe and suction tube

Calculus

- Review the treatment and preparation with the patient and his family. (See *Understanding extracorporeal shock wave lithotripsy*, page 224.)
- Verify that the patient has signed an appropriate consent form.
- Explain postprocedure care. If ESWL will be done for gallstones, explain that the patient may have mild pain afterward.
- Arrange for the patient to see the ESWL device before treatment if possible.
- An I.V. line, possible indwelling urinary catheter, and ECG electrodes are placed.

- Administer medications, including antibiotics, as ordered.
- Maintain a patent indwelling urinary catheter, if indicated, and an I.V. line.
- Strain urine for renal calculi fragments, and send the specimen to the laboratory.
- Report frank or persistent bleeding.
- Encourage ambulation as early as possible.
- Increase the patient's fluid intake as ordered.
- Provide comfort measures.

   WARNING *Immediately report severe unremitting pain, persistent hematuria, inability to void, fever and chills, or recurrent nausea and vomiting. These may include continued stone obstruction, internal bleeding, or infection.*

- Monitor vital signs, intake and output, complications, and urine color and pH.
- Assess the patient for pain and provide an analgesic as ordered.
- Provide nephrostomy tube care as ordered.
- Prepare the patient for recurrent treatment with the same or other type of lithotripsy, or for surgical treatment if required.

(continued)

Understanding extracorporeal shock wave lithotripsy

Dear Patient:

Your health care provider has ordered a special procedure called extracorporeal shock wave lithotripsy to get rid of your kidney or urinary system stones.

During this procedure, a machine will direct shock waves through water or a water-filled cushion and send them into your body, where they will crush the stone.

Keep in mind that the energy from these shock waves is targeted at the stone and shouldn't damage your body tissues. Here's what to expect.

BEFORE THE PROCEDURE

On the night before the procedure, don't eat or drink anything after midnight. The next day when you arrive at the hospital at your scheduled time, a nurse will take a blood sample and urine specimen. She may also perform an electrocardiogram to evaluate your heart function.

Then a nurse will start an I.V. line in your arm or hand so you can receive fluids and drugs. You'll be given a sedative to prevent pain and help you remain still during the procedure. A technician will X-ray your kidneys, ureters, and bladder to find out the size and location of your stone.

DURING THE PROCEDURE

You'll sit in a special chair and be secured with a belt. Next you may be lowered into a tub of lukewarm water that reaches to your shoulders. If necessary, you'll be shifted in the chair so you're in the best position for your treatment. You may also lie on a stretcher that's positioned over a water-filled cushion to receive your treatment.

Throughout the procedure, you'll be asleep or feel drowsy.

AFTER THE PROCEDURE

You're usually allowed to go home right after the procedure unless a fever or other complications develop. Expect your health care provider to give you prescriptions for medication to relieve pain and prevent infection.

Because internal bleeding is possible, don't take aspirin or other anti-inflammatory medicines for 7 to 10 days after the procedure. These drugs could worsen bleeding.

Expect blood-tinged urine and bruising, especially on your back, for several days. If these signs continue for longer, or if you experience fever or excessive pain, call your health care provider immediately.

For several days after the procedure, drink extra fluids, and strain your urine, saving the stone fragments for your practitioner to examine. Make an appointment for follow-up X-rays and blood studies.

PATIENT TEACHING

GENERAL

- Review medication administration, dosing, and possible adverse reactions with the patient.
- Tell the patient about possible complications.
- Stress the importance of daily oral fluid intake of 3 to 4 qt (3 to 4 L) for about 1 month after treatment.
- Instruct the patient to strain urine for the first week after renal calculi removal, to save fragments in the container provided, and to bring the container to the first follow-up visit.
- Discuss expected adverse effects of ESWL, including pain in the treated side as fragments pass, slight redness or bruising on the treated side, blood-tinged urine for several days after treatment (after removal of renal calculi), and mild GI upset. Reassure the patient that these effects are normal. However, tell him to report severe unremitting pain, persistent hematuria, inability to void, fever and chills, or recurrent nausea and vomiting.
- Tell the patient to limit activity as instructed by the practitioner. Encourage the patient to resume normal activities, including exercise and work, as soon as he's able unless the practitioner instructs otherwise. Explain that physical activity will enhance the passage of calculi fragments.
- Stress the importance of complying with special dietary or drug regimens designed to reduce the risk of formation of new calculi.
- Discuss ways to prevent new calculi formation.
- Stress the need for follow-up care.

RESOURCES

Organizations
American Association of Clinical Urologists: *www.aacuweb.org*
American College of Surgeons: *www.facs.org*
American Medical Association: *www.ama-assn.org*

Selected references
Clayman, R. "Randomized Controlled Study of Mechanical Percussion, Diuresis, and Inversion Therapy to Assist Passage of Lower Pole Renal Calculi After Shock Wave Lithotripsy," *Journal of Urology* 175(2):585, February 2006.

Honeck, P., et al. "Shock Wave Lithotripsy Versus Ureteroscopy for Distal Ureteral Calculi: A Prospective Study," *Urological Research* 34(3):190-192, June 2006.

Lahme, S. "Shockwave Lithotripsy and Endourological Stone Treatment in Children," *Urological Research* 34(2): 112-117, April 2006.

Liver resection

- Surgical removal of a portion of the liver usually done to remove a tumor and appropriate surrounding liver tissue, leaving no evidence of cancer
- May not be possible if tumors are located near critical liver blood vessels

INDICATIONS

- Liver cancer (hepatocellular cancer)
- Tumors (one or two) of the liver that are 3 cm or less with excellent hepatic function, without associated cirrhosis
- Metastasis from other sites, such as breast, kidney, lung, selected tumors of the pancreas and small intestine, and sarcomas

PROCEDURE

- The patient receives general anesthesia, and the surgeon makes an abdominal incision.
- Several types of liver resections can be performed ranging from resection of a lobe (left or right) to segments (or small portions) of the liver.
- Resection of liver segments (also called *segmentectomy*) is done to treat multiple liver tumors. Segments may be resected to preserve the normal liver. Other treatments may be performed, such as a hepatic intra-arterial catheter for postoperative chemotherapy. To be effective, all tumors must be removed with a margin of ½″ (1.3 cm) of normal liver to ensure removal of microscopic cancer cells that may surround the main tumor.
- The surgeon may place abdominal drains and will then close the abdomen with sutures.

COMPLICATIONS

- Liver failure
- Infection
- Bleeding, hemorrhage
- Disseminated intravascular coagulation

NURSING DIAGNOSES

- Deficient fluid volume
- Ineffective gas exchange
- Risk for infection

EXPECTED OUTCOMES

The patient will:

- maintain adequate fluid volume as evidenced by adequate intake and output
- maintain patent airway and adequate oxygenation as evidenced by arterial blood gas levels within normal limits
- be free from signs and symptoms of infection.

PRETREATMENT CARE

- Explain that when a portion of a normal liver is removed, the remaining liver can regenerate to the original size within 1 or 2 weeks; however, a cirrhotic liver can't regenerate.
- Make sure that preoperative tests and studies have been completed and documented. Before resection, biopsies are usually done to determine if there's associated cirrhosis. Routine tests may include a colonoscopy (if the patient has had colon cancer) or a computer tomography scan of the abdomen, pelvis, or chest.
- Review the procedure with the patient and what to expect postoperatively.
- Verify that a consent form has been signed.
- Make sure the patient takes nothing by mouth after midnight and that any preoperative preparation has been done.

POSTTREATMENT CARE

- Maintain patent airway and adequate oxygenation.
- Monitor vital signs and intake and output.
- Assess for complications, such as bleeding and liver failure.
- Assist with turning, coughing, and deep-breathing exercises; encourage use of incentive spirometry.
- Administer pain medication and assess for effect.
- Monitor cardiovascular and neurologic status.
- Administer blood products as ordered.
- Monitor pulse oximetry.
- Assess for signs of decreased tissue perfusion.
- Monitor results of coagulation studies.
- Administer medications as ordered.
- Provide adequate I.V. hydration.
- Monitor for signs of infection.

PATIENT TEACHING

GENERAL

- Review the disorder, diagnostic studies, and treatment with the patient.
- Discuss all procedures and their purpose with the patient.
- Review medication administration, dosages, and possible adverse effects, with the patient.
- Teach pre- and postoperative care.
- Stress the need for follow-up care.
- Refer the patient to appropriate resources and support services.

RESOURCES

Organizations
American Liver Foundation:
www.liverfoundation.org
American Medical Association:
www.ama-assn.org

Selected references
Aloia, T.A., et al. "Solitary Colorectal Liver Metastasis: Resection Determines Outcome," Archives of Surgery 141(5):400-467, May 2006.

Cahill, B.A. "Management of Patients who have Undergone Hepatic Artery Chemoembolization," *Clinical Journal of Oncology Nursing* 9(1):69-75, February 2005.

Charatcharoenwitthaya, P., and Lindor, K.D. "Current Concepts in the Pathogenesis of Primary Biliary Cirrhosis," *Annals of Hepatology* 4(3):161-75, July-September 2005.

Lobectomy, cerebral

OVERVIEW

- Removal of a portion of the frontal, occipital, parietal, or temporal lobes of the brain
- Temporal lobectomy: most common and successful form of cerebral lobectomy for epilepsy
- Frontal lobectomy: second most common type of epilepsy surgery, but less successful and may cause changes in personality, motivation, organization ability, and social behaviors

INDICATIONS

- Tumors
- Epilepsy with an identified lobe as focus
- Hematoma

PROCEDURE

- The anesthetist starts a peripheral I.V. line, a central venous pressure line, and an arterial line; the patient receives local or general anesthesia.
- A lobectomy requires exposing an area of the brain using a craniotomy. (See *Comparison of cranial surgical approaches.*)
- The surgeon makes an incision in the scalp, removes a piece of bone and pulls back a section of the dura. He uses preoperative information to help identify abnormal brain tissue and to avoid areas of the brain responsible for vital functions.
- Part of the surgery may be performed with the patient awake so that contact with vital areas of the brain is avoided. Probes are used to stimulate different areas of the brain while the patient counts, identifies pictures, or performs other tasks.
- After the brain tissue is removed, the dura and bone are fixed back into place, and the scalp is closed using stitches or staples.

COMPLICATIONS

- Infection
- Vasospasm
- Hemorrhage
- Air embolism
- Respiratory compromise
- Increased intracranial pressure (ICP)
- Syndrome of inappropriate antidiuretic hormone
- Failure to relieve seizures
- Nerve damage
- Language or verbal deficits
- Meningitis

Comparison of cranial surgical approaches

SUPRATENTORIAL (above the tentorium)
Incision is made above the area to be operated on; is usually located behind the hairline.

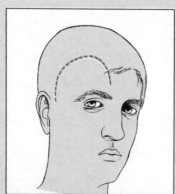

INFRATENTORIAL (below the tentorium, brain stem)
Incision is made at the nape of the neck, around the occipital lobe.

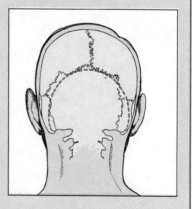

NURSING DIAGNOSES

◆ Impaired gas exchange
◆ Ineffective breathing pattern
◆ Ineffective tissue perfusion: Cardio-pulmonary, cerebral

EXPECTED OUTCOMES
The patient will:
◆ maintain adequate ventilation as evidenced by arterial blood gas levels within normal limits
◆ exhibit normal breathing pattern
◆ maintain tissue perfusion as evidenced by blood pressure and cardiac rhythm within normal limits and improved Glasgow Coma Scale score.

PRETREATMENT CARE

◆ Make sure that preoperative evaluation has been completed (seizure monitoring, electroencephalography, and magnetic resonance imaging) to help pinpoint the location of the lesion and confirm source of the seizures.
◆ Review the treatment as well as pretreatment and posttreatment nursing care.
◆ Verify that an appropriate consent form has been signed.
◆ Tell the patient that his head will be shaved in the operating room.
◆ Explain the intensive care unit and equipment the patient will see postoperatively.
◆ Perform a complete neurologic assessment.

POSTTREATMENT CARE

◆ Position the patient on his side with the head of the bed elevated 15 to 30 degrees; turn the patient carefully every 2 hours.
◆ Encourage coughing and deep-breathing exercises; suction gently as needed.
◆ Ensure a quiet, calm environment.
◆ Maintain seizure precautions.
◆ Monitor vital signs, intake and output, level of consciousness, respiratory status, ICP, heart rate and rhythm, and hemodynamic values.
◆ Assess fluid and electrolyte balance and urine specific gravity.
◆ Monitor drain patency, surgical wound and dressings, and drainage.
◆ Maintain a patent airway.
◆ Administer prescribed oxygen.
◆ Take steps to ensure the patient's safety.
◆ Administer medications as ordered.
◆ Monitor the patient for complications.

⚡ **WARNING** *Notify the practitioner immediately if you detect a worsening mental status, pupillary changes, or focal signs such as increasing weakness in an arm or leg. These findings may indicate increased ICP.*

PATIENT TEACHING

GENERAL
◆ Review medications and possible adverse reactions with the patient.
◆ Review care of the surgical wound with the patient.
◆ Tell the patient that headache and facial swelling will likely occur for 2 or 3 days after surgery.
◆ Review postoperative deep-breathing exercises with the patient.
◆ Review the use of antiembolism stockings as ordered.
◆ Review the signs and symptoms of infection, possible complications, and when the patient should notify the practitioner.
◆ Advise the patient to avoid alcohol and smoking.
◆ If the patient has been on seizure medication preoperatively, inform him that he will likely need to continue taking it; once seizure control is established, his medications may be reduced or eliminated.
◆ Tell the patient that scalp numbness, nausea, feelings of tiredness or depression, headaches, difficulty speaking, or remembering or finding words are temporary adverse effects that should subside.
◆ Stress the importance of follow-up care.

RESOURCES
Organizations
American Academy of Neurology: *www.aan.com*
American Medical Association: *www.ama-assn.org*
Epilepsy Therapy Development Project: *www.epilepsy.com*

Selected references
Gallo, B.V. "Epilepsy, Surgery, and the Elderly," *Epilepsy Research* 68(Suppl 1):83-86, January 2006.
Khoury, J.S., et al. "Predicting Seizure Frequency After Epilepsy Surgery," *Epilepsy Research* 67(3):89-99, December 2005.
Nolan, S. "Traumatic Brain Injury: A Review," *Critical Care Nursing Quarterly* 28(2):188-94, April-June 2005.

Loop electrosurgical excision

OVERVIEW

- Loop electrosurgical excision procedure (LEEP): performed with a thin, low-voltage electrified wire loop to remove abnormal cervical tissue
- Performed after abnormal Papanicolaou (Pap) test results have been confirmed by colposcopy and cervical biopsy
- After LEEP: specimen examined again for cancerous cells
- Can be as effective as cryotherapy or laser treatment
- Also known as *large loop excision of the transformation zone*

INDICATIONS

- Removal of abnormal cervical tissue
- Removal of abnormal tissue high in the cervical canal that can't be seen during colposcopy; may be done instead of a cone biopsy
- Microinvasive cervical cancer
- Abnormal Pap test

PROCEDURE

- LEEP is usually performed as an outpatient procedure.
- A cervical block is injected to anesthetized the cervix; in addition an oral or I.V. pain medication may also be used.
- An acetic acid or iodine solution, which makes abnormal cells more visible, may be applied to the cervix before the procedure.
- The patient is placed in the lithotomy position and the practitioner inserts a speculum to examine the vagina and cervix.

COMPLICATIONS

- Uterine perforation
- Bleeding
- Infection
- Cervical stenosis
- Infertility
- Decreased cervical mucus
- Cervical incompetence

NURSING DIAGNOSES

- Acute pain
- Anxiety
- Deficient knowledge (disorder and treatment)

EXPECTED OUTCOMES

The patient will:

- express and demonstrate relief of discomfort
- express feelings of decreased anxiety
- verbalize understanding of the disorder and treatment regimen.

PRETREATMENT CARE

◆ Explain the treatment and preparation to the patient.
◆ Verify that the patient has signed an appropriate consent form.
◆ Provide emotional support.
◆ Obtain and document results of diagnostic studies, medical history, and physical examination; notify the practitioner of abnormalities.
◆ Make sure the patient has fasted and used an enema preoperatively as ordered.
◆ Administer I.V. fluids as ordered.

POSTTREATMENT CARE

◆ Administer analgesics as ordered.
◆ Institute safety precautions.

⚡ **WARNING** *Be sure to report continuous, sharp abdominal pain that doesn't respond to analgesics; this indicates possible uterine perforation—a potentially life-threatening complication.*

◆ Monitor vital signs and intake and output.
◆ Monitor type and amount of vaginal drainage, and observe for signs of infection.

PATIENT TEACHING

GENERAL

◆ Review medications and possible adverse reactions with the patient.
◆ Discuss with the patient the possibility of postoperative abdominal cramping and pain in the pelvis and lower back.
◆ Inform the patient that postoperative vaginal drainage may appear dark brown during the first week and that discharge or spotting may occur for approximately 3 weeks. Instruct her to use sanitary napkins instead of tampons for 3 weeks.
◆ Advise the patient to avoid sexual intercourse for 3 weeks. Also, tell her to avoid douching.
◆ Tell the patient to report increased bleeding to the practitioner.
◆ Tell the patient about the signs and symptoms of infection.
◆ Inform the patient that activity should be limited; also, tell her that the recovery time depends on the extent of the procedure. Most patients return to normal activities within 1 to 3 days.
◆ Instruct the patient to notify the practitioner if she develops a fever, spots or bleeds longer than 1 week, bleeds heavier than her normal menses, or has increasing pelvic pain or a foul-smelling, yellowish vaginal discharge (indicating an infection).
◆ Stress the need for follow-up care.
◆ Inform the patient that menses may be heavier-than-normal for the first two or three menstrual cycles after the procedure.

RESOURCES

Organizations

American College of Obstetrics and Gynecology: *www.acog.org*
Obstetrics, Gynecology, Infertility and Women's Health: *www.obgyn.net*

Selected references

Brewster, W.R., et al. "Feasibility of Management of High-Grade Cervical Lesions in a Single Visit: A Randomized Controlled Trial," *JAMA* 294(17):2182-87, November 2005.
Huff, B.C. "Can Advanced Practice Clinicians Perform Loop Electrosurgical Excision Procedures and Cryotherapy?" *Journal of Lower Genital Tract Diseases* 9(3):143-44, July 2005.
Szymanski, L.M., et al. "Post-Loop Electrosurgical Excision Procedure Sepsis in a Human Immunodeficiency Virus-Infected Woman," *Obstetrics and Gynecology* 107(2):496-98, February 2006.

Lung volume reduction surgery

OVERVIEW

- Removal of diseased portion of the lung increasing chest cavity space
- Can alter flattened diaphragm of a patient with emphysema to assume a more normal shape, making the diaphragm function better
- Results in diminished shortness of breath, greater exercise tolerance, and better quality of life

INDICATIONS
- Severe chronic obstructive pulmonary disease (COPD)

PROCEDURE

- The patient receives general anesthesia.
- Portions of one or both of the patient's lungs are removed surgically by opening the chest wall or by thoracoscopy.
- One or more chest tubes are placed during surgery to prevent lung tissue collapse.

THORACOSCOPY (UNILATERAL OR BILATERAL)
- Thoracoscopy is a minimally invasive technique (sometimes called *VATS* or *video-assisted thoracic surgery*).
- The patient is positioned supine but is slightly raised on the affected side, with the arm held above his head.
- Three small (about 1″ [2.5-cm]) incisions are made between the ribs.
- A videoscope is placed through one of the incisions. A stapler and grasper are inserted in the other incisions to remove damaged areas and to reseal the remaining lung.
- Sutures are used to close the incisions.
- The patient may be repositioned and the procedure performed on the other side.

STERNOTOMY (BILATERAL)
- An incision is made through the breastbone to expose both lungs.
- Both lungs are reduced at the same time.
- The chest bone is wired together and the skin is closed.
- This is the most invasive technique and is used when thoracoscopy isn't appropriate.
- It's used only for patients with upper lobe disease.

THORACOTOMY (UNILATERAL)
- For the thoracotomy technique, an incision is made between the ribs and the ribs are separated with retractors. The incision is about 5″ to 12″ (13 to 30 cm) long.
- The lung is reduced as required.
- The muscle and skin are closed by sutures.
- Thoracotomy is commonly used when the surgeon can't visualize the lung clearly through the thoracoscope or when dense scar tissue exists.

COMPLICATIONS
- Subcutaneous crepitus, which may indicate tracheal or bronchial perforation or pneumothorax
- Hypoxemia
- Cardiac arrhythmias
- Bleeding
- Infection
- Bronchospasm
- Air leakage
- Pneumonia
- Stroke
- Bleeding
- Myocardial infarction

NURSING DIAGNOSES

- Impaired gas exchange
- Ineffective breathing pattern
- Ineffective tissue perfusion: Cardiopulmonary

EXPECTED OUTCOMES
The patient will:

- maintain adequate ventilation as evidenced by arterial blood gas levels within normal limits
- exhibit normal breathing pattern
- maintain adequate tissue perfusion as evidenced by blood pressure and heart rate within normal limits.

PRETREATMENT CARE

- Review with the patient the surgeon's description of the technique to be used, and explain pretreatment and posttreatment nursing care.
- Verify that an appropriate consent form has been signed.
- Note and document patient allergies.
- Instruct the patient to fast for 6 to 12 hours before the test.
- Obtain vital signs and results of preprocedure studies; report abnormal findings.
- An I.V. sedative may be given.
- Remove the patient's dentures.

POSTTREATMENT CARE

- Monitor vital signs, pulse oximetry, and intake and output.
- Maintain a patent airway and adequate oxygenation.
- Monitor patency of chest tubes, assess respiratory status and characteristics of sputum, measure drainage, and auscultate for crepitus and decreased breath sounds.
- Position the patient to promote chest expansion postoperatively.
- Observe the patient for bleeding.
- Provide pulmonary rehabilitation; suctioning, deep breathing, percussion, incentive spirometry, and respiratory treatments as ordered.
- Provide measures for pain control.
- Check the follow-up chest X-ray for pneumothorax.

⚡ **WARNING** *Immediately report subcutaneous crepitus around the patient's face, neck, or chest because these may indicate tracheal or bronchial perforation or pneumothorax.*

PATIENT TEACHING

GENERAL

- Instruct the patient about coughing, use of an incentive spirometer, and other pulmonary rehabilitation measures as directed by the practitioner.
- Review the signs of complications with the patient, such as increased shortness of breath, hemoptysis, or chest pain.
- Review medications and possible adverse reactions with the patient.
- Teach the patient how to care for the incision site.
- Tell the patient about the signs and symptoms of infection.
- Advise the patient to limit his activity as instructed by the practitioner.

RESOURCES
Organizations
American College of Surgeons: *www.facs.org*
American Lung Association: *www.lungusa.org*
American Medical Association: *www.ama-assn.org*

Selected references
Benditt, J.O. "Surgical Options for Patients With COPD: Sorting Out the Choices," *Respiratory Care* 51(2):173-82, February 2006.
Mineo, T.C., et al. "Awake Nonresectional Lung Volume Reduction Surgery," *Annals of Surgery* 243(1):131-36, January 2006.
Smith, B. "The Nursing of a Patient Following Lung Volume Reduction Surgery," *Nursing Times* 101(6):61-63, February 2005.

Mastectomy

- Breast excision done primarily to remove malignant breast tissue and regional lymphatic metastasis
- May involve one of various procedures (see *Types of mastectomy*)
- May be combined with radiation and chemotherapy

INDICATIONS

- Breast cancer
- Family history of breast cancer (prophylactic)

Types of mastectomy

If a tumor is confined to breast tissue and no lymph node involvement is detected, a lumpectomy or total (simple) mastectomy may be performed. A total mastectomy may also be used palliatively for advanced, ulcerative cancer and for extensive benign disease.

A modified radical mastectomy—the standard surgery for stages I and II lesions—removes small, localized tumors. It has replaced radical mastectomy as the most widely used surgical procedure for treating breast cancer. Besides causing less disfigurement than a radical mastectomy, it reduces postoperative arm edema and shoulder problems.

A radical mastectomy controls the spread of larger, metastatic lesions. Later, breast reconstruction may be performed using a portion of the latissimus dorsi. Rarely, an extended radical mastectomy may be used to treat cancer in the medial quadrant of the breast or in subareolar tissue. This procedure is done to prevent possible metastasis to the internal mammary lymph nodes.

PROCEDURE

- The patient receives general anesthesia.
- The surgeon makes an incision, usually in the shape of an oval, around the nipple, running across the width of the breast.

TOTAL MASTECTOMY

- The entire breast is removed without dissecting the lymph nodes.
- A skin graft may be applied if necessary.

MODIFIED RADICAL MASTECTOMY

- The entire breast is removed.
- Axillary lymph nodes are resected and the pectoralis major is left intact.
- The pectoralis minor may be removed.
- If the patient has small lesions and no metastasis, breast reconstruction may follow immediately or a few days later.

RADICAL MASTECTOMY

- The entire breast, axillary lymph nodes, underlying pectoral muscles, and adjacent tissues are removed.
- Skin flaps and exposed tissue are covered with moist packs.
- The chest wall and axilla are irrigated before closure.

EXTENDED RADICAL MASTECTOMY

- The breast, underlying pectoral muscles, axillary contents, and upper internal mammary (mediastinal) lymph node chain are removed.
- After closure of the mastectomy site, a drain or catheter may be inserted.
- Large pressure dressings may be applied if a drain isn't inserted.

COMPLICATIONS

- Infection
- Delayed healing
- Lymphedema
- Change in self-concept

NURSING DIAGNOSES

- Acute pain
- Disturbed body image
- Risk for infection

EXPECTED OUTCOMES

The patient will:

- verbalize or demonstrate feelings of comfort
- verbalize feelings of increased self-esteem
- show no signs of infection.

PRETREATMENT CARE

- Explain the treatment and preparation to the patient and her family.
- Verify that the patient has signed an appropriate consent form.
- Explain postoperative care.
- Take baseline arm measurements on both sides.
- Perform a preoperative assessment and complete the surgical verification process.
- Restrict food and fluids as ordered.
- If the patient will have a radical mastectomy, explain that skin on the anterior surface of one thigh may be shaved and prepared in case she needs a graft.
- Provide emotional support.

POSTTREATMENT CARE

- Administer medications as ordered.
- Elevate the patient's arm on a pillow.
- Regularly check the suction tubing to ensure proper functioning.
- Initiate flexion and extension arm exercises as ordered.
- Place a sign in the patient's room indicating that no blood pressure readings, injections, or venipunctures should be performed on the affected arm.
- Gently encourage the patient to look at the operative site.
- Encourage her to express her feelings.
- Arrange a fitting for a temporary breast pad after 2 or 3 days.
- Monitor the patient's vital signs and intake and output.
- Assess for complications, such as abnormal bleeding and infection.
- Monitor drainage and surgical wound and dressings.
- Assess emotional response and provide reassurance as appropriate.

PATIENT TEACHING

GENERAL

- Review the medications and possible adverse reactions with the patient.
- Discuss the signs and symptoms of infection with the patient.
- Inform the patient about complications of the procedure.
- Instruct the patient about signs and symptoms of infection and when to notify the practitioner.
- Teach the patient how to prevent infection.
- Tell the patient about the importance of using the affected arm as much as possible.
- Instruct the patient about range-of-motion exercises and other postoperative exercises. (See *Exercises to strengthen your arm and shoulder,* pages 236 and 237.)
- Tell the patient to use a temporary breast prosthesis if she feels one is needed.
- Instruct the patient to avoid blood pressure readings, injections, and venipunctures on the affected arm.
- Tell the patient to avoid keeping the affected arm in a dependent position for a prolonged period.
- Instruct the patient to protect the affected arm from injury.
- Advise the patient to take adequate rest periods.
- Advise the patient to perform monthly breast self-examinations.
- Stress the importance of follow-up care.
- Inform the patient that a permanent prosthesis can be fitted 3 to 4 weeks after surgery.
- Refer the patient to the American Cancer Society and Reach to Recovery.

RESOURCES

Organizations

American College of Obstetricians and Gynecologists: *www.acog.org*

National Cancer Institute: *www.nci.nih.gov/cancerinfo*

Obstetrics, Gynecology, Infertility, Pregnancy, Birth, and Women's Health: *www.obgyn.net*

Selected references

Armer, J., and Fu, M.R. "Age Differences in Post-Breast Cancer Lymphedema Signs and Symptoms," *Cancer Nursing* 28(3): 200-207; quiz 208-209, May-June 2005.

Boehmk, M.M., and Dickerson, S.S. "Symptom, Symptom Experiences, and Symptom Distress Encountered by Women with Breast Cancer Undergoing Current Treatment Modalities," *Cancer Nursing* 28(5):382-89, September-October 2005.

Romanek, K.M., et al. "Age Differences in Treatment Decision Making for Breast Cancer in a Sample of Healthy Women: The Effects of Body Image and Risk Framing," *Oncology Nursing Forum* 32(4):799-806, July 2005.

(continued)

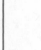
Exercises to strengthen your arm and shoulder

Dear Patient:

After your mastectomy, you'll need to strengthen your arm and shoulder muscles. When permitted by your health care provider, do the exercises below daily. They'll help increase your mobility by preventing your arm and shoulder muscles from stiffening and becoming shorter. Daily exercise will also help maintain your muscle tone and improve your circulation.

Follow these instructions, doing each exercise as many times as directed.

WALL CLIMB

Stand facing a wall, with your toes as close to the wall as possible and your feet apart. Bend your elbows slightly. Then place your palms against the wall at shoulder level.

Flexing your fingers, work your hands up the wall until you fully extend your arms. Then work your hands back down to the starting point.

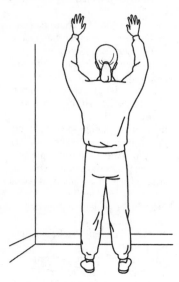

PENDULUM SWINGS

1. Place your unaffected arm on the back of a chair. Bend forward from the waist, and let your affected arm hang loosely.

2. Swing your arm from left to right in front of you. Make sure the movement comes from your shoulder joint and not from your elbow.

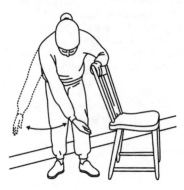

3. Maintain the same position and trace small circles with your arm. Again, make sure the motion comes from your shoulder joint. (As your arm relaxes, the size of the circle will probably increase.) Then circle in the opposite direction.

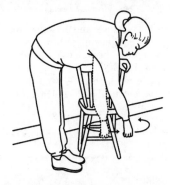

4. Swing your arm forward and backward from your shoulder, within your range of comfort.

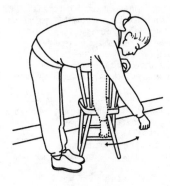

PULLEY

Drape a rope over your shower curtain rod (or through an overhead pulley, hook, or loop). Hold the opposite ends of the rope in each hand.

With your arm outstretched, use a seesaw motion to slide the rope back and forth over the rod.

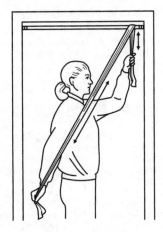

ROPE TURNS

Tie a rope to a doorknob; then stand facing the door. Hold the rope's free end in the hand of your affected side. Place your other hand on your hip. Extend your affected arm slightly to the side away from your body. Now turn the rope, making as wide a swing as possible. Start slowly, and increase your speed as your arm grows stronger.

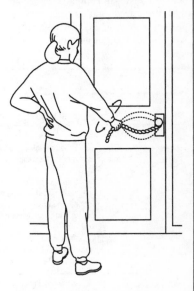

Mechanical ventilation

- Uses a machine that generates a controlled flow of oxygen in and out of lungs
- May use positive or negative pressure

POSITIVE-PRESSURE VENTILATOR

- Causes inspiration while increasing tidal volume (although doesn't ensure adequate gas exchange)
- Inspiratory cycles: vary in volume, pressure, or time
- Volume-cycled ventilator (most commonly used): delivers a preset volume of air each time, regardless of amount of lung resistance
- Pressure-cycled ventilator: generates flow until the machine reaches a preset pressure regardless of the volume delivered or the time required to achieve the pressure
- Time-cycled ventilator: generates flow for a preset amount of time
- High-frequency ventilator: uses high respiratory rates and low tidal volume (V_T) to maintain alveolar ventilation

NEGATIVE-PRESSURE VENTILATOR

- Pulls the thorax outward, allowing air to flow into lungs
- Examples of ventilators: iron lung, cuirass (chest shell), and body wrap

INDICATIONS FOR POSITIVE-PRESSURE VENTILATOR

- Central nervous system disorders, such as cerebral hemorrhage and spinal cord transection
- Acute respiratory distress syndrome
- Pulmonary edema
- Chronic obstructive pulmonary disease
- Flail chest
- Acute hypoventilation

INDICATIONS FOR NEGATIVE-PRESSURE VENTILATOR

- Neuromuscular disorders

PROCEDURE

- Put on gloves and personal protective equipment.
- Connect the endotracheal tube to the ventilator.
- Observe for chest expansion and auscultate for bilateral breath sounds.

Responding to ventilator alarms

SIGNAL	POSSIBLE CAUSE	NURSING INTERVENTIONS
Low-pressure alarm	• Tube disconnected from ventilator • Endotracheal (ET) tube displaced above vocal cords or tracheostomy tube extubated	• Reconnect tube to ventilator. • Check tube placement and reposition if needed. If extubation or displacement has occurred, ventilate patient manually and call practitioner immediately.
	• Leaking tidal volume from low cuff pressure (from an underinflated or ruptured cuff or a leak in the cuff or one-way valve) • Ventilator malfunction	• Listen for a whooshing sound around tube, indicating an air leak. If you hear one, check cuff pressure. If you can't maintain pressure, call the practitioner; he may need to insert a new tube. • Disconnect the patient from the ventilator and ventilate him manually if necessary. Obtain another ventilator.
	• Leak in ventilator circuitry (from loose connection or hole in tubing, loss of temperature-sensitive device, or cracked humidification jar)	• Make sure all connections are intact. Check for holes or leaks in tubing and replace if necessary. Check the humidification jar and replace if cracked.
High-pressure alarm	• Increased airway pressure or decreased lung compliance caused by worsening disease • Patient biting on oral ET tube	• Auscultate the lungs for evidence of increasing lung consolidation, barotrauma, or wheezing. Call practitioner if indicated. • Insert a bite block if needed. • Consider an analgesic or sedation if appropriate.
	• Secretions in airway	• Look for secretions in the airway. To remove them, suction the patient or have him cough.
	• Condensate in large-bore tubing • Intubation of right mainstem bronchus	• Check tubing for condensate and remove any fluid. • Auscultate the lungs for evidence of diminished or absent breath sounds in the left lung fields. • Check tube position. If it has slipped, call the practitioner; he may need to reposition it.
	• Patient coughing, gagging, or attempting to talk	• If the patient fights the ventilator, the practitioner may order a sedative or neuromuscular blocking agent.
	• Chest wall resistance	• Reposition the patient to improve chest expansion. If repositioning doesn't help, administer the prescribed analgesic.
	• Failure of high-pressure relief valve • Bronchospasm	• Have faulty equipment replaced. • Assess the patient for the cause. Report to the practitioner, and treat as ordered.

- Monitor the patient's arterial blood gas (ABG) values after initial ventilator setup (usually 20 to 30 minutes), after any changes in ventilator settings, and as the patient's clinical condition warrants.
- Adjust ventilator settings depending on ABG analysis.
- Check ventilator tubing for condensation.
- Drain the condensate into a collection trap and empty. Don't drain the condensate into the humidifier.
- Monitor the in-line thermometer to ensure air is close to body temperature.
- When monitoring vital signs, count spontaneous and ventilator-delivered breaths.
- Change, clean, or dispose of ventilator tubing and equipment every 48 to 72 hours to reduce risk of bacterial contamination.
- When ordered, begin to wean the patient from the ventilator.

COMPLICATIONS
- Tension pneumothorax
- Decreased cardiac output
- Oxygen toxicity
- Fluid volume excess
- Infection
- Stress ulcers

NURSING DIAGNOSES

- Impaired gas exchange
- Ineffective breathing pattern
- Ineffective tissue perfusion: Cardiopulmonary

EXPECTED OUTCOMES
The patient will:
- maintain adequate ventilation
- exhibit normal breathing pattern
- maintain tissue perfusion.

PRETREATMENT CARE

- In most facilities, respiratory therapists set up and maintain the ventilator.
- In most cases, add sterile distilled water to the humidifier and connect the ventilator to the appropriate gas source.

POSTTREATMENT CARE

WARNING *Make sure ventilator alarms are on at all times. (See* Responding to ventilator alarms.*)*
- If the problem can't be identified, disconnect the patient from the ventilator and use a handheld resuscitation bag to ventilate him.
- Provide emotional support to reduce anxiety, even if the patient is unresponsive.
- Unless contraindicated, turn the patient from side to side every 1 or 2 hours.
- Perform active or passive range-of-motion exercises.
- If permitted, position the patient upright at regular intervals.
- Prevent condensation in the tubing from flowing into the lungs.
- Provide care for the patient's artificial airway as needed.
- Assess peripheral circulation and monitor urine output.
- Watch for fluid volume excess or dehydration.
- Place the call bell within reach.
- Establish a method of communication such as a communication board.
- Give a sedative or neuromuscular blocking drug as ordered to relax the patient and prevent spontaneous breathing efforts that interfere with the ventilator's action.
- Reassure the patient and his family that the paralysis is temporary.
- Closely observe a patient with inability to breathe or talk.
- Make sure that emergency equipment is readily available.
- Explain procedures and ensure patient safety.

- Make sure that the patient gets adequate rest and sleep.
- Provide subdued lighting and low noise, and restrict staff movement around the patient.
- Observe for signs of hypoxia when weaning the patient.
- With patient's input, schedule weaning around daily regimen.
- As weaning progresses, encourage the patient to get out of bed.
- Suggest diversionary activities to take his mind off breathing.

PATIENT TEACHING

GENERAL
- For use at home, provide a teaching plan that covers ventilator care and settings, artificial airway care, suctioning, respiratory therapy, communication, nutrition, therapeutic exercise, signs and symptoms of infection, and troubleshooting minor equipment malfunctions.
- Have the caregiver demonstrate the ability to use the equipment.
- Refer the patient to a home health agency and durable medical equipment vendor.
- Refer the patient to community resources.

RESOURCES
Organizations
American College of Emergency Physicians: *www.acep.org*
American Medical Association: *www.ama-assn.org*

Selected references
American Association for Respiratory Care. "AARC Clinical Practice Guideline: Care of the Ventilator Circuit," *Respiratory Care* 48(9):869-79, September 2003.
Christine, N. "Caring for the Mechanically Ventilated Patient: Part One," *Nursing Standards* 20(17):55-64; quiz 66, January 2006.
Manno, M.S. "Managing Mechanical Ventilation," *Nursing* 35(12):36-41; quiz 41-42, December 2005.

Meckel's diverticulectomy

OVERVIEW

- Excision of a Meckel's diverticulum
- Performed by laparoscopy or open surgical procedure

INDICATIONS

- Infection or inflammation of Meckel's diverticulum

PROCEDURE

- The patient receives general anesthesia.
- The surgeon makes an incision in the right side of the lower abdomen. The small intestine is located and the diverticulum is removed. The intestine is repaired and the incision is closed. (See *Meckel's diverticulectomy.*)
- A small segment of the intestine may sometimes need to be removed with the diverticulum, in which case the adjoining ends of the intestine are sewn back together.

COMPLICATIONS

- Hemorrhage
- Sepsis
- Ileus
- Fluid and electrolyte imbalance
- Pelvic abscess
- Bleeding or leakage from the anastomosis site
- Peritonitis
- Postresection obstruction
- Wound infection

NURSING DIAGNOSES

- Acute pain
- Ineffective tissue perfusion: GI
- Risk for infection

EXPECTED OUTCOMES

The patient will:

- demonstrate or express feelings of increased comfort
- regain normal bowel function
- remain free from signs and symptoms of infection.

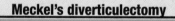

Meckel's diverticulectomy

Meckel's diverticulum is found and removed during surgery; the intestine is repaired.

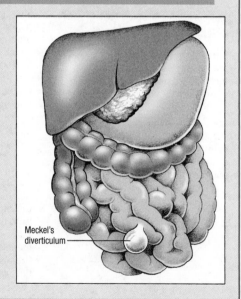

Meckel's diverticulum

PRETREATMENT CARE

- Explain preoperative and postoperative procedures and equipment to the patient and his family.
- Discuss postoperative analgesia.
- Make sure the patient or responsible family member has signed an appropriate consent form.
- Provide total parenteral nutrition as ordered.
- Administer antibiotics and other medications as ordered.
- Monitor vital signs, nutritional status, fluid and electrolyte status, intake and output, and daily weight
- Administer an enema to clean the patient's bowel as ordered.

POSTTREATMENT CARE

- Provide meticulous wound care.
- Administer analgesics as ordered.
- Maintain I.V. replacement therapy as ordered.
- Keep nasogastric tube patent and monitor drainage.
- Encourage the patient to express feelings and concerns.
- Monitor vital signs and intake and output.
- Assess for dehydration and electrolyte imbalance.
- Monitor for signs of infection, peritonitis, or sepsis.

WARNING *Immediately report excessive bleeding or draining from the incision, which could indicate hemorrhage or infection.*

- Encourage deep-breathing and coughing exercises. Encourage splinting of the incision site as necessary.
- Monitor bowel sounds; encourage oral fluid intake when the patient is able, and give stool softeners and laxatives as ordered.

WARNING *Monitor for and immediately report signs and symptoms of anastomotic leakage, including low-grade fever, malaise, slight leukocytosis, abdominal distention, tenderness, hemorrhage, hypovolemic shock, bloody stools, or wound drainage.*

PATIENT TEACHING

GENERAL

- Tell the patient of dietary restrictions.
- Instruct the patient to have a high fluid intake if not contraindicated.
- Advise the patient to avoid alcohol, laxatives, and diuretics (unless approved by the practitioner).
- Review the signs and symptoms of inflammation and infection.
- Discuss any complications with the patient and inform the patient when to notify the practitioner.
- Advise the patient to seek follow-up care.

RESOURCES
Organizations
American College of Gastroenterology: *www.acg.gi.org*
American Gastroenterological Association: *www.gastro.org*
American Medical Association: *www.ama-assn.org*
American Society of Colon and Rectal Surgeons: *www.ascrs.affiniscape.com*

Selected references

Alufohai, E., et al. "Surgical Complications of Meckel's Diverticulae: A Review of Seven Cases," *Journal of Medicine and Biomedical Research* 4(1): 88-91, June 2005.
Holland, A.J. "Diverticulectomy is Inadequate Treatment for Short Meckel's Diverticulum with Heterotopic Mucosa," *Journal of Pediatric Surgery* 40(7):1215, July 2005.

Minimally invasive direct coronary artery bypass

- Minimally invasive direct coronary artery bypass (MIDCAB): newer procedure available for performing coronary artery bypass grafting (CABG)
- Restores normal blood flow to the myocardium
- More difficult than CABG because the surgeon must maneuver through an incision that's about one-third the size of the incision in conventional CABG; requires more skill and manual dexterity than conventional CABG because surgeon is operating on a beating heart
- Variations of MIDCAB: port access bypass surgery, off-pump bypass surgery, keyhole or buttonhole surgery or laparoscopic bypass, and robotic visualization techniques

INDICATIONS
- Left anterior descending blockage
- Right coronary artery blockage
- Patients at high-risk for traditional CABG
- Contraindicated in patients with multivessel coronary artery disease

PROCEDURE

- Once the patient is anesthetized, the surgeon makes a 4″ (10.2 cm) long transverse incision on the front of the chest, toward the left side. This incision is then deepened to divide the pectoral muscles. A small portion of the front of the rib is removed.
- Once the chest has been opened and retracted, an internal mammary artery, (IMA) is harvested from the subclavian arteries. After the IMA is harvested, the frame for the MIDCAB instrumentation is fitted onto the incision. The heart stabilizer limits the movement of the heart to within 1 mm of motion, thereby permitting the surgeon to operate. A site blower removes blood from the field of operation, providing a clear view and a site light provides illumination while a site manipulator moves the heart.
- Once the IMA has been collected and the MIDCAB instrumentation is in place, the surgeon makes an incision in the pericardium, thereby exposing the left anterior descending coronary artery (LAD). One end of the IMA is attached to the artery of the beating heart—before the blockage—with sutures, and the other end is sutured to the LAD after the blockage. The IMA diverts blood around the clogged section of coronary artery. Once the IMA is in place, the MIDCAB instrumentation is removed and the incision is sutured.

COMPLICATIONS
- Cardiac arrhythmias
- Hypertension or hypotension
- Cardiac tamponade
- Thromboembolism
- Hemorrhage
- Postpericardiotomy syndrome
- Myocardial infarction
- Stroke
- Postoperative depression or emotional instability
- Pulmonary embolism
- Infection

NURSING DIAGNOSES

- Decreased cardiac output
- Ineffective tissue perfusion: Cardiopulmonary
- Risk for infection

EXPECTED OUTCOMES
The patient will:
- maintain adequate cardiac output
- maintain hemodynamic stability
- remain free from signs and symptoms of infection.

PRETREATMENT CARE

- Explain the treatment and preparation and verify that an appropriate consent form has been signed.
- Explain what to expect during the immediate postoperative period, including endotracheal tube and mechanical ventilator, cardiac monitor, nasogastric tube, chest tube, indwelling urinary catheter, arterial line, possibly epicardial pacing wires, and pulmonary artery catheter.
- Institute cardiac monitoring.
- The evening before surgery, have the patient shower with antiseptic soap as ordered and restrict food and fluids after midnight as ordered.
- Provide sedation as ordered and assist with pulmonary artery catheterization and insertion of arterial lines.

POSTTREATMENT CARE

◆ Keep emergency resuscitative equipment immediately available.
◆ Maintain arterial pressure within the limits set by the practitioner.
◆ Adjust ordered I.V. medications according to facility protocol.
◆ Assist with weaning the patient from the ventilator as appropriate.
◆ Promote chest physiotherapy; encourage coughing, deep breathing, and use of incentive spirometry.
◆ Assist the patient with range-of-motion (ROM) exercises.
◆ Monitor vital signs and intake and output.
◆ Assess heart rate and rhythm, heart sounds, peripheral vascular status, electrocardiogram and hemodynamic values, and cardiovascular status.
◆ Monitor for complications.
◆ Assess nutritional status.
◆ Monitor arterial blood gas values, and assess respiratory status and breath sounds.
◆ Monitor neurologic status.
◆ Monitor renal function.
◆ Assess surgical wounds and dressings.
◆ Monitor for electrolyte imbalances.

PATIENT TEACHING

GENERAL

◆ Review the medications and possible adverse reactions with the patient.
◆ Teach the patient how to perform incentive spirometry.
◆ Teach the patient to perform ROM exercises.
◆ Teach the patient how to care for the incision site.
◆ Review the signs and symptoms of infection, arterial reocclusion, and postpericardiotomy syndrome with the patient.
◆ Instruct the patient about how to identify and cope with postoperative depression.
◆ Discuss complications with the patient and when to notify the practitioner.
◆ Inform the patient of dietary restrictions.
◆ Tell the patient to restrict activity and to have adequate rest periods; also, tell him to follow his prescribed exercise program.
◆ Advise the patient to stop smoking.
◆ Refer the patient to the Mended Hearts Club and American Heart Association for information and support.

RESOURCES
Organizations
American College of Cardiology:
   www.acc.org
American Medical Association:
   www.ama-assn.org
HeartCenterOnline:
   www.heartcenteronline.com
Heart Surgery USA:
   www.heartsurgery-usa.com

Selected references

Bonatti, J., et al. "Ongoing Procedure Development in Robotically Assisted Totally Endoscopic Coronary Artery Bypass Grafting (TECAB)," *Heart Surgery Forum* 8(4):E287-91, August 2005.

Boodhwani, M., et al. "Minimally Invasive Direct Coronary Artery Bypass for the Treatment of Isolated Disease of the Left Anterior Descending Coronary Artery," *Canadian Journal of Surgery* 48(4):307-10, August 2005.

Egerod, I., and Hansen, G.M. "Evidence-Based Practice among Danish Cardiac Nurses: A National Survey," *Journal of Advanced Nursing* 51(5):465-73, September 2005.

Hartford, K. "Telenursing and Patients' Recovery from Bypass Surgery," *Journal of Advanced Nursing* 50(5):459-68, June 2005.

Reid, T., et al. "Psychosocial Interventions for Panic Disorder after Coronary Artery Bypass Graft: A Case Study," *Dimensions of Critical Care Nursing* 24(4):165-70, July-August 2005.

Mohs' microsurgery

OVERVIEW

◆ Highly specialized treatment for total removal of skin cancers—also called *Mohs' surgery,* or formerly, *chemosurgery*
◆ Performed by a team of medical personnel that includes physicians, nurses, and technicians

INDICATIONS
◆ Basal cell carcinoma

PROCEDURE

◆ A local anesthetic is applied and the tumor is scraped using a curette. A thin piece of tissue is then surgically removed around the scraped skin and carefully divided into pieces that fit on a microscope slide. The edges are marked with colored dyes; a careful map or diagram of the removed tissue is made; and the tissue is frozen by the technician.
◆ Most bleeding is controlled using pressure; occasionally, a small blood vessel needs to be tied using suture material. A pressure dressing is then applied, and the patient is asked to wait while the slides are being processed.
◆ The surgeon studies the slides microscopically to tell if any tumor is still present. If cancer cells exist, they can be located by referring to the map. Another layer of tissue is then removed, and the procedure is repeated until the surgeon is satisfied that the entire base and sides of the wound have no cancer cells. It usually takes removal of two or three layers of tissue (called *stages*) to complete the surgery.

COMPLICATIONS
◆ Bleeding
◆ Infection
◆ Temporary or permanent numbness
◆ Scarring of the area
◆ Return of skin cancer

NURSING DIAGNOSES
◆ Disturbed body image
◆ Impaired tissue integrity
◆ Risk for infection

EXPECTED OUTCOMES
The patient will:
◆ verbalize positive self-esteem
◆ demonstrate skin that's intact and healing
◆ show no signs of infection.

PRETREATMENT CARE

◆ Review the procedure with the patient and answer questions.
◆ Verify that a consent form has been signed.
◆ A biopsy may be done before the procedure to confirm skin cancer.
◆ The patient may need to stop taking aspirin or aspirin-containing products at least 1 week before the surgery because it may interfere with the normal blood clotting mechanism.

POSTTREATMENT CARE

◆ Monitor vital signs.
◆ Assess wound for drainage.
◆ Provide skin care as ordered.
◆ If stitches are present, provide care as ordered.
◆ Provide pain medication as ordered and assess for effect.
◆ Apply ice to affected area.
◆ Series of transections made into the brain's cerebral cortex, interrupting fibers that connect other parts of the brain and stopping seizure impulses by cutting horizontal nerve fibers in the gray matter, but sparing the vital functions located in the white matter
◆ Can help to reduce or eliminate seizures arising from vital functional areas of the cerebral cortex; may be done alone or with the removal of a section of brain tissue

INDICATIONS
◆ The patient who doesn't respond to antiseizure medication and whose seizures arise in areas of vital brain function
◆ Landau-Kleffner syndrome

PATIENT TEACHING

GENERAL
◆ Review skin care with the patient.
◆ Tell the patient the signs of complications, such as persistent bleeding or signs of infection, and when to notify the practitioner.
◆ If the patient has a significant scar or requires plastic surgery, explain that this will be done on follow-up appointments as appropriate.
◆ Instruct the patient to use ice packs.
◆ Review the medications prescribed and their purpose, dose, and adverse effects.
◆ Instruct the patient about how to care for the skin to prevent skin cancer. (See *Preventing recurrence of skin cancer.*)
◆ Advise the patient to seek follow-up care.

RESOURCES
Organizations
American Academy of Dermatology: *www.aad.org*
National Cancer Institute: *www.nci.nih.gov/cancerinfo*

Selected references
Bielan, B. "What's Your Assessment? Melanomas," *Dermatological Nursing* 17(4):285, 315, August 2005.
Demierre, M.F., et al. "New Treatments for Melanoma," *Dermatological Nursing* 17(4):287-95, August 2005.
Ferguson, K. "Melanoma," *Journal of Continuing Education in Nursing* 36(6): 242-43, November-December 2005.
Hill, M.J. "Sun and Skin: Still a Burning Issue," *Dermatological Nursing* 17(3): 178, June 2005.

Preventing recurrence of skin cancer

Dear Patient:

After having developed skin cancer, statistics say that you have a higher chance of developing another occurrence. The damage your skin has already received from the sun can't be reversed, but you can take precautions to prevent further skin cancer.

• Avoid exposure to the sun as much as possible. Avoid excessive sunshine if possible; avoid going outdoors during the peak hours of the sun (11 a.m. to 3 p.m.) when the sun's rays are the strongest.

• Use a sunscreen, applying it at least 10 minutes before exposure to sunlight. The sunscreens' strengths are labeled; the higher numbers are more protective. Usually a sunscreen with a sun protection factor of 15 or higher is recommended. Remember to put sunscreen on all skin surfaces exposed to the sun.

• Reapply sunscreen after swimming or sweating.

• Wear a wide-brimmed hat, long-sleeved shirt, and other protective clothing as appropriate when going outdoors; white or light colors help reflect the sun's rays.

• Don't use tanning booths or sunlamps.

• Check your skin every month for signs of skin cancer. If you notice an area on your skin that looks unusual, ask your health care provider about it.

CHECKING YOUR SKIN

• Use a full-length mirror and a hand-held mirror to check every inch of your skin.

• Know where your birthmarks, moles, and blemishes are and what they look like. Check for anything new, such as a change in the size, texture, or color of a mole, or a sore that doesn't heal.

• Remember to check the front and back of your body in the mirror, then raise your arms and look at the left and right sides. Don't forget to check your arms and legs, buttocks, and genitals.

• Sit and closely examine your feet, including the bottoms of your feet and the spaces between your toes.

• Remember to check your face, neck, and scalp. You may need to use a comb to move hair so that you can examine the scalp and back of the neck areas better.

By checking yourself regularly, you'll get familiar with what's normal for you. If you find anything unusual, see your health care provider.

Multiple subpial transection

OVERVIEW

- Treatment for partial seizures in parts of the brain that can't be removed safely, including areas that that control movement, sensation, language, and memory

PROCEDURE

- The patient is anesthetized, the surgeon makes an incision in the scalp, removes a piece of the cranium, and pulls back a section of the dura creating a "window" through which he will insert instruments. Information gathered during preoperative brain imaging will help to identify the area of abnormal brain tissue and areas of the brain responsible for vital brain functions to avoid.
- The surgeon uses a microscope to make a series of parallel transections in the gray matter, just below the pia mater (subpial), over the area that's been identified as the location of the seizures.
- After the transections are made, he places the dura and bone back to their original positions, and closes the scalp using stitches or staples.

COMPLICATIONS

- Mild impairment of language function if transection is in language area of the brain
- Neurologic complications, such as lack of awareness of one side of the body, loss of coordination, problems with speech, such as stuttering, difficulty speaking, or remembering information
- Infection
- Bleeding
- Allergic reaction to anesthesia
- Increased intracranial pressure (ICP)
- Scalp numbness
- Tiredness or depression
- Headaches
- Failure to relieve seizures

NURSING DIAGNOSES

- Disturbed sensory perception (all)
- Risk for infection
- Risk for injury

EXPECTED OUTCOMES

The patient will:
- exhibit improved or normal neurologic status
- exhibit no signs of infection
- exhibit no large amounts of bleeding.

PRETREATMENT CARE

- A preoperative evaluation is completed that includes several tests such as seizure monitoring, EEG, magnetic resonance imaging, and positron emission tomography. The tests help to locate the area in the brain where the seizures are occurring and determine if surgery is possible.
- EEG-video monitoring, in conjunction with EEG monitoring, may be done to record seizures as they're occurring. In some cases, invasive monitoring (use of electrodes that are placed inside the skull over a specific area of the brain) might also be used to identify the tissue that's causing the seizures.
- Review the surgical procedure with the patient and his family and ensure that a consent form has been signed.
- Review the patient's history, laboratory test results, and medications.
- The evening or morning before the surgery, have the patient take a bath and wash his hair.
- Tell the patient and his family that the face may appear bruised and swollen a few days after the surgery, but that this will gradually disappear.

POSTTREATMENT CARE

- Monitor vital signs, daily weight, and intake and output.
- Monitor level of consciousness, respiratory status, and for signs of increased ICP.
- Monitor heart rate, rhythm, and hemodynamic values.
- Monitor fluid and electrolyte balance.
- Monitor urine specific gravity.
- Maintain patency of any drains present; monitor surgical wound and dressings; note drainage and monitor for signs of complications.
- Assess effectiveness of pain medication.
- Maintain seizure precautions.
- Maintain oxygenation; encourage the patient to take deep breaths and cough; suction as indicated.
- Give drugs, as ordered.

PATIENT TEACHING

GENERAL

- Tell the patient that activities will return gradually to normal within 2 or 3 months.

 AGE FACTOR *Inform parents that their child may need to be home from school for about 6 weeks after the surgery.*

- Stress the need for follow-up and continuing care.
- Tell the family it's unlikely that the patient's medications will be changed for at least 6 months.
- Tell the patient that hair will grow back and hide the surgical scar.
- Review the medications, dosage, and adverse effects with the patient and tell him that he'll continue to take antiseizure medication.

RESOURCES

Organizations

American Academy of Neurology: *www.aan.com*
Epilepsy.com: *www.epilepsy.com/epilepsy/multiple_subpial.html*
MedicineNet.com: *www.medicinenet.com*

Selected references

Cross, C. "Seizures. Regaining Control," *RN* 67(12):44-50; quiz 51, December 2004.
Dhar, R., et al. "Long-term Seizure Outcomes Following Epilepsy Surgery: A Systematic Review and Meta-analysis," *Brain* 128(Pt 5):1188-98, May 2005.
Mikati, M.A., and Shamseddine, A.N. "Management of Landau-Kleffner Syndrome," *Paediatric Drugs* 7(6):377-89, November-December 2005.

Myringotomy

OVERVIEW

- Surgical creation of a small incision in the eardrum to drain accumulated fluids
- May involve placing tympanostomy tubes in the eardrum at the same time

INDICATIONS

- Fluid buildup behind the eardrum for 4 months or longer, and hearing loss or other risk of developmental problems
- Acute ear infections
- Repeated hyperbaric oxygen therapy
- Barotrauma from flying or deep-sea diving

  AGE FACTOR *Myringotomy may be done at the surgeon's discretion, based on the child's condition.*

PROCEDURE

- While the child is under general anesthesia, a small incision is made in the eardrum.
- Fluid, usually thickened secretions, is suctioned out.
- In most situations, a tympanostomy tube will be inserted into the eardrum to keep the middle ear aerated for a prolonged time. This small tube allows air to flow in and fluid to continuously flow out of the middle ear.
- Usually, drops will be placed in the ear, and a cotton plug inserted in the ear canal.
- The procedure usually takes less than 15 minutes.
- The incision heals on its own, without the need for sutures. The hole closes and the ear tubes usually fall out naturally, after an average of 14 months.

COMPLICATIONS

- Infection
- Scarring of the eardrum
- Chronic drainage from the ear
- Failure to resolve the ear infections
- Persistent perforation after the tube falls out of the eardrum
- Need for further and more aggressive surgery such as tonsil, adenoid, sinus, or ear surgery
- Hearing loss
- Foreign body reaction to the tube itself—for example, an allergic reaction to the tube material (rare)

NURSING DIAGNOSES

- Acute pain
- Anxiety
- Disturbed sensory perception (auditory)

EXPECTED OUTCOMES

The patient will:
- express feelings of comfort
- express feelings and concerns
- regain hearing function.

PRETREATMENT CARE

- Review the patient's medical history before surgery and verify that a consent form has been signed.
- If the practitioner has ordered preoperative laboratory studies, ensure that these are completed.

  AGE FACTOR *It's advised that the parents be honest and direct with the child as they explain the surgery. Let the child know that he'll be safe and that the parents will be close by. A calming and reassuring attitude will ease the child's anxiety.*
- Note allergies.
- Tell the patient (or parents) not to eat anything before surgery to avoid anesthetic complications.
- Review the procedure with the family and answer questions.

POSTTREATMENT CARE

- Monitor vital signs, pulse oximetry, and intake and output.
- Assess the ear for drainage.
- Monitor for signs of infection or bleeding.
- Monitor for pain and assess effect of pain medication.
- Use comfort measures.
- Once the patient is awake, offer fluids as ordered; monitor for nausea and vomiting.

PATIENT TEACHING

GENERAL

- Inform the parents that the ventilating tubes remain in place for 6 months to several years; eventually, they extrude out of the eardrum and fall into the ear canal. Tell them that the practitioner can remove the tube during an office visit in the future or that it may fall out of the ear without the child realizing it.
- Tell the parents to monitor for ear infections; if ear infections return after the first tubes fall out, the procedure can be repeated. Tell them that a profuse, foul-smelling discharge from the ear suggests an infection.
- Instruct the parents not to let the child swim unless special earplugs are worn; also tell them that the child should wear a cap while showering for several days or weeks after the procedure.
- Tell the parents which signs of infection to report to the practitioner.
- Stress the importance of follow-up care; inform the parents that an audiogram is usually performed after the ear has healed.
- Review the medications prescribed, how to administer them (for example, ear drops), and possible adverse reactions.
- Review what to expect postoperatively: Tell the parents that ear drainage may occur immediately after the procedure or when the tubes are in place; yellow, clear fluid or mucus may drain for several days to weeks after the surgery; and that a bloody discharge may occur after surgery.
- Tell the parents that cotton wool may be kept in the ear canal and should be changed as needed to keep the ear dry.

RESOURCES

Organizations

American Academy of Pediatrics: *www.aap.org*
American Association of Otolaryngology: *www.entnet.org*
American College of Surgeons: *www.facs.org*
American Medical Association: *www.ama-assn.org*
MedicineNet.com: *www.medicinenet.com*

Selected references

D'Eredita, R., and Marsh, R.R. "Tympanic Membrane Healing Process and Biocompatibility of an Innovative Absorbable Ventilation Tube," *Otology and Nuerotology* 27(1):65-70, January 2006.

Kay, N.J. "Nasal Surgery and Eustachian Tube Function: Effects on Middle Ear Ventilation," *Clinical Otolaryngology* 31(1):80, February 2006.

Montgomery, D. "A New Approach to Treating Acute Otitis Media," *Journal of Pediatric Health Care* 19(1):50-52, January-February 2005.

Nephrectomy

OVERVIEW

- Surgical removal of a kidney
- May be unilateral or bilateral
- Partial nephrectomy: resection of a portion of the kidney
- Simple nephrectomy: removal of the entire kidney
- Radical nephrectomy: resection of the entire kidney and surrounding fat tissue
- Laparoscopic nephrectomy: used with simple and partial nephrectomies to procure a donor kidney for transplantation

INDICATIONS

- Renal cell carcinoma
- Renal trauma or infection
- Hypertension, if conservative treatment fails
- Hydronephrosis
- Inoperable renal calculi
- Procurement of a healthy kidney for transplantation

PROCEDURE

- The patient receives general anesthesia.

TRADITIONAL NEPHRECTOMY

- The surgeon makes a flank incision (thoracicoabdominal or transthoracic) to expose the kidney.
- The kidney is freed from fat and adhesions.
- The lower pole of the kidney is released.
- The upper one-third of the ureter is freed, double-clamped, cut between the clamps, and ligated on both ends.
- The vascular pedicle is freed and double-clamped.
- The renal artery and the renal vein are clamped.
- The kidney is removed distal to the clamps.
- The surrounding perinephric fat and ureter are resected.
- A flank catheter and Penrose drain may be inserted.
- The wound is sutured closed.

LAPAROSCOPIC NEPHRECTOMY

- The surgeon makes four or five ½″ incisions.
- Narrow surgical instruments are inserted into the abdomen through the previously made incisions.
- The surgeon uses a small camera to help visualize inside the abdomen to clamp the vasculature.
- The surgeon makes a 2½″ incision and removes the kidney.
- The incisions are closed with sutures.

COMPLICATIONS

- Infection
- Hemorrhage
- Atelectasis
- Pneumonia
- Deep vein thrombosis
- Pulmonary embolism

NURSING DIAGNOSES

- Deficient fluid volume
- Ineffective tissue perfusion: Renal
- Risk for infection

EXPECTED OUTCOMES

The patient will:

- maintain adequate fluid volume
- maintain adequate urine output and blood pressure within normal limits and demonstrate normal results of blood and electrolyte tests
- remain free from infection.

PRETREATMENT CARE

- Explain the treatment and preparation to the patient and his family.
- Verify that the patient has signed an appropriate consent form.
- Explain postoperative care.
- Restrict oral intake as ordered.
- Administer I.V. fluids as ordered.

POSTTREATMENT CARE

- Administer medications as ordered.
- Provide care for the I.V. line, nasogastric tube, and indwelling urinary catheter.
- Notify the practitioner if urine output falls below 50 ml/hour.
- Maintain drain patency; assess character and amount of drainage, redress drain site (per protocol), and assess for infection.
- Monitor the surgical wound and dressings; assess for abnormal bleeding and drainage.
- Change dressings as ordered.
- Assess respiratory status.
- Encourage coughing, deep breathing, incentive spirometry, and changes in position.
- Encourage early and regular ambulation.
- Apply antiembolism stockings as ordered.
- Monitor the patient's vital signs, daily weight, and intake and output.
- Monitor bowel sounds, and resume oral intake when sounds return. Administer stool softener, as needed, to promote regular movement without discomfort.
- Assess for complications, such as hemorrhage, shock, and infection, and report changes to the practitioner.

PATIENT TEACHING

GENERAL

- Advise the patient to cough and perform deep-breathing exercises.
- Review the signs and symptoms of infection with the patient.
- Tell the patient about potential complications and instruct him when to notify the practitioner.
- Teach the patient how to monitor his intake and output.
- Inform the patient about prescribed fluid intake and dietary restrictions.
- Tell the patient about any prescribed activity restrictions.
- Stress the need for follow-up care.
- Emphasize the importance of wearing medical identification at all times.

RESOURCES

Organizations
American Medical Association: *www.ama-assn.org*
American Trauma Society: *www.amtrauma.org*

Selected references
Galli, B., et al. "Laparoscopic Radical Nephrectomy in Renal Cell Carcinoma," *Urologic Nursing* 25(2):83-86, 133, April 2005.
Reisiger, K.E., et al. "Laparoscopic Renal Surgery and the Risk of Rhabdomyolysis: Diagnosis and Treatment," *Urology* 66(5 Suppl):29-35, November 2005.
Warnock, D.G. "Towards a Definition and Classification of Acute Kidney Injury," *Journal of the American Society of Nephrology* 16(11):3149-150, November 2005.

Nerve block

OVERVIEW

- Injections of medication—local anesthetics, corticosteroids, and opioids—onto or near nerves
- In cases of severe pain: nerve may be destroyed with injections of phenol or pure ethanol, or by using needles that freeze or heat the nerves
- Injections into joints also referred to as "blocks"
- Spinal injections to the lumbar, cervical, or thoracic spine areas: possibly given for pain from disc herniation, spinal stenosis, or herpes zoster; injections possibly given to facet joints
- Peripheral nerve blocks: directed to sensory and motor nerves; given to the occipital nerves, intercostal nerves, ilioinguinal nerve
- Sympathetic nerve block: directed to nerves that control gland function, sweating, and vasoconstriction and dilation; may be given to the stellate ganglion, lumbar sympathetic nerves, sympathetic nerves in front of the sacrum, or celiac plexus
- May be part of comprehensive pain management strategy

INDICATIONS

- Acute pain
- Chronic pain
- Nerve and joint inflammation
- Determination of pain source

PROCEDURE

- The patient is given a local anesthetic.
- Under fluoroscopy or computed tomography scanning, the practitioner locates the spinal nerve root.
- A straight or curved needle is introduced through the skin into the area adjacent to the nerve root.
- An anesthetic, corticosteroid, or opioid is then injected into the area bathing the nerve root.

COMPLICATIONS

- Allergic reaction
- Infection
- Trauma to site
- Partial loss of motor or sensory function

NURSING DIAGNOSES

- Acute pain
- Impaired physical mobility
- Ineffective tissue perfusion: Peripheral

EXPECTED OUTCOMES

The patient will:
- express feelings of increased comfort
- attain the highest degree of mobility possible within the confines of injury
- exhibit adequate tissue perfusion and pulses distally.

PRETREATMENT CARE

- Explain the procedure to the patient and answer questions.
- Verify that a consent form has been signed.
- Note patient history and allergies.
- Perform a neurologic assessment and assess vital signs.

POSTTREATMENT CARE

- The patient must assess his pain relief over the first 3 or 4 hours after the injection and report this to the anesthesiologist.
- Assess vital signs and neurologic status.
- Assess for pain relief, utilizing pain rating scales as appropriate.
- Monitor for complications.
- With cervical blocks, the patient can expect hoarseness, redness of the eye, drooping of the eyelid, and pupillary constriction for 4 to 8 hours after the injection.

PATIENT TEACHING

GENERAL

- Tell the patient that he may note redness distal to the injection site and have a warm feeling.
- Inform the patient that although pain relief may be noted immediately, the duration of relief is variable.

RESOURCES

Organizations

American College of Surgeons: *www.facs.org*
American College of Surgeons Oncology Group: *www.acosog.org*
American Medical Association: *www.ama-assn.org*

Selected references

Cole, A. "Nurse-Administered Femoral Nerve Block after Hip Fracture," *Nursing Times* 101(37):34-36, September 2005.

Niskanen, R.O., and Strandberg, N. "Bedside Femoral Block Performed on the First Postoperative Day after Unilateral Total Knee Arthroplasty: A Randomized Study of 49 Patients," *Journal of Knee Surgery* 18(3):192-96, July 2005.

Williams, B.A., et al. "Reduction of Verbal Pain Scores after Anterior Cruciate Ligament Reconstruction with 2-Day Continuous Femoral Nerve Block: A Randomized Clinical Trial," *Anesthesiology* 104(2):315-27, February 2006.

Noninvasive positive airway pressure

- Delivery of ventilatory support without need for an invasive artificial airway; may be given by a volume ventilator, a pressure-controlled ventilator, a bilevel positive airway pressure (BiPAP) device, or a continuous positive airway pressure (CPAP) device
- Noninvasive positive pressure ventilation (NPPV): used as an intermittent mode of assistance or as instantaneous and continuous support given to patients in acute respiratory distress
- CPAP: delivers continuous positive air pressure that improves breathing by counteracting intrinsic positive end-expiratory pressure decreasing preload and afterload, improving lung compliance, and decreasing the work of breathing
- CPAP devices: consist of a mask, tubes, and a fan that use air pressure to push the tongue forward and open the throat, which allows air to pass through the throat, and keeps the airways from being blocked, reducing snoring and preventing apnea
- BiPAP: delivers CPAP but also senses when an inspiratory effort is being made, thus delivers a higher pressure during inspiration; when flow stops, pressure returns to CPAP level; this positive pressure wave during inspiration unloads diaphragm, decreasing the work of breathing

INDICATIONS

- Sleep apnea
- Sleep-related breathing disorders
- Obstructive and mixed apnea
- Hypoxia
- Hypercapnia
- Acute or chronic respiratory failure
- Heart failure
- Acute pulmonary edema
- Acute asthma
- Cystic fibrosis
- Restrictive thoracic disorders

⚡ **WARNING** *If the patient has a decreased level of consciousness, copious secretions, can't protect his airway, or is hemodynamically unstable, an intubation is needed.*

- Choose the correct size of mask and initiate ventilator at CPAP of 0 cm water with a pressure support of 10 cm water.
- Hold the mask gently on the patient's face until the patient is comfortable and in full synchrony with the ventilator.
- Apply wound care dressing on the patient's nasal bridge and other pressure points, as appropriate.
- Secure the mask with head straps, but avoid a tight fit.
- Slowly increase CPAP to more than 5 cm water.
- Increase pressure support (that is, inspired positive airway pressure, 10 to 20 cm water) to achieve maximal exhaled tidal volume (10 to 15 ml/kg).
- Evaluate that ventilatory support is adequate, which is indicated by an improvement in dyspnea, a decreased respiratory rate, achievement of desired tidal volume, and good comfort for the patient.
- Oxygen supplementation is achieved through NPPV machine-to-machine oxygen saturation of greater than 90%.
- A backup rate may be provided in case the patient becomes apneic.
- In patients with hypoxemia, increase CPAP in increments of 2 or 3 cm water until the fraction of inspired oxygen is less than 0.6.
- Set the ventilator alarms and backup apnea parameters.
- Ask the patient to call for needs, and provide reassurance and encouragement.
- Monitor with oximetry, and adjust ventilator settings after obtaining arterial blood gas results.

COMPLICATIONS

◆ Skin irritation
◆ Nose dryness and stuffiness
◆ Eye irritation
◆ Sinus pain or congestion
◆ Barotrauma
◆ Adverse hemodynamic effects, such as preload reduction and hypotension

NURSING DIAGNOSES

◆ Impaired gas exchange
◆ Ineffective breathing pattern
◆ Ineffective tissue perfusion: Cardiopulmonary

EXPECTED OUTCOMES

The patient will:
◆ maintain pulse oximetry or arterial blood gas levels within normal limits
◆ exhibit normal breathing pattern
◆ maintain normal vital signs, blood pressure, capillary refill, and lung sounds.

PRETREATMENT CARE

◆ Explain the procedure to the patient and the intended effect.
◆ Verify that a consent form has been signed.
◆ Make sure the patient meets the criteria for the device and that use of the device isn't contraindicated.
◆ Monitor the patient's vital signs, pulse oximetry level, and hemodynamics if present.
◆ Perform an assessment and obtain patient history.

POSTTREATMENT CARE

◆ Monitor vital signs, hemodynamics, and pulse oximetry.
◆ Assess cardiac rate and rhythm.
◆ Monitor respiratory and cardiovascular status.
◆ Assess intake and output.
◆ Monitor for complications.
◆ Monitor laboratory test results.
◆ Suction patient, as indicated, and assist with deep-breathing and coughing exercises.

(continued)

Using continuous positive airway pressure

Dear Patient:

When you sleep, your tongue or relaxed fatty tissue in your throat blocks your breathing. To help you breathe more easily, a continuous positive airway pressure (also called *CPAP*) unit has been ordered to keep the fatty tissue out of your airway.

HOW CPAP WORKS

While you sleep, you'll wear a mask that fits snugly over your nose or a nasal prong that fits into your nose and supplies pressurized air. A flow generator feeds compressed air through this mask. You'll regulate the air pressure with a valve that you'll set for the level that will prevent your apnea.

Before using CPAP, you'll undergo a sleep study. This will help to calculate the pressure level that's right for you. Then a custom-fitted CPAP unit will be prescribed for your use at home.

USING CPAP

Your equipment supplier will show you how to set the machine for the prescribed pressure, how to check for leaks or kinks, and how to clean the mask and change the air filter. Some machines are also available that automatically regulate the pressure, as well as having humidified air.

Your symptoms should subside quickly after you start CPAP. Remember to keep using the device every night, even after you feel better. Otherwise, sleep apnea could recur.

TROUBLESHOOTING

Keep the names and telephone numbers of your health care provider and your equipment supplier handy.

◆ If your mask doesn't fit properly, your skin may become red and chafed, and escaping air may irritate your eyes. Call your equipment supplier and ask for a new mask. There are many types available.

◆ If you suspect the CPAP device may be giving you an earache, runny nose, or sinus pain, consult your health care provider. Also, report symptoms that recur or don't subside.

◆ If you have any mechanical or electrical problems with the equipment, let your equipment supplier know at once.

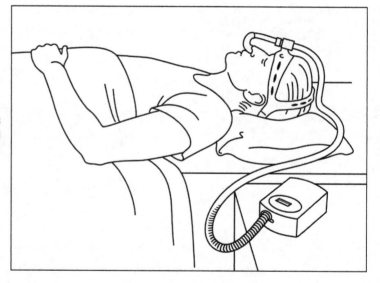

PATIENT TEACHING

GENERAL

◆ Stress the importance of follow-up care.
◆ Review the use and care of the airway device. (See *Using continuous positive airway pressure.*)
◆ Tell the patient that it may be necessary to try several masks to provide effective ventilation that's comfortable to him.
◆ Show the patient how to remove the mask in case of panic or vomiting.
◆ Tell the patient that because the mask must fit firmly over the nose and cheeks, it may irritate the skin; a different size or kind of mask may help. Also, there are special skin moisturizers made for users of CPAP devices. Some petroleum-based products can damage the mask, so tell the patient to check with the manufacturer or supplier.
◆ Discuss the use of nasal pillows that fit into the nostrils and relieve pressure on the bridge of the nose as appropriate. Suggest that the alternative use of a CPAP mask one night and nasal pillows the next night may increase comfort.
◆ Discuss the use of a chin strap to help hold up the jaw to prevent air escape.
◆ Tell the patient that it may be difficult to wear the mask all night long, every night, from the beginning. Tell him to keep trying, even if he can only use the mask for 1 hour per night at first, then gradually increase it.

RESOURCES

Organizations

American Medical Association: *www.ama-assn.org*
National Heart, Lung, and Blood Institute: *www.nhlbi.nih.gov*

Selected references

Dickerson, S.S., and Kennedy, M.C. "CPAP Devices: Encouraging Patients with Sleep Apnea," *Rehabilitation Nursing* 31(3):114-22, May-June 2006.
Loredo, J.S. et al. "Effect of Continuous Positive Airway Pressure versus Supplemental Oxygen on Sleep Quality in obstructive Sleep Apnea: A Placebo–CPAP-controlled Study," *Sleep* 29(4): 564-71, April 2006.
Pirret, A.M., et al. "Local Experience with the Use of Nasal Bubble CPAP in Infants with Bronchiolitis Admitted to a Combined Adult/Paediatric Intensive Care Unit," *Intensive and Critical Care Nursing: The Official Journal of the British Society of Critical Care Nurses* 21(5):314-19, October 2005.

Oophorectomy and salpingectomy

- Oophorectomy: surgical removal of one or both ovaries
- Bilateral oophorectomy: may be performed during a hysterectomy if disease has spread to ovaries
- Salpingectomy: surgical removal of one or both fallopian tubes
- Salpingo-oophorectomy: when oophorectomy and salpingectomy are performed together
- May be performed laparoscopically

INDICATIONS
Oophorectomy
- Ovarian cysts
- Ovarian cancer
- Estrogen-dependent tumor
- Endometriosis

Salpingectomy
- Salpingitis
- Severe pelvic inflammatory disease
- Endometriosis
- Ectopic pregnancy
- Permanent contraception

- After the patient receives general anesthesia, a transverse or vertical incision is made through the abdominal wall.
- After the internal reproductive organs are located, one or both ovaries, one or both fallopian tubes, or both ovaries and both fallopian tubes are excised.
- When the procedure is done with a hysterectomy, the uterus is also removed.
- The abdominal incision is closed with sutures or staples, and a sterile dressing is applied.

COMPLICATIONS
- Hemorrhage
- Infection
- Atelectasis
- Pulmonary embolism
- Physical changes related to estrogen loss
- Change in self-concept

- Acute pain
- Deficient fluid volume
- Situational low self-esteem

EXPECTED OUTCOMES
The patient will:
- express relief of pain
- maintain adequate fluid volume
- express positive statements about self.

PRETREATMENT CARE

◆ Explain the treatment and preparation to the patient and her family.
◆ Verify that the patient has signed an appropriate consent form.
◆ Explain postoperative care.
◆ Encourage the patient to discuss her feelings.
◆ Insert a urinary catheter and connect it to gravity drainage.

POSTTREATMENT CARE

◆ Administer medications as ordered.
◆ Encourage coughing and deep-breathing exercises.
◆ Help the patient splint the incision with a pillow.
◆ Assist the patient out of bed.
◆ Encourage ambulation as ordered.
◆ Administer I.V. therapy until the patient can tolerate oral intake.
◆ Monitor the patient's vital signs and intake and output.
◆ Monitor the surgical wound and dressings.
◆ Perform dressing changes and incision care as ordered.
◆ Remove the urinary catheter, as ordered, and reassess voiding patterns and urine characteristics.
◆ Monitor vaginal drainage for odor, color, and amount; report signs of excessive bleeding or infection to the practitioner.

PATIENT TEACHING

GENERAL

◆ Review the medications and possible adverse reactions with the patient.
◆ Teach the patient the signs and symptoms of infection.
◆ Tell the patient about possible complications and instruct her when to notify the practitioner.
◆ Tell the patient about activity restrictions ordered by the practitioner.
◆ Stress the need for follow-up care.

RESOURCES

Organizations

American Board of Obstetrics and Gynecology: *www.abog.org*
American Medical Association: *www.ama-assn.org*

Selected references

Agostini, A., et al. "Value of Laparoscopic Assistance for Vaginal Hysterectomy With Prophylactic Bilateral Oophorectomy," *American Journal of Obstetrics and Gynecology* 194(2):351-54, February 2006.

Chung-Park, M. "Anxiety Attacks Following Surgical Menopause: A Case Report," *Holistic Nursing Practice* 19(5): 236-40, September-October 2005.

Lozeau, A.M., and Potter, B. "Diagnosis and Management of Ectopic Pregnancy," *American Family Physician* 72(9): 1707-14, November 2005.

Open reduction and internal fixation of fractures

OVERVIEW

- Involves using an implanted fixation device (consisting of nails, screws, pins, wires, or rods, possibly used with metal plates) to stabilize a fracture (also known as *surgical reduction*)
- Used to treat fractures of the face and jaw, spine, bones of the arms and legs, and joints (usually hip)
- May involve keeping the device in the body indefinitely unless the patient has adverse reactions after healing process is complete (see *Types of internal fixation devices*)
- Permits earlier mobilization and shorter hospitalization, which is particularly beneficial in elderly patients with hip fractures

INDICATIONS
- Fracture

PROCEDURE

- After the patient receives general anesthesia, the surgeon makes an incision at the fracture site, or above and below depending on the site and type of fracture.
- The surgeon manipulates the bone ends into their correct position and then fixes them with steel plates and screws. Rods may be inserted through the bone shaft to stabilize the fracture. This is called *open reduction and internal fixation.*
- A fine plastic drainage tube may be placed from the wound to drain any residual blood from the surgery.
- The skin wound is then closed with stitches.

COMPLICATIONS

- Wound infection, especially involving metal fixation device (may require reopening the incision, draining the suture line, and removing the fixation device)
- Malunion
- Nonunion
- Fat or pulmonary embolism
- Neurovascular impairment

  AGE FACTOR *If the fracture is near the growth plate of the bone, the child will need to be followed carefully to ensure proper healing and to avoid complications.*
- Chronic pain

Types of internal fixation devices

Choice of a specific internal fixation device depends on the fracture's location, type, and configuration.

In trochanteric or subtrochanteric fractures, the surgeon may use a hip pin or nail, with or without a screw plate. A pin or plate with extra nails stabilizes the fracture by impacting the bone ends at the fracture site.	In an uncomplicated fracture of the femoral shaft, the surgeon may use an intramedullary rod. This device permits early ambulation with partial weight bearing.	Another choice for fixation of a long-bone fracture is a screw plate, shown here on the tibia.	In an arm fracture, the surgeon may fix the involved bones with a plate, rod, or nail. Most radial and ulnar fractures may be fixed with plates, whereas humeral fractures are commonly fixed with rods.

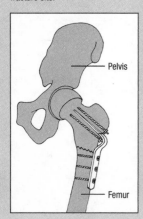

Pelvis
Femur

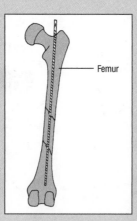

Femur

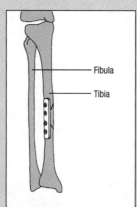

Fibula
Tibia

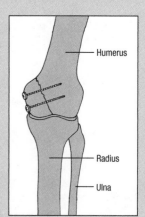

Humerus
Radius
Ulna

- Acute pain
- Impaired physical mobility
- Risk for infection

EXPECTED OUTCOMES
The patient will:
- express feelings of increased comfort
- attain the highest degree of mobility possible within the confines of injury
- remain free from infection.

PRETREATMENT CARE

- Explain the procedure to the patient.
- Assess neurovascular status in the affected extremity.
- Verify that the patient has signed an appropriate consent form.

POSTTREATMENT CARE

- After the procedure, monitor the patient's vital signs every 2 to 4 hours for 24 hours, then every 4 to 8 hours, according to your facility's protocol.

  ⚡ **WARNING** *Changes in vital signs may indicate hemorrhage or infection.*

- Monitor fluid intake and output every 4 to 8 hours.
- Perform neurovascular checks every 2 to 4 hours for 24 hours, then every 4 to 8 hours as appropriate. Assess color, motion, sensation, digital movement, edema, capillary refill, and pulses of the affected area.
- Compare findings with the unaffected side.
- Apply an ice bag to the surgical site to reduce swelling, relieve pain, and lessen bleeding.
- Give analgesics or opioids before exercising or mobilizing the affected area. If the patient is using patient-controlled analgesia, instruct him to give himself a dose before exercising or mobilizing.

- Monitor the patient for pain unrelieved by analgesics or opioids and for burning, tingling, or numbness, which may indicate infection or impaired circulation.
- Elevate the affected limb on a pillow, if appropriate, to minimize edema.
- Check surgical dressings for excessive drainage or bleeding.
- Check the incision site for signs of infection (such as erythema, drainage, edema, or unusual pain).
- Help the patient perform range-of-motion and other muscle-strengthening exercises to promote circulation, improve muscle tone, and maintain joint function.
- Gradually and progressively teach the patient to move and walk, helped by use of an overhead frame with trapeze, crutches, or a walker.
- To avoid the complications of immobility after surgery, have the patient use an incentive spirometer.
- Apply elastic stockings and sequential compression device, as appropriate.
- Check to see if the patient needs a pressure-relief mattress.

PATIENT TEACHING

GENERAL
- Tell the patient what to expect during postoperative assessment and monitoring, teach him how to use an incentive spirometer, and prepare him for proposed exercise and progressive ambulation regimens if needed.
- Instruct the patient to report pain to the practitioner.
- Before discharge, teach the patient and his family how to care for the incision site.
- Explain to the patient the signs and symptoms of wound infection.
- Teach the patient and his family about giving medications for pain.
- Advise the patient about following an exercise regimen, as appropriate.
- Teach the patient how to use crutches or a walker, as appropriate.

RESOURCES
Organizations
American Academy of Orthopaedic Surgeons: *www.aaos.org*
American Academy of Pediatrics: *www.aap.org*

Selected references
DiFazio, R., and Atkinson, C.C. "Extremity Fractures in Children: When Is It an Emergency?" *Journal of Pediatric Nursing* 20(4):298-304, August 2005.

Gortzak, Y., et al. "Pediatric Olecranon Fractures: Open Reduction and Internal Fixation with Removable Kirschner Wires and Absorbable Sutures," *Journal of Pediatric Orthopaedics* 26(1):39-42, January-February 2006.

Leung, Y.F., et al. "The Crisscross Injury Mechanism in Forearm Injuries," *Archives of Orthopaedic and Trauma Surgery* 125(5):298-303, June 2005.

Schmittenbecher, P.P. "State-of-the-Art Treatment of Forearm Shaft Fractures," *Injury* 36(Suppl 1):A25-34, February 2005.

Orchiectomy

OVERVIEW

- Removal of one or both testicles
- May be performed as abdominal surgery or local surgery in surgeon's office

INDICATIONS
- Testicular cancer

PROCEDURE

- Depending on the surgeon's preference and the patient's condition, an abdominal or testicular approach may be used.
- With the abdominal approach the patient will receive general anesthesia. The surgeon makes a 4" (10.2-cm) incision through the lower abdomen on the affected side, then pushes the testicle up through the pelvic region and removes it. The area is then sutured and the wound closed.
- Alternatively, with the testicular approach, local anesthesia is used and the surgeon makes an incision along the testicle, which is pulled free from the surrounding area. The spermatic cord is clamped and ligated with an appropriate type of suture material. The cord is ligated twice with this suture to prevent bleeding when it's cut. The ligated end of the spermatic cord is checked for bleeding and then released back into the body. The other testicle is located and removed in the same manner. The subcutaneous tissues and skin are closed with appropriate suture material and technique.
- Before closing, the surgeon may place a testicular prosthesis.

COMPLICATIONS
- Bleeding
- Infection
- Emotional adjustment
- Sexual dysfunction
- Pain
- Nerve injury

NURSING DIAGNOSES

- Impaired urinary elimination
- Risk for infection
- Risk for situational low self-esteem

EXPECTED OUTCOMES
The patient will:
- demonstrate normal elimination patterns
- exhibit no signs of infection
- express feelings of positive self-worth.

PRETREATMENT CARE

- Review the procedure with the patient and answer any questions.
- Verify that a consent form has been signed.
- Review preoperative laboratory blood work and diagnostic testing; make sure that the practitioner's history and physical examination are completed.
- Note allergies.
- Provide emotional support.
- Provide a baseline nursing assessment.
- Complete the surgical verification process.

POSTTREATMENT CARE

- Monitor the patient's vital signs and intake and output.
- Assess for signs of complications, such as bleeding and infection.
- Maintain patency of I.V. tubes and monitor hydration status.
- Monitor blood studies.
- Encourage the patient to deep breathe and cough; assist with ambulation.
- Provide pain medication and assess for effect.
- Assess for edema and bruising; ice may be applied and the area elevated while the patient is in bed as ordered.

PATIENT TEACHING

GENERAL
- Tell the patient about administration, dosage, and possible adverse reactions to his medications.
- Inform the patient that he'll have discomfort as he begins to ambulate, but that this should improve.
- Instruct the patient to wear comfortable clothing, such as nonrestrictive sweatpants, until healing occurs.
- Tell the patient that there may be numbness of the skin around the incision, but that should eventually dissipate.
- Review the symptoms to report to the practitioner such as complications.
- Instruct the patient to seek follow-up care.
- Tell the patient to restrict activity, such as avoiding driving or lifting heavy objects, as directed by the practitioner. (See *Recovering from testicular surgery.*)

RESOURCES
Organizations
American Urological Association: *www.auanet.org*
National Cancer Institute: *www.nci.nih.gov/cancerinfo*

Selected references
Fleer, J., et al. "Quality of Life of Testicular Cancer Survivors and the Relationship with Sociodemographics, Cancer-related Variables, and Life Events," *Supportive Care in Cancer* 14(3):251-59, March 2006.

Haga, K., et al. "Adult Paratesticular Rhabdomyosarcoma," *Natural Clinical Practice Urology* 2(8):398-402, August 2005.

Kaplan, M., and Klein, E.A. "Bilateral Metachronous Testicular Seminoma," *Natural Clinical Practice Urology* 2(9):457-60, September 2005.

Recovering from testicular surgery

Dear Patient:

As with most operations, you'll need a few weeks to recover completely from testicular surgery. During this time, follow these guidelines to minimize your discomfort and speed recuperation.

CARE FOR YOUR INCISION PROPERLY

Before you leave the hospital, you'll be shown how to clean the incisional area and change the dressing. When you go home, refer to the following instructions:

◆ Keep the incision dry at all times. Change the dressing if it gets wet during bathing or feels damp from perspiration.

◆ Never reuse cotton-tipped swabs or gauze pads. Discard them after you have changed the dressing.

◆ If your skin becomes irritated from the adhesive tape, consult your health care provider, who may recommend substituting a protective dressing or using a protective wipe or spray to create a barrier between your skin and the adhesive.

◆ Call your health care provider at once if the incision opens or bleeds heavily.

RECOGNIZE AND REPORT INFECTION

Take your temperature daily for the first week. Immediately report a fever above 100.5° F (38° C). Also, notify your health care provider at once if you have chills, if you notice drainage from the incision, or if your incision becomes painful, red, or swollen.

SPECIAL INSTRUCTIONS

◆ Wear a scrotal support to reduce pain and to protect the scrotum.

◆ Avoid strenuous physical activity until your incision is completely healed. Walking is a safe way to exercise without overdoing.

◆ Eat properly and drink plenty of fluids. If you have less of an appetite than usual, try eating small, frequent meals instead of three large meals.

◆ Report pain that persists more than 10 days after surgery.

Ovarian cystectomy

- Removal of ovarian cysts
- Performed only for benign cysts and when the patient wishes to salvage the ovary
- Performed laparoscopically or through a conventional incision; former approach results in less pain and disfigurement and faster recuperation

INDICATIONS
- Ovarian cysts

PROCEDURE

- The patient receives general anesthesia.
- Laparoscopy can remove the ovarian cysts safely and effectively, without affecting the healthy ovarian tissue. The cysts, regardless of their size, can be removed intact because they're carefully dissected free from the ovary and removed from the body via collapsible laparoscopic bags. Cysts that are suspicious for cancer may be sent for immediate pathologic examination during the surgery and appropriate steps taken based on the diagnosis.
- In the conventional approach, a transverse or vertical incision is made through the abdominal wall. After the internal reproductive organs are located, one or both ovaries are examined and the cysts removed. The abdominal incision is closed with sutures or staples, and a sterile dressing is applied.

COMPLICATIONS
- Hemorrhage
- Infection
- Pulmonary embolism
- Infertility if both ovaries are damaged
- Adhesions

NURSING DIAGNOSES

- Acute pain
- Deficient fluid volume
- Risk for infection

EXPECTED OUTCOMES
The patient will:
- express relief of pain
- maintain adequate fluid volume
- exhibit no signs or symptoms of infection.

PRETREATMENT CARE

- Explain the treatment and preparation to the patient and her family.
- Verify that the patient has signed an appropriate consent form.
- Explain postoperative care.
- Encourage the patient to discuss her feelings.
- Insert a urinary catheter and connect it to gravity drainage.

POSTTREATMENT CARE

- Administer medications as ordered.
- Perform dressing changes and incision care as ordered.
- Encourage coughing and deep-breathing exercises.
- Help the patient splint the incision with a pillow.
- Assist the patient out of bed.
- Encourage ambulation as ordered.
- Administer I.V. therapy until the patient can tolerate oral intake.
- Monitor the patient's vital signs and intake and output.
- Assess for complications, such as presence of abnormal bleeding or infection.
- Monitor the surgical wound and dressings.
- Assess drainage.

PATIENT TEACHING

GENERAL

- Review the medications and possible adverse reactions with the patient.
- Tell the patient the signs and symptoms of infection.
- Discuss possible complications of the procedure with the patient and when to notify the practitioner.
- Review activity restrictions with the patient; tell her that she may return to normal activities within 1 or 2 weeks.
- Stress the need for follow-up care.

RESOURCES
Organizations
American Board of Obstetrics and Gynecology: *www.abog.org*
American Medical Association: *www.ama-assn.org*

Selected references
Candiani, M., et al. "Ovarian Recovery after Laparoscopic Enucleation of Ovarian Cysts: Insights from Echographic Short-Term Postsurgical Follow-up," *Journal of Minimally Invasive Gynecology* 12(5):409-14, September-October 2005.

Tinelli, R., et al. "Conservative Surgery for Borderline Ovarian Tumors: A Review," *Gynecologic Oncology* 100(1):185-91, January 2006.

Pacemaker insertion

OVERVIEW

- Pacemaker: battery-operated generator that controls heart rate by emitting timed electrical signals, which trigger contraction of the heart muscle; may be temporary or permanent
- Capabilities of pacemakers: described by a five-letter coding system, although three letters are more commonly used
- First letter: identifies the heart chamber being paced—V (ventricle), A (atrium), D (dual, ventricle and atrium), or O (none)
- Second letter: identifies the heart chamber where pacemaker senses intrinsic activity—V (ventricle), A (atrium), D (dual, ventricle and atrium), or O (none)
- Third letter: indicates pacemaker's mode of response to the intrinsic activity that it senses in atrium or ventricle—T (triggered), I (inhibited), D (dual, triggered or inhibited), or O (none)
- Fourth letter: indicates the pacemaker's programmability—P (basic function programmability), M (multiprogrammable), C (communicating functions such as telemetry), R (rate responsiveness or modulation), or O (none)
- Fifth letter: denotes special tachyarrhythmia functions and identifies how the pacemaker will respond to a tachyarrhythmia—P (pacing ability), S (shock), D (dual, can shock and pace), or O (none)

INDICATIONS
Temporary pacemaker
- Emergency treatment of symptomatic bradycardia
- Bridge to permanent pacemaker implantation or to determine the effect of pacing on cardiac function
- Open-heart surgery

Permanent pacemaker
- Symptomatic bradycardia
- Advanced symptomatic atrioventricular block
- Sick sinus syndrome
- Sinus arrest
- Sinoatrial block
- Stokes-Adams syndrome
- Tachyarrhythmias
- Arrhythmias caused by antiarrhythmic drugs

PROCEDURE

- Insertion or application of a temporary pacemaker varies, depending on the device. (See *Types of temporary pacemakers.*)

PERMANENT PACEMAKER
- The pacemaker is implanted using a transvenous endocardial approach (requiring local anesthesia).
- The patient is sedated and the chest or abdomen is prepared.
- A 3″ to 4″ (7.5- to 10-cm) incision is made in the selected site.
- The electrode catheter is inserted through a vein and guided by fluoroscopy to the heart chamber appropriate for the pacemaker type.
- Pacemaker leads are inserted.
- A pacing system analyzer is used to set the pulse generator to the proper stimulating and sensing thresholds.
- The pulse generator is attached to the leads and implanted into a pocket of muscle in the chest wall.
- The incision is closed, and a tight occlusive dressing is applied.

COMPLICATIONS
- Infection
- Venous thrombosis, embolism
- Pneumothorax
- Pectoral or diaphragmatic muscle stimulation from the pacemaker
- Arrhythmias
- Cardiac tamponade
- Heart failure
- Pacemaker malfunction
- Microshock (temporary)

Types of temporary pacemakers

Temporary pacemakers come in three types: transcutaneous, transvenous, and epicardial. They're used to pace the heart after cardiac surgery, during cardiopulmonary resuscitation, and when sinus arrest, symptomatic sinus bradycardia, or complete heart block occurs.

TRANSCUTANEOUS PACEMAKER
Completely noninvasive and easily applied, a transcutaneous pacemaker proves especially useful in an emergency. To perform pacing with the device, the practitioner places pacing electrodes at heart level on the patient's chest and back and connects them to a pulse generator.

TRANSVENOUS PACEMAKER
This balloon-tipped pacing catheter is inserted via the subclavian or jugular vein into the right ventricle. The procedure can be done at the bedside or in the cardiac catheterization laboratory. A transvenous pacemaker offers better control of the heartbeat than a transcutaneous pacemaker. However, electrode insertion takes longer, limiting its usefulness in emergencies.

EPICARDIAL PACEMAKER
Implanted during open-heart surgery, an epicardial pacemaker permits rapid treatment of postoperative complications. During surgery, the surgeon attaches the leads to the heart and runs them out through the abdominal wall. Afterward, the leads are coiled on the patient's chest, insulated, and covered with a dressing. If pacing is needed, the leads are simply uncovered and attached to a pulse generator. When pacing is no longer needed, the leads can be easily removed.

NURSING DIAGNOSES

- Activity intolerance
- Decreased cardiac output
- Risk for infection

EXPECTED OUTCOMES
The patient will:
- carry out activities of daily living without excess fatigue or decreased energy
- maintain adequate cardiac output
- remain free from infection.

PRETREATMENT CARE

- Explain the treatment and preparation to the patient and his family.
- Verify that the patient or a responsible family member has signed an appropriate consent form.
- Explain postoperative care.
- Obtain baseline vital signs and a 12-lead electrocardiogram (ECG).
- Restrict food and fluids as ordered.
- Establish an I.V. if not already in place so that emergency medications can be administered if needed.

POSTTREATMENT CARE

- Administer medications as ordered.
- Maintain continuous cardiac monitoring.
- Monitor for cardiac arrhythmias.

- Document the type of pacemaker inserted, lead system, pacemaker mode, and pacing guidelines.
- If the patient requires defibrillation, place paddles at least 4″ (10.2 cm) from the pulse generator; avoid anteroposterior paddle placement.
- After the first 24 hours, begin passive range-of-motion exercises on the affected arm if ordered.
- Monitor the patient's vital signs and intake and output.
- Assess for complications, such as abnormal bleeding and infection.

WARNING *Watch for signs and symptoms of a perforated ventricle, with resultant cardiac tamponade: persistent hiccups, distant heart sounds, pulsus paradoxus, hypotension with narrow pulse pressure, increased venous pressure, cyanosis, distended jugular veins, decreased urine output, restlessness, or complaints of fullness in the chest. Notify the practitioner immediately if the patient develops any of these conditions.*

- Assess the surgical wound and dressing.
- Monitor drainage.
- Assess pacemaker function. (See *Assessing pacemaker function.*)

If the patient has had a temporary pacemaker inserted, complete the following:

- After insertion of a temporary pacemaker, assess the patient's vital signs, skin color, level of consciousness, and peripheral pulses to determine the effectiveness of the paced rhythm.
- Perform a 12-lead ECG to serve as a baseline, and then perform additional 12-lead ECGs daily or with clinical changes. Also, if possible, obtain a rhythm strip before, during, and after pacemaker placement; any time pacemaker settings are changed; and whenever the patient receives treatment because of a complication due to the pacemaker.
- Continuously monitor the ECG reading, noting capture, sensing, rate, intrinsic beats, and competition of paced and intrinsic rhythms. If the pacemaker is sensing correctly, the

---

Assessing pacemaker function

After a pacemaker has been inserted, follow these steps to assess its function:

1. Determine the pacemaker's mode and settings.
2. Review the patient's 12-lead electrocardiogram (ECG).
3. Select a monitoring lead that clearly shows the pacemaker spikes.
4. Consider the pacemaker mode and whether symptoms of decreased cardiac output are present when evaluating the ECG.
5. Look for information that tells you which chamber is paced. Ask:
– Is there capture?
– Is there a P wave or QRS complex after each atrial or ventricular spike?
– Do P waves and QRS complexes stem from intrinsic activity?
– If intrinsic activity is present, what's the pacemaker's response?
6. Determine the rate by quickly counting the number of complexes in a 6-second ECG strip or, more accurately, by counting the number of small boxes between complexes and dividing by 1,500.

Pacemaker impulses are visible on an ECG tracing as spikes. Large or small, pacemaker

spikes appear above or below the isoelectric line. The illustration below shows an atrial and ventricular pacemaker spike.

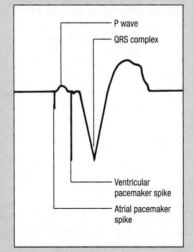

P wave
QRS complex
Ventricular pacemaker spike
Atrial pacemaker spike

(continued)

sense indicator on the pulse generator should flash with each beat.

- Watch for oversensing. If the pacemaker is too sensitive, it can misinterpret muscle movements or other events in the cardiac cycle as intrinsic cardiac electrical activity. Pacing won't occur when it's needed, and the heart rate and atrioventricular synchrony won't be maintained.
- When using a transcutaneous pacemaker, don't place the electrodes over a bony area because bone conducts current poorly. With a female patient, place the anterior electrode under the patient's breast but not over her diaphragm. If the physician inserts the electrode through the brachial or femoral vein, immobilize the patient's arm or leg to avoid putting stress on the pacing wires.
- If the patient has epicardial pacing wires in place, clean the insertion site as per facility policy and change the dressing daily. At the same time, monitor the site for signs of infection. Always keep the pulse generator nearby in case pacing becomes necessary.
- Institute precautions to prevent microshock; this includes warning the patient not to use any electrical equipment that isn't grounded, such as telephones, electrical shavers, televisions, or lamps.
- Place a plastic cover supplied by the manufacturer over the pacemaker controls to avoid an accidental setting change. Also, insulate the pacemaker by covering exposed metal parts, such as electrode connections and pacemaker terminals, with nonconducting tape, or place the pacing unit in a dry, rubber surgical glove.
- If the patient is disoriented or uncooperative, use restraints as necessary to prevent accidental removal of pacemaker wires. If the patient needs emergency defibrillation, make sure the pacemaker can withstand the procedure. If you're unsure, disconnect the pulse generator to prevent damage.

PATIENT TEACHING

GENERAL

- Discuss the possible complications and when to notify the practitioner.
- Tell the patient about any diet or activity restrictions ordered by the practitioner.
- Teach the patient how to monitor the heart rate and rhythm.
- Instruct the patient to avoid placing excessive pressure over the insertion site, making sudden moves, or extending his arms over his head for 4 weeks after discharge.
- Emphasize the importance of informing medical personnel of the implanted pacemaker before undergoing certain diagnostic tests.
- Stress the need for follow-up care. (See *Caring for your permanent pacemaker*.)
- Advise the patient to notify the practitioner if he experiences signs of pacemaker failure, such as palpitations, a fast heart rate, a slow heart rate (5 to 10 beats less than the pacemaker's setting), dizziness, fainting, shortness of breath, swollen ankles or feet, anxiety, forgetfulness, or confusion.
- Provide the patient with an identification card that lists the pacemaker type and manufacturer, serial number, pacemaker rate setting, date implanted, and practitioner's name. Also instruct the patient in measures for daily care, safety and activity guidelines, and special precautions.

RESOURCES
Organizations
American College of Cardiology: *www.acc.org*
American Heart Association: *www.americanheart.org*

Selected references
Barrett, L.O., and Sticco, C.C. "Delayed Cardiac Tamponade by Iatrogenic Aortic Perforation with Pacemaker Implantation," *Journal of Thoracic and Cardiovascular Surgery* 131(2):480-81, February 2006.
Hall, M.C., and Todd, D.M. "Modern Management of Arrhythmias," *Postgraduate Medical Journal* 82(964):117-25, February 2006.
Overbay, D., and Criddle, L. "Mastering Temporary Invasive Cardiac Pacing," *Critical Care Nurse* 24(3):25-32, June 2004.

Caring for your permanent pacemaker

Dear Patient:

After your permanent pacemaker has been placed, you will need to perform daily care. In addition, there are safety and activity measures and special precautions you should know about.

Follow these instructions and contact your health care provider if you have any questions.

DAILY CARE

◆ Clean your pacemaker site gently with soap and water when you take a shower or a bath. Leave the incision exposed to the air.

◆ Inspect your skin around the incision. A slight bulge is normal, but call your health care provider if you feel discomfort or notice swelling, redness, a discharge, or other problems.

◆ Check your pulse for 1 minute as your nurse or health care provider showed you—on the side of your neck, inside your elbow, or on the thumb side of your wrist. Your pulse rate should be the same as your pacemaker rate or faster. Contact your health care provider if you think your heart is beating too fast or too slow.

◆ Take your medications, including those for pain, as prescribed. Even with a pacemaker, you still need the medication your health care provider ordered.

SAFETY AND ACTIVITY

◆ Keep your pacemaker instruction booklet handy, and carry your pacemaker identification card at all times. This card has your pacemaker model number and other information needed by health care personnel who treat you.

◆ You can resume most of your usual activities when you feel comfortable doing so, but don't drive until your health care provider gives you permission. Also avoid heavy lifting and stretching exercises for at least 4 weeks or as directed by your health care provider.

◆ Try to use both arms equally to prevent stiffness. Check with your health care provider before you golf, swim, play tennis, or perform other strenuous activities.

ELECTROMAGNETIC INTERFERENCE

◆ Today's pacemakers are designed and insulated to eliminate most electrical interference. You can safely operate common household electrical devices, including microwave ovens, razors, and sewing machines. You can ride in or operate a motor vehicle without it affecting your pacemaker.

◆ Take care to avoid direct contact with large running motors, high-powered CB radios and other similar equipment, welding machinery, and radar devices.

◆ If your pacemaker activates the metal detector in an airport, show your pacemaker identification card to the security official.

◆ Because the metal in your pacemaker makes you ineligible for certain diagnostic studies, such as magnetic resonance imaging, be sure to inform your health care providers, dentist, and other health care personnel that you have a pacemaker.

◆ When using a cellular phone, use it on the side opposite your pacemaker.

SPECIAL PRECAUTIONS

◆ If you feel light-headed or dizzy when you're near any electrical equipment, moving away from the device should restore normal pacemaker function. Ask your health care provider about particular electrical devices.

◆ Notify your health care provider if you experience signs of pacemaker failure, such as palpitations, a fast heart rate, a slow heart rate (5 to 10 beats less than the pacemaker's setting), dizziness, fainting, shortness of breath, swollen ankles or feet, anxiety, forgetfulness, or confusion.

CHECKUPS

◆ Be sure to schedule and keep regular checkup appointments with your health care provider.

◆ If your health care provider checks your pacemaker status by telephone, keep your transmission schedule and instructions in a handy place.

Pallidotomy

- Involves destruction of part of the globus pallidus (part of the brain involved with the control of movement); may help to restore the balance required for normal movement
- May be unilateral or bilateral
- Unilateral pallidotomy: improves the side of the body opposite the lesioned side of the brain
- Bilateral pallidotomy: improves dyskinesias further, but also increases risk of worsened effects on cognition, swallowing, and speech, thus, it's rarely performed

INDICATIONS

- Dyskinesias
- Dystonia
- Tremor
- Rigidity
- Bradykinesia
- Gait disturbance

- A local anesthetic is applied to the scalp area, and the patient is awake during the surgery.
- Through a small hole drilled in the skull, the surgeon inserts a hollow probe to the target location; placement is confirmed by electrical tests. The area is then destroyed using either heat or cold.
- With heat destruction, the probe heats surrounding tissue by emission of radio waves. The heat destroys nearby tissue. Effects of the surgery are apparent almost immediately.
- With cold destruction, an extremely cold substance, liquid nitrogen, is circulated inside the probe. The cold probe destroys the targeted brain tissue. The probe is then removed, and the wound is closed.

COMPLICATIONS

- Hemorrhage
- Infection
- Seizures
- Visual deficits
- Temporary facial paralysis
- Weakness, loss of sensation, or paralysis on one side of the body
- Loss or slurred speech and difficulty swallowing
- Temporary problems with balance
- Numbness around the mouth and in the hands
- Problems with thought and memory
- Stroke
- Death

- Disturbed sensory perception (all)
- Risk for infection
- Risk for injury

EXPECTED OUTCOMES

The patient will:

- exhibit improved or normal neurologic status
- exhibit no signs of infection
- not have any falls.

PRETREATMENT CARE

- Before surgery, detailed brain scans using magnetic resonance imaging are done to identify the precise location for treatment.
- Review the surgical procedure with the patient and his family and ensure that a consent form has been signed.
- Review the patient's history, medications, and laboratory test results.
- The evening or morning before the surgery, have the patient take a bath and wash his hair.
- Assess the patient's neurologic status for baseline level.

POSTTREATMENT CARE

- Monitor the patient's vital signs, intake and output, and daily weight.
- Monitor level of consciousness and respiratory status.
- Monitor for signs of increased intracranial pressure.
- Monitor hemodynamic values and heart rate and rhythm.
- Monitor fluid and electrolyte balance.
- Monitor urine specific gravity.
- Monitor surgical wound and dressings; note drainage and monitor for signs of complications.
- Assess effectiveness of pain medication.
- Maintain oxygenation; encourage the patient to take deep breaths and cough; suction as indicated.
- Assess the patient's neurologic status every 2 hours or as ordered.

PATIENT TEACHING

GENERAL

- Tell the patient he will be able to gradually return to normal activities.
- Emphasize need for follow-up and continuing care.
- Tell the family it's unlikely that the patient's medications will be stopped immediately, but will be tapered or changed based on the patient's recovery.

RESOURCES

Organizations

American Academy of Neurology: *www.aan.com*
MedicineNet, Inc.: *www.medicinenet.com*

Selected references

Farrell, A., et al. "Effects of Neurosurgical Management of Parkinson's Disease on Speech Characteristics and Oromotor Function," *Journal of Speech, Language, and Hearing Research* 48(1):5-20, February 2005.

Murat, I., et al. "Destructive Stereotactic Surgery for Treatment of Dystonia," *Surgical Neurology* 64(Suppl 2):S89-94; discussion S94-95, November 2005.

Pancreaticoduodenectomy

- Surgical removal of the pancreas with resection, drainage procedure, and anastomoses to treat pancreatic diseases when more conservative techniques have failed
- Carries a high risk of complications
- Also called *Whipple procedure*

INDICATIONS
- Pancreatic cancer
- Chronic pancreatitis
- Islet cell tumor or insulinoma

- The patient receives anesthesia and the surgeon makes an abdominal incision.
- The rest of the procedure is based on evaluation of the pancreas, liver, gallbladder, and common bile duct.
- The surgeon removes the head of the pancreas, the entire duodenum, a portion of the jejunum, the distal third of the stomach, and the lower half of the common bile duct, with the reestablishment of continuity of the biliary, pancreatic, and GI tract systems.
- The surgeon inserts two drains into the abdomen and closes the wound.

COMPLICATIONS
- Hemorrhage
- Fistula formation
- Abscess
- Type 1 diabetes
- Delayed gastric emptying
- Pancreatic anastomotic leak

- Acute pain
- Imbalanced nutrition: Less than body requirements
- Risk for infection

EXPECTED OUTCOMES
The patient will:
- express feelings of comfort
- maintain or achieve ideal body weight
- remain free from signs and symptoms of infection.

PRETREATMENT CARE

- Explain the treatment and preparation to the patient and his family.
- Verify that the patient has signed an appropriate consent form.
- Explain postoperative care.
- Provide emotional support.
- Administer analgesics as ordered.
- Arrange for required diagnostic studies as ordered.
- Provide enteral or parenteral nutrition before surgery if ordered.
- Provide low-fat, high-calorie feedings as ordered.
- Administer oral hypoglycemic agents or insulin as ordered.
- Administer mechanical and antibiotic bowel preparation as well as prophylactic systemic antibiotics as ordered.
- Assist with nasogastric tube and indwelling urinary catheter insertion.
- Monitor the patient's vital signs and intake and output.
- Monitor blood and urine glucose levels.

POSTTREATMENT CARE

- Administer medications as ordered.
- Administer plasma expanders and I.V. fluids as ordered.
- Administer oxygen as ordered.
- Encourage deep breathing, coughing, and use of incentive spirometry.
- Maintain the patency of drainage tubes.
- Change dressings, and provide incision care as ordered.
- Use a wound pouching system to contain drainage as needed.

⚡ **WARNING** *Monitor for and report absent bowel sounds, severe abdominal pain, vomiting, or fever, which may indicate a fistula or paralytic ileus.*

- Monitor the patient's vital signs.
- Assess hemodynamic values.
- Monitor intake and output.
- Assess nutritional status.
- Monitor pulmonary status.
- Monitor for complications, such as infection and abnormal bleeding.
- Assess the surgical wound and dressing.
- Monitor drainage.
- Assess for metabolic alkalosis or acidosis.
- Monitor serum glucose and calcium levels.

PATIENT TEACHING

GENERAL

- Review medications and possible adverse reactions with the patient.
- Teach the patient how to care for the incision site.
- Tell the patient about the signs and symptoms of infection.
- Review possible complications with the patient and about when to notify the practitioner.
- Teach the patient about how to monitor blood glucose levels at home.
- Tell the patient how to recognize and manage hypoglycemia and hyperglycemia.
- Inform the patient about dietary and activity restrictions ordered by the practitioner.
- Tell the patient about pancreatic enzyme replacement if necessary.
- Stress the need for follow-up care.

RESOURCES
Organizations
American College of Gastroenterology: *www.acg.gi.org*

Selected references
Huerta, S., et al. "Predictors of Morbidity and Mortality in Patients with Traumatic Duodenal Injuries," *The American Surgeon* 71(9):763-67, September 2005.

Marrache, F., et al. "Severe Cholangitis following Pancreaticoduodenectomy for Pseudotumoral Form of Lymphoplasmacytic Sclerosing Pancreatitis," *American Journal of Gastroenterology* 100(12):2808-813, December 2005.

Tani, M., et al. "Improvement of Delayed Gastric Emptying in Pylorus-preserving Pancreaticoduodenectomy. Results of a Prospective, Randomized, Controlled Trial," *Annals of Surgery* 243(3): 316-20, March 2006.

Paracentesis

- Abdominal paracentesis: performed at the bedside; involves aspiration of fluid from the peritoneal space through a needle, trocar, or cannula inserted in the abdominal wall
- Helps determine cause of ascites while relieving pressure created by it
- May precede other procedures, including radiography, peritoneal dialysis, and surgery

INDICATIONS
- Massive ascites resistant to other therapy
- Intra-abdominal bleeding after traumatic injury
- To obtain a peritoneal fluid specimen for laboratory analysis

- Help the patient sit up in bed, on the side of the bed, or in a chair so that fluid accumulates in the lower abdomen.
- Expose the patient's abdomen from diaphragm to pubis.
- Cover the rest of the patient to avoid chills.
- Place a linen-saver pad under the patient.
- Remind the patient to stay as still as possible during the procedure.
- Wash your hands; put on a gown and goggles.
- Open the paracentesis tray using sterile technique.
- Put on gloves.
- The practitioner will prepare the patient's abdomen with povidone-iodine solution, drape the operative site with sterile drapes, and administer the local anesthetic.
- A small incision may be made before inserting the needle or trocar and cannula (usually 1″ to 2″ [2.5 to 5 cm] below the umbilicus).
- Listen for a popping sound; this signifies that the needle or trocar has pierced the peritoneum.
- Assist the practitioner in collecting specimens in proper containers.
- If the practitioner orders substantial drainage, connect the three-way stopcock and tubing to the cannula.
- Run the other end of the tubing to a large sterile Vacutainer, or aspirate the fluid with a three-way stopcock and 50-ml syringe.
- Help the patient remain still throughout the procedure.
- If the patient shows signs of hypovolemic shock, reduce the vertical distance between the needle or the trocar and cannula and the drainage collection container to slow the drainage rate. If necessary, stop the drainage.
- Verify suction in the Vacutainer collection bottle when you connect it to the drainage tubing. Use macrodrip tubing without a backflow device.
- Gently turn the patient from side to side to enhance drainage.
- As the fluid drains, monitor the patient's vital signs every 15 minutes.
- The incision may be sutured after the needle or trocar and cannula are removed.
- Wearing sterile gloves, apply the dry, sterile pressure dressing and povidone-iodine ointment to the site.

COMPLICATIONS
- Hypotension
- Oliguria
- Hyponatremia
- Perforation of abdominal organs
- Wound infection
- Peritonitis
- If excessive fluid (more than 2 L) is removed, ascitic fluid tends to form again

- Ineffective breathing pattern
- Risk for deficient fluid volume
- Risk for infection

EXPECTED OUTCOMES
The patient will:
- exhibit a breathing pattern within normal limits
- have fluid volume that remains within normal limits
- remain free from signs and symptoms of infection.

PRETREATMENT CARE

- Explain the procedure to the patient.
- Instruct the patient that he need not restrict fluid and food intake.
- Reassure the patient that he won't feel pain, but may feel a stinging sensation and pressure.
- Verify that a signed consent has been obtained.
- Have the patient void before the procedure.
- If the patient can't void, insert an indwelling urinary catheter, if ordered.
- Identify and record baseline values: vital signs, weight, and abdominal girth. Indicate the abdominal area measured with a felt-tipped marking pen. Baseline data will be used to monitor the patient's status.
- Provide support to decrease the patient's anxiety during the procedure.

POSTTREATMENT CARE

- Help the patient assume a comfortable position.
- Monitor the patient's vital signs and check the dressing for drainage every 15 minutes for 1 hour, every 30 minutes for 2 hours, every hour for 4 hours, and then every 4 hours for 24 hours to detect delayed reactions to the procedure.
- Note color, amount, and character of drainage.
- Label the Vacutainer specimen tubes, and send them to the laboratory with request forms.
- If the patient is receiving antibiotics, note this on the request form.
- Remove and dispose of all equipment properly.
- After the procedure, observe for peritoneal fluid leakage; notify the practitioner if this develops.
- Maintain daily patient weight and abdominal girth records and compare these values with the baseline figures.
- Watch closely for vertigo, faintness, diaphoresis, pallor, heightened anxiety, tachycardia, dyspnea, and hypotension—especially if more than 1,500 ml of peritoneal fluid was aspirated at one time, which may induce a fluid shift and hypovolemic shock. Immediately report signs of shock to the practitioner.
- Salt-poor albumin may be ordered I.V. to prevent hypovolemia and a decline in renal function.

PATIENT TEACHING

GENERAL
- Review medication administration, dosages, and potential adverse reactions with the patient.
- Instruct the patient that he may not need to restrict food and fluids after the procedure.
- Explain that ascitic fluid may recur, thus the patient may require repeated procedures.
- Teach the patient with ascites to weigh himself daily and report sudden gains to the practitioner.

RESOURCES
Organizations
American College of Gastroenterology: *www.acg.gi.org*
American College of Surgeons: *www.facs.org*
American Gastroenterological Association: *www.gastro.org*
American Medical Association: *www.ama-assn.org*

Selected references
Almakdisi, T., et al. "Lymphomas and Chylous Ascites: Review of the Literature," *Oncologist* 10(8):632-35, September 2005.
Khuroo, M.S., et al. "Budd-Chiari Syndrome: Long-Term Effect on Outcome with Transjugular Intrahepatic Portosystemic Shunt," *Journal of Gastroenterology and Hepatology* 20(10):1494-502, October 2005.
Wright, A.S., and Rikkers, L.F. "Current Management of Portal Hypertension," *Journal of Gastrointestinal Surgery* 9(7):992-1005, September-October 2005.

Parathyroidectomy

- Surgical removal of one or more of the four parathyroid glands
- Number of glands removed dependent on the underlying cause of excessive parathyroid hormone secretion

INDICATIONS
- Primary hyperparathyroidism
- Adenoma
- Glandular hyperplasia
- Intrathyroid lesion

- After the patient is anesthetized, the surgeon makes a cervical neck incision and exposes the thyroid gland.
- The four parathyroid glands are located and tagged.
- If a gland can't be located, a cervical thymectomy and thyroid lobectomy are done on the side where the gland is missing, and a specimen is sent for an immediate frozen section.
- If the missing gland isn't found in the removed tissue, the procedure may be stopped and localization studies done before a second surgery.
- Alternatively, the sternum may be opened and the mediastinum explored for the missing gland.
- When all four parathyroids are found, they're examined for hyperplasia and the affected glands are removed.
- The surgeon tags the remaining glands or any remnant of a gland that wasn't removed.
- A Penrose drain or closed wound drainage device is inserted, and the wound is sutured.

COMPLICATIONS
- Hemorrhage
- Infection
- Recurrent damage to the laryngeal nerve
- Hypoparathyroidism

- Acute pain
- Deficient fluid volume
- Disturbed sensory perception (all)

EXPECTED OUTCOMES
The patient will:
- express feelings of comfort
- maintain adequate fluid volume
- exhibit improved neurologic status.

- Explain the treatment and preparation to the patient and his family.
- Verify that the patient has signed an appropriate consent form.
- Explain postoperative care, including the likelihood that talking and swallowing will be painful for the first few days after surgery.
- Administer I.V. fluids and medications, such as diuretics and antihypercalcemic agents as ordered.

POSTTREATMENT CARE

- Administer medications as ordered.
- Keep the patient in high Fowler's position.
- Encourage the patient to cough, breathe deeply, and use an incentive spirometer.
- Provide surgical wound care as ordered.
- Keep a tracheotomy tray at the bedside for the first 24 hours after surgery.
- Monitor the patient's vital signs, intake and output, and complications.
- Monitor the surgical wound, dressings, and drainage.
- Assess for abnormal bleeding and infection.
- Monitor respiratory status.
- Assess voice quality and speaking ability.
- Monitor serum calcium levels.

⚡ **WARNING** *Watch for and report signs and symptoms of increased neuromuscular excitability, including positive Chvostek's and Trousseau's signs, numbness and tingling of the fingers and toes or around the mouth, muscle cramps, and tetany.*

PATIENT TEACHING

GENERAL

- Teach the patient how to care for the incision site.
- Inform the patient about the signs and symptoms of infection.
- Tell the patient of possible complications and about when to notify the practitioner.
- Instruct the patient to cough and to perform deep-breathing exercises.
- Advise the patient to use an incentive spirometer.
- Stress the need for follow-up care.
- Emphasize the importance of consulting the practitioner before taking nonprescription drugs, especially magnesium-containing laxatives and antacids, mineral oil, and vitamins A and D.
- Advise the patient to maintain a high-calcium, low-phosphorus diet as ordered after total parathyroidectomy.
- Teach the patient the signs and symptoms of hypercalcemia and hypocalcemia.
- Tell the patient of activity restrictions as ordered by the practitioner.

RESOURCES
Organizations
American Medical Association: *www.ama-assn.org*
The Hormone Foundation of the Endocrine Society: *www.hormone.org*

Selected references
Cetani, F., et al. "Genetic Analyses in Familial Isolated Hyperparathyroidism: Implication for Clinical Assessment and Surgical Management," *Clinical Endocrinology* 64(2):146-52, February 2006.

Conroy, S., and O'Malley, B. "Hypercalcaemia in Cancer," *British Medical Journal* 331(7522):954, October 2005.

Florez, J.C., et al. "Hypercalcemia and Local Production of Parathyroid Hormone-Related Protein by a Perisellar Rhabdomyosarcoma after Remote Pituitary Irradiation," *Endocrine Practice* 11(3):184-89, May-June 2005.

Richards, M.L., et al. "Parathyroidectomy in Secondary Hyperparathyroidism: Is There an Optimal Operative Management?" *Surgery* 139(2):174-80, February 2006.

Penile implant

- Allows achievement of sexual intercourse with no complications
- Penile prostheses:
- semi-rigid prosthesis—allows an erection sufficient for penetration and better suited for patients with less manual dexterity
- rigid prostheses—associated with a low mechanical failure rate, but may produce a noticeably unsightly erection and interfere with urination
- malleable rods—few mechanical parts and low risk of malfunction; very easy to use; may produce visible erection even in the flaccid position

AGE FACTOR *The rigid prosthesis is good for men with poor hand mobility who are elderly or don't want the increased risk of malfunction that can result from moving parts.*

- Inflatable penile prostheses:
- one-piece prosthesis—doesn't become as erect as rigid one and doesn't deflate as much as the multicomponent inflatable; also limited to the "average-sized penis"
- multicomponent prosthesis—gives the best appearance when erect and is the softest when deflated
- May complicate potential prostate surgery

INDICATIONS
- Erectile dysfunction

PROCEDURE

- The type of implant surgery is usually based on the surgeon's experience and the type of device chosen, but can include a perineal (under the scrotum) approach, a penoscrotal (at the base of the penis on top of the scrotum) approach, in the penile shaft, or an infrapubic (above the penis) incision.
- A catheter is inserted and a self-retaining circular retractor with elastic hooks is placed over the patient's genitalia. The surgeon makes 1″ (2.5-cm) incision at the penoscrotal junction at the mid-raphe to the superficial/dartos fascia to divide the area.
- He then sprays antibiotic solution over the site and the prosthesis to reduce infection. He checks the prosthesis for integrity and function.
- The surgeon brings the distal half of the cylinder through the distal corporal body and inserts the device and sutures the area.
- Next, the surgeon places an abdominal reservoir, depending on the patient's history of radiation, and fills it to the correct volume (60 to 100 ml). Then he brings the tubing to the pump, trims it to the appropriate length, and connects it to the pump.
- The surgeon then checks the prosthesis for inflation, deflation, and leaks. To help stop potential bleeding and hold the tissue in correct shape, the prosthesis is left in a semirigid state.
- Last, the surgeon inserts the pump in a scrotal pouch and sets the penis as symmetrical as possible. He closes the skin and connects the catheter to dependent drainage.

COMPLICATIONS
- Infection
- Perforation of the corporal body in the area where the prosthesis is held, which can cause migration of the device
- Perforation into the urethra or glans penis
- Tubing kinks
- Fluid leaks
- Aneurysm
- Dilation of the cylinders
- Breakage of the wire
- Silicone spillage
- Loss of rigidity to the prosthesis
- Erosion of the reservoir
- Spontaneous deflation
- Spontaneous inflation
- Penile curvature, which is a variant of Peyronie's disease
- Pump or pump reservoir migration
- Phimosis or paraphimosis, both of which may require circumcision

NURSING DIAGNOSES

◆ Impaired urinary elimination
◆ Risk for infection
◆ Risk for situational low self-esteem

EXPECTED OUTCOMES
The patient will:
◆ demonstrate normal elimination patterns
◆ exhibit no signs of infection
◆ express feelings of positive self-worth.

PRETREATMENT CARE

◆ Review the risks and benefits of the procedure with the patient as requested.
◆ The surgeon should discuss the surgery, frequency and ramifications of potential complications, and appropriate expectations following surgery with the patient.
◆ Inform the patient that the prosthesis will allow him to achieve a rigid erection on demand and will likely have little effect on his libido, but will *not* lengthen his penis.
◆ Verify that a consent form has been signed.

POSTTREATMENT CARE

◆ Monitor the patient's vital signs and intake and output.
◆ Assess laboratory values.
◆ Monitor for complications.
◆ Provide comfort measures.
◆ Assess for pain and monitor effect of pain medication.

PATIENT TEACHING

GENERAL
◆ Review the disorder, diagnostic studies, and treatment with the patient.
◆ Teach the patient about the signs of infection.
◆ Stress the importance of follow-up.
◆ Tell the patient of activity restrictions.
◆ Teach the patient about the use and care of the penile implant.

RESOURCES
Organizations
American Urological Association: *www.auanet.org*

Selected references
Morey, A.F. "Use of Rectus Fascia Graft for Corporeal Reconstruction During Placement of Penile Implant," *Journal of Urology* 175(2):594, February 2006.

Wolter, C.E., and Hellstrom, W.J. "The Hydrophilic-Coated Inflatable Penile Prosthesis: 1-Year Experience," *Journal of Sexual Medicine* 1(2):221-24, September 2004.

Zermann, D.H., et al. "Penile Prosthetic Surgery in Neurologically Impaired Patients: Long-Term Follow-up," *Journal of Urology* 175(3):1041-1044, March 2006.

Percutaneous ethanol injection of liver

OVERVIEW

- Involves injection of pure alcohol into liver cells to induce tumor destruction by dehydrating tumor cells
- During treatment: tumor location relative to adjacent blood vessels and bile ducts identified to avoid bleeding, bile duct inflammation, bile leakage
- Optimal results dependent on radiologist experience in scanning techniques and if facility has percutaneous needle insertion under real-time visualization
- For best results: requires well-defined tumors less than 3 cm in diameter and surrounded by scar tissue

INDICATIONS
- Ablation of tumors
- Debulk or downsize tumors
- Devascularize tumors before surgery
- Ablation of hepatic cysts

PROCEDURE

- The area is prepared and a local anesthetic is injected. The patient may be given a sedative.
- Using a thin needle with ultrasound or computer topographic visual guidance, the practitioner injects the alcohol percutaneously into the tumor. This could take five to six sessions to completely destroy the cancer cells.

COMPLICATIONS
- Alcohol leakage (onto the surface of the liver and into the abdominal cavity) causing pain and fever
- Bleeding
- Bile duct leakage
- Pain
- Liver failure
- Infection
- Hypotension

NURSING DIAGNOSES

- Ineffective breathing pattern
- Risk for deficient fluid volume
- Risk for infection

EXPECTED OUTCOMES
The patient will:
- have a breathing pattern within normal limits
- have fluid volume that remains within normal limits
- have no signs or symptoms of infection.

PRETREATMENT CARE

- Explain the procedure to the patient.
- Reassure him that he shouldn't feel pain, but may feel a stinging sensation and pressure.
- Verify that a signed consent has been obtained.
- Have the patient void before the procedure.
- If the patient can't void, insert an indwelling urinary catheter, if ordered.
- Assess the patient's respiratory and abdominal status, and record assessment for baseline levels.
- Monitor the patient's liver function tests, and notify the practitioner of abnormalities.

POSTTREATMENT CARE

- Help the patient assume a comfortable position.
- Monitor the patient's vital signs and check the dressing for drainage.
- Note color, amount, and character of drainage.
- Remove and dispose of all equipment properly.
- Observe for fluid leakage; notify the practitioner if this occurs.
- Monitor the patient for infection.

PATIENT TEACHING

GENERAL

- Review the disorder, diagnostic studies, and treatment with the patient.
- Review the administration, dosage, and possible adverse effects of the medication with the patient.
- Explain the procedure to the patient.
- Instruct the patient that he need not restrict fluid and food intake.
- Provide support to decrease the patient's anxiety during the procedure.

RESOURCES
Organizations
American College of Gastroenterology: *www.acg.gi.org*
American College of Surgeons: *www.facs.org*
American Gastroenterological Association: *www.gastro.org*
American Medical Association: *www.ama-assn.org*

Selected references

Blum, H.E. "Hepatocellular Carcinoma: Therapy and Prevention," *World Journal of Gastroenterology* 11(47):7391-400, December 2005.

Castroagudin, J.F., et al. "Safety of Percutaneous Ethanol Injection as Neoadjuvant Therapy for Hepatocellular Carcinoma in Waiting List Liver Transplant Candidates," *Transplant Proceedings* 37(9):3871-873, November 2005.

Luo, B.M., et al. "Percutaneous Ethanol Injection, Radiofrequency and their Combination in Treatment of Hepatocellular Carcinoma," *World Journal of Gastroenterology* 11(40):6277-280, October 2005.

Pericardiocentesis

OVERVIEW

- Needle aspiration of pericardial fluid for analysis
- Therapeutic and diagnostic; most useful as an emergency measure to relieve cardiac tamponade
- Fluid specimen used to confirm and identify cause of pericardial effusion and determine therapy
- Excess pericardial fluid: may accumulate after inflammation, cardiac surgery, rupture, or penetrating trauma to the pericardium
- Rapidly forming effusions: may induce cardiac tamponade, a potentially lethal syndrome marked by increased intrapericardial pressure that prevents complete ventricular filling and reduces cardiac output
- Slowly forming effusions: pose less immediate danger and allow the pericardium more time to adapt to accumulating fluid
- Pericardial effusions: typically classified as transudates or exudates (see *Pericardial effusions: Transudates and exudates*)

INDICATIONS

- Cardiac tamponade
- Pericardial effusion

Pericardial effusions: Transudates and exudates

Transudates are protein-poor effusions that usually arise from mechanical factors altering fluid formation or resorption, such as increased hydrostatic pressure, decreased plasma oncotic pressure, or obstruction of the pericardial lymphatic drainage system by a tumor.

Most exudates result from inflammation and contain large amounts of protein. Inflammation damages the capillary membrane, allowing protein molecules to leak into the pericardial fluid.

Both effusion types occur in pericarditis, neoplasms, acute myocardial infarction, tuberculosis, rheumatoid disease, and systemic lupus erythematosus.

PROCEDURE

- The skin is cleaned by the physician with sterile gauze pads soaked in povidone-iodine solution and an anesthetic is injected.
- The physician attaches a 50-ml syringe to one end of a three-way stopcock and the cardiac needle to the other.
- The V_1 lead (precordial leadwire) of the electrocardiogram (ECG) may be attached to the hub of the aspirating needle using the alligator clips to help determine if the needle is in contact with the epicardium during the procedure.
- An echocardiogram may also be used to help guide needle placement.
- The physician inserts the needle through the chest wall into the pericardial sac, maintaining aspiration until fluid appears in the syringe.
- The needle should be angled 35 to 45 degrees toward the tip of the right scapula between the left costal margin and the xiphoid process; this minimizes the risk of lacerating the coronary vessels or the pleura.
- Observe the ECG tracing when the cardiac needle is being inserted; ST-segment elevation indicates that the needle has reached the epicardial surface and should be retracted slightly.

    WARNING *An abnormally shaped QRS complex may indicate perforation of the myocardium. Premature ventricular contractions usually indicate that the needle has touched the ventricular wall. Watch for grossly bloody fluid aspirate, which may indicate inadvertent puncture of a cardiac chamber.*

- After the needle is positioned, the physician attaches a Kelly clamp to the skin surface so it won't advance further.
- Assist the physician by labeling and numbering the specimen tubes, and cleaning the top of the tube used for culture and sensitivity with povidone-iodine solution. (See *Aspirating pericardial fluid.*)
- A pericardial catheter may be connected to a drainage bag or to low-suction drainage.
- The insertion site is cleaned and dressed.

COMPLICATIONS

- Laceration of a coronary artery or the myocardium (potentially fatal)
- Vasovagal arrest
- Infection
- Cardiac arrhythmias
- Myocardial perforation
- Respiratory distress

NURSING DIAGNOSES

- Acute pain
- Decreased cardiac output
- Ineffective tissue perfusion: Cardiopulmonary

EXPECTED OUTCOMES

The patient will:
- verbalize feelings of comfort
- maintain adequate cardiac output
- maintain blood pressure, capillary refill, pulses, vital signs, lung sounds, and respiratory rate with normal limits.

PRETREATMENT CARE

- Explain the procedure to the patient and answer questions.
- Tell the patient that the anesthetic may cause brief burning and local pain.
- Verify that a consent form has been signed.
- Tell the patient that he may feel pressure when the needle is inserted into the pericardial sac.

- Inform the patient that he'll be monitored closely during and after the procedure.
- Instruct the patient to be still during the procedure; tell him that a sedative may be administered to help him relax.
- Connect the patient to the bedside monitor, set to read lead V_1.
- Make sure that a defibrillator and emergency drugs are nearby.
- Provide adequate lighting at the puncture site.
- Adjust the height of the patient's bed to allow the physician to perform the procedure comfortably.
- Put the patient in the supine position with his thorax elevated 60 degrees.
- Wash your hands and put on gloves and protective eyewear.
- Open the equipment tray on an overbed table, being careful not to contaminate the sterile field.

WARNING *To minimize the risk of complications, echocardiography should precede pericardiocentesis to determine the effusion site.*

POSTTREATMENT CARE

- If bacterial culture and sensitivity tests are scheduled, record on the laboratory request any antimicrobial drugs the patient is receiving.
- If anaerobic organisms are suspected, consult the laboratory about proper collection technique to avoid exposing the aspirate to air.
- Send specimens to the laboratory immediately.
- Check blood pressure, pulse, respirations, oxygen saturation, and heart sounds every 15 minutes until stable, then every half hour for 2 hours, every hour for 4 hours, and every 4 hours thereafter. Your facility may require more frequent monitoring.
- Monitor continuously for cardiac arrhythmias. Document rhythm strips according to facility policy.
- Return all equipment to the proper location. Dispose of equipment according to facility policy.
- After the procedure, be alert for respiratory and cardiac distress.
- Watch especially for signs of cardiac tamponade: muffled and distant heartbeat, jugular vein distention, paradoxical pulse, and shock.

PATIENT TEACHING

GENERAL
- Teach the patient the signs and symptoms of recurent effusion, infection, and cardiac arrhythmia to report to the practitioner.
- Review medication administration, dosages, and possible adverse reactions with the patient.

RESOURCES
Organizations
American College of Emergency Physicians: *www.acep.org*
American College of Surgeons: *www.facs.org*
Trauma.org: *www.trauma.org*

Selected references
Ashraf, A., et al. "Etiology, Management, and Outcome of Patients with Pericardial and Pleuro-Pericardial Effusions," *Journal of Medical Sciences* 13(2):96-100, July 2005.
Krantz, M.J., and Rowan, S.R. "Paradoxical Decrease in Blood Pressure After Relief of Cardiac Tamponade: The Role of Sympathetic Activity," *Medical Science Monitor* 12(2):CS16-19, February 2006.
Nakata, A., et al. "A Patient with Graves' Disease Accompanied by Bloody Pericardial Effusion," *Internal Medicine* 44(10):1064-1068, October 2005.

Aspirating pericardial fluid

In pericardiocentesis, a needle and syringe are inserted through the chest wall into the pericardial sac (as shown below). Electrocardiographic (ECG) monitoring, with a leadwire attached to the needle and electrodes placed on the limbs (right arm [RA], left arm [LA], and left leg [LL]), helps ensure proper needle placement and avoids damage to the heart.

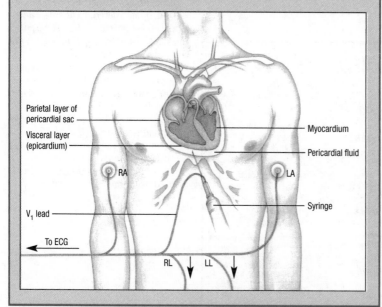

Parietal layer of pericardial sac
Visceral layer (epicardium)
RA
V_1 lead
To ECG
RL   LL
Myocardium
Pericardial fluid
LA
Syringe

Peritoneal dialysis

- Performed by specially trained nurses, either manually or using an automatic or semiautomatic cycle machine
- Dialysate (solution instilled into the peritoneal cavity by a catheter): draws waste products, excess fluid, and electrolytes from the blood across semipermeable peritoneal membrane, removing impurities with it (see *How peritoneal dialysis works*)
- Procedure repeated (using new dialysate) until waste removal is complete and fluid, electrolyte, and acid-base balance is restored

INDICATIONS

- Chronic renal failure with cardiovascular instability
- Vascular access problems that prevent hemodialysis
- Fluid overload
- Electrolyte imbalances

WARNING *Contraindications to peritoneal dialysis include extensive abdominal or bowel surgery, extensive abdominal trauma, severe vascular disease, obesity, and respiratory distress.*

- The physician cleans the patient's abdomen with povidone-iodine solution, drapes it with a sterile drape, and then anesthetizes a small area of the patient's abdomen below the umbilicus. He makes a small incision with the scalpel, inserts the catheter into the peritoneal cavity—using the stylet to guide the catheter—and sutures or tapes the catheter in place. (See *Comparing peritoneal dialysis catheters.*)
- If the catheter is already in place, clean the site with povidone-iodine solution in a circular outward motion before each dialysis treatment.
- Connect the catheter to the administration set, using strict sterile technique to prevent contamination of the catheter and solution, which may cause peritonitis.
- Remove your gloves.
- Put on a new pair of sterile gloves, place the drain dressings around the catheter, cover them with the gauze pads, and tape them securely.
- Unclamp the lines to the patient. Rapidly instill 500 ml of dialysate into the peritoneal cavity to test the catheter's patency.

- Clamp the lines to the patient and immediately unclamp the lines to the drainage bag to allow fluid to drain into the bag. Outflow should be brisk.
- Having established the catheter's patency, clamp the lines to the drainage bag and unclamp the lines to the patient to infuse the prescribed volume of solution over a period of 5 to 10 minutes. As soon as the dialysate container empties, clamp the lines to the patient to prevent air from entering the tubing.
- Allow the solution to dwell in the peritoneal cavity for the prescribed time (10 minutes to 4 hours).
- Warm the solution for the next infusion.
- At the end of the prescribed dwell time, unclamp the line to the drainage bag and allow the solution to drain from the peritoneal cavity into the drainage bag (usually 20 to 30 minutes).
- Repeat the infusion-dwell-drain cycle immediately after outflow until the prescribed number of fluid exchanges have been completed.
- If the practitioner or the facility protocol requires a dialysate specimen, collect one after every 10 infusion-dwell-drain cycles (always during the drain phase), after every 24-hour period, or as ordered. To do this, attach the 10-ml syringe to the needle and insert it into the injection port on the drainage line, using strict sterile technique, and aspirate the drainage specimen and transfer to the specimen container. Label it and send it to the laboratory with a request form.
- Monitor the patient and his response to treatment during dialysis.
- Monitor the patient's vital signs every 10 to 15 minutes for the first 1 to 2 hours of exchanges, then every 2 to 4 hours, or more frequently if necessary.

How peritoneal dialysis works

Peritoneal dialysis works through a combination of diffusion and osmosis.

DIFFUSION

In diffusion, particles move through a semipermeable membrane from an area of high-solute concentration to an area of low-solute concentration.

In peritoneal dialysis, the water-based dialysate being infused contains glucose, sodium chloride, calcium, magnesium, acetate or lactate, and no waste products. Therefore, the waste products and excess electrolytes in the blood cross through the semipermeable peritoneal membrane into the dialysate. Removing the waste-filled dialysate and replacing it with fresh solution keeps the waste concentration low and encourages further diffusion.

OSMOSIS

In osmosis, fluids move through a semipermeable membrane from an area of low-solute concentration to an area of high-solute concentration. In peritoneal dialysis, dextrose is added to the dialysate to give it a higher solute concentration than the blood, creating a high osmotic gradient. Water migrates from the blood through the membrane at the beginning of each infusion, when the osmotic gradient is highest.

- Ensure that all personnel in the room wear masks whenever the dialysis system is opened or entered.
- To prevent respiratory distress, position the patient for maximal lung expansion and promote lung expansion through turning and deep-breathing exercises.

⚡ **WARNING** *If the patient suffers severe respiratory distress during the dwell phase of dialysis, drain the peritoneal cavity and notify the practitioner.*
- Assess fluid balance at the end of each infusion-dwell-drain cycle.

- Patient discomfort at the start of the procedure is normal. If the patient experiences pain during the procedure, determine when it occurs, its quality and duration, and whether it radiates to other body parts. Notify the practitioner as necessary. Pain during infusion usually results from a

---

Comparing peritoneal dialysis catheters

The first step in any type of peritoneal dialysis is insertion of a catheter to allow instillation of dialyzing solution. The surgeon may insert one of the three catheters described here.

TENCKHOFF CATHETER

To implant a Tenckhoff catheter, the surgeon inserts the first 6¾" (17 cm) of the catheter into the patient's abdomen. The next 2¾" (7 cm) segment, which may have a Dacron cuff at one or both ends, is imbedded subcutaneously. Within a few days after insertion, the patient's tissues grow around the cuffs, forming a tight barrier against bacterial infiltration. The remaining 3⅞" (10 cm) of the catheter extends outside of the abdomen and is equipped with a metal adapter at the tip that connects to dialyzer tubing.

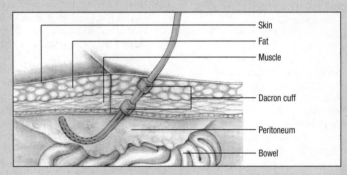

FLANGED-COLLAR CATHETER

To insert this kind of catheter, the surgeon positions its flanged collar just below the dermis so that the device extends through the abdominal wall. He keeps the distal end of the cuff from extending into the peritoneum, where it could cause adhesions.

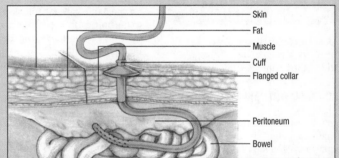

COLUMN-DISK PERITONEAL CATHETER

To insert a column-disk peritoneal catheter (CDPC), the surgeon rolls up the flexible disk section of the implant, inserts it into the peritoneal cavity, and retracts it against the abdominal wall. The implant's first cuff rests just outside the peritoneal membrane, and its second cuff rests just underneath the skin.

Because the CDPC doesn't float freely in the peritoneal cavity, it keeps inflowing dialyzing solution from being directed at the sensitive organs, which increases patient comfort during dialysis.

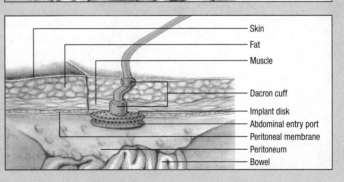

(continued)

dialysate that's too cool or acidic or from rapid inflow. Slowing the inflow rate may reduce the pain. Severe, diffuse pain with rebound tenderness and cloudy effluent may indicate peritoneal infection. Pain that radiates to the shoulder commonly results from air accumulation under the diaphragm. Severe perineal or rectal pain can result from improper catheter placement.

COMPLICATIONS
- Peritonitis
- Protein depletion
- Respiratory distress
- Constipation
- Hypovolemia
- Hypotension
- Shock
- Blood volume expansion
- Hypertension
- Peripheral edema
- Pulmonary edema
- Heart failure
- Electrolyte imbalance
- Hyperglycemia

NURSING DIAGNOSES

- Deficient fluid volume
- Impaired gas exchange
- Risk for infection

EXPECTED OUTCOMES
The patient will:
- maintain adequate fluid volume
- maintain patent airway and adequate oxygenation
- remain free from signs and symptoms of infection.

PRETREATMENT CARE

- Warm the solution to body temperature with a heating pad or commercial warmer. Don't warm the solution in a microwave oven.
- Explain the procedure to the patient.
- Assess and record vital signs, weight, and abdominal girth to establish baseline levels.
- Review recent laboratory values (blood urea nitrogen, creatinine, sodium, potassium, and complete blood count).
- Have the patient try to urinate. If he can't urinate and you suspect his bladder isn't empty, obtain an order for straight catheterization to empty his bladder.
- Put the patient in the supine position and have him put on a sterile face mask.
- Put on a sterile face mask. Prepare the dialysis fluid and administration set. Close the clamps on all lines. Place the drainage bag below the patient to facilitate gravity drainage, and connect the drainage line to it. Connect the dialysate infusion lines to the bottles or bags of dialysate using sterile technique. Hang the bottles or bags on the I.V. pole at the patient's bedside. Prime the tubing then close all clamps.

POSTTREATMENT CARE

- After completing the prescribed number of exchanges, clamp the catheter, and put on sterile gloves. Disconnect the administration set from the peritoneal catheter. Place the sterile protective cap over the catheter's distal end. Dispose of used equipment appropriately.
- Change the dressing at least every 24 hours or whenever it becomes wet or soiled. Frequent dressing changes prevent skin excoriation from leakage.
- To prevent protein depletion, the practitioner may order a high-protein diet or a protein supplement and he'll also monitor albumin levels.

WARNING *Dialysate is available in three concentrations—4.25% dextrose, 2.5% dextrose, and 1.5% dextrose. The 4.25% solution removes the largest amount of fluid from the blood. If the patient receives this concentrated solution, monitor him carefully to prevent excess fluid loss. Some of the glucose in the 4.25% solution may enter the patient's bloodstream, causing hyperglycemia severe enough to require an insulin injection or an insulin addition to the dialysate.*
- Patients with low potassium levels may require the addition of potassium to the dialysate solution to prevent further losses.
- Monitor fluid volume balance, blood pressure, and pulse.
- Notify the practitioner if the patient retains 500 ml or more of fluid for three consecutive cycles or loses at least 1 L of fluid for three consecutive cycles.
- Weigh the patient daily to help determine fluid loss. Note the time and variations in the weighing technique.
- If inflow and outflow are slow or absent, check the tubing for kinks, raise the I.V. pole, or reposition the patient to increase the inflow rate. Repositioning the patient or applying manual pressure to the lateral aspects of the patient's abdomen may help increase drainage. If these maneuvers fail, notify the practitioner. Improper positioning of the catheter or an accumulation of fibrin may obstruct the catheter.

WARNING *Always examine outflow fluid (effluent) for color and clarity. If the effluent remains pink-tinged or is grossly bloody, suspect bleeding into the peritoneal cavity and notify the practitioner. Notify the practitioner if the outflow contains feces, which suggests bowel perforation, or if it's cloudy, which suggests peritonitis. Obtain a sample for culture and Gram stain. Send the sample in a labeled container to the laboratory with a laboratory request form.*
- Obtain a referral for home health care services after discharge.

Learning about peritoneal dialysis

Dear Patient:

Your health care provider has ordered peritoneal dialysis for you. This procedure removes impurities from your blood when your kidneys aren't working properly.

BEFORE DIALYSIS

The nurse will take your blood pressure twice—once while you're standing and once while you're lying down. She'll also weigh you and measure your abdomen. Then she'll tell you to urinate to make you feel more comfortable and to protect your bladder.

Next, your health care provider will create an opening in your peritoneal cavity, which is near your stomach. (First, the area will be numbed with an anesthetic.) Then a slender tube called a catheter will be inserted into the opening. (See the illustration.)

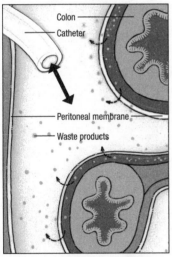

Colon
Catheter
Peritoneal membrane
Waste products

The catheter is used to transfer a special warmed solution into your peritoneal cavity. The solution collects impurities that cross through your peritoneum (a membrane that acts like a filter). After a specified time, the solution is drained from your body.

You and the nurse (or the dialysis technician) will wear masks during dialysis to prevent infection. After the nurse connects the inflow and the drainage tubings, she'll hang the solution bag above you on a bedside pole and the drainage bag below your bed.

DURING DIALYSIS

To start dialysis, the nurse will open a clamp to allow the solution to flow into your peritoneal cavity where it will remain for a prescribed time. Then it will drain into the collection bag. The procedure will be repeated until the right amount of solution has been instilled for the prescribed number of cycles.

To ensure your progress, the nurse will take your blood pressure, check your breathing, examine the tubing, and change your catheter dressing whenever it's soiled or wet.

AFTER DIALYSIS

The nurse will disconnect the tubing and cover the catheter with a sterile, protective cap. She'll apply ointment and bandage the catheter site.

Call your health care provider if you notice signs of infection (such as redness or swelling) or fluid imbalance (such as a sudden weight gain, or swollen arms or legs). As the nurse has taught you, take your vital signs regularly and change the catheter dressing. Be sure to keep all your follow-up appointments.

GENERAL

◆ Review medication administration, dosages, and possible adverse reactions with the patient.
◆ Alert the patient that a lot of assistance may be needed in his daily care.
◆ To minimize discomfort, instruct the patient to perform daily care during a drain phase in the cycle, when his abdomen is less distended.
◆ Explain the procedure to the patient and review all steps; perform return demonstrations if the patient is to continue this at home. (See *Learning about peritoneal dialysis.* See also *Performing a solution exchange,* pages 288 to 290.)
◆ Teach the patient how to prevent infection; tell him the signs to report to the practitioner. (See *Preventing peritonitis,* page 291.)
◆ Provide the name and contact information for the home health care service provider to the patient.

RESOURCES
Organizations
American College of Emergency Physicians: *www.acep.org*
American College of Surgeons: *www.facs.org*
American Medical Association: *www.ama-assn.org*

Selected references

Bonifati, C. "Antimicrobial Agents and Catheter-related Interventions to Prevent Peritonitis in Peritoneal Dialysis: Using Evidence in the Context of Clinical Practice," *International Journal of Artificial Organs* 29(1):41-49, January 2006.
Kanagasundaram, N.S., and Paganini, P. "Acute Renal Failure on the Intensive Care Unit," *Clinical Medicine* 5(5):435-40, September-October 2005.
Peritoneal Dialysis Special Interest Group. "The Peritoneal Equilibration Test," *Nephrology Nursing Journal* 32(4):452-53, July-August 2005.

(continued)

Performing a solution exchange

Dear Patient:

You and your health care provider have chosen continuous ambulatory peritoneal dialysis (CAPD) for your dialysis program. CAPD is easier to do at home than other forms of dialysis, but when you perform a CAPD solution exchange at home, you must guard against bacteria entering the dialysis system. The following instructions tell how to drain the used solution and replace it with a fresh one so you don't contaminate the system.

GATHER THE EQUIPMENT

First, gather the prescribed bag of peritoneal dialysate solution of the correct volume and dextrose concentration, two outlet port clamps, and a sterile CAPD prep kit. This kit contains povidone-iodine (Betadine) sponges, sterile 4″ × 4″ gauze pads (you can also use a shell clamp on the connection between the solution spike and the dialysate outflow port), hypoallergenic tape, and a mask. If you must inject medication into the solution, you'll also need the necessary number of 25G needles, 10-ml syringes, and the medication itself.

BEFORE YOU BEGIN

If you want to warm the dialysate solution, place it in a basin of warm water directly from the faucet. Warming the solution isn't essential, but it should be done if you feel cramps during infusion. Keep the protective wrap on the bag until it's ready to be used. Remember to wash your hands thoroughly before removing the outer wrap and handling the bag. You may also warm the solution by wrapping it in a heating pad set at mild heat.

DRAINING THE OLD SOLUTION

1. Remove the empty solution bag from inside your clothing. Check to make sure that the shell clamp or povidone-iodine-saturated dressing is still in place. If it has become dislodged, apply a gauze dressing covered with povidone-iodine to the connection and cover it with a dry sterile dressing.

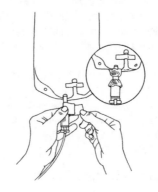

2. Put on your mask and place the bag in the drainage position below your stomach. Open the clamp on the drainage tubing. Allow about 15 to 20 minutes for the solution to drain from your abdomen into the bag.

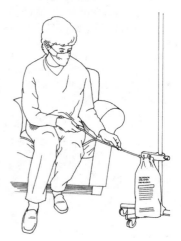

CHECKING THE NEW SOLUTION BAG

Meanwhile, remove the dialysate bag wrapping. Is the solution clear? If it isn't, don't use it. Read the concentration information on the label to make sure you have the right solution, and check the expiration date. Squeeze the bag firmly to test for leaks.

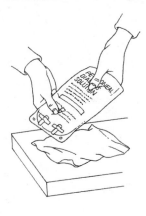

ADDING MEDICATION

If your health care provider has told you to add medication to the new bag, wipe the injection port with a sponge saturated with povidone-iodine and allow the solution to dry for a few minutes. Draw up the prescribed amount of medication. Then insert the needle through the rubber stopper of the injection port, as shown below, and inject the medication. To mix the medication in the solution, turn the bag and squeeze it several times. Tape the injection port so it's out of the way.

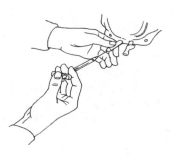

DOUBLE-CHECKING THE BAGS

When the solution has finished draining, close the clamp on the tubing and place the drainage bag on a flat surface, next to the new bag. Position the used solution bag with its clear side up, so you can check the fluid for cloudiness or particles.

Position the new bag with its label side up, so you can double-check the concentration and the expiration date. Arrange the bags so that their ends extend over the edge of the work surface. Place a clamp on the new bag's outlet port.

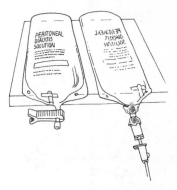

(continued)

SETTING UP THE NEW BAG

1. Remove the povidone-iodine dressing or shell clamp from the used bag's outlet port tubing junction. Clamp the used bag's outlet port, making sure that it remains a safe distance from the spike junction.

2. Remove the cover from the new bag's outlet port without touching the port. Now you're ready to transfer the tubing spike.

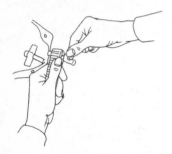

3. Grasp the finger grip on the tubing spike in the drainage-bag outlet port. With your free hand, hold the clamp on the used bag's outlet port. Twist and pull the used bag's spike to remove it from the port. Take care not to touch anything with the spike tip.

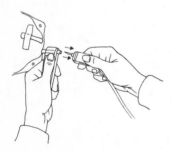

4. Immediately insert the spike into the new bag's outlet port. Apply a shell clamp or povidone-iodine dressing to the junction of the outlet port and tubing. Then remove the outlet port clamp.

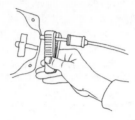

5. Hang the new bag on an I.V. pole. Then open the roller clamp on the tubing to allow the solution to drain into your abdomen. After about 5 minutes, when almost all the solution has drained from the bag, close the clamp. Leaving a little fluid in the bag will make it easier to fold.

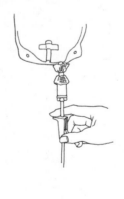

6. Remove the bag from the pole and place it in front of you. Fold over the connection between the spike and outlet port so it's centered on the bag. Then coil the tubing over this connection. Next, fold the other end of the bag over the connection and tubing and place the bag inside a pouch, if you use one. Put the pouch inside your clothing.

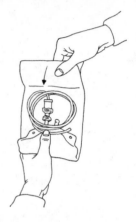

If your health care provider has ordered a drainage sample, take the used bag to the hospital laboratory for analysis. Otherwise, carefully empty the used solution into the toilet and discard the empty bag in a trash can.

Preventing peritonitis

Dear Patient:

Because you'll be using peritoneal dialysis at home, you must guard against peritonitis—an infection that occurs when harmful bacteria enter the dialysis system. Follow these tips to help prevent peritonitis.

AVOID CONTAMINATION

◆ Wash your hands with soap and water before opening the dialysis system, handling the dialysis solution, or changing the dressing over your catheter.

◆ Change the dressing over your catheter every day and whenever it becomes wet or soiled.

◆ Cover your mouth or nose with a surgical mask whenever you open the dialysis system—for example, to perform a solution exchange.

◆ Perform solution exchanges in a clean, dry room with the doors and windows closed. Don't do them in the bathroom.

◆ Check dialysate drainage for cloudiness or particles—possible signs of infection.

◆ Always make sure that you have the equipment you'll need to do the exchange before you get started.

◆ Ask your family to handle phone calls and other interruptions while you're doing your exchange. Otherwise, ignore distractions until you're done.

◆ Don't use fresh dialysate solution that has excessive moisture on the outside of the bag. This could indicate a leak in the bag and possible contamination.

◆ Take showers instead of tub baths to prevent bacteria from entering the dialysis system. Tape a plastic cover over the insertion site to prevent contamination of the connections.

◆ Follow other instructions or restrictions recommended by your nurses and health care provider.

WHEN TO SEEK HELP

◆ Call your continuous ambulatory peritoneal dialysis (CAPD) unit or health care provider if the skin around the peritoneal catheter becomes red, warm, or painful or if you note drainage. Also report leakage around the catheter insertion site.

◆ Follow the instructions you were given for care of the dialysate tubing spike should it become contaminated by contact with your hand or some other surface. This will necessitate a tubing change, which is usually done in the CAPD unit.

◆ Notify your CAPD unit or health care provider if you detect signs of peritonitis, such as abdominal distention or pain, cloudy dialysate, fever, chills, nausea, vomiting, or diarrhea.

Prostatectomy

OVERVIEW

- Surgical removal of the prostate
- Transurethral resection of the prostate (TURP): removal of the prostate via insertion of a resectoscope into the urethra
- May be performed by an open surgical approach, such as suprapubic prostatectomy, retropubic prostatectomy (which allows pelvic lymph node dissection for prostate cancer staging), or perineal prostatectomy (safer for obese patients and those who have had lower abdominal or pelvic surgery)

INDICATIONS
- Prostate cancer
- Obstructive benign prostatic hyperplasia

PROCEDURE

TURP
- The patient is placed in a lithotomy position and is given anesthesia.
- The surgeon introduces a resectoscope into the urethra and advances it to the prostate.
- A clear irrigating solution is instilled, and the obstruction is visualized.
- The resectoscope's cutting loop is used to resect prostatic tissue and restore the urethral opening.

SUPRAPUBIC PROSTATECTOMY
- The patient receives a general anesthetic and is placed in a supine position.
- The surgeon makes a horizontal incision just above the pubic symphysis.
- Fluid is instilled into the bladder.
- A small incision is made in the bladder wall to expose the prostate.
- The surgeon shells out prostatic tissue with a finger.
- The obstruction is cleared and bleeding points are ligated.
- A suprapubic drainage tube and Penrose drain are inserted.

RETROPUBIC PROSTATECTOMY
- The patient is anesthetized and placed in a supine position.
- A horizontal suprapubic incision is made.
- The prostate is approached from between the bladder and pubic arch.
- Another incision is made in the prostatic capsule, and the obstructing tissue is removed.
- Bleeding is controlled.
- A suprapubic tube and Penrose drain are inserted.

PERINEAL PROSTATECTOMY
- The patient is anesthetized and placed in an exaggerated lithotomy position.
- The surgeon makes an inverted U-shaped incision in the perineum.
- The entire prostate is removed, along with the seminal vesicles.
- The urethra is anastomosed to the bladder.
- The incision is closed, leaving a Penrose drain in place.

COMPLICATIONS
- Hemorrhage
- Infection
- Urine retention and incontinence
- Impotence

NURSING DIAGNOSES

- Acute pain
- Impaired urinary elimination
- Risk for infection

EXPECTED OUTCOMES
The patient will:
- demonstrate signs of comfort
- demonstrate normal elimination patterns
- show no signs of infection.

PRETREATMENT CARE

- Explain the treatment and preparation to the patient and his family.
- Veify that the patient or a family member has signed an appropriate consent form.
- Explain postoperative care.
- Administer an enema as ordered.
- Restrict foods and fluids as ordered.
- Offer emotional support to the patient.

POSTTREATMENT CARE

- Administer medications as ordered.
- Maintain urinary catheter and suprapubic tube patency as ordered.
- Keep the urinary collection container below the bladder level.
- Administer antispasmodics and analgesics as ordered.
- Offer sitz baths.
- Arrange for psychological and sexual counseling as needed.

⚡ **WARNING** *Never administer medication rectally in a patient who has had a total prostatectomy.*

- Monitor for and report signs and symptoms of dilutional hyponatremia, such as altered mental status, muscle twitching, and seizures.
- Monitor vital signs, urine characteristics, and intake and output.
- Monitor for complications, such as abnormal bleeding and infection.
- Assess surgical wound and dressings.
- Monitor drainage.
- Monitor fluid and electrolyte status.
- Monitor for and report signs and symptoms of epididymitis, including fever, chills, groin pain, and a swollen, tender epididymis.

PATIENT TEACHING

GENERAL
- Teach the patient how to care for the incision site.
- Tell the patient the signs and symptoms of infection and abnormal bleeding.
- Tell the patient about possible complications and when to notify the practitioner.
- Stress the importance of drinking 12 8-oz glasses of water daily and urinating at least every 2 hours. (See *Speeding your recovery after prostate surgery*.)

- Discuss with the patient the likelihood of experiencing transient urinary frequency and dribbling after catheter removal.
- Teach the patient how to perform Kegel exercises.
- Instruct the patient to avoid caffeine-containing beverages.
- Advise the patient to take sitz baths.
- Stress the importance of follow-up care.

- Advise the patient to have annual prostate-specific antigen tests.

RESOURCES
Organizations
American College of Emergency Physicians: *www.acep.org*
American Urological Association: *www.auanet.org*

Selected references
Burt, J., et al. "Radical Prostatectomy: Men's Experiences and Postoperative Needs," *Journal of Clinical Nursing* 14(7):883-90, August 2005.

Mason, T.M. "Information Needs of Wives of Men following Prostatectomy," *Oncology Nursing Forum* 32(3):557-63, May 2005.

Willener, R., and Hantikainen, V. "Individual Quality of Life following Radical Prostatectomy in Men with Prostate Cancer," *Urologic Nursing* 25(2):88-90, 95-100, April 2005.

PATIENT-TEACHING AID

Speeding your recovery after prostate surgery

Dear Patient:

Here's what you can expect after prostate surgery, along with directions for caring for yourself.

EXPECT TROUBLE URINATING

At first, you may have a feeling of heaviness in the pelvic area, burning during urination, a frequent need to urinate, and loss of some control over urination. Don't worry; these symptoms will disappear with time.

If you notice blood in your urine during the first 2 weeks after surgery, drink fluids and lie down to rest. The next time you urinate, the bleeding should decrease.

Let your health care provider know right away if you continue to see blood in your urine or if you can't urinate at all.

Also let your health care provider know immediately if you develop a fever.

PREVENT CONSTIPATION

Eat a well-balanced diet and drink 12 8-oz glasses of fluid daily, unless your health care provider directs otherwise. Don't strain to have a bowel movement. If you become constipated, take a mild laxative.

Don't use an enema or place anything, such as a suppository, into your rectum for at least 4 weeks after surgery.

CUT BACK ON ACTIVITIES

Take only short walks and avoid climbing stairs as much as possible. Don't lift heavy objects. Also, don't drive for at least 2 weeks, and don't exercise strenuously for at least 3 weeks.

STRENGTHEN YOUR PERINEAL MUSCLES

Perform this exercise to strengthen your perineal muscles after surgery: Press your buttocks together, hold this position for a few seconds, and then relax. Repeat this 10 times.

Perform this exercise as many times daily as your health care provider orders.

WAIT TO HAVE INTERCOURSE

Don't have intercourse for at least 4 weeks after surgery because sexual activity can cause bleeding.

When you have intercourse, most of the semen (the fluid that contains sperm) will pass into your bladder rather than out through your urethra. This won't affect your ability to have an erection or an orgasm. However, it will decrease your fertility.

Don't be alarmed if the semen in your bladder causes cloudy urine the first time you urinate after intercourse.

ASK ABOUT WORK

During your next appointment with your health care provider, ask when you can return to work. The timing will vary depending on the type of surgery you had, the kind of work you do, and your general health.

SCHEDULE AN ANNUAL CHECKUP

Continue to have an annual examination so your health care provider can check the prostate area that wasn't removed during surgery.

Proton beam therapy

OVERVIEW

- Procedure that deposits radiation at the point of greatest beam penetration in tissue (also known as *Bragg peak*); exact depth dependent on the proton beam's energy
- Used to treat various solid tumors
- Delivers high doses to a localized area, avoiding normal tissues

INDICATIONS

- Pediatric cancers
- Head and neck cancers
- Brain and cranial base tumors
- Eye tumors
- Sarcomas
- Prostate cancer
- Spine tumors
- Thoracic cancers
- GI cancers

PROCEDURE

- Radiation penetration depth is calculated based on the tumor's location.
- A cyclotron energizes protons, which are then directed to the tumor by magnetic fields.
- The protons enter the body and release their energy into the tumor, delivering a precalculated dose of radiation.
- Therapy is conducted daily for 15 days.

COMPLICATIONS

- Local skin reactions
- Anorexia
- Fatigue
- Bone marrow suppression
- Increased risk of bleeding and infection
- Dysfunction or structural change in body parts within the irradiated area:
- Alopecia from scalp irradiation
- Stomatitis and esophagitis from head and neck irradiation
- Pneumonitis, pericarditis, and upper GI distress from thoracic irradiation
- Lower GI and genitourinary problems from abdominopelvic irradiation

AGE FACTOR *Adverse effects depend on the patient's age, medical history, diagnosis, and the tumor's size and location.*

NURSING DIAGNOSES

- Disturbed sensory perception (all)
- Risk for infection
- Situational low self-esteem

EXPECTED OUTCOMES

The patient will:

- exhibit improved or normal neurologic status
- exhibit no signs of infection
- verbalize positive feelings about self.

PRETREATMENT CARE

- Explain the treatment and preparation to the patient and his family.
- Verify that the patient has signed an appropriate consent form.
- Take the patient on a tour of the radiation department.
- Obtain a thorough patient history.
- Obtain baseline white blood cell (WBC) and platelet counts.
- Before proton treatment imaging studies are reviewed, ensure that proton therapy is appropriate.
- Before treatment, the patient undergoes a simulation process that helps with the actual treatment. Using a custom immobilization device (helping the patient maintain a steady body position), treatment planning X-ray images are obtained that help identify the lesions or target areas within the body.

- When the patient comes for proton treatment, images are taken using state-of-the-art X-ray or ultrasound technology; these pretreatment images are compared with the planning images to ensure high-precision alignment.

POSTTREATMENT CARE

- Administer medications as ordered.
- Implement measures to control bleeding and prevent infection.
- Provide meticulous skin care.
- Provide comfort measures and supportive care.
- Monitor vital signs.
- Monitor WBC and platelet counts.
- Assess for complications, such as abnormal bleeding and infection.
- Monitor breath sounds.
- Monitor drainage.

PATIENT TEACHING

GENERAL

- Review the therapy and possible adverse reactions with the patient.
- Review skin care at the radiation site with the patient.
- Advise the patient about sperm banking if appropriate.
- Tell the patient to avoid applying lotions, medications, deodorants, perfumes, and powders to the site during treatment.
- Tell the patient to wear comfortable, loose clothing over the treated area.
- Advise the patient to avoid sun exposure for 1 year after treatment.
- Stress the importance of using a sunblock with a sun protection factor of 15 or higher.
- Inform the patient about how to manage adverse effects at home, such as eating small, frequent meals to minimize GI distress and drinking adequate amounts of fluid to help minimize genitourinary complications.
- Review the signs and symptoms of infection with the patient.
- Tell the patient about possible complications and about when to notify the practitioner.
- Stress the importance of follow-up care.
- Refer the patient to support groups such as the American Cancer Society.

RESOURCES
Organizations
American Academy of Neurology:
 www.aan.com
American Cancer Society:
 www.cancer.org
National Association for Proton Therapy:
 www.proton-therapy.org

Selected references
DeLaney, T.F. "Proton Beam Radiation Therapy," *Cancer Investigations* 24(2):199-208, March 2006.
Jones, B. "The Case for Particle Therapy," *British Journal of Radiology* 79(937):24-31, January 2006.
Nihei, K., et al. "High-Dose Proton Beam Therapy for Stage I Non-Small-Cell Lung Cancer," *International Journal of Radiation Oncology, Biology, Physics* 65(1):107-111, May 2006.

Radiation, external

OVERVIEW

- Delivery of high levels of radiation (externally) to a specific body area
- Destroys ability of cancer cells to grow and multiply by either decreasing the mitosis rate or impairing synthesis of deoxyribonucleic or ribonucleic acid
- Also called *external beam radiation* or *teletherapy*

INDICATIONS
- Curative or palliative treatment for cancer
- Extensive skin disease

PROCEDURE

- External radiation treatments are given in the radiation department.
- The radiation oncologist may mark precise treatment areas on the patient's skin with tiny tattoo dots of semipermanent ink.
- The patient is placed on the treatment table and is instructed to lie immobile.
- A large machine directs radiation at the target site for the prescribed period, usually 1 or 2 minutes.

COMPLICATIONS
- Local skin reactions
- Anorexia
- Fatigue
- Bone marrow suppression
- Increased risk of bleeding and infection
- Dysfunction or structural change in body parts within the irradiated area:
- Alopecia from scalp irradiation
- Stomatitis and esophagitis from head and neck irradiation
- Pneumonitis, pericarditis, and upper GI distress from thoracic irradiation
- Lower GI and genitourinary problems from abdominopelvic irradiation

NURSING DIAGNOSES

- Disturbed sensory perception (all)
- Risk for infection
- Situational low self-esteem

EXPECTED OUTCOMES
The patient will:
- exhibit improved or normal neurologic status
- exhibit no signs of infection
- verbalize positive feelings about self.

PRETREATMENT CARE

- Explain the treatment and preparation to the patient and his family.
- Verify that the patient or responsible family member has signed an appropriate consent form.
- Take the patient on a tour of the radiation department.
- Obtain a thorough patient history.
- Obtain baseline white blood cell (WBC) and platelet counts.

POSTTREATMENT CARE

- Implement measures to control bleeding and prevent infection.
- Provide meticulous skin care.
- Provide comfort measures and supportive care.
- Monitor the patient's vital signs.
- Monitor WBC and platelet counts.
- Assess for complications, such as abnormal bleeding and infection.
- Monitor breath sounds.
- Monitor drainage.

PATIENT TEACHING

GENERAL

- Review medications and possible adverse reactions with the patient.
- Review care of the skin at the radiation site with the patient.
- Advise the patient about sperm banking if appropriate.
- Tell the patient to avoid applying lotions, medications, deodorants, perfumes, and powders to the site during treatment.
- Advise the patient to wear comfortable, loose clothing over the treated area.
- Tell the patient to avoid sun exposure for 1 year after treatment.
- Stress the importance of using a sunblock with a sun protection factor of 15 or higher.
- Advise the patient how to manage adverse effects at home.
- Review the signs and symptoms of infection with the patient.
- Inform the patient about possible complications and when to notify the practitioner.
- Stress the importance of follow-up care.
- Refer the patient to support groups such as the American Cancer Society.

RESOURCES
Organizations
American Academy of Neurology: *www.aan.com*
American Cancer Society: *www.cancer.org*

Selected references
Cady, J. "Navigating External Beam Radiation Therapy for Head and Neck Cancer," *Clinical Journal of Oncology Nursing* 9(3):362-66, June 2005.

D'Antonio, J. "Chronic Myelogenous Leukemia," *Clinical Journal of Oncology Nursing* 9(5):535-38, October 2005. Review. Erratum in: *Clinical Journal of Oncology Nursing.* 9(6):672, December 2005.

Thompson, N., et al. "MammoSite Radiation Therapy System," *Clinical Journal of Oncology Nursing* 9(3):375-77, June 2005.

Radiation, internal

- Delivery of high levels of radiation (internally) to a specific body area; also called *brachytherapy*
- May be administered locally or systemically, using various approaches
- Interstitial approach: direct implantation of radioactive substance sealed in an applicator (such as a mold, needle, bead, seed, or ribbon) in the tumor or surrounding tissue, or applicator placement on top of a body surface
- Intracavitary approach: use of unsealed radioactive substance for temporary delivery into a hollow body cavity (such as the vagina, abdomen, or pleura); may involve use of a remote afterloader, with radiation delivered at very high doses to a specific area daily for 3 to 5 days
- Intraoperative radiation: delivery of a large dose of external radiation to the tumor and surrounding tissue during surgery
- Radiolabeled antibodies: delivery of radiation directly to the cancer site where, after injection, the antibodies actively seek out the cancer cells and destroy them, which may lessen the risk of damage to healthy cells
- Systemic applications: systemic delivery of radiation using radioactive material in a solution or colloidal suspension given orally or I.V.; used for primary and metastatic thyroid cancer

INDICATIONS
- Primary cancer
- Metastatic cancer

- The proper precautions should be taken against radiation contamination.

INTERSTITIAL OR INTRACAVITARY APPROACH
- The surgeon usually inserts the applicator for the radioactive source in the operating room, with the patient under anesthesia.
- To minimize exposure of facility personnel, the radioactive source is placed in the applicator after the patient returns to his room.
- If the radioactive source isn't permanent, it's left in place for 24 to 72 hours and then removed in the patient's room.
- If a remote afterloader is used, the patient is treated in an inpatient or outpatient department.

I.V., ORAL, OR INTRACAVITARY INSTILLATION
- This is usually performed in the radiation therapy department.
- After intracavitary instillation of a suspension, the patient lies on a flat surface and is rotated every 15 minutes for 2 or 3 hours to distribute the suspension.

COMPLICATIONS
- Localized skin burns
- Hemorrhage
- Neurologic dysfunction
- Leukemia and other cancers
- Cataracts
- Alopecia
- Xerostomia
- Thrombocytopenia
- Genetic mutation and sterility (if radiation directed at gonads)
- Radiation reaction

- Activity intolerance
- Ineffective protection
- Risk for infection

EXPECTED OUTCOMES
The patient will:
- exhibit improved tolerance of activity
- demonstrate use of protective measures, including conserving energy, maintaining a balanced diet, and getting adequate rest
- experience no chills, fever, or other signs and symptoms of infection

PRETREATMENT CARE

- Explain the treatment and preparation to the patient and his family.
- Verify that the patient or a family member has signed an appropriate consent form.
- Obtain a thorough patient history.
- Obtain baseline white blood cell and platelet counts.
- Evaluate the patient for possible problems in positioning, range of motion, and comfort.
- Prepare the patient for a temporary change in appearance if the implant is placed in a visible area, such as the neck or breast.

POSTTREATMENT CARE

- Reassure the patient that normal activities can be resumed after the temporary radiation source has been removed or the permanent source has decayed.
- Report and properly store a dislodged radioactive implant, according to facility policy.
- Follow facility policy regarding radiation precautions.
- Monitor the patient's vital signs and intake and output.
- Assess for complications.
- Monitor for abnormal bleeding.
- Monitor for signs of infection.

PATIENT TEACHING

GENERAL

- Review radiation therapy and potential adverse effects with the patient. (See *Learning about an internal radiation implant,* pages 300 and 301.)
- Advise about the home management of adverse effects, such as adequate fluid intake and not using creams or lotions on the affected skin.
- Tell the patient about possible complications and when to notify the practitioner.
- Inform the patient that the full benefits of treatment may not occur for several months.
- Stress the need for temporary isolation after ingestion or instillation of a radioactive source.
- Review activity restrictions related to applicator location as appropriate.
- Tell the patient that visits by children and pregnant women aren't allowed.
- Stress the importance of follow-up care.
- Refer the patient to support groups such as the American Cancer Society.

RESOURCES

Organizations

American Academy of Neurology:
www.aan.com
American Academy of Pediatrics:
www.aap.org
American Cancer Society:
www.cancer.org

Selected references

Jani, A.B., et al. "Role of External Beam Radiotherapy with Low-Dose-Rate Brachytherapy in Treatment of Prostate Cancer," *Urology* (67)5:1007-11, May 2006.

Mayers, G.L. "Targeted Molecular Brachytherapy," *Drug Development Research* 67(1):94-106, January 2006.

Shaikh, R.U., et al. "Selective Internal Radiation Therapy (SIRT) with Y-90 Microspheres: Preferential Tumor Uptake," *Clinical Nuclear Medicine* 31(2):115, February 2006.

(continued)

Learning about an internal radiation implant

Dear Patient:

You're scheduled to have an internal radiation implant. This therapy treats cervical cancer by temporary insertion of a radioisotope (contained inside a special holder) in your vagina. When in place, the implant will destroy cancer cells in your cervix with X-rays, while at the same time exposing healthy tissues to minimal radiation.

Expect to stay in the hospital about 3 or 4 days, with the implant in place for about 2 or 3 days.

BEFORE THE IMPLANT PROCEDURE

The day before or the morning of the implant procedure, you'll be admitted to the hospital and given a private room. Once the implant is in place, you'll be isolated from other patients and the hospital staff to protect them from unnecessary radiation exposure.

The evening before the procedure you'll have a low-fiber or liquid dinner, and your health care provider may order an enema to clean your bowels. If you'll have a general anesthetic, don't eat or drink after midnight the night before the procedure.

Before going to the operating room, you may receive a douche with an antiseptic solution.

DURING THE IMPLANT PROCEDURE

In the operating room, you'll receive a local or general anesthetic. You'll also have a catheter placed in your bladder to drain urine.

Next, the holding device for the radioisotope will be implanted, and packing will be added to secure it in place. This will take about 20 minutes. Then X-rays will be taken to confirm that the holder is in the right position. Parts of the holder will be visible outside your vagina.

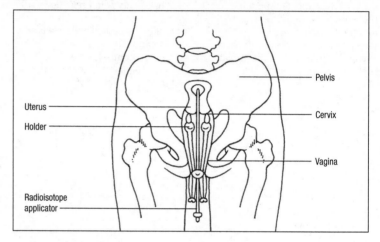

Then you'll go to the postanesthesia care unit. You'll be monitored closely for 1 or 2 hours until you recover from the anesthesia.

When you return to your room, the radioisotope will be inserted into the holder. This takes a few minutes and doesn't hurt.

You may have markings drawn on your inner thighs. These landmarks will be checked periodically to make sure that the implant doesn't move out of place.

Support stockings may be placed on your legs to improve your circulation while you're confined to bed.

SAFETY PRECAUTIONS

Once the radioisotope is in the holder, the hospital staff will implement safety measures to avoid exposure to unnecessary radiation. You'll notice that:

◆ hospital workers who come into your room will wear a film badge to measure their radiation exposure

◆ hospital staff members and visitors will limit their time in your room because radiation exposure increases with time

◆ lead shields may surround your bed to protect the staff from radiation

◆ staff members may stand some distance away from your bed while talking to you. The farther away they stand, the less radiation they'll receive.

Learning about an internal radiation implant _(continued)_

WHILE THE IMPLANT IS IN PLACE

For the next 2 or 3 days, you'll lie on your back while the implant does its work. Try not to move around too much—you don't want to risk dislodging it.

The head of your bed may be raised slightly at mealtimes, and you may be served a liquid or a low-fiber diet. This will help prevent you from having gas and bowel movements. You may also be given medicine to prevent bowel movements.

Expect some discomfort. Ask the nurse for medicine if you feel sick to your stomach or if you have pain.

Also expect to have vaginal drainage while the implant is in place. The nurse will place pads beneath you and change them frequently to keep you dry and clean. She won't change your bed linens because the movement might dislodge the implant.

Practice breathing deeply and coughing hourly while you're awake. Also, exercise your feet and ankles to stimulate your circulation. If you aren't sure how to perform these exercises, ask the nurse.

AFTER THE IMPLANT IS REMOVED

You'll probably go home on the day that the implant and bladder catheter are removed.

As you recuperate, here are some tips for coping with side effects:
◆ Try to rest frequently during the day because you may feel tired for several weeks.

◆ Douche once per day with a solution of 2 tablespoons (30 milliliters) of vinegar (or povidone-iodine [Betadine]—available at the drugstore) to 1 quart (1 liter) of water. This helps minimize the odor from vaginal discharge, which may last for 2 or more weeks.
◆ Follow a low-fiber diet. Eat small frequent meals, and avoid coffee, tea, and cocoa. These measures may relieve diarrhea, which may continue for about 2 weeks.
◆ As comfort permits, resume regular sexual intercourse to counteract a narrowed vagina that may result from scar tissue, or inquire about using a dilator.

WHEN TO CALL YOUR HEALTH CARE PROVIDER

Promptly report these symptoms:
◆ inability to urinate within 6 to 8 hours of having your catheter removed
◆ burning when you urinate
◆ bloody urine
◆ bowel problems, such as constipation, diarrhea, or rectal bleeding
◆ extreme nausea or vomiting
◆ fever over 100° F (37.8° C)
◆ persistent or unusual pain.

Radical neck dissection

- Surgical removal of neck node cancer
- Several different classifications of surgery, depending on extent of resection
- Classic radical neck dissection: removal of all ipsilateral lymphatic structures from the mandible to the clavicle and the infrahyoid muscles to the anterior border of the trapezius
- Modified radical neck dissection type I: preserves the spinal accessory nerve
- Modified radical neck dissection type II: preserves the internal jugular vein and spinal accessory nerve
- Modified radical neck dissection type III: preserves the sternocleidomastoid muscle, the internal jugular vein, and the spinal accessory nerve
- Extended radical neck dissection: removal of lymph node groups or additional structures (not included in the classic neck dissection)

INDICATIONS

- Oral cavity cancer
- Pharyngeal cancer
- Laryngeal cancer
- Thyroid cancer
- Cutaneous malignancies

- The patient is given general anesthesia, and a tracheotomy is performed. The anesthetist may also perform an orotracheal intubation.
- Place the patient in the supine position. The neck and upper chest are prepared and draped.
- The surgeon makes an incision in the neck region, and fatty tissue is removed. He ligates the facial artery and submandibular duct and removes the submandibular nodes.
- Next, he incises the sternocleidomastoid muscle above the clavicle. He removes the spinal accessory nerve; however the phrenic nerve and brachial plexus are preserved. The surgical specimen is then separated from the carotid and vagus nerve.
- The surgeon inserts a drain and closes the wound in layers with staples or sutures.
- A compression dressing might be used for unilateral neck dissection; however, compressive dressings aren't used for bilateral neck dissections.

COMPLICATIONS

- Hemorrhage
- Hypotension (due to carotid sinus stimulation)
- Pneumothorax
- Air embolus
- Embolism
- Nerve damage
- Chylous fistula
- Hematoma
- Wound infection
- Skin flap loss
- Salivary fistula
- Facial edema
- Electrolyte disturbances
- Carotid artery rupture
- Horner's sundrome
- Difficulty with feeding, swallowing, and speaking
- Vocal cord paralysis

- Impaired gas exchange
- Ineffective breathing pattern
- Ineffective tissue perfusion: Cardiopulmonary

EXPECTED OUTCOMES

The patient will:
- maintain adequate ventilation
- exhibit normal breathing pattern
- maintain tissue perfusion.

PRETREATMENT CARE

- Review the procedure and preoperative care with the patient and his family, and answer any questions that they may have.
- Assess the patient's neurologic, cardiovascular, and respiratory status.
- Obtain the patient's weight and assess his nutritional status.
- Perform an electrocardiogram as indicated.
- Verify that an appropriate consent form has been signed.
- Make sure the patient takes nothing by mouth after midnight before the surgery.
- Know that preoperative antibiotics are required if the procedure involves going through the neck into the upper aerodigestive tract.
- Tell the patient what to expect postoperatively (such as a feeding tube, neck edema, drains to help reduce the swelling, ventilator, and inability to speak).
- Arrange a visit with someone who has had a radical neck dissection, if possible.
- Arrange for the speech-language pathologist to meet with the patient and his family before surgery.
- Help the patient choose a temporary way to communicate such as writing, alphabet board, or sign language.

POSTTREATMENT CARE

- Make sure the patient's head is elevated at a 30-degree angle.
- Monitor the patient's vital signs and intake and output.
- Ensure that constant humidification, suctioning, and cleaning of the tracheotomy tube are maintained.
- Maintain oxygenation status as ordered.
- Suction the patient as indicated; assess breath sounds and pulse oximetry; monitor response to ventilator settings; and assist with weaning as indicated.
- Assist the patient to turn, cough, and deep breathe after extubation.
- Give pain medications as needed.
- Ensure that drains are functioning properly and maintain suction as ordered.
- Make sure there's a spare tracheotomy tube at the patient's bedside that's the same size as his tube.
- Monitor for bleeding and edema at the wound site; assess for wound dehiscence; monitor dressings and drainage; and provide wound care.
- Administer fluids as ordered.
- Maintain the patency of the nasogastric tube; begin tube feedings or parenteral therapy as ordered.
- Provide mouth care.
- Provide emotional support.
- Keep a means of communication always available for the patient.
- Administer medications as ordered.
- Monitor for signs of infection or formation of a hematoma.
- Encourage early ambulation with assistance and perform passive range-of-motion exercises to the affected areas as ordered.
- Monitor for possible fistula if the oral or upper digestive tract was opened.
- Monitor hemodynamic status.
- Assess neurologic status and monitor the surgery's effects on nerves.
- Monitor ability to swallow; consult with a speech therapist if needed.
- Monitor laboratory studies.
- Obtain a referral for home health care services.

PATIENT TEACHING

GENERAL

- Teach the patient the signs and symptoms of complications and when to notify the practitioner.
- Provide information about coping with dry mouth, skin irritations or wounds, and nerve damage as appropriate.
- Review medication administration, dosages, and adverse effects with the patient.
- Review physical therapy exercises for the shoulder.
- Stress the need for follow-up care and checkups as scheduled.
- Tell the patient that sutures or clips are usually removed at 7 to 14 days; however, they should remain in place for at least 10 days after the surgery if radiation therapy has been administered.
- Provide the name and contact information for the home health care service provider.

RESOURCES
Organizations
American Academy of Otolaryngology—Head and Neck Surgery:
www.entnet.org
American Cancer Society:
www.cancer.org

Selected references
Rodriguez, C.S., et al. "Pain Measurement in Older Adults with Head and Neck Cancer and Communication Impairments," *Cancer Nursing* 27(6):425-33, November-December 2004.
Spector, J.G., et al. "Management of T3N1 Glottic Carcinoma: Therapeutic Outcomes," *Laryngoscope* 116(1):106-10, January 2006.
Stenson, K.M., et al. "Planned Post-Chemoradiation Neck Dissection: Significance of Radiation Dose," *Laryngoscope* 116(1):33-36, January 2006.

Radioactive iodine therapy

OVERVIEW

- Therapeutic administration of the radioisotope iodine 131 (^{131}I)
- Initially causes acute radiation thyroiditis and gradual thyroid atrophy
- Eventually reduces thyroid hormone levels
- Rarely requires an inpatient stay after administration, unless the patient received a large radioiodine dose (30 mCi or greater)

INDICATIONS
- Hyperthyroidism
- Thyroid cancer

PROCEDURE

- In the nuclear medicine or radiation therapy department, the patient receives an oral dose of ^{131}I or ^{123}I.
- A larger dose is given for thyroid cancer than for hyperthyroidism.
- To treat hyperthyroidism, the dose depends on thyroid size and the gland's degree of radiosensitivity.

COMPLICATIONS
- Hypothyroidism
- Radiation thyroiditis
- Dysphagia
- Salivary gland inflammation
- Thyroid crisis

NURSING DIAGNOSES

- Activity intolerance
- Ineffective protection
- Risk for infection

EXPECTED OUTCOMES
The patient will:
- exhibit improved tolerance of activity
- demonstrate use of protective measures
- experience no chills, fever, or other signs and symptoms of infection.

PRETREATMENT CARE

- Explain the treatment and patient preparation to the patient and his family.
- Verify that the patient has signed an appropriate consent form.
- Discontinue thyroid hormone antagonists 4 to 7 days before ^{131}I administration as ordered.
- Make sure the patient isn't taking the antiarrhythmic drug amiodarone (Cordarone).

POSTTREATMENT CARE

- Encourage increased oral fluid intake for the first 48 hours after treatment.
- Instruct the patient to flush the toilet three times after each use for the first 48 hours.
- Provide disposable eating utensils if the patient requires hospitalization.
- Caution the patient against close contact with young children and pregnant women for 7 days after treatment.
- Monitor the patient's vital signs and intake and output.
- Assess for complications.

PATIENT TEACHING

GENERAL
- Review the adverse effects and complications of treatment with the patient.
- Tell the patient that urine and saliva will be slightly radioactive for 24 hours and that vomitus will be highly radioactive for 6 to 8 hours after treatment. (See *Precautions after radioactive iodine therapy.*)
- Instruct the patient about proper disposal of excrement.
- Tell the patient that the maximum effects of treatment may not occur for 3 months.
- Tell the patient to take the prescribed thyroid hormone antagonists.
- Advise the patient to have periodic laboratory tests for serum thyroid hormone.
- Review the signs and symptoms of hypothyroidism and hyperthyroidism with the patient.
- Review the signs and symptoms of radiation thyroiditis with the patient.
- Tell the patient to avoid taking salicylates.
- Emphasize to a woman of childbearing age to avoid conception for several months after therapy.
- Stress the need for follow-up care.

Precautions after radioactive iodine therapy

RESOURCES
Organizations
American Academy of Neurology:
www.aan.com
American Cancer Society:
www.cancer.org
American Thyroid Association:
www.thyroid.org

Dear Patient:

You've received a dose of radioactive iodine to help treat your thyroid condition. This treatment won't affect your other body tissues. Although this is a safe treatment, you'll need to follow these instructions to prevent harm to you or others.

EATING AND DRINKING

You can eat what you like, but be sure to use disposable plates, cups, and utensils for the next 48 hours. Drink plenty of fluids (about 2 quarts or liters) for the next 48 hours to help remove the radioactive iodine from your body.

USING THE BATHROOM

Your urine, feces, saliva, and perspiration will be slightly radioactive for 48 hours after therapy. You may use your family bathroom to urinate or defecate, but flush the toilet three times to make certain all waste is discarded. Wash your hands thoroughly afterward.

WASHING YOURSELF

If you take a shower or bath within 48 hours after treatment, remember to rinse the shower stall or tub after each use. Wash your clothes, towels, and washcloths separately from those of your family.

You can brush your teeth and resume other normal mouth care. Just make sure you rinse and drain the sink when you've finished.

LIVING ARRANGEMENTS

Avoid close contact with infants, children, and pregnant women for 1 week after therapy. For safety's sake, sleep alone and avoid kissing or sexual intimacy for 48 hours after your treatment. After that, you may resume your normal relationship unless your health care provider gives you other instructions.

If you're breast-feeding, you must stop. Your health care provider will tell you when you can start again.

WHEN TO CALL YOUR HEALTH CARE PROVIDER

If you vomit within 12 hours after therapy, call your health care provider immediately. Flush the vomit down the toilet and, if possible, wear gloves while cleaning up. (Discard the gloves in a plastic bag after use.) Discourage other people from coming in contact with the vomit. If they do, however, tell them to wash their hands thoroughly.

If you get a fever and feel restless or upset within 48 hours of therapy, call your health care provider right away. Also call him if your neck feels tender. He may prescribe medicine to make you more comfortable.

Selected references
Cooper, D.S., et al. "Management Guidelines for Patients with Thyroid Nodules and Differentiated Thyroid Cancer: The American Thyroid Association Guidelines Taskforce," *Thyroid* 16(2):109-43, February 2006.
Rivkees, S.A. "The Management of Hyperthyroidism in Children with Emphasis on the Use of Radioactive Iodine," *Pediatric Endocrinology Reviews* 1(Suppl 2):212-21; discussion 221-22, December 2004.
Robbins, R.J., and Schlumberger, M.J. "The Evolving Role of ^{131}I for the Treatment of Differentiated Thyroid Carcinoma," *The Journal of Nuclear Medicine* 46(1):285-375, January 2005.

Radiofrequency ablation of tumors

- Insertion of radiofrequency ablation (RFA) energy through needle to destroy tumor
- Highly successful, less expensive, and preferred treatment
- Minimally invasive procedure; most patients can return home on same day of procedure
- May also be performed with laparoscopy or during open surgery; percutaneous approach preferred by most radiologists because it's less invasive and produces fewer complications
- Able to destroy a tumor and a small rim of normal tissue around the liver's edges without affecting most of the normal liver; however, not used to treat liver tumors if there's active metastasis
- Used when surgery isn't possible or if the patient is a poor surgical risk

INDICATIONS
- Liver tumors
- Kidney tumors
- Pain management for small bone cancer

⚡ **WARNING** *RFA can destroy small liver tumors (less than 5 cm in diameter) but it can't eliminate microscopic-sized tumors.*

- A local anesthetic is injected into the site and the patient is sedated by I.V. injection.
- The physician guides a special needle through the skin and into the tumor by images from ultrasound or computed tomography (CT) scanning.
- When properly positioned, a plunger is advanced so that the electrodes extend from the needle tip. When fully extended, the electrodes resemble an open umbrella. (See *Radiofrequency ablation.*)
- Insulated wires to the needle electrodes and to grounding pads are placed on the patient's back or thigh, to connect the radiofrequency generator. It produces alternating electric current in the range of radiofrequency waves.
- The needle sends RFA current from the hollow core of the needle to penetrate and destroy the tumor. In addition, heat from radiofrequency energy closes up small blood vessels, reducing the risk of bleeding.

COMPLICATIONS
- Injury to adjacent organs and tissues (such as gallbladder, bile ducts, diaphragm, and bowel loops) requiring surgical correction
- Shoulder pain
- Gallbladder inflammation
- Thermal damage to the bowel or adjacent tissues
- Postablation syndrome
- Bleeding

⚡ **WARNING** *To control severe bleeding, an additional procedure or surgery may be necessary.*

- Ineffective breathing pattern
- Risk for deficient fluid volume
- Risk for infection

EXPECTED OUTCOMES
The patient will:
- have a breathing pattern within normal limits
- have fluid volume that remains within normal limits
- remain free from signs and symptoms of infection.

PRETREATMENT CARE

- Explain the procedure to the patient.
- Verify that an appropriate consent form has been signed.
- Ensure that the patient has taken nothing by mouth from midnight the evening before treatment.
- Know that medications may need to be restricted before treatment, such as aspirin (usually stopped 10 days before) or blood thinners (such as warfarin [Coumadin]).
- Have the patient void before the procedure.
- Identify and record baseline laboratory values.
- Perform a baseline nursing assessment.

POSTTREATMENT CARE

- Help the patient assume a comfortable position.
- Monitor the patient's vital signs and check the dressing for drainage.
- Note color, amount, and character of drainage.
- Remove and dispose of all equipment properly.
- Monitor for complications.
- Assess for pain and nausea as the sedation wears off.
- Make sure the patient has a computed tomography (CT) scan or magnetic resonance imaging (MRI) of the liver scheduled within a few hours to 1 week after RFA to ensure that all tumor tissue has been destroyed and to detect complications.

PATIENT TEACHING

GENERAL

- Tell the patient that a radiologist will interpret the CT scan or MRI and determine if the entire liver tumor appears to have been eliminated. Tell the patient that a repeat CT scan may be done every 3 months to check for new tumors.
- Discuss postablation syndrome—flu-like symptoms that appear 3 to 5 days after the procedure and usually last 5 days, but can last a few weeks.
- Teach the patient about possible complications and when to notify the practitioner.

RESOURCES
Organizations
American College of Gastroenterology: *www.acg.gi.org*
American College of Surgeons: *www.facs.org*
American Gastroenterological Association: *www.gastro.org*
Society of Interventional Radiology: *www.sirweb.org*

Selected references
Blum, H.E. "Hepatocellular Carcinoma: Therapy and Prevention," *World Journal of Gastroenterology* 11(47):7391-400, December 2005.
Brillet, P.Y., et al. "Percutaneous Radiofrequency Ablation for Hepatocellular Carcinoma before Liver Transplantation: A Prospective Study with Histopathologic Comparison," *American Journal of Roentgenology* 186(5 Suppl):S296-305, May 2006.
Luo, B.M., et al. "Percutaneous Ethanol Injection, Radiofrequency and their Combination in Treatment of Hepatocellular Carcinoma," *World Journal of Gastroenterology* 11(40):6277-80, October 2005.

Radiofrequency ablation

A special needle shaped like an umbrella is used to ablate the tumor. Once the needle is in place, the current is directed toward the tumor and the tumor is destroyed.

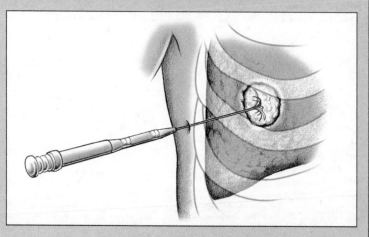

Restrictive gastric surgeries

- Combination of procedures that use both restriction and malabsorption methods to produce weight loss
- Types include adjustable gastric banding and vertical banded gastroplasty
- Results in a smaller stomach so the patient feels fuller faster, thus significantly reduces caloric intake
- Not as successful as other types of gastric surgeries

INDICATIONS

- Body mass index (BMI) of 40 or more (a patient with a BMI of 40 or more is at least 100 pounds over his recommended weight; normal BMI is between 18.5 and 25)
- A BMI of 35 or more with a life-threatening illness that can be improved with weight loss, such as sleep apnea, type 2 diabetes, and heart disease

NURSING DIAGNOSES

- Activity intolerance
- Chronic low self-esteem
- Imbalanced nutrition: More than body requirements

EXPECTED OUTCOMES
The patient will:
- be able to perform activities of daily living
- express feelings of positive self-worth
- have laboratory values that return to within normal limits and exhibit weight loss.

PRETREATMENT CARE

- A complete medical examination is done to evaluate overall health. A psychological evaluation is also done to determine if the patient will be adhering to the new lifestyle.
- Extensive nutritional counseling is done with the patient.
- Explain the treatment and preparation to the patient and his family.
- Verify that the patient has signed an appropriate consent form.
- Obtain serum samples for hematologic studies as ordered.
- Begin I.V. fluid replacement and total parenteral nutrition (TPN) as ordered.
- Prepare the patient for abdominal X-rays as ordered.
- Explain postoperative care and equipment.
- Monitor the patient's vital signs, intake and output, nutritional status, and laboratory test results.

PROCEDURE

- The surgery is performed with the patient under anesthesia.
- The small stomach pouch is created using bands (gastric banding), staples (stomach stapling), or a combination. The surgeon leaves a narrow passage in the newly created pouch so that food can still go through the remainder of the stomach and small intestines, except it does so more slowly. (See *Gastric banding and stapling*.)

COMPLICATIONS

- Bleeding
- Infections
- Bowel obstruction
- Peritonitis
- Gallstones
- Gastritis
- Vomiting
- Dumping syndrome

Gastric banding and stapling

An alternative gastric surgery is adjustable gastric banding in which a band is placed over the stomach to change its size. It may be adjusted over time. Stomach stapling may also be done to reduce the size of the stomach.

ADJUSTABLE GASTRIC BANDING
Stomach opening can be tightened or loosened over time to change the passage size.

VERTICAL BANDED GASTROPLASTY
Band and staples create a smaller stomach pouch.

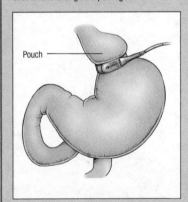

Pouch

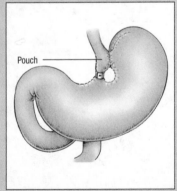

Pouch

Source: www.health.allrefer.com/health/gastric-bypass-adjustable-gastric-banding.html

POSTTREATMENT CARE

- Maintain I.V. replacement therapy as ordered.
- Keep the nasogastric tube patent, but don't reposition it.
- Provide wound care as indicated, and monitor wound drainage.
- Monitor respiratory status and encourage regular coughing and deep-breathing exercises.
- Encourage splinting of the incision site as needed.
- Monitor the patient's vital signs, intake and output, and daily weight.
- Report signs of dehydration, peritonitis, sepsis, infection, or postresection obstruction.

⚡ ***WARNING*** *Monitor for and immediately report signs and symptoms of anastomotic leakage, including low-grade fever, malaise, slight leukocytosis, abdominal distention, tenderness, hemorrhage, hypovolemic shock, and bloody stools or wound drainage.*

- Administer medications as ordered.
- Assess for abdominal pain and for abdominal cramps or shoulder pain; explain that bloating or abdominal fullness from laparoscopy will subside as gas is absorbed.
- Provide comfort measures.
- Place the patient in low or semi-Fowler's position.

⚡ ***WARNING*** *Watch for hypotension, bradycardia, and respiratory changes; these may signal hemorrhage and shock.*

- Administer tube feedings or TPN as ordered.
- Assess for complications, and monitor laboratory test results.
- Monitor for abnormal bleeding.
- Monitor bowel sounds.

⚡ ***WARNING*** *Monitor for and report weakness, nausea, flatulence, and palpitations occurring within 30 minutes after a meal. These findings suggest that the patient has dumping syndrome.*

PATIENT TEACHING

GENERAL

- Instruct the patient to report abnormal bleeding.
- Review the signs and symptoms of infection with the patient.
- Review the signs and symptoms of obstruction or perforation with the patient.
- Tell the patient about possible complications and when to notify the practitioner.
- Tell the patient to continue performing coughing and deep-breathing exercises.
- Tell the patient about splinting of the incision site.
- Teach the patient how to care for the surgical wound.
- Inform the patient about dumping syndrome and how to prevent it.
- Tell the patient that an average of 10 lb (4.5 kg) per month is usually lost and that a stable weight occurs 18 to 24 months after surgery. Also, tell him that the greatest rate of weight loss occurs at the very beginning.
- Advise the patient that he'll need follow-up care often during the first year; these visits will address his physical and mental health status, change in weight, and nutritional needs.
- Inform the patient that to achieve weight loss and avoid complications he should exercise and eat properly.
- Tell the patient that he may remain on restricted food for several weeks after the surgery. Even after that time, he'll feel full very quickly because the stomach holds less food but will eventually expand.
- Inform the patient that because he may need replacement of iron, calcium, vitamin B_{12}, or other nutrients, the practitioner may prescribe supplements such as a multivitamin with minerals.

- Inform the patient that once his diet begins to include solid food, he'll need to chew each bite very slowly and thoroughly. Also, tell him to eat small meals frequently during the day rather than large meals.
- Advise the patient that he may need to separate fluid and food intake by at least 30 minutes. Instruct him to only sip fluids.
- Tell the patient that he may not be able to tolerate large amounts of fat, alcohol, or sugar; he should reduce his intake of fat (especially fast-food, deep-fried, and high-fat foods) and foods that are high in sugar, such as cakes, cookies, and candy.

RESOURCES
Organizations
American College of Gastroenterology: *www.acg.gi.org*
American Gastroenterological Association: *www.gastro.org*
American Society for Bariatric Surgery: *www.asbs.org*

Selected references
Blackwood, H.S. "Help Your Patient Downsize with Bariatric Surgery," *Nursing* Suppl:4-9, Fall 2005.
Parkes, E. "Nutritional Management of Patients after Bariatric Surgery," *The American Journal of Medical Sciences* 331(4):207-13, April 2006.
Smith, B.L. "Bariatric Surgery. It's No Easy Fix," *RN* 68(6):58-63; quiz 64, June 2005.

Scleral buckling

OVERVIEW

- Surgical procedure in which a silicone sponge brings two layers of retina back together after a retinal tear
- Sponge: forms a "buckle" that pushes the sclera toward the middle of the eye, relieving the pull on the retina; pressure of the two layers of retina being pushed together also removes fluid under the retina; buckle may be permanent or temporary
- Most common treatment for retinal detachment

INDICATIONS

- Retinal detachment due to a tear, hole, or break in the retina (rhegmatogenous detachment)

PROCEDURE

- Either local or general anesthesia is used during the procedure, which may be done in an inpatient or outpatient facility.
- The surgeon places a piece of silicone sponge, rubber, or semi-hard plastic against the eye's outer surface. Or, he may cut into the sclera to place the material.
- The material is sewn to the eye to keep it in place. (See *Scleral buckling*.)
- Such methods as extreme cold (cryopexy), heat (diathermy), or light (laser photocoagulation) may be used to scar the retina holding it in place to form a seal. This helps to hold the layers of the eye together and prevent fluid from getting between them.
- A gas bubble may also be injected into the eye to prevent fluid from passing through.

COMPLICATIONS

- Detachment of the choroid
- Increased intraocular pressure
- Change in the shape of the eye
- Refractive error
- Bleeding
- Infection
- Swelling or inflammation of the macula, other parts of the retina, or the membranes surrounding the retina
- Misaligned eyes (strabismus)
- Double vision (diplopia)
- Cataract formation
- Loss of sight in affected eye
- Loss of eye
- Scarring

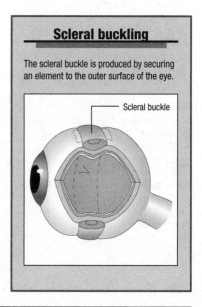

Scleral buckling

The scleral buckle is produced by securing an element to the outer surface of the eye.

Scleral buckle

NURSING DIAGNOSES

- Anxiety
- Deficient knowledge (disorder and treatment)
- Disturbed sensory perception (visual)

EXPECTED OUTCOMES
The patient will:
- verbalize feelings of decreased anxiety
- verbalize understanding of diagnosis and comply with treatment
- regain visual function.

PRETREATMENT CARE

- Before the surgery, both eyes may be patched and the patient placed on bed rest to avoid worsening the detachment.
- Eyedrops are instilled to dilate the pupils.
- Verify that an appropriate consent form has been signed.
- Note any allergies and medications the patient is taking.

POSTTREATMENT CARE

- Monitor vital signs.
- Assess for pain, swelling, redness, or tenderness; also, assess effect of pain medication.
- Administer eyedrops as ordered.
- Give medications as ordered.
- Assist with visual acuity testing.
- Administer comfort measures as indicated.

PATIENT TEACHING

GENERAL
- Instruct the patient about the use of eyedrops he may need to use.
- Instruct on eye care.
- Teach the patient about what to expect as he recovers—that pain and swelling may persist for a few weeks.
- Tell the patient he may have to wear a patch over the affected eye for 1 or more days.
- Have the patient follow up with a vision examination after about 6 months to check for changes in vision. Glasses, contact lenses, or a new prescription may be needed to correct the changes.
- Teach the patient about signs and symptoms that require immediate medical attention, such as sudden vision change or eye pain.
- Teach the patient the signs and symptoms of infection and when to report it to the practitioner.

RESOURCES
Organizations
American Academy of Ophthalmology: *www.aao.org*
American Medical Association: *www.ama-assn.org*

Selected references
Mennel, S., et al. "Transient Serous Retinal Detachment in Classic and Occult Choroidal Neovascularization after Photodynamic Therapy," *American Journal of Ophthalmology* 140(4):758-60, October 2005.

Montrone, L., et al. "Regional Assessment of Cone System Function following Uncomplicated Retinal Detachment Surgery," *Documenta Ophthalmologica* 110(1):103-10, January 2005.

Prasad, S. "The Urgency and Site of Retinal Detachment Surgery," *Eye*, November 4, 2005. [Online]

Sclerotherapy

OVERVIEW

- Injection of a sclerosant into swollen veins or surrounding tissue resulting in fibrosis and local edema, thus compressing the vessel
- Eradicates varices and variceal bleeding and prevents rebleeding
- Cosmetically improves legs' appearance when used for leg varicosities
- Also known as *endoscopic injection sclerotherapy*

INDICATIONS

- Bleeding esophageal varices
- Leg varicosities
- Hemorrhoids

PROCEDURE

ESOPHAGEAL VARICES

- The patient receives I.V. sedation.
- The patient's throat is sprayed with a topical anesthetic.
- The practitioner performs sclerotherapy with esophagogastric duodenoscopy.
- After oral passage of the endoscope, the bleeding varices are identified.
- The practitioner injects 2 ml of a sclerosing agent through a flexible needle injector into each bleeding varix.
- The needle is withdrawn into the sheath, and the site is observed.
- If bleeding doesn't stop within 2 to 5 minutes, a second injection is made below the bleeding site, and the procedure is repeated until bleeding stops.
- Prophylactic sclerotherapy may be done on other distended, nonbleeding varices.

LEG VARICOSITIES

- The sclerosing agent is injected directly into the vein.
- One injection is administered for every inch of vein.
- After the injections are finished, compression tape and a cotton ball are applied to the leg.

COMPLICATIONS

- Transient noncardiac chest pain
- Dysphagia
- Allergic reaction to the sclerosing agent
- Ulceration at the injection site
- Pulmonary complications
- Esophageal stricture
- Bacteremia
- Traumatic esophageal perforation and hemorrhage
- Scarring of legs
- Peripheral edema

NURSING DIAGNOSES

- Activity intolerance
- Anxiety
- Ineffective tissue perfusion: Cardiopulmonary

EXPECTED OUTCOMES

The patient will:
- carry out activities of daily living without excess fatigue or decreased energy
- verbalize decreased anxiety
- maintain hemodynamic stability.

PRETREATMENT CARE

- ◆ Explain the treatment and preparation to the patient and his family.
- ◆ Verify that the patient has signed an appropriate consent form.

ESOPHAGEAL VARICES
- ◆ Have the patient remove dentures and empty his bladder.
- ◆ Obtain baseline vital signs.
- ◆ Establish and maintain vascular access.
- ◆ Administer sedatives as ordered.
- ◆ The patient should take nothing by mouth for 6 to 8 hours before surgery.

LEG VARICOSITIES
- ◆ Instruct the patient to discontinue aspirin products 1 week before surgery.
- ◆ Advise the patient to not apply lotions on the affected leg on the day of surgery.

POSTTREATMENT CARE

ESOPHAGEAL VARICES
- ◆ Administer medications as ordered.
- ◆ Administer I.V. fluids as ordered.
- ◆ Administer supplemental oxygen as ordered.
- ◆ Institute safety precautions.
- ◆ Monitor the patient's vital signs and intake and output.
- ◆ Assess respiratory status.
- ◆ Monitor for complications such as abnormal bleeding.
- ◆ Monitor level of consciousness.
- ◆ Assess for return of normal cough and gag reflexes.

LEG VARICOSITIES
- ◆ The patient should apply compression stockings after the procedure.
- ◆ Instruct the patient to resume activities, but to avoid prolonged standing or sitting or high-impact activities.

PATIENT TEACHING

GENERAL
- ◆ Review the medications and adverse reactions with the patient.
- ◆ Tell the patient about possible complications and when to notify the practitioner.
- ◆ Inform the patient about dietary restrictions.
- ◆ Stress the need for follow-up care.
- ◆ For leg varicosities, instruct the patient to continue the use of compression stockings for 7 to 10 days after surgery and up to 6 weeks, if possible.

RESOURCES
Organizations
American College of Surgeons: *www.facs.org*
American Medical Association: *www.ama-assn.org*
American Society of Plastic Surgeons: *www.plasticsurgery.org*

Selected references
Bergan, J., et al. "Venous Disorders: Treatment with Sclerosant Foam," *Journal of Cardiovascular Surgery* 47(1):9-18, February 2006.

Itha, S., and Yachha, S.K. "Endoscopic Outcome beyond Esophageal Variceal Eradication in Children with Extrahepatic Portal Venous Obstruction," *Journal of Pediatric Gastroenterology and Nutrition* 42(2):196-200, February 2006.

Nagler, H.M. "Is Antegrade Sclerotherapy a Valid Alternative for the Treatment of Varicocele?" *Natural Clinical Practice: Urology* 2(9):424-25, September 2005.

Skin grafting

- Surgical procedure in which healthy skin is taken either from the patient (autograft), donor (allograft), or animal (xenograft) to resurface an area of the patient's body damaged by burns, traumatic injury, or surgery
- Types of grafts include:
  – pinch graft—quarter inch pieces of skin placed over wound sites; not affected by poor blood supply
  – split-thickness graft—includes the epidermis and part of the dermis
  – full-thickness graft—includes the epidermis and entire dermis
  – pedicle graft—full-thickness graft that also includes subcutaneous blood vessels; however, part of the donor site remains attached to the donor area until blood supply is established at the recipient site
- Successful grafting dependent on clean wound granulation with adequate vascularization, complete contact of the graft with the wound bed, sterile technique to prevent infection, adequate graft immobilization, and skilled care
- Usually occurs after wound debridement; with enzymatic debridement, grafting performed 5 to 7 days after debridement is complete; with surgical debridement, grafting performed same day as surgery

INDICATIONS
- Burns
- Reconstructive surgical procedures requiring grafting
- Extensive wounds

PROCEDURE

- The patient is usually given general anesthesia, but for minor grafting, local anesthesia and sedation may be given.
- The grafting donor site is predetermined before surgery; it's usually a site that's hidden under clothing. The skin must be healthy, with a good blood supply.
- The surgeon then cleans the wound site and removes dead tissue. Then he either injects epinephrine, or applies pressure to the area surrounding the wound to decrease blood flow to the area.
- The donor site is then marked—3% to 5% larger than the wound site—and cleaned.
- For split-thickness grafts, the surgeon uses a dermatome to "shave" the donor tissue. The tissue may be applied as a sheet or a mesh (tissue is thinned and enlarged through the use of a special machine).
- For full-thickness grafts, a scalpel is used to cut the donor tissue; the tissue is then removed with a special hook and any fatty tissue is removed before attaching to the recipient site.

- The donor tissue is spread over the wound, then covered with a gentle pressure dressing. Small sutures may also be used to keep the graft intact.
- The donor site for split-thickness grafts is covered with a sterile, nonadherent dressing. The donor site for full-thickness grafts must be surgically closed.

COMPLICATIONS
- Infection
- Graft rejection
- Bleeding

   WARNING *Graft failure may result from traumatic injury, hematoma or seroma formation, infection, an inadequate graft bed, rejection, or compromised nutritional status.*

NURSING DIAGNOSES

- Deficient fluid volume
- Disturbed body image
- Impaired gas exchange
- Risk for infection

EXPECTED OUTCOMES
The patient will:
- maintain adequate fluid volume
- demonstrate acceptance of graft through participation in graft care

---

Evacuating fluid from a sheet graft

When small pockets of fluid (called *blebs*) accumulate beneath a sheet graft, evacuate the fluid using a sterile scalpel and sterile cotton-tipped applicators. First, carefully perforate the center of the bleb with the scalpel.

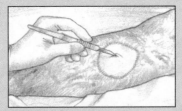

Gently express the fluid with the cotton-tipped applicators.

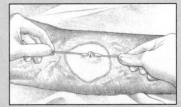

Never express fluid by rolling the bleb to the edge of the graft. This disturbs healing in other areas.

- maintain a patent airway and adequate oxygenation
- remain free from signs and symptoms of infection.

PRETREATMENT CARE

- Explain the procedure to the patient and answer questions.
- Verify that an appropriate consent form has been signed.

Caring for donor graft site

Autografts are usually taken from another area of the patient's body with a dermatome, an instrument that cuts uniform, split-thickness skin portions (typically, about 0.013-cm to 0.05-cm thick). Autografting makes the donor site a partial-thickness wound, which may bleed, drain, and cause pain.

This site needs scrupulous care to prevent infection, which could change the site to a full-thickness wound. Depending on the graft's thickness, tissue may be obtained from the donor site again in as few as 10 days.

Usually, Xeroflo gauze is applied postoperatively. The outer gauze dressing can be taken off on the first postoperative day; the Xeroflo will protect the new epithelial proliferation.

Care for the donor site as you care for the autograft, using dressing changes at the initial stages to prevent infection and promote healing. Follow the guidelines below.

DRESSING THE WOUND

- Wash your hands and put on sterile gloves.
- Remove the outer gauze dressings within 24 hours. Inspect the Xeroflo for signs of infection; then leave the wound open to the air to speed drying and healing.
- Leave small amounts of fluid accumulation alone. Using asceptic technique, aspirate larger amounts through the dressing with a small-gauge needle and syringe.
- Apply a lanolin-based cream daily to completely healed donor sites to keep skin tissue pliable and to remove crusts.

- The patient should take nothing by mouth after midnight before surgery as appropriate.
- Provide wound care, as indicated, using sterile technique.

POSTTREATMENT CARE

- Provide adequate I.V. hydration as ordered.
- Administer medications as ordered.
- Provide emotional support.
- Monitor the patient's vital signs and pulse oximetry level.

⚡ **WARNING** *To protect the graft, avoid using a blood pressure cuff over the graft, don't tug or pull dressings during dressing changes, and keep the patient from lying on the graft.*

- Monitor peripheral pulses and signs of decreased tissue perfusion.
- Assess pain level and response to analgesics.
- Monitor for signs and symptoms of complications.
- Don't remove the dressings unless ordered. The graft dressings usually stay in place for 3 to 5 days after surgery to avoid disturbing the graft site.
- Provide graft care as ordered or per facility protocol.

⚡ **WARNING** *To avoid dislodging the graft, hydrotherapy is usually discontinued for 3 to 4 days after grafting.*

- If the patient dislodges the graft, apply sterile skin compresses to keep the area moist until the surgeon reapplies the graft.
- If the graft affects an arm or a leg, elevate the affected extremity to reduce postoperative edema and check for bleeding and signs of neurovascular impairment.
- Maintain bedrest or activity restrictions, as ordered, based on graft location.

- Inspect a sheet graft frequently for blebs and evacuate them carefully with a sterile scalpel if ordered. (See *Evacuating fluid from a sheet graft.*)
- Clean completely healed areas and apply a moisturizing cream to them to keep the skin pliable and to retard scarring.
- Provide donor graft site care. (See *Caring for donor graft site.*)

PATIENT TEACHING

GENERAL
- Review the administration, dosage, and adverse effects of medications with the patient.
- Teach the patient how to perform skin graft care.
- Tell the patient about the signs and symptoms to report.

RESOURCES
Organizations
American Medical Association: *www.ama-assn.org*
Burn Foundation: *www.burnfoundation.org*
The Burn Resource Center: *www.burnsurvivor.com*

Selected references
Cubison, T.C., and Gilbert, P.M. "So Much for Percentage, but What About the Weight?" *Emergency Medicine Journal* 22(9):643-45, September 2005.
Hohlfeld, J., et al. "Tissue Engineered Fetal Skin Constructs for Paediatric Burns," *Lancet* 366(9488):840-42, September 2005.
Singer, A.J., et al. "Octylcyanoacrylate for the Treatment of Small, Superficial, Partial-Thickness Burns: A Pilot Study," *Academic Emergency Medicine* 12(9):900-904, September 2005.

Somnoplasty

- Minimally invasive procedure for treatment of upper-airway obstruction
- Controlled, low-power radiofrequency energy: creates submucosal volumetric lesions to reduce tissue volume and stiffen remaining tissue in the desired area
- Lesions healing over 6 to 8 weeks
- More than one treatment usually needed to achieve optimal results; considered safer than other treatments

INDICATIONS
- Chronic nasal obstruction
- Obstructive sleep apnea
- Habitual snoring

PROCEDURE

- The procedure is usually performed at an outpatient facility
- A local anesthetic is used; the uvula and palate are anesthetized.
- A radiofrequency control unit is inserted into the mouth. An electrode on the unit is inserted into the tissue and heat is applied to the area creating a coagulative lesion. The surface area isn't affected by the heat, and more than one lesion may be created.
- Over 3 to 8 weeks, the lesion is absorbed, and collagen in the treated area contracts until the tissue stiffens and the obstruction is reduced.

COMPLICATIONS
- Swelling
- Sore throat
- Infection
- Bleeding

NURSING DIAGNOSES

- Disturbed sleep pattern
- Impaired gas exchange
- Ineffective breathing pattern

EXPECTED OUTCOMES
The patient will:
- feel rested after sleeping
- maintain adequate ventilation
- exhibit normal breathing pattern.

PRETREATMENT CARE

◆ Explain the procedure to the patient and answer any questions.
◆ Verify that an appropriate consent form has been signed.
◆ Instruct the patient to avoid aspirin and aspirin-containing products for 10 days before surgery.
◆ Explain to the patient that dietary restrictions aren't necessary, but if he smokes, he should stop.
◆ Complete the history and physical examination and note allergies.

POSTTREATMENT CARE

◆ Ensure adequate humidification.
◆ Administer medications as ordered.
◆ Place the patient in a comfortable position that facilitates breathing.
◆ Monitor the patient's vital signs and pulse oximetry level.
◆ Assess for bleeding.
◆ Monitor for complications.

PATIENT TEACHING

GENERAL

◆ Teach the patient the signs of infection.
◆ Stress the need for follow-up care.
◆ Inform the patient that for pain relief, he can take over-the-counter analgesics for up to 3 days; however, analgesics may also be prescribed.
◆ If treatment is performed for snoring, tell the patient that initially snoring may worsen, but should improve within 1 to 2 weeks.

RESOURCES
Organizations
American College of Surgeons: *www.facs.org*
American Medical Association: *www.ama-assn.org*
Somnoplasty: *www.somnoplasty.com*

Selected references
Can, M., et al. "Serum Cardiovascular Risk Factors in Obstructive Sleep Apnea," *Chest* 129(2):233-37, February 2006.
Carroll, T., et al. "Alternative Surgical Dissection Techniques," *Otolaryngology Clinics of North America* 38(2):397-411, April 2005.
Edwards, N., et al. "Severity of Sleep-Disordered Breathing Improves following Parturition," *Sleep.* 28(6):737-41, June 2005.

Spinal surgery: arthrodesis

OVERVIEW

- Surgical procedure to graft bone chips between the vertebral spaces to stabilize the spine
- Used when conservative treatments (such as prolonged bed rest, traction, and use of a back brace) are ineffective
- Also called *spinal fusion*

INDICATIONS

- Herniated disk
- Vertebral fracture
- Vertebral dislocation
- Spinal cord tumor
- Vertebrae seriously weakened by trauma or disease
- Deformity correction

PROCEDURE

- The patient receives a general anesthetic.
- For cervical fusion, the anterior approach is usually used; for lumbar and thoracic fusion, the posterior approach is used.
- The surgeon exposes the affected vertebrae.
- If a bone graft is used, an incision is made in the donor's hip and pieces or chips of the bone are removed, usually from the iliac crest.
- Bone chips, bone bank, or both are shaped and inserted into the defect.
- Wire, spinal plates, rods, or screws are used to secure bone grafts into several vertebrae surrounding the unstable area.
- The incision is closed and a dressing, splint, or cast is applied.
- External traction, such as a halo device, may be applied if surgery involved the cervical spine.

COMPLICATIONS

- Herniation relapse
- Arachnoiditis
- Chronic neuritis
- Immobility
- Nerve or muscle damage
- Infection

NURSING DIAGNOSES

- Activity intolerance
- Acute pain
- Disturbed sensory perception (all)

EXPECTED OUTCOMES

The patient will:
- demonstrate improved mobility
- verbalize feelings of comfort
- exhibit improved neurologic status.

PRETREATMENT CARE

- Explain the treatment and preparation to the patient and his family.
- Verify that the patient has signed an appropriate consent form.
- Discuss postoperative recovery and rehabilitation. Reassure the patient that analgesics and muscle relaxants will be available during recovery.
- Tell the patient that he'll return from surgery with a dressing over the incision and that there may be activity restrictions.
- Just before surgery, perform a baseline assessment of motor function and sensation in the patient's lower trunk, legs, and feet as well as upper extremities and fingers for cervical involvement. Carefully document the results for comparison with postoperative findings.

POSTTREATMENT CARE

- Administer medications as ordered.
- Maintain activity restrictions as ordered
- Assist the surgeon with the initial dressing change.
- Monitor the patient's vital signs and intake and output.
- Assess the surgical wound and dressings.
- Monitor for drainage and bleeding.
- Assess motor and neurologic function; compare the results with baseline findings.

PATIENT TEACHING

GENERAL

- Review the medications and possible adverse reactions with the patient.
- Show the patient how to care for the incision site. (See *Recovering from spinal surgery.*)
- Teach the patient the signs and symptoms of infection.
- Tell the patient about possible complications and when to notify the practitioner.
- Review activity restrictions with the patient.
- Instruct the patient to perform prescribed exercises.
- Tell the patient about proper body mechanics.

Recovering from spinal surgery

Dear Patient:

Your surgeon has asked that you follow these instructions as you recover from your spinal surgery.

HOW TO CARE FOR YOUR INCISION

◆ Check your incision site often for signs of infection, such as increased pain and tenderness, redness, swelling, and changes in the amount and character of drainage.
◆ Report such signs to your surgeon immediately.
◆ Avoid soaking your stitches in a bathtub until healing is complete.
◆ Shower with your incision facing away from the stream of water until healing is complete.

ACTIVITY GUIDELINES

◆ Avoid sitting for prolonged periods.
◆ Avoid lifting heavy objects or bending over until instructed.
◆ Don't climb long flights of stairs until instructed.
◆ Resume activity gradually after surgery. Start with short walks and slowly progress to longer distances.
◆ Do your prescribed exercises daily or as instructed (pelvic tilt, leg raises, toe pointing, _____
_____).
◆ Rest frequently and avoid overexertion.
◆ Driving instructions: _____
_____

HOW TO USE PROPER BODY MECHANICS

◆ When in bed, lie on your back with your knees propped up with pillows or on your side with your knees bent and a pillow between your legs.
– Don't lie on your stomach or on your back with your legs flat.
– Sleep on a moderately firm mattress. If necessary, purchase a new one or insert a bed board between your existing mattresses.
◆ When sitting, place your feet on a low stool to elevate your knees above hip level.
  Use a firm, straight-backed chair and sit up straight with your lower back pressed flat against the chair back.
◆ When standing for prolonged periods, alternate placing each foot on a low stool to straighten your lower back and relieve strain.
◆ When bending, keep your spine straight and bend at your knees and hips rather than at your waist.
  Call your surgeon promptly if you develop increasing pain or signs of infection, or have any questions about your recovery. Keep your follow-up office visit on _____.

RESOURCES

Organizations

American Academy of Neurology: *www.aan.com*
American Academy of Orthopaedic Surgeons: *www.aaos.org*
American College of Surgeons: *www.facs.org*
American Medical Association: *www.ama-assn.org*

Selected references

Bajnoczy, S. "Artificial Disc Replacement—Evolutionary Treatment for Degenerative Disc Disease," *AORN Journal* 82(2):192, 195-202, 205-206; quiz 207-12, August 2005.
Deyo, R.A., and Mirza, S.K. "Trends and Variations in the Use of Spine Surgery," *Clinical Orthopaedics and Related Research* 443:139-46, February 2006.
Rodts, M.F. "Total Disc Replacement Arthroplasty," *Orthopaedic Nursing* 23(3):216-19, May-June 2004.
Strayer, A. "Lumbar Spine: Common Pathology and Interventions," *Journal of Neuroscience Nursing* 37(4):181-93, August 2005.

Spinal surgery: kyphoplasty

OVERVIEW

- Minimally invasive surgical procedure providing support to vertebral bodies and decreasing pain
- Utilizes cementlike substance that's injected into vertebrae under fluoroscopy
- Similar to vertebroplasty procedure, with added step of balloon inflation of vertebrae elevating vertebrae before cement injection

INDICATIONS
- Compression fracture
- Vertebral dislocation
- Vertebrae seriously weakened by trauma or disease (osteoporosis)

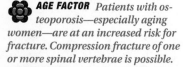 **AGE FACTOR** *Patients with osteoporosis—especially aging women—are at an increased risk for fracture. Compression fracture of one or more spinal vertebrae is possible.*

PROCEDURE

- The patient receives general or local anesthesia and is placed in a prone position. The procedure is performed with fluoroscopy.
- After a small incision is made in the back, a narrow tube is inserted into the affected area, and a balloon inserted and inflated. This inflation creates a cavity inside the vertebrae as well as elevates the fracture to return the vertebrae to a normal position.
- After the balloon is removed, the cavity is filled with a cementlike material that hardens quickly to stabilize the bone.
- This procedure is repeated for all involved vertebrae.
- A dressing is then applied to the incision site when the procedure is complete.

COMPLICATIONS
- Herniation relapse
- Arachnoiditis
- Chronic neuritis
- Immobility
- Nerve or muscle damage
- Leakage of cement
- Spinal compression

NURSING DIAGNOSES

- Activity intolerance
- Acute pain
- Disturbed sensory perception (all)

EXPECTED OUTCOMES
The patient will:
- demonstrate improved mobility
- verbalize feelings of comfort
- exhibit improved neurologic status.

PRETREATMENT CARE

- Explain the treatment and preparation to the patient and his family.
- Verify that the patient has signed an appropriate consent form.
- Discuss postoperative recovery and rehabilitation. Reassure the patient that analgesics and muscle relaxants will be available during recovery.
- Tell the patient that he'll return from surgery with a dressing over the incision and that there may be activity restrictions.
- Just before surgery, perform a baseline assessment of motor function and sensation in the patient's lower trunk, legs, and feet, and upper extremities and fingers for cervical involvement. Carefully document the results for comparison with postoperative findings.

POSTTREATMENT CARE

- Administer medications as ordered.
- Maintain activity restrictions.
- Assist the surgeon with the initial dressing change.
- If the patient doesn't void within 8 to 12 hours after surgery, notify the practitioner, and prepare to insert a urinary catheter.
- Monitor the patient's vital signs and intake and output.
- Assess the surgical wound and dressings.
- Monitor for drainage and bleeding.
- Assess motor and neurologic function, Also, assess motor and neurologic function in the patient's trunk and lower extremities and upper extremities and fingers for cervical involvement; compare the results with baseline findings.

PATIENT TEACHING

GENERAL
- Review the medications and possible adverse reactions with the patient.
- Show the patient how to care for the incision site.
- Teach the patient the signs and symptoms of infection.
- Tell the patient of possible complications and when to notify the practitioner.
- Instruct the patient to shower with the incision facing away from the stream of water.
- Review activity restrictions with the patient. (See *Dealing with osteoporosis.*)
- Instruct the patient to perform prescribed exercises.
- Tell the patient about proper body mechanics.
- Advise the patient to avoid lying on his stomach or on his back with legs flat.
- Stress the need for follow-up care.

Dealing with osteoporosis

Dear Patient:

After kyphoplasty, it's important to prevent further damage to the spine. Here are some measures to help you manage your osteoporosis.

◆ Use proper body mechanics at all times. When bending, keep your spine straight and bend at your knees and hips rather than at your waist. Avoid twisting movements and prolonged bending.

◆ Eat a diet rich in calcium. Calcium-rich foods include milk, yogurt, cheese, sardines (with bones), canned salmon, broccoli, tofu, turnip greens, and kale. You should eat or use supplements to reach a calcium intake of 1,200 mg daily with vitamin D intake of 400 to 800 international units daily.

◆ Avoid smoking and excessive alcohol use.

◆ Engage in regular weight-bearing and muscle-strengthening exercise as instructed by your health care provider.

◆ If you're taking estrogen, perform breast self-examination at least once per month. Report any lumps immedi-ately to your health care provider. Also be sure to have yearly gynecologic ex-aminations. Report abnormal vaginal bleeding promptly to your gynecolo-gist.

◆ If you're taking a calcium supple-ment, maintain a liberal fluid intake. This will maintain adequate urine out-put and help avoid kidney stones, ex-cess calcium in the urine, and excess calcium in the blood.

◆ Report any new pain sites immedi-ately to your health care provider, es-pecially after trauma.

◆ Sleep on a moderately firm mat-tress and avoid excessive bed rest.

◆ If you use a back brace, follow the manufacturer's and surgeon's instruc-tions on proper usage.

RESOURCES

Organizations

American Academy of Neurology: *www.aan.com*
American Academy of Orthopaedic Sur-geons: *www.aaos.org*
American College of Surgeons: *www.facs.org*
American Medical Association: *www.ama-assn.org*
Spine-Health.com: *www.spine-health.com*

Selected references

Bajnoczy, S. "Artificial Disc Replace-ment—Evolutionary Treatment for De-generative Disc Disease," *AORN Jour-nal* 82(2):192, 195-202, 205-206; quiz 207-12, August 2005.

Deyo, R.A., and Mirza, S.K. "Trends and Variations in the Use of Spine Surgery," *Clinical Orthopaedics and Related Re-search* 443:139-46, February 2006.

Fowler, S.B., et al. "Health-Related Quality of Life in Patients Undergoing Anterior Cervical Discectomy Fusion," *Journal of Neuroscience Nursing* 37(2):97-100, April 2005.

Lemke, D.M. "Vertebroplasty and Kypho-plasty for Treatment of Painful Osteo-porotic Compression Fractures," *Jour-nal of American Academy of Nurse Practitioners* 17(7):268-76, July 2005.

Rodts, M.F. "Total Disc Replacement Arthroplasty," *Orthopaedic Nursing* 23(3):216-19, May-June 2004.

Strayer, A. "Lumbar Spine: Common Pathology and Interventions," *Journal of Neuroscience Nursing* 37(4):181-93, August 2005.

Spinal surgery: laminectomy

OVERVIEW

- Surgical procedure to remove one or more of the bony laminae that cover the vertebrae; typically done to relieve pressure on the spinal cord or spinal nerve roots
- After removal of several laminae, spinal fusion (grafting of bone chips between vertebral spaces) commonly performed to stabilize the spine

INDICATIONS

- Herniated disk
- Compression fracture
- Vertebral dislocation
- Spinal cord tumor
- Vertebrae seriously weakened by trauma or disease

PROCEDURE

- The patient receives a general anesthetic and is placed in a prone or side-lying position.
- A midline vertical incision is made.
- The fascia and muscles are stripped off the bony laminae.
- One or more sections of laminae are removed to expose the spinal defect (herniated disk, bone spur, disk fragment).

COMPLICATIONS

- Infection
- Bleeding
- Spinal fluid leakage
- Nerve or muscle damage

NURSING DIAGNOSES

- Activity intolerance
- Acute pain
- Disturbed sensory perception (all)

EXPECTED OUTCOMES

The patient will:
- demonstrate improved mobility
- verbalize feelings of comfort
- exhibit improved neurologic status.

PRETREATMENT CARE

- Explain the treatment and preparation to the patient and his family.
- Verify that the patient has signed an appropriate consent form.
- Discuss postoperative recovery and rehabilitation. Reassure the patient that analgesics and muscle relaxants will be available during recovery.
- Tell the patient that he'll return from surgery with a dressing over the incision and that there may be activity restrictions. Show him the logrolling method of turning, and explain that he'll use this method later to get in and out of bed by himself.
- Just before surgery, perform a baseline assessment of motor function and sensation in the patient's lower trunk, legs, and feet as well as upper extremities and fingers for cervical involvement. Carefully document the results for comparison with postoperative findings.
- Tell the patient to discontinue aspirin and aspirin-containing products for 7 to 10 days before surgery.
- Instruct the patient not to have anything to eat or drink after midnight before the procedure.
- If the patient smokes, advise him to stop.

POSTTREATMENT CARE

- Administer medications as ordered; instruct the patient on the use of patient-controlled analgesia if appropriate.
- Keep the head of the bed flat or elevated no more than 45 degrees for at least 24 hours after surgery.
- Maintain activity restrictions.
- Assist the surgeon with the initial dressing change.
- Monitor the patient's vital signs and intake and output.
- Assess the surgical wound and dressings.
- Monitor for drainage and bleeding.
- Monitor for cerebrospinal fluid leakage.
- Assess motor and neurologic function. Compare the results with baseline findings.

PATIENT TEACHING

GENERAL

- Review the medications and possible adverse reactions with the patient.
- Show the patient how to care for the incision site.
- Teach the patient the signs and symptoms of infection.
- Tell the patient of possible complications and when to notify the practitioner.
- Instruct the patient to shower with his back facing away from the stream of water.
- Review activity restrictions with the patient.
- Instruct the patient to perform prescribed exercises.
- Tell the patient about proper body mechanics.
- Advise the patient to use a firm, straight-backed chair.
- Advise the patient to sleep only on a firm mattress or insert a bed board between the mattress and box spring.
- Stress the need for follow-up care.

RESOURCES
Organizations
American Academy of Neurology: *www.aan.com*
American Academy of Orthopaedic Surgeons: *www.aaos.org*
American College of Surgeons: *www.facs.org*
American Medical Association: *www.ama-assn.org*

Selected references
Bajnoczy, S. "Artificial Disc Replacement—Evolutionary Treatment for Degenerative Disc Disease," *AORN Journal* 82(2):192, 195-202, 205-206; quiz 207-12, August 2005.

Deyo, R.A., and Mirza, S.K. "Trends and Variations in the Use of Spine Surgery," *Clinical Orthopaedics and Related Research* 443:139-46, February 2006.

Fowler, S.B., et al. "Health-Related Quality of Life in Patients Undergoing Anterior Cervical Discectomy Fusion," *Journal of Neuroscience Nursing* 37(2):97-100, April 2005.

Lemke, D.M. "Vertebroplasty and Kyphoplasty for Treatment of Painful Osteoporotic Compression Fractures," *Journal of American Academy of Nurse Practitioners* 17(7):268-76, July 2005.

Rodts, M.F. "Total Disc Replacement Arthroplasty," *Orthopaedic Nursing* 23(3):216-19, May-June 2004.

Strayer, A. "Lumbar Spine: Common Pathology and Interventions," *Journal of Neuroscience Nursing* 37(4):181-93, August 2005.

Spinal surgery: laminoplasty

OVERVIEW

- Surgical procedure involving reconstruction of the lamina—bony plate that covers the posterior arch of a vertebra—to increase the amount of space available for the neural tissue
- Performed to relieve the symptoms of spinal stenosis
- Also called *open-door laminoplasty*

INDICATIONS

- Compression fracture
- Spinal cord tumor
- Spinal stenosis

AGE FACTOR *Laminoplasty effectively treats neurologic deficits in younger patients with congenital spinal stenosis.*

PROCEDURE

- The patient receives a general anesthetic and is placed in a prone position.
- A midline vertical incision is made. One side of the vertebrae is cut to form a "hinge" and the other side is cut all the way through.
- Small titanium miniplates and pieces of bone are then inserted and the vertebrae are put back in place with an increased spinal space.
- This increased space allows for decompression of spinal cord and nerve roots. (See *Looking at laminoplasty.*)

COMPLICATIONS

- Infection
- Bleeding
- Spinal fluid leakage
- Unstable spinal column
- Nerve or muscle damage

NURSING DIAGNOSES

- Activity intolerance
- Acute pain
- Disturbed sensory perception (all)

EXPECTED OUTCOMES

The patient will:
- demonstrate improved mobility
- verbalize feelings of comfort
- exhibit improved neurologic status.

PRETREATMENT CARE

- Explain the treatment and preparation to the patient and his family.
- Verify that the patient has signed an appropriate consent form.
- Discuss postoperative recovery and rehabilitation. Reassure the patient that analgesics and muscle relaxants will be available during recovery.
- Tell the patient that he'll return from surgery with a dressing over the incision and that there may be some activity restrictions. If the cervical vertebrae are involved, tell the patient

Looking at laminoplasty

During laminoplasty, the surgeon removes the damaged lamina (see illustrations 1 and 2). The lamina is repaired using an allographic bone material and then secured with titanium screws and plates (see illustrations 3 and 4).

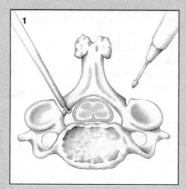
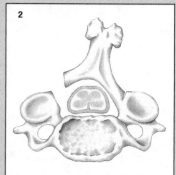
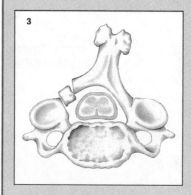
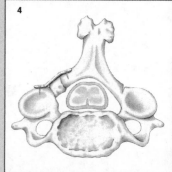

that he'll need to wear a soft cervical collar for 6 weeks.
- Just before surgery, perform a baseline assessment of motor function and sensation in the patient's lower trunk, legs, and feet as well as upper extremities and fingers for cervical involvement. Carefully document the results for comparison with postoperative findings.

POSTTREATMENT CARE

- Administer medications as ordered.
- Assist the surgeon with the initial dressing change.
- Monitor the patient's vital signs and intake and output.
- Assess the surgical wound and dressings.
- Monitor for drainage and bleeding.
- Monitor for cerebrospinal fluid leakage.
- Assess motor and neurologic function; compare the results with baseline findings.

PATIENT TEACHING

GENERAL
- Review the medications and possible adverse reactions with the patient.
- Show the patient how to care for the incision site.
- Teach the patient the signs and symptoms of infection.
- Tell the patient of possible complications and when to notify the practitioner.
- Instruct the patient to shower with his incision facing away from the stream of water.
- Review activity restrictions with the patient.
- Instruct the patient to perform prescribed exercises.
- Tell the patient about proper body mechanics.
- Advise the patient to use a firm, straight-backed chair.
- Advise the patient to sleep only on a firm mattress or insert a bed board between the mattress and box spring.
- Stress the need for follow-up care.

RESOURCES
Organizations
American Academy of Neurology: *www.aan.com*
American Academy of Orthopaedic Surgeons: *www.aaos.org*
American College of Surgeons: *www.facs.org*
American Medical Association: *www.ama-assn.org*
SpineUniverse: *www.spineuniverse.com*

Selected references
Bajnoczy, S. "Artificial Disc Replacement—Evolutionary Treatment for Degenerative Disc Disease," *AORN Journal* 82(2):192, 195-202, 205-206; quiz 207-12, August 2005.
Deyo, R.A., and Mirza, S.K. "Trends and Variations in the Use of Spine Surgery," *Clinical Orthopaedics and Related Research* 443:139-46, February 2006.
Fowler, S.B., et al. "Health-Related Quality of Life in Patients Undergoing Anterior Cervical Discectomy Fusion," *Journal of Neuroscience Nursing* 37(2):97-100, April 2005.
Lemke, D.M. "Vertebroplasty and Kyphoplasty for Treatment of Painful Osteoporotic Compression Fractures," *Journal of American Academy of Nurse Practitioners* 17(7):268-76, July 2005.
Rodts, M.F. "Total Disc Replacement Arthroplasty," *Orthopaedic Nursing* 23(3):216-19, May-June 2004.
Strayer, A. "Lumbar Spine: Common Pathology and Interventions," *Journal of Neuroscience Nursing* 37(4):181-93, August 2005.

Spinal surgery: microdiskectomy

OVERVIEW

- Minimally invasive surgical procedure that's an alternative to laminectomy for decompressing and repairing damaged lumbar disks
- Typically used for smaller, less severe disk abnormalities
- Carries a 50% success rate

INDICATIONS
- Herniated disk
- Cauda equina syndrome

PROCEDURE

- The procedure may be performed on an outpatient basis; the patient receives local anesthesia.
- Under guided X-ray visualization, the surgeon locates the damaged disk and removes the nerve root and injured disk tissues.
- The incision is stapled and may be covered with a dressing.

COMPLICATIONS
- Herniation relapse
- Spinal fluid leakage
- Nerve or root damage

NURSING DIAGNOSES

- Activity intolerance
- Acute pain
- Disturbed sensory perception (all)

EXPECTED OUTCOMES
The patient will:
- demonstrate improved mobility
- verbalize feelings of comfort
- exhibit improved neurologic status.

PRETREATMENT CARE

- Explain the treatment and preparation to the patient and his family.
- Verify that the patient has signed an appropriate consent form.
- Discuss postoperative recovery and rehabilitation. Reassure the patient that analgesics and muscle relaxants will be available during recovery.
- Tell the patient that he'll return from surgery with a dressing over the incision and that there may be activity restrictions.
- Just before surgery, perform a baseline assessment of motor function and sensation in the patient's lower trunk, legs, and feet as well as upper extremities and fingers for cervical involvement. Carefully document the results for comparison with postoperative findings.

POSTTREATMENT CARE

◆ Administer medications as ordered.
◆ Assist the surgeon with the initial dressing change.
◆ Monitor the patient's vital signs and intake and output.
◆ Assess the surgical wound and dressings.
◆ Monitor for drainage and bleeding.
◆ Monitor for cerebrospinal fluid leakage.
◆ Assess motor and neurologic function; compare the results with baseline findings.

PATIENT TEACHING

GENERAL

◆ Review the medications and possible adverse reactions with the patient.
◆ Show the patient how to care for the incision site.
◆ Teach the patient the signs and symptoms of infection.
◆ Tell the patient of possible complications and when to notify the practitioner.
◆ Instruct the patient to shower with his incision facing away from the stream of water.
◆ Review activity restrictions with the patient.
◆ Instruct the patient to perform prescribed exercises.
◆ Tell the patient about proper body mechanics.
◆ Stress the need for follow-up care.

RESOURCES
Organizations
American Academy of Neurology: *www.aan.com*
American Academy of Orthopaedic Surgeons: *www.aaos.org*
American College of Surgeons: *www.facs.org*
American Medical Association: *www.ama-assn.org*

Selected references
Bajnoczy, S. "Artificial Disc Replacement—Evolutionary Treatment for Degenerative Disc Disease," *AORN Journal* 82(2):192, 195-202, 205-206; quiz 207-12, August 2005.
Deyo, R.A., and Mirza, S.K. "Trends and Variations in the Use of Spine Surgery," *Clinical Orthopaedics and Related Research* 443:139-46, February 2006.
Fowler, S.B., et al. "Health-Related Quality of Life in Patients Undergoing Anterior Cervical Discectomy Fusion," *Journal of Neuroscience Nursing* 37(2):97-100, April 2005.
Lemke, D.M. "Vertebroplasty and Kyphoplasty for Treatment of Painful Osteoporotic Compression Fractures," *Journal of American Academy of Nurse Practitioners* 17(7):268-76, July 2005.
Rodts, M.F. "Total Disc Replacement Arthroplasty," *Orthopaedic Nursing* 23(3):216-19, May-June 2004.
Strayer, A. "Lumbar Spine: Common Pathology and Interventions," *Journal of Neuroscience Nursing* 37(4):181-93, August 2005.

Spinal surgery: rod implantation

OVERVIEW

- Surgical attachment of hooks, rods, and wires to redistribute stress to the spine and keep the bones in proper alignment
- Provides a stable, rigid column that encourages bones to fuse after surgery, corrects deformity, and provides stability to the spine
- Types of spinal instrumentation: Luque rod, Drummond instrumentation, Cotrel-Dubousset instrumentation, Zeilke instrumentation, Kaneda device, Harrington rods, and Wisconsin instrumentation
- Endoscopic implantation of rods performed in certain circumstances
- Choice of instrumentation based on the type of disorder, age and health of the patient, and the surgeon's particular experience with the spinal instrumentation device

INDICATIONS
- Scoliosis
- Birth defects
- Fractures
- Marfan syndrome
- Neurofibromatosis
- Neuromuscular diseases
- Severe injuries
- Tumors

PROCEDURE

- The procedure is performed by a neurology or orthopedic surgical team usually under general anesthesia.
- The surgery is usually done at the same time as spinal fusion.
- The surgeon can use a posterior or anterior approach.
- The surgeon strips the muscles away from the surgical site and the bone surface is peeled away. This helps the bone graft to fuse better.
- In some cases, the vertebral disc is removed to provide a larger area for the spinal fusion.
- Rods, hooks, and wires are inserted and secured to stabilize the area and the incision is closed.

COMPLICATIONS
- Nerve damage
- Paralysis
- Infection
- Inflammatory reaction caused by foreign material in the body
- Serious infection of the membranes covering the spinal cord and brain
- Psychological problems

   AGE FACTOR This type of surgery may be emotionally difficult to endure in young people. Patients who have had spinal instrumentation must avoid contact sports and eliminate situations that will abnormally put stress on their spines.

NURSING DIAGNOSES

- Acute pain
- Risk for infection
- Situational low self-esteem

EXPECTED OUTCOMES
The patient will:
- express feelings of comfort
- be free from signs and symptoms of infection
- verbalize positive feelings about self.

PRETREATMENT CARE

- Make sure the patient has undergone tests to determine the nature and exact location of his condition; these may include X-rays, magnetic resonance imaging (MRI), computed tomography (CT) scanning, and myelograms.
- Make sure the patient has had preoperative laboratory blood and urine tests and, possibly, an electrocardiogram.
- Explain the treatment and preparation to the patient and his family.
- Verify that the patient or a responsible family member has signed an appropriate consent form.
- Explain postoperative care and equipment.
- Monitor the patient's vital signs, intake and output, nutritional status, and laboratory test results.

POSTTREATMENT CARE

- ◆ Monitor neurologic status and vital signs.
- ◆ Change the patient's position often while on bed rest.
- ◆ Have a physical therapist assist the patient in learning self-care and in performing strengthening and range-of-motion exercises.

◆ **AGE FACTOR** *The length of the hospital stay depends on the age and health of the patient as well as the specific problem that was corrected. Tell the patient that he can expect to remain under a practitioner's care for many months.*

- ◆ Provide care of the surgical wound, and assess for infection.
- ◆ Encourage regular coughing and deep-breathing exercises and use of incentive spirometry.
- ◆ Monitor the patient's daily weight and intake and output.
- ◆ Monitor drainage from wound.
- ◆ Administer medications as ordered.
- ◆ Provide comfort measures.
- ◆ Monitor the patient's vital signs and intake and output.

◆ **WARNING** *Watch for hypotension, bradycardia, and changes in respiration; these may signal hemorrhage and shock.*

- ◆ Assess for complications and monitor laboratory test results.
- ◆ Monitor for abnormal bleeding.
- ◆ Encourage the patient to verbalize his feelings regarding the surgery.

PATIENT TEACHING

GENERAL

- ◆ Review medications and possible adverse reactions with the patient.
- ◆ Inform the patient about possible complications.
- ◆ Encourage the patient to perform frequent deep-breathing and coughing exercises.
- ◆ Teach the patient's family or caregiver how to care for the surgical wound.
- ◆ Review signs and symptoms of infection and when to notify the practitioner.
- ◆ Tell the patient that the repaired spine should be kept in proper position to maintain alignment.
- ◆ Teach the patient how to move properly and how to reposition, sit, stand, and walk. Teach the patient to use the logrolling technique to turn in bed.
- ◆ Inform the patient that movement will be limited for some time; review activity restrictions.
- ◆ Tell the patient that he may need to wear a brace after the cast is removed.

RESOURCES
Organizations
American Academy of Neurology: *www.aan.com*
American Medical Association: *www.ama-assn.org*
American Trauma Society: *www.amtrauma.org*

Selected references
Dickerman, R.D., et al. "Spinal Cord Injury in a 14-Year-Old Male Secondary to Cervical Hyperflexion with Exercise," *Spinal Cord* August 30, 2005. [Epub ahead of print]

Foster, M.R. "A Functional Classification of Spinal Instrumentation," *Spine Journal* 5(6):682-94, November-December 2005.

Shehu, B.B., and Ismail, N.J. "Successful Conservative Management of Traumatic Cervical Spine Fracture-Dislocation," *British Journal of Neurosurgery* 19(1):79, February 2005.

Shem, K.L. "Late Complications of Displaced Thoracolumbar Fusion Instrumentation Presenting as New Pain in Individuals with Spinal Cord Injury," *Journal of Spinal Cord Medicine* 28(4):326-29, April 2005.

Spinal surgery: vertebroplasty

- Minimally invasive procedure that picks up the pieces of a fracture and supports the vertebral body by cementing it back into a solid unit
- Cementlike material injected into the fractured bone to stabilize the fracture, providing immediate pain relief

INDICATIONS

- Compression fracture
- Vertebral dislocation
- Vertebrae seriously weakened by trauma or disease (osteoporosis)

AGE FACTOR *People with osteoporosis—especially aging women—are at an increased risk for fracture. Compression fracture of one or more spinal vertebrae is possible.*

- The patient receives a local anesthetic and is placed in a prone position.
- A small incision is made in the back through which the surgeon threads a narrow tube.
- Using fluoroscopy to guide it to the correct position, the tube creates a path through the back into the fractured vertebrae.
- The cavity is filled with a cementlike material that hardens quickly, stabilizing the bone.
- The incision is closed and a dressing is applied.

COMPLICATIONS

- Infection
- Bleeding
- Increased back pain
- Nerve or muscle damage

- Activity intolerance
- Acute pain
- Disturbed sensory perception (all)

EXPECTED OUTCOMES
The patient will:
- demonstrate improved mobility
- verbalize feelings of comfort
- exhibit improved neurologic status.

- Explain the treatment and preparation to the patient and his family.
- Verify that the patient has signed an appropriate consent form.
- Discuss postoperative recovery and rehabilitation. Reassure the patient that analgesics and muscle relaxants will be available during recovery.
- Just before surgery, perform a baseline assessment of motor function and sensation. Carefully document the results for comparison with postoperative findings.

POSTTREATMENT CARE

◆ Administer medications as ordered.
◆ Monitor the patient's vital signs and intake and output.
◆ Assess the surgical wound and dressings; monitor for drainage.
◆ Assess for abnormal bleeding.
◆ Monitor for cerebrospinal fluid leakage.
◆ Assess motor and neurologic function; compare the results with baseline findings.
◆ Give analgesics and muscle relaxants, as ordered.

PATIENT TEACHING

GENERAL

◆ Review the medications and possible adverse reactions with the patient.
◆ Show the patient how to care for the incision site.
◆ Teach the patient the signs and symptoms of infection.
◆ Tell the patient of possible complications and about when to notify the practitioner.
◆ Instruct the patient to shower with his incision facing away from the stream of water.
◆ Review activity restrictions with the patient.
◆ Instruct the patient to perform prescribed exercises.
◆ Tell the patient about proper body mechanics.
◆ Stress the need for follow-up care.

RESOURCES
Organizations

American Academy of Neurology: *www.aan.com*
American Academy of Orthopaedic Surgeons: *www.aaos.org*
American College of Surgeons: *www.facs.org*
American Medical Association: *www.ama-assn.org*

Selected references

Bajnoczy, S. "Artificial Disc Replacement—Evolutionary Treatment for Degenerative Disc Disease," *AORN Journal* 82(2):192, 195-202, 205-206, quiz 207-12, August 2005.

Deyo, R.A., and Mirza, S.K. "Trends and Variations in the Use of Spine Surgery," *Clinical Orthopaedics and Related Research* 443:139-46, February 2006.

Fowler, S.B., et al. "Health-Related Quality of Life in Patients Undergoing Anterior Cervical Discectomy Fusion," *Journal of Neuroscience Nursing* 37(2):97-100, April 2005.

Lemke, D.M. "Vertebroplasty and Kyphoplasty for Treatment of Painful Osteoporotic Compression Fractures," *Journal of American Academy of Nurse Practitioners* 17(7):268-76, July 2005.

Rodts, M.F. "Total Disc Replacement Arthroplasty," *Orthopaedic Nursing* 23(3):216-19, May-June 2004.

Strayer, A. "Lumbar Spine: Common Pathology and Interventions," *Journal of Neuroscience Nursing* 37(4):181-93, August 2005.

Splenectomy

OVERVIEW

- Surgical removal of part or entire spleen
- Procedure performed based on severity of condition suggesting spleen removal; may be performed by open surgery or laparascopically
- Long-term treatment with antibiotics possibly prescribed following surgery

INDICATIONS

- Traumatic splenic rupture
- Hypersplenism
- Hereditary spherocytosis
- Chronic idiopathic thrombocytopenic purpura
- Hodgkin's disease
- Cancer of spleen
- Splenic abscess
- Hereditary elliptocytosis
- Splenic artery rupture
- Hemolytic disorders
- Myelofibrosis

PROCEDURE

- The patient is placed under general anesthesia.
- The peritoneal cavity is exposed through a left rectus paramedial or subcostal incision.
- The splenic artery, vein, and ligaments are ligated.
- The spleen is removed.
- After carefully checking for bleeding, the abdomen is closed.
- A drain may be placed in the left subdiaphragmatic space.
- The incision site is sutured and dressed.

LAPAROSCOPIC

- For laparoscopic removal, a small incision is made, and the abdominal cavity is injected with carbon dioxide.
- The spleen is detached and removed in pieces. A drain is then placed.
- All incisions are sutured closed and dressings applied.

COMPLICATIONS

- Pancreatic inflammation
- Bleeding
- Infection

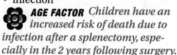 **AGE FACTOR** *Children have an increased risk of death due to infection after a splenectomy, especially in the 2 years following surgery.*

NURSING DIAGNOSES

- Acute pain
- Deficient fluid volume
- Risk for infection

EXPECTED OUTCOMES

The patient will:

- verbalize feelings of comfort
- maintain adequate fluid volume
- remain free from signs and symptoms of infection.

PRETREATMENT CARE

- Explain the treatment and preparation to the patient and his family.
- Verify that the patient has signed an appropriate consent form.
- Report abnormal results of blood studies.
- Administer blood products, vitamin K, or fresh frozen plasma as ordered.
- Obtain vital signs, and perform a baseline respiratory assessment.
- Notify the practitioner if you suspect respiratory infection; surgery may be delayed.
- Explain postoperative care.
- Administer antibiotics before the procedure as ordered.

POSTTREATMENT CARE

- Administer medications and I.V. fluids as ordered.
- Assist with early ambulation.
- Encourage coughing, deep breathing, and incentive spirometer use.
- Administer analgesics as needed and ordered.
- Provide comfort measures.
- Provide incision site care as ordered.
- Change dressings as ordered.
- Maintain patency of drains.
- Monitor the patient's vital signs and intake and output.
- Assess for complications, such as abnormal bleeding and infection.
- Assess the surgical wound and dressings.
- Monitor drainage.
- Monitor hematologic studies.
- Administer vaccinations as ordered

PATIENT TEACHING

GENERAL

- Review the medications and possible adverse reactions with the patient.
- Tell the patient to continue to perform coughing and deep-breathing exercises.
- Teach the patient the signs and symptoms of infection.
- Tell the patient of possible complications and when to notify the practitioner.
- Tell the patient how to prevent infection.
- Explain about long-term antibiotic therapy if indicated. Stress the importance of following prescribed therapy.
- Teach the patient how to care for the incision site.
- Stress the need for follow-up care.

RESOURCES

Organizations

American Academy of Pediatrics:
www.aap.org
American Medical Association:
www.ama-assn.org
American Trauma Society:
www.amtrauma.org

Selected references

Eckert, K.L. "Penetrating and Blunt Abdominal Trauma," *Critical Care Nursing Quarterly* 28(1):41-59, January-March 2005.

Hornor, G. "Physical Abuse: Recognition and Reporting," *Journal of Pediatric Health Care* 19(1):4-11, January-February 2005.

Landau, A., et al. "Liver Injuries in Children: The Role of Selective Non-Operative Management," *Injury* 37(1):66-71, January 2006.

Shen, H.B., et al. "Clinical Application of Laparoscopic Spleen-Preserving Operation in Traumatic Spleen Rupture," *Chinese Journal of Traumatology* 8(5):293-96, October 2005.

Stapedectomy

- Microsurgical procedure (through the ear canal) to remove the stapes, incus, and malleus; after removal, a prosthesis is inserted into the ear
- Procedure performed to prevent progressive hearing loss

INDICATIONS
- Otosclerosis

AGE FACTOR *Otosclerosis (ear bone degeneration) most commonly develops during the adolescent or early adult years.*

- The patient is given either general or local anesthesia.
- The surgeon makes an incision in the ear canal near the tympanic membrane and it's raised so that a microscope can be used to view the structures.
- The bones of the middle ear are evaluated. The surgeon tests and separates the stapes from the incus, allowing the incus and malleus to move. Next, he uses a laser or other microinstrument to vaporize the tendon and the arch of the stapes, and remove the stapes. The window joining the middle ear to the inner ear, which serves as a platform for the stapes bone, is opened.
- The laser, on a very low power setting, is then directed at the window and a small opening is made. The surgeon places the prosthesis (made of platinum or stainless steel) onto the incus bone and attaches it. He uses a piece of fat or other tissue from a small incision behind the ear lobe and uses it to help seal the hole in the window and the space around the prosthesis.
- The surgeon folds back the ear drum into its normal position and holds it down with a small gelatin sponge.

COMPLICATIONS
- Perforation of the tympanic membrane
- Injury to facial nerves
- Cochlear deafness
- Infection
- Vertigo
- Tinnitus
- Changes in taste
- Dry mouth

- Acute pain
- Anxiety
- Disturbed sensory perception (auditory)

EXPECTED OUTCOMES
The patient will:
- express feelings of comfort
- express feelings and concerns
- regain or maintain hearing function.

- Review the procedure with the patient and his family and answer any questions.
- Verify that an appropriate consent form has been signed.
- Make sure that preoperative blood work and testing has been done and the results are available.
- If the patient has a perforated tympanic membrane due to a middle ear infection, it must be cleared and the membrane healed before stapedectomy.
- Assess the patient for signs of upper airway infection or sore throat. If present, the surgery should be postponed.

- Monitor the patient's vital signs.
- Assess response to treatment, and monitor hearing acuity as indicated.
- Monitor dressings.
- Give medications as ordered.
- Administer pain medication as ordered.
- Encourage the patient's family to express concerns related to the condition.
- Provide comfort measures as indicated.

GENERAL

- Teach the patient how to care for the ear after surgery.
- Tell the patient to immediately report severe dizziness or vertigo to the practitioner because it may indicate a break in the seal between fluids of the middle and inner ear.
- Review activity restrictions. For 2 to 3 days after the procedure, the patient should avoid blowing his nose, swimming underwater, lifting heavy objects, and flying on a plane.
- Tell the patient to avoid loud noise because the ear will be extra sensitive after the procedure.
- Stress the need to keep the affected ear dry until it's healed. The patient should wear an earplug while showering and dry the entire ear when done.
- Stress the need for follow-up care.

RESOURCES

Organizations

American Academy of Otolaryngology—
  Head and Neck Surgery:
  www.entnet.org
American Academy of Pediatrics:
  www.aap.org
Ear Surgery Information Center:
  www.earsurgery.org

Selected references

Huettenbrink, K.B., and Beutner, D. "A New Crimping Device for Stapedectomy Prostheses," *Laryngoscope* 115(11):2065-2067, November 2005.
Kujala, J., et al. "Video-Oculography Findings in Patients with Otosclerosis," *Otology and Neurotology* 26(6):1134-137, November 2005.
Yung, M.W., et al. "The Learning Curve in Stapes Surgery and its Implication to Training," *Laryngoscope* 116(1):67-71, January 2006.

Stent placement

OVERVIEW

- Procedure in which a small, flexible tube made of medical grade plastic or wire mesh is implanted in a vessel or duct to treat several medical conditions
- Can open blocked or narrowed blood vessels caused by peripheral arterial disease or other conditions; hospitalization and general anesthesia usually aren't required
- Generally less traumatic than surgical implantation because it involves smaller incisions, less pain, and shorter hospital stays
- Newer stents coated with medications to prevent restenosis; more effective (than standard stents) in preventing the artery from closing again

INDICATIONS

- Peripheral vascular disease or peripheral artery disease
- Renal procedures
- Hemodialysis access maintenance
- Carotid stenosis
- Coronary artery disease
- Abdominal aortic aneurysm
- Esophageal stricture
- Biliary disease
- Coronary artery blockage

PROCEDURE

- The patient receives anesthesia appropriate to the stent being placed. Local anesthesia is generally used with some analgesia; general anesthesia may be indicated in other conditions, especially if the procedure is anticipated to be painful.
- The procedure is done in a specially equipped suite with emergency equipment and staffing. The patient's electrocardiogram and oxygenation are monitored during the procedure.
- Two of the more common stenting procedures are the cardiac stent and liver stent.
- Interventional radiologist makes a pencil-tip–size incision in the skin. The stent, which is placed on the end of a catheter, is threaded under X-ray guidance to the area of treatment.

CARDIAC STENT

- Angioplasty is performed by a cardiologist who inserts a very small balloon attached to a catheter into a blood vessel through a small incision in the skin. The catheter is threaded under X-ray guidance to the site of the blocked artery. The balloon is inflated to open the artery. Sometimes, a small stent is inserted; it expands to hold the artery open and is usually placed at the narrowed section.

LIVER STENT

- A transjugular intrahepatic portosystemic shunt is inserted to treat portal hypertension.
- The interventional radiologist threads a catheter through a small incision in the skin near the neck and guides it to the blocked blood vessels in the liver. Under X-ray guidance, a tunnel is created in the liver through which the blocked blood can flow. The tunnel is held open by the insertion of a small metal stent. (See *Viewing a liver stent.*)

COMPLICATIONS

- Bleeding or bruising at the catheter-insertion site
- Restenosis of the artery
- Infection
- Stent migration
- Shunt failure or closure
- Death

NURSING DIAGNOSES

- Activity intolerance
- Ineffective tissue perfusion: Cardiopulmonary
- Risk for fluid imbalance

EXPECTED OUTCOMES

The patient will:

- carry out activities of daily living without excess fatigue or decreased energy
- maintain adequate cardiac perfusion
- maintain adequate blood volume as evidenced by stable vital signs and absence of bleeding.

PRETREATMENT CARE

- Ensure that preliminary evaluation is done as ordered, depending on the type of stent to be placed.
- Ensure that diagnostic testing has been completed, including computer tomography, magnetic resonance imaging, ultrasound, X-rays, or tests to check the patency of the vessels as ordered.
- Review the procedure with the patient and answer any questions.
- Verify that an appropriate consent form has been signed.
- Review with the patient what to expect postoperatively.
- Perform a baseline assessment and verify pulse quality.
- Make sure the patient doesn't take anything by mouth after midnight before the procedure.
- Note if the patient has allergies or is taking any medications.

POSTTREATMENT CARE

- Monitor the patient's vital signs and peripheral pulses.
- Monitor intake and output.
- Assess respiratory function and monitor pulse oximetry.
- Monitor the patient's electrocardiogram.
- Maintain patency of I.V.s and provide hydration as ordered.
- Administer medications as ordered.
- Assess dressings and distal pulses; if a compression device is applied to the catheter site, assess the site for bleeding and provide care.
- Encourage the patient to breathe deeply and to cough as indicated; assist with incentive spirometry.
- Assist with ambulation as ordered.
- Monitor for signs of complications.

⚡ **WARNING** *Report signs of hypovolemic shock, renal failure, sepsis, or respiratory failure immediately.*

PATIENT TEACHING

GENERAL

- Tell the patient if there are restrictions regarding exercise and driving.
- Teach the patient how to recognize signs of complications and what to report to the practitioner.
- Review the medications, dosage, and adverse effects with the patient.
- If the patient is prescribed a blood thinner, instruct him about the signs of bleeding and how to minimize it.
- Teach the patient how to use an incentive spirometer.
- Inform the patient that regardless of which artery is blocked, angioplasty doesn't reverse or cure arteriosclerosis. Stress the importance of following a healthy, low-fat diet, getting adequate exercise, and not smoking. Tell the patient with diabetes, hypertension, or high cholesterol to follow the treatment plan prescribed by his practitioner.
- Advise the patient to avoid lifting heavy objects, performing strenuous exercise, and smoking for at least 24 hours.
- Instruct the patient to notify the practitioner if pain, a warm feeling in the area where the catheter was inserted, or a change in the color of the leg occurs.

RESOURCES
Organizations
American College of Cardiology: *www.acc.org*
American College of Surgeons: *www.facs.org*
American Heart Association: *www.americanheart.org*
American Medical Association: *www.ama-assn.org*

Selected references
Benson, L.M., et al. "Determining Best Practice: Comparison of Three Methods of Femoral Sheath Removal after Cardiac Interventional Procedures," *Heart & Lung* 34(2):115-21, March-April 2005.
Cepero, K. "The Latest in Cardiac Care," *Nursing Management* 36:14-16, May 2005.
Oliver, B., et al. "How Drug-Eluting Stents Keep Coronary Blood Flowing," *Nursing* 35(2):36-41; quiz 41-42, February 2005.

Viewing a liver stent

Stents are placed for various conditions. Below is an illustration of a liver stent.

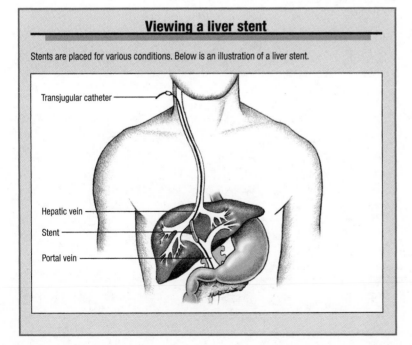

Transjugular catheter

Hepatic vein

Stent

Portal vein

Stereotactic radiosurgery

- Stereotactic radiosurgery (SRS): non-invasive delivery of single high dose of radiation (1-day session) to an area of the brain to treat abnormalities, tumors, or other functional disorders
- May be the primary treatment; used with inaccessible tumors or as an adjunct to other treatments with recurring or malignant tumor
- Forms of SRS:
  – particle beam (proton) and cobalt60 based (gamma knife)—used for small tumors
  – linear accelerator based—used for larger tumors (greater than 3.5 cm)
- Fractionated stereotactic radiotherapy: radiation administered over several days or weeks by the same procedure; larger total radiation dose
- Three-dimensional computer-aided planning and high degree of immobilization allowing for minimal amount of radiation to healthy brain tissue

INDICATIONS

- Brain tumors (benign and malignant)
- Trigeminal neuralgia
- Essential tremor
- Parkinson's tremor or rigidity
- Arteriovenous malformations

- Before performing SRS, the patient is fitted with a stereotactic frame that allows for precise delivery of radiation to the required area. For fractionated radiotherapy, the frame is attached to a rigid plastic mask that contours to the patient's skeletal frame and is reused. The frame for single use is bolted to the patient's head with metal bolts.
- The patient doesn't require anesthesia, although local anesthesia may be used to attach the frame to the patients head.
- Radiation is then aimed at the tumor from various directions. The amount of radiation required directly correlates to the exact size and location of the tumor, as determined by magnetic resonance imaging and computed-tomography scanning.
- The frame is detached when the procedure is complete.

COMPLICATIONS

- Headache
- Recurrence of tumor
- Nausea and vomiting
- Fatigue

- Anxiety
- Disturbed body image
- Fear

EXPECTED OUTCOMES

The patient will:
- exhibit maintain a calm demeanor during the procedure
- exhibit acceptance of treatment and follow-up care
- express a reduction in fear when the procedure is complete.

PRETREATMENT CARE

- Explain the treatment and preparation to the patient and his family.
- Verify that the patient has signed an appropriate consent form.
- Answer questions about pretreatment studies or these procedures and remind the patient that the frame will be applied for the procedure, but removed when the procedure is complete.
- Obtain baseline vital signs.
- Provide reassurance.

POSTTREATMENT CARE

- Administer medications as ordered.
- Provide comfort measures and supportive care.
- Monitor the patient's vital signs.

PATIENT TEACHING

GENERAL

- Teach the patient how to manage adverse effects at home.
- Discuss possible complications with the patient and when to notify the practitioner.
- Stress the importance of follow-up care.
- Refer the patient to support groups such as the American Cancer Society.

RESOURCES

Organizations

American Academy of Neurology:
www.aan.com
American Cancer Society:
www.cancer.org

Selected references

Lau, L.I., et al. "Paradoxical Worsening with Superior Ophthalmic Vein Thrombosis after Gamma Knife Radiosurgery for Dural Arteriovenous Fistula of Cavernous Sinus: A Case Report Suggesting the Mechanism of the Phenomenon," *Eye,* February 17, 2006. [Online]

Oskouian, R.J., et al. "The Craniopharyngioma," *Frontiers of Hormone Research,* 34:105-26, 2006.

Sheehan, J.P., et al. "Stereotactic Radiosurgery for Pituitary Adenomas: A Review of the Literature and Experience," *Frontiers of Hormone Research,* 34:185-205, 2006.

Sympathectomy

- Surgical procedure that cauterizes a portion of the sympathetic nerve chain, which is located parallel to the spinal cord
- Aims to increase blood flow to narrowed vessels; may be performed to decrease excessive sweating or blushing
- Performed using a fiber-optic camera and small surgical instruments

INDICATIONS
- Reflex sympathetic dystrophy
- Raynaud's phenomenon
- Hyperhidrosis
- Excessive facial blushing

- The procedure may be done in an outpatient setting under general anesthesia.
- After a small incision is made behind the pectoralis fold in the armpit, carbon dioxide is injected into the thoracic cavity and the lung is deflated.
- Using an endoscopic instrument, the surgeon locates and cuts or coagulates the appropriate ganglia.
- In facial hyperhidrosis and facial blushing, it's sufficient to sharply divide the sympathetic fibers.
- In the treatment of palmar hyperhidrosis, which requires thermocoagulation of the second ganglion, care should be taken not to cause spreading of thermal energy along the nervous trunk.
- Eventually, the carbon dioxide is reaspirated and the incision closed.
- The procedure is repeated on the other side.

COMPLICATIONS
- Horner's syndrome
- Treatment failure
- Pneumothorax
- Compensatory sweating (sweating in areas other than original location)
- Gustatory sweating (sweating after eating certain foods)

- Activity intolerance
- Acute pain
- Disturbed body image

EXPECTED OUTCOMES
The patient will:
- exhibit improved tolerance of activity
- remain free from pain
- develop a positive self-image.

PRETREATMENT CARE

- Explain the procedure to the patient and answer any questions.
- Verify that an appropriate consent form has been signed.
- Note allergies and patient history.
- Perform a neurologic assessment and assess vital signs.
- Pretesting with a nerve block to the affected area should be performed before the procedure to determine if treatment will be effective.
- Instruct the patient not to eat or drink after midnight before the procedure.
- Tell the patient that he'll probably be able to return to normal activities after 2 to 3 days.
- Tell the patient that there may be some pain after the procedure, but medication will be available to relieve discomfort.

POSTTREATMENT CARE

- Administer medication as ordered.
- Assess the patient's vital signs and neurologic status.
- Assess for effects of surgery.
- Monitor for complications.

PATIENT TEACHING

GENERAL

- Tell the patient that compensatory sweating may appear and that it tends to decrease within the first 6 to 12 months; however, it's almost irreversible if it persists for longer than 1 year.
- Teach the patient how to recognize signs of complications and what to report to the practitioner.
- Review activity restrictions.
- Encourage follow-up care.

RESOURCES
Organizations
American Academy of Neurology: *www.aan.com*
American Medical Association: *www.ama-assn.org*
American Sympathectomy Institute: *www.umm.edu/sympathectomy*

Selected references
Cavazza, S., et al. "Iatrogenic Horner's Syndrome," *European Journal of Ophthalmology* 15(4):504-506, July-August 2005.

"Horner Syndrome," *Mayo Clinic Womens Healthsource* 9(10):6, October 2005.

Moya, J., et al. "Thoracic Sympathicolysis for Primary Hyperhidrosis: A Review of 918 Procedures," *Surgical Endoscopy* 20(4):598-602, April 2006.

Ozel, S.K., and Kazez, A. "Horner Syndrome Due to First Rib Fracture after Major Thoracic Trauma," *Journal of Pediatric Surgery* 40(10):e17-19, October 2005.

Pather, N., et al. "Cervico-Thoracic Ganglion: Its Clinical Implications," *Clinical Anatomy* 19(4):232-26, May 2006.

Temporal lobe resection

OVERVIEW

- Surgery on the portion of the temporal lobe of the brain where seizure activity initiates
- Appropriate only for patients with seizures originating in the anterior or middle portions of the temporal lobe
- Generally a unilateral procedure
- Damage from brain diseases, frequent seizures, or surgery to the temporal lobes possibly affecting hearing, language, and memory as well as movement and sensation

  AGE FACTOR *The temporal lobes are the most common source of seizures in teenagers and those in early adulthood.*

- Recommended only for patients with disabling seizures uncontrolled by medication, or those who can't take anticonvulsants due to severe adverse reactions

INDICATIONS

- Localized disease in the temporal lobe with or without seizures, such as gliomas or hippocampal sclerosis
- Epilepsy with an identified temporal focus

PROCEDURE

- The patient may receive either local anesthesia with some mild preoperative sedation (required when the patient must be able to communicate and follow commands so the focal area can be more accurately mapped before resection) or general anesthesia.
- The anesthetist obtains peripheral I.V. access, and may also insert a central venous pressure line and an arterial line.
- The head is shaved and the patient is positioned according to the surgeon's direction.
- The surgeon makes incisions in the scalp to create a flap of skin, then cuts out a section of the underlying bone.
- The dural covering is then retracted. A small microscope is used to magnify the tissues as the surgeon enters and resects the affected area of the lobe.
- After the affected tissues are removed, the dura is replaced and the bone piece is fitted back into place. The scalp tissues are closed using sutures or staples.

COMPLICATIONS

- Infection
- Vasospasm
- Hemorrhage
- Air embolism
- Respiratory compromise
- Increased intracranial pressure (ICP)
- Diabetes insipidus
- Syndrome of inappropriate antidiuretic hormone
- Failure to relieve seizures
- Neurologic damage

NURSING DIAGNOSES

- Disturbed sensory perception (all)
- Ineffective breathing pattern
- Risk for infection

EXPECTED OUTCOMES

The patient will:

- exhibit improved or normal neurologic status
- maintain adequate ventilation
- exhibit no signs of infection.

PRETREATMENT CARE

- Check that presurgery testing has been completed, including seizure monitoring, electroencephalography, magnetic resonance imaging or positron emission tomography, and single photon emission computed tomography.
- Review the basic procedure and preoperative and postoperative nursing care with the patient.
- Verify that an appropriate consent form has been signed.
- Tell the patient that a portion of his head will be shaved in the operating room.
- Explain the intensive care unit and equipment the patient will see postoperatively.
- Perform a complete neurologic and cardiopulmonary assessment and obtain baseline vital signs.

POSTTREATMENT CARE

- Position the patient on his side with the head of the bed elevated 15 to 30 degrees; assist the patient in turning every 2 hours.
- Encourage careful deep breathing and coughing; suction gently as needed.
- Ensure a quiet, calm environment.
- Monitor vital signs, neurologic vital signs, intake and output, respiratory status, heart rate and rhythm, and hemodynamic and ICP measurements if monitored.
- Assess fluid and electrolyte balance, urine specific gravity, and daily weight.
- Monitor drain patency if present, the surgical wound and dressings, and drainage.
- Maintain a patent airway.
- Administer prescribed oxygen if required.
- Administer medications as ordered, including anticonvulsants and analgesics.
- Provide support to family members.
- Monitor the patient for complications.

⚡ **WARNING** *Notify the practitioner immediately if there's a deterioration in level of consciousness, pupillary changes, or increasing weakness in an arm or leg that might indicate increased ICP.*

PATIENT TEACHING

GENERAL

- Review medications and possible adverse reactions with the patient.
- Teach the patient and his family how take care of the surgical wound.
- Tell the patient that headache, nausea, scalp numbness around the incision, fatigue, continued auras, and difficulty with word finding or speech may occur postoperatively but generally improve spontaneously.
- Review postoperative leg and deep-breathing exercises with the patient.
- Instruct the patient to use antiembolism stockings until full activity is resumed, to prevent deep vein thrombosis.
- Review the signs and symptoms of infection, other complications, and when to notify the practitioner.
- Suggest the use of a wig, hat, or scarf until the patient's hair grows back as appropriate.
- Advise the patient to avoid alcohol and smoking.
- Tell the patient that resumption of usual activities generally occurs 6 to 8 weeks after surgery, but must be approved by the surgeon.
- Inform the patient that he'll likely need to continue taking antiseizure medication for about 2 years, and that, once the degree of seizure control is known, these may be reduced or eliminated.
- Stress the importance of follow-up care with the surgeon and treating neurologist.

RESOURCES

Organizations

American Academy of Neurology: *www.aan.com*
American Medical Association: *www.ama-assn.org*
Epilepsy Therapy Development Project: *www.epilepsy.com*

Selected references

Dunn, D. "Preventing Perioperative Complications in Special Populations," *Nursing* 35(11):36-43, November 2005.
Gallo, BV. "Epilepsy, Surgery, and the Elderly," *Epilepsy Research* 68(Suppl 1):83-86, January 2006.
Khoury, J.S., et al. "Predicting Seizure Frequency After Epilepsy Surgery," *Epilepsy Research* 67(3):89-99, December 2005.

Thalamotomy

OVERVIEW

- Precise destruction of a portion of the thalamus that controls tremors
- Usually performed to reduce tremors associated with Parkinson's disease but having no impact on other movement dysfunctions characteristic of the disease
- Rarely performed now due to risk and development of deep brain stimulation techniques that are safer and don't destroy tissue
- **AGE FACTOR** *Thalamotomy is usually performed on patients younger than age 65 with normal intellectual function and recent memory. It provides more sustained relief when performed relatively early in the disease process.*
- Most effective for tremors of the arms rather than legs
- Because the thalamus acts on the opposite side of the body from its position in the brain, surgery required to the left thalamus in those with more severe right-sided tremors

INDICATIONS

- Severe tremors unresponsive to other therapies, which cause difficulty in functional activities

PROCEDURE

- The anesthetist obtains peripheral I.V. access.
- The area of the scalp to be opened is shaved, and the patient positioned comfortably but with the head immobilized.
- The neurosurgeon injects a local anesthetic into the scalp at the incision site.
- The surgeon makes an incision in the scalp to expose the bone, then drills a small hole in the skull and retracts the dura.
- Information is gathered during presurgical three-dimensional brain imaging and coordinate mapping (stereotaxic imaging) is used to locate the thalamus. A thin stereotaxic probe is inserted to the designated coordinates. The surgeon then gently touches various locations and works with the patient to determine the specific area that requires destruction in order to stop the tremor.
- When the correct area is identified, the surgeon inserts a hollow probe through which extremely cold liquid nitrogen is circulated into the targeted brain tissue. This procedure ablates the cells of the area.
- The probe is removed, the dura and bone piece is replaced, and the scalp is closed with sutures or staples.

COMPLICATIONS

- Infection
- Weakness, loss of sensation, or paralysis
- Hemorrhagic stroke
- Numbness around the mouth (leading to drooling) and in the hands
- Visual loss

NURSING DIAGNOSES

- Impaired physical mobility
- Risk for deficient fluid volume
- Risk for infection

EXPECTED OUTCOMES

The patient will:

- exhibit improved ability to perform self-care activities
- maintain adequate intravascular fluid volume without signs or symptoms of abnormal bleeding
- exhibit no signs or symptoms of infection.

PRETREATMENT CARE

- Check that preoperative testing has been completed, including stereotaxic X-rays.
- Review the basic procedure and nursing care to expect before and after it.
- Verify that an appropriate consent form has been signed.
- Tell the patient that a portion of his head will be shaved in the operating room.
- Perform a complete neurologic and cardiopulmonary assessment and obtain baseline vital signs and a description of usual visual acuity level.

POSTTREATMENT CARE

- Position the patient on his side with the head of the bed elevated 15 to 30 degrees; assist the patient to turn carefully every 2 hours.
- Encourage careful deep breathing and coughing.
- Ensure a quiet, calm environment.
- Monitor vital signs, neurologic vital signs, visual complaints, intake and output, respiratory status, heart rate and rhythm, and hemodynamic and intracranial pressure (ICP) measurements (if monitored).
- Assess fluid and electrolyte balance, urine specific gravity, and daily weight.
- Monitor drain patency, surgical wound and dressings, and drainage.
- Monitor the patient for complications.

WARNING Notify the practitioner immediately if there's a deterioration of level of consciousness, pupillary changes, or increasing weakness in an arm or leg that might indicate increased ICP.

PATIENT TEACHING

GENERAL

- Review medications and possible adverse reactions with the patient.
- Teach the patient how to care for the surgical wound, and to identify the signs and symptoms of infection.
- Tell the patient that headache and scalp numbness in the area of the incision usually remit spontaneously.
- Review the signs and symptoms of infection and other complications, and tell the patient to notify the practitioner promptly if new changes in vision, balance, or extremity strength are noted.
- Suggest the use of a wig, hat, or scarf until the patient's hair grows back as appropriate.
- Advise the patient to avoid alcohol and smoking.
- Inform the patient that although surgery can stop or decrease the tremors, it doesn't affect other motor symptoms of the disease or drug therapy.
- Tell the patient that his antiparkinsonian drugs will be continued and adjusted as needed.
- Stress the importance of follow-up care with the surgeon and neurologist.

RESOURCES
Organizations
American Academy of Neurology: *www.aan.com*
American Medical Association: *www.ama-assn.org*
National Parkinson Foundation: *www.parkinson.org*

Selected references
Duval, C., et al. "The Impact of Ventrolateral Thalamotomy on Tremor and Voluntary Motor Behavior in Patients with Parkinson's Disease," *Experimental Brain Research* 170(2):160-71, April 2006.
Katayama, Y., et al. "Difference in Surgical Strategies Between Thalamotomy and Thalamic Deep Brain Stimulation for Tremor Control," *Journal of Neurology* 252(Suppl 4):IV17-22, October 2005.

Thoracentesis

- Relieves pulmonary compression and respiratory distress by removing accumulated air or fluid from pleural space
- Resolves an excess of fluid (hemothorax or pleural effusion), air (pneumothorax), or both in the pleural space that changes intrapleural pressure and causes partial or complete lung collapse
- Allows instillation of chemotherapeutic agents or other drugs into pleural space
- May involve chest tube insertion to allow drainage of air or fluid from pleural space
- May also be used as a diagnostic tool to provide a specimen of pleural fluid or tissue for analysis for malignant cells or pathogens
- Also known as *pleural fluid aspiration*

INDICATIONS

- Excess pleural fluid or air due to trauma or other pulmonary disease
- Lung or pleural malignancy requiring local chemotherapy

⚡ **WARNING** *Thoracentesis is contraindicated in patients with uncorrected bleeding disorders or anticoagulant therapy.*

PROCEDURE

- Position the patient seated and leaning forward on a support, to widen the intercostal spaces and allow easier access to the pleural cavity. If the patient can't sit up, position him on the unaffected side with the arm on the affected side elevated.
- The practitioner will determine the insertion site. For tension pneumothorax, the midclavicular second to third intercostal space is the usual insertion site because air rises to the top of the intrapleural space. For hemothorax or pleural effusion, the eighth to ninth posterior intercostal spaces are commonly used because fluid settles to the lower levels of the intrapleural space. For removal of air and fluid, chest tubes are inserted into a high and a low site. (See *Performing needle thoracentesis.*)
- Prepare and drape the site.
- A local anesthetic is injected into the subcutaneous tissue and the thoracentesis needle is inserted.
- When the needle reaches the pocket of fluid, it's attached to a 50-ml syringe or a vacuum bottle and the fluid is removed.
- During aspiration, monitor the patient for signs of respiratory distress and hypotension.

⚡ **WARNING** *The procedure will be stopped if the patient has sudden chest tightness or begins coughing. Signs of acute pulmonary edema are rarely associated with lung reexpansion.*

- Note pleural fluid characteristics and total volume.
- After the needle is withdrawn, apply pressure until hemostasis is obtained then apply a small dressing.
- Alternatively, one or more chest tubes may be inserted and connected to a thoracic drainage system, the tubes are sutured in place and dressings are applied. Immediately after the drainage system is connected, instruct the patient to take a deep breath, hold it momentarily, and slowly exhale to assist drainage of the pleural space and lung reexpansion.
- Place fluid specimens obtained in proper containers, label appropriately, and send them to the laboratory immediately; pleural fluid for pH determination must be collected anaer-

---

Performing needle thoracentesis

For a patient with life-threatening tension pneumothorax, needle thoracentesis temporarily relieves pleural pressure until a practitioner can insert a chest tube.

HOW NEEDLE THORACENTESIS WORKS

A needle attached to a flutter valve is inserted into the affected pleural space. (If no flutter valve is available, one can be made from a perforated finger cot or glove attached with a rubber band.) When the patient exhales, trapped air escapes via the flutter valve instead of being retained under pressure. The flutter valve also prevents more air from entering the involved lung during inhalation.

HOW TO PERFORM THE PROCEDURE

You may need to assist the practitioner in performing the procedure. Here's how to proceed:
- Clean the skin around the second intercostal space at the midclavicular line with antiseptic solution. Use a circular motion, starting at the center and working outward.
- The practitioner inserts a sterile 16G (or larger) needle over the superior portion of the rib and through the tissue covering the pleural cavity. The vein, artery, and nerve lie behind the rib's inferior border.
- Listen for a hissing sound. This signals the needle's entry into the pleural cavity.
- If a flutter valve is used, it's secured to the needle. The arrow on the valve indicates the direction of airflow. A sterile glove is placed on the distal end of the valve to collect drainage.
- The needle is left in place until a chest tube can be inserted.

obically, heparinized, kept on ice, and analyzed promptly.

COMPLICATIONS

- Pneumothorax
- Infection
- Pain
- Cough
- Failure to access the pleural air or fluid site
- Subcutaneous hematoma or laceration of intercostals artery
- Reexpansion pulmonary edema (RPE)

NURSING DIAGNOSES

- Deficient fluid volume
- Impaired gas exchange
- Ineffective tissue perfusion: Cardiopulmonary

EXPECTED OUTCOMES

The patient will:
- maintain adequate fluid volume
- maintain patent airway and adequate oxygenation
- maintain hemodynamic stability.

PRETREATMENT CARE

- Verify that an appropriate consent form has been signed.
- Reinforce the practitioner's explanation of the procedure and describe the nursing care that will be provided. (See *Learning about thoracentesis*, pages 348 and 349.)
- Note and report allergies and record baseline vital signs.
- If the patient will receive sedation in addition to local anesthesia, restrict food and fluids.
- Explain that pleural fluid may be located by chest X-ray or ultrasound and that he'll receive a local anesthetic before the trocar is inserted.

- Instruct the patient to avoid coughing, deep breathing, or moving during the treatment.
- Explain chest tube drainage equipment and how to turn in bed safely with device to avoid kinking or obstructing the tubes.

POSTTREATMENT CARE

- Elevate the head of the bed to facilitate breathing.
- Obtain a chest X-ray as ordered.
- Tell the patient to immediately report difficulty breathing or chest pain.
- Immediately report signs and symptoms of pneumothorax, tension pneumothorax, and pleural fluid reaccumulation.
- Monitor the patient for RPE and other complications.
- Monitor vital signs, pulse oximetry, and breath sounds.
- Observe the puncture site for drainage, inflammation or signs of infection, and change the dressings as ordered.
- If chest tubes are inserted, securely tape the junction of the chest tube and the drainage tube to prevent their separation. Check the status of the drainage tubing. Make sure that the tubing remains at the level of the patient and that there are no dependent loops. Monitor and record the drainage in the drainage collection chamber.
- Remember that routine clamping of the chest tube isn't recommended because of the risk of tension pneumothorax.
- During patient transport, keep the thoracic drainage system below the patient's chest level.

WARNING *If the chest tube comes out, cover the site immediately with 4" × 4" gauze pads and tape them in place. Stay with the patient, and monitor his vital signs every 10 minutes. Observe him for signs and symptoms of tension pneumothorax (such as hypotension, distended jugular veins, absent breath sounds, tracheal shift, hypoxemia, weak and rapid pulse, dyspnea, tachypnea, diaphoresis, and chest pain). Have another staff member notify the practitioner, and gather equipment needed to reinsert the tube.*

- Place the rubber-tipped clamps at the bedside.
- If the drainage system cracks, or a tube disconnects, clamp the chest tube momentarily as close to the insertion site as possible. Because no air or liquid can escape from the pleural space while the tube is clamped, observe the patient closely for signs and symptoms of tension pneumothorax while the clamp is in place. Or, submerge the distal end of the tube in a container of normal saline solution to create a temporary water seal while the drainage system is being replaced. Follow facility policy.
- The tube may be clamped for several hours before removal. This allows time to observe the patient for signs and symptoms of respiratory distress, an indication that air or fluid remains trapped in the pleural space.
- A chest tube is usually removed within 7 days of insertion to prevent infection in the tube tract.

(continued)

PATIENT TEACHING

GENERAL

- Encourage the patient to perform coughing and deep-breathing exercises, and to use an incentive spirometer until usual lung function resumes.
- Teach the patient and his family how to use and read a finger pulse oximetry device at home if ordered by the practitioner, and which readings to report to the practitioner immediately.
- Review medication administration, dosages, and possible adverse effects with the patient.
- Refer the patient to appropriate resources and support services.

RESOURCES
Organizations

American Lung Association:
www.lungsusa.org
American Medical Association:
www.ama-assn.org
National Foundation for Trauma Care:
www.traumafoundation.org

Selected references

Bass, J., and White, D.A. "Thoracentesis in Patients with Hematologic Malignancy: Yield and Safety," *Chest* 127(6): 2101-105, June 2005.

Black, H., et al. "A 25-Year-Old Patient with Spontaneous Hemothorax," *Chest* 128(4):3080-83, October 2005.

Sharma, O.P., et al. "Prevalence of Delayed Hemothorax in Blunt Thoracic Trauma," *American Surgeon* 71(6):481-86, June 2005.

Yamamoto, L., et al. "Thoracic Trauma: The Deadly Dozen," *Critical Care Nursing Quarterly* 28(1):22-40, January-March 2005.

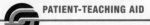

Learning about thoracentesis

Dear Patient:

Thoracentesis has been ordered to help you breathe more easily. In this procedure, a needle is used to remove extra fluid from the area around your lung, called *the pleural space*. A sample of this fluid will be sent to the laboratory, where it will be studied to find out what's causing your disorder.

The procedure is usually done in your hospital room, and it takes about 10 or 15 minutes.

GETTING READY

First, you'll put on a hospital gown that opens down the back so the correct location for the procedure can be easily reached.

Then your vital signs—temperature, pulse rate, respiratory rate, and blood pressure—will be checked.

Next, your back and chest will be examined and an area for inserting the needle will be chosen. Then that area will be shaved and cleaned.

Just before the procedure begins, you'll be asked to assume a special position (you'll be assisted, if necessary). If a fluid sample is to be taken from your back, you'll be asked to sit on the edge of the bed and lean forward on your overbed table. You'll rest your arms on a pillow and your feet on a stool (as shown here).

Alternatively, you may be asked to straddle a chair (as shown here).

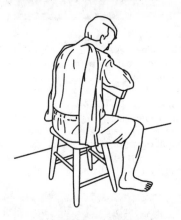

If a fluid sample is obtained from your chest instead, you'll sit up in bed with the head of your bed raised. This is called *semi-Fowler's position*.

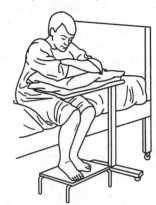

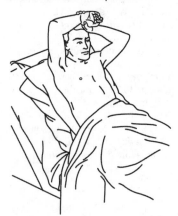

DURING THE PROCEDURE

Immediately before thoracentesis, your chest or back will be cleaned with a cold antiseptic solution. Then the area will be numbed with a local anesthetic injection. This may cause a slight stinging or burning sensation.

Then thoracentesis will begin with the insertion of a special needle between your ribs and into your chest cavity where the fluid lies.

You shouldn't feel much discomfort, but you may feel some pressure when the needle is inserted.

Don't move, and don't breathe deeply or cough when the needle is in place because this could damage your lung.

Be sure to report if you feel short of breath, dizzy, weak, or sweaty or if your heart is racing.

Now, the needle and a syringe will be used to withdraw excess pleural fluid. If you have a lot of fluid, a suction device may also be used. If your lung holds more than 2 L of fluid, you may need thoracentesis again later.

AFTER THE PROCEDURE

When the needle is removed, you may feel the urge to cough. (Go ahead. It's safe to do so.) Then pressure will be applied to the site and a snug bandage will be applied to the wound.

Immediately after thoracentesis, you'll have an X-ray to monitor your progress and check for complications. Your vital signs will be monitored frequently for the next few hours.

If a lot of fluid was removed, you may notice that you're breathing more easily.

WHAT TO WATCH FOR

Report if you feel faint. You may need oxygen. Be sure to report any other discomfort, such as difficult breathing, chest pain, or uncontrollable coughing—these can signal complications.

Thoracotomy

OVERVIEW

- Surgical incision into the thoracic cavity, usually performed to remove part or all of a lung and spare healthy lung tissue from disease
- May involve pneumonectomy, lobectomy, segmental resection, or wedge resection (see *Understanding types of lung excision*)
- Exploratory thoracotomy used diagnostically to examine the chest and pleural space for chest trauma and tumors
- Decortication removes fibrous membrane covering the visceral pleura; helps reexpand the lung in empyema
- Thoracoplasty involving removal of part or all of one rib to reduce size of chest cavity, decreasing the risk of mediastinal shift; may be done when tuberculosis has reduced lung volume

INDICATIONS

- Diseased lung tissue requiring removal

PROCEDURE

- The patient receives general anesthesia.
- In posterolateral thoracotomy, the incision begins in the submammary fold of the anterior chest, is drawn below the scapular tip and along the ribs, and then curves posteriorly and up to the scapular spine.
- In anterolateral thoracotomy, the incision begins below the breast and above the costal margins, extending from the anterior axillary line and then turning downward to avoid the axillary apex.
- In median sternotomy, a straight incision is made from the suprasternal notch to below the xiphoid process; the sternum must be transected with an electric or air-driven saw.
- After the incision is made, the surgeon may remove tissue for a biopsy.
- Bleeding sources are tied off.
- Injuries within the thoracic cavity are located and repaired.
- The ribs may be spread and the lung exposed for excision.

PNEUMONECTOMY

- The surgeon ligates and severs the pulmonary arteries.
- The mainstem bronchus leading to the affected lung is clamped.
- The bronchus is divided and closed with nonabsorbable sutures or staples.
- The lung is removed.
- To ensure airtight closure, a pleural flap is placed over the bronchus and closed.

- The phrenic nerve is severed on the affected side.
- After air pressure in the pleural cavity stabilizes, the chest is closed.

LOBECTOMY

- The surgeon resects the affected lobe.
- Appropriate arteries, veins, and bronchial passages are ligated and severed.
- One or two chest tubes are inserted for drainage and lung re-expansion.

Understanding types of lung excision

Lung excision may be total (pneumonectomy) or partial (lobectomy, segmental resection, or wedge resection), depending on your patient's condition. These illustrations show the extent of each surgery for the right lung.

PNEUMONECTOMY

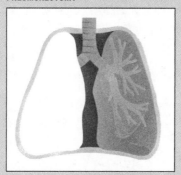

SEGMENTAL RESECTION

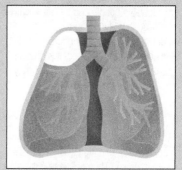

LOBECTOMY

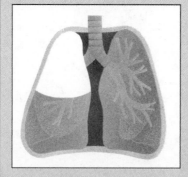

WEDGE RESECTION

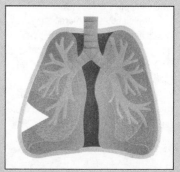

SEGMENTAL RESECTION

◆ The surgeon removes the affected lung segment.
◆ The appropriate artery, vein, and bronchus are ligated and severed.
◆ Two chest tubes are inserted to aid lung re-expansion.

WEDGE RESECTION

◆ The affected area is clamped, excised, and sutured.
◆ The surgeon inserts two chest tubes to aid lung re-expansion.
◆ After completing the procedure requiring the thoracotomy, the surgeon closes the chest cavity and applies a dressing.

COMPLICATIONS

◆ Hemorrhage
◆ Infection
◆ Tension pneumothorax
◆ Bronchopleural fistula
◆ Empyema
◆ Persistent air space that the remaining lung tissue doesn't expand to fill

NURSING DIAGNOSES

◆ Deficient fluid volume
◆ Impaired gas exchange
◆ Ineffective tissue perfusion: Cardiopulmonary

EXPECTED OUTCOMES

The patient will:
◆ maintain adequate fluid volume
◆ maintain patent airway and adequate oxygenation per pulse oximetry or arterial blood oxygen saturation testing
◆ maintain vital signs, blood pressure, capillary refill time, skin color, and peripheral pulses within normal limits.

PRETREATMENT CARE

◆ Explain the treatment and preparation to the patient and his family.
◆ Verify that the patient has signed an appropriate consent form.
◆ Explain postoperative care.

◆ Arrange for laboratory studies and tests; report abnormal results.
◆ Withhold food and fluids as ordered.

POSTTREATMENT CARE

◆ Administer medications as ordered.
◆ After pneumonectomy, make sure the patient lies only on the operative side or his back until he's stabilized.
◆ Make sure chest tubes are patent and functioning.
◆ Provide comfort measures.
◆ Encourage coughing, deep breathing, and incentive spirometry use.
◆ Have the patient splint the incision as needed.
◆ Perform passive range-of-motion (ROM) exercises, progressing to active ROM exercises.
◆ Perform incision site care and dressing changes as ordered.
◆ Monitor the patient's vital signs and intake and output.
◆ Assess for complications.
◆ Monitor respiratory status, and assess breath sounds.
◆ Monitor the surgical wound and dressings.
◆ Assess drainage.
◆ Monitor for abnormal bleeding.

⚡ *WARNING Monitor for and immediately report if dyspnea, chest pain, hypotension, irritating cough, vertigo, syncope, anxiety, subcutaneous emphysema, or tracheal deviation from the midline occurs. These findings indicate tension pneumothorax.*

PATIENT TEACHING

GENERAL

◆ Review medications and possible adverse reactions with the patient.
◆ Encourage the patient to perform coughing and deep-breathing exercises, and to use an incentive spirometer.
◆ Teach the patient how to care for the incision and to change dressings.
◆ Review the signs and symptoms of infection with the patient.

◆ Describe the signs and symptoms of possible complications to the patient, and tell him to notify the practitioner if any of these develop.
◆ Show the patient how to monitor sputum characteristics.
◆ Encourage the patient to perform ROM exercises.
◆ Advise the patient to balance physical activity and rest as directed by the practitioner.
◆ Teach the patient ways to prevent infection.
◆ Advise the patient to stop smoking and provide resources for assistance if appropriate.
◆ Arrange for home health care services if ordered and provide the patient with the agency's name and telephone number.
◆ Stress the importance of regular follow-up care.

RESOURCES
Organizations
American Lung Association:
www.lungsusa.org
American Medical Association:
www.ama-assn.org
National Foundation for Trauma Care:
www.traumafoundation.org

Selected references
Mattioli, G., et al., "Muscle-Sparing Thoracotomy Combined With Mechanically Stapled Lung Resection for Benign Lung Disorders: Functional Results and Quality of Life," *Pediatric Surgery International* 22(6):4911-95, June 2006.
Roviaro, G., et al. "Tracheal Sleeve Pneumonectomy: Long-Term Outcome," *Lung Cancer* 52(1):105-10, April 2006.
Tashima, T., et al., "Comparison of Video-assisted Minithoracotomy and Standard Open Thoracotomy for the Treatment of Non-small Cell Lung Cancer," *Minimally Invasive Therapy and Allied Technologies* 14(3): 203-208, March 2005.

Thrombolytic therapy

- Administration of thrombolytic drug, such as streptokinase (Streptase), alteplase (Activase), tenecteplase (TNKase), or reteplase (Retavase), to rapidly correct acute and extensive thrombotic disorders
- Involves conversion of plasminogen to plasmin by thrombolytic drugs, which leads to lysis of thrombi, fibrinogen, and other plasma proteins

INDICATIONS

- Thromboembolic disorders
- Deep vein thrombosis
- Peripheral arterial occlusion
- Acute myocardial infarction
- Acute pulmonary emboli
- Failing or failed atrioventricular fistulas

- Thrombolytic therapy may be administered in various settings, such as the interventional radiology department, intensive care unit, emergency department, or cardiac catheterization laboratory.
- Most thrombolytic agents are given by I.V. bolus, with I.V. infusion given at a specific rate in a separate I.V. line.
- Selected thrombolytics can be given by intracoronary infusion.
- Thrombolytics can also be given locally or directly into the thrombus (as in pulmonary embolism).

COMPLICATIONS

- Bleeding
- Adverse reactions to the thrombolytic
- Streptokinase resistance (with repeated use of drug)
- Arrhythmias

- Activity intolerance
- Decreased cardiac output
- Ineffective tissue perfusion: Cardiopulmonary

EXPECTED OUTCOMES

The patient will:

- carry out activities of daily living without excess fatigue or decreased energy
- maintain adequate cardiac output
- maintain vital signs, blood pressure, and peripheral pulses within normal limits.

PRETREATMENT CARE

- Explain the treatment and preparation to the patient and his family.
- Make sure the patient has signed an appropriate consent form.
- Explain posttreatment care.
- Obtain samples for blood typing and crossmatching and for coagulation studies.
- Obtain a baseline electrocardiogram and serum electrolyte, arterial blood gas, blood urea nitrogen, creatinine, and cardiac enzyme levels as ordered.

POSTTREATMENT CARE

- Administer medications as ordered.
- Minimize invasive procedures and venipunctures.
- Administer anticoagulants as ordered.
- Provide comfort measures.
- Provide supplemental oxygen as ordered.
- Restrict physical activity as ordered.
- Monitor vital signs and intake and output.
- Assess for complications, such as hypersensitivity reactions and abnormal bleeding.
- Monitor heart rate and rhythm, and assess peripheral pulses.
- Assess motor and sensory function.
- Monitor respiratory status.
- Monitor results of coagulation studies.

PATIENT TEACHING

GENERAL

- Review medications and possible adverse reactions with the patient.
- Tell the patient to promptly report abnormal or prolonged bleeding to the practitioner.
- Review the signs and symptoms of thrombus formation and thromboembolic events with the patient.
- Instruct the patient to call the practitioner if he develops new irregular heart beats, palpitations, or chest pain or discomfort.
- Teach the patient how to prevent thrombotic events.
- Encourage the patient to stop smoking.
- Stress the need for follow-up care.

RESOURCES
Organizations
American College of Cardiology: *www.acc.org*
American Heart Association: *www.americanheart.org*

Selected references
O'Donnell, S., et al. "In-Hospital Care Pathway Delays: Gender and Myocardial Infarction," *Journal of Advanced Nursing* 52(1):14-21, October 2005.
Quinn, T. "The Role of Nurses in Improving Emergency Cardiac Care," *Nursing Standard* 19(48):41-48, August 2005.
Qureshi, A.I., et al. "Time to Hospital Arrival, Use of Thrombolytics, and In-Hospital Outcomes in Ischemic Stroke," *Neurology* 64(12):2115-20, June 2005.
Tough, J. "Thrombolytic Therapy in Acute Myocardial Infarction," *Nursing Standard* 19(37):55-64, May 2005.

Thyroidectomy

- Surgical removal of all or part of the thyroid gland

INDICATIONS
- Hyperthyroidism
- Respiratory obstruction caused by goiter
- Thyroid cancer

- The patient is anesthetized.
- The surgeon extends the patient's neck fully and determines the incision line by measuring bilaterally from each clavicle.
- The surgeon cuts through the skin, fascia, and muscle and raises skin flaps from the strap muscles.
- The muscles are separated at midline, revealing the isthmus of the thyroid.
- The thyroid artery and veins are ligated to help prevent bleeding.
- The surgeon locates and views the laryngeal nerves and parathyroid glands.
- He dissects and removes the thyroid tissue.
- A Penrose drain or a closed wound drainage device is inserted, and the wound is closed.

COMPLICATIONS
- Hemorrhage
- Parathyroid damage
- Hypocalcemia
- Tetany
- Laryngeal nerve damage
- Vocal cord paralysis
- Thyroid storm

- Activity intolerance
- Decreased cardiac output
- Ineffective tissue perfusion: Cardiopulmonary

EXPECTED OUTCOMES
The patient will:
- carry out activities of daily living without excess fatigue or decreased energy
- maintain adequate cardiac output
- maintain vital signs, blood pressure, and peripheral pulses within normal limits.

- Explain the treatment and preparation to the patient and his family.
- Verify that the patient has signed an appropriate consent form.
- Explain postoperative care.
- Inform the patient that some hoarseness and a sore throat will occur after surgery.
- Make sure the patient has followed the preoperative drug regimen as ordered.
- Collect blood samples for serum thyroid hormone measurement.
- Obtain a 12-lead electrocardiogram.

POSTTREATMENT CARE

- Administer medications as ordered.
- Keep the patient in high Fowler's position.
- Evaluate the patient's speech for signs of laryngeal nerve damage.
- Keep a tracheotomy tray at the bedside for 24 hours after surgery.
- Provide surgical wound care and dressing changes as ordered.
- Provide comfort measures.
- Maintain patency of drains.
- Monitor the patient's vital signs and intake and output.
- Assess the surgical wound and dressings.
- Monitor drainage.
- Assess for abnormal bleeding.
- Monitor respiratory status.
- Assess for hypocalcemia (such as Chvostek's and Trousseau's signs).
- Monitor for thyroid storm.

PATIENT TEACHING

GENERAL

- Review medications and possible adverse reactions with the patient.
- Review the signs and symptoms of respiratory distress with the patient.
- Explain the signs and symptoms of hypothyroidism and hyperthyroidism.
- Review the signs and symptoms of infection and hypocalcemia with the patient and tell him to notify the practitioner promptly if these develop.
- Tell the patient to call the practitioner if abnormal or excessive bleeding occurs.
- Instruct the patient to take the prescribed thyroid hormone replacement therapy and return for annual blood testing once the dosage has been stabilized.
- Tell the patient to take calcium supplements as indicated.
- Show the patient how to care for the incision site and how to change dressings.
- Stress the need for follow-up care.

RESOURCES
Organizations
American Association of Clinical Endocrinologists: *www.aace.com*
American College of Surgeons: *www.facs.org*
American Thyroid Association: *www.thyroid.org*

Selected references
Aloumanis, K., et al. "Urgent Thyroidectomy for Acute Airway Obstruction Caused by a Goiter in a Euthyroid Pregnant Woman," *Thyroid* 16(1):85-88, January 2006.

Amer, K.S. "Advances in Assessment, Diagnosis, and Treatment of Hyperthyroidism in Children," *Journal of Pediatric Nursing* 20(2):119-26, April 2005.

Besic, N., et al. "Aggressiveness of Therapy and Prognosis of Patients with Hurthle Cell Papillary Thyroid Carcinoma," *Thyroid* 16(1):67-72, January 2006.

Grimes, C.M., et al. "Intraoperative Thyroid Storm: A Case Report," *American Nephrology Nurses' Association Journal* 72(1):53-55, February 2004.

Tonsillectomy and adenoidectomy

OVERVIEW

- Surgical removal of the tonsils and adenoids

INDICATIONS

- Frequently recurrent or chronic tonsil and adenoid infection
- Obstructive sleep apnea
- Peritonsillar abscess
- Recurrent middle ear infections due to tonsil enlargement

PROCEDURE

- The patient is given a general anesthetic and an I.V. is initiated.
- The surgeon resects the tonsils and adenoids through the mouth.
- Then he electrocauterizes the base of the tonsils and adenoids to stop the bleeding.

COMPLICATIONS

- Bleeding
- Infection
- Dehydration
- Permanent voice changes
- Nasal regurgitation (rare)
- Failure to improve the nasal airway or resolve snoring, sleep apnea, or breathing through the mouth

NURSING DIAGNOSES

- Anxiety
- Ineffective airway clearance
- Risk for deficient fluid volume

EXPECTED OUTCOMES

The patient will:

- express feelings of comfort and demonstrate decreased anxiety
- maintain adequate ventilation
- have no signs or symptoms of bleeding and maintain adequate intake and output.

PRETREATMENT CARE

- Instruct the patient to take nothing by mouth for 6 hours preoperatively.
- Verify that an appropriate consent form has been signed.

AGE FACTOR *Provide additional comfort to a child by giving him his favorite toy, stuffed animal, or blanket.*

- Check to see that preoperative laboratory testing has been completed.
- Make sure that the patient hasn't taken aspirin or aspirin-containing products within 10 days of surgery. Nonsteroidal anti-inflammatory drugs (such as ibuprofen) shouldn't be taken within 7 days of surgery. Tell the patient that it's important to check medications carefully because many over-the-counter products contain aspirin or ibuprofen-related drugs.

AGE FACTOR *Encourage parents to be honest with their child when they explain the surgery. Advise them to tell the child that the procedure is being done to make him healthier and reassure him that the hospital and staff are safe. Parents also must reinforce that they'll always be nearby. Have them also tell the child that he may experience some pain such as a sore throat for a short time, but he can take medicines for it. Suggest that the parents and child visit the surgical facility before surgery, and work together with the many books and activity brochures designed to explain common hospital procedures to children.*

POSTTREATMENT CARE

- Maintain a patent airway.
- Prevent aspiration by positioning the patient on his side.
- Keep suction equipment readily available.
- Provide water after the gag reflex returns. Encourage nonirritating oral fluids like cold noncitrus juices, or water ice.

⚡ **WARNING** *Avoid giving the patient milk products and salty or irritating foods. Also, don't give red-colored fluids because they mask signs of bleeding.*

- Provide analgesics for pain relief.
- Encourage deep-breathing exercises.
- Monitor the patient's vital signs, hydration status, and intake and output.
- Assess frequently for signs of bleeding.
- Monitor respiratory status.

⚡ **WARNING** *Immediately report excessive bleeding, increased pulse rate, or decreased blood pressure.*

PATIENT TEACHING

GENERAL

- Stress the importance of completing the entire course of antibiotics, if ordered.
- Tell the patient to avoid irritating foods and fluids, including mouthwashes.
- Emphasize the need for soft foods for about 3 weeks after surgery to decrease the risk of rebleeding.
- Review medication administration, dosages, and possible adverse effects with the patient.
- Explain that throat discomfort and minor bleeding may occur after surgery.
- Tell the patient to expect a white scab to form in his throat 5 to 10 days after surgery.
- Stress the need to report continued or excessive bleeding, ear discomfort, or a fever that lasts for 3 days or longer.

⚡ **WARNING** *The greatest risk of bleeding occurs 7 to 10 days postoperatively.*

RESOURCES
Organizations
American Academy of Allergy, Asthma, and Immunology: *www.aaaai.org*
American Academy of Otolaryngology-Head and Neck Surgery: *www.entnet.org*
National Institute of Allergy and Infectious Disease: *www.niad.nih.gov*

Selected references
Ewah, B.N., et al. "Postoperative Pain, Nausea and Vomiting Following Paediatric Day-Case Tonsillectomy," *Anaesthesia* 61(2):116-22, February 2006.

Kheirandish, L., et al. "Intranasal Steroids and Oral Leukotriene Modifier Therapy in Residual Sleep-Disordered Breathing after Tonsillectomy and Adenoidectomy in Children," *Pediatrics* 117(1): e61-66, January 2006.

Mitchell, R.B., and Kelly, J. "Child Behavior after Adenotonsillectomy for Obstructive Sleep Apnea Syndrome," *Laryngoscope* 115(11):2051-55, November 2005.

Ray, R.M., and Bower, C.M. "Pediatric Obstructive Sleep Apnea: The Year in Review," *Current Opinion in Otolaryngology and Head and Neck Surgery* 13(6): 360-65, December 2005.

Trabeculectomy

OVERVIEW

- Creation of a new passageway by which the aqueous fluid inside the eye can escape, thereby lowering the intraocular pressure (IOP)
- Used in glaucoma patients where the Canal of Schlemm is blocked, to reduce IOP and prevent visual field loss
- Procedure depends on type of glaucoma, degree of advancement, general health of patient and ability to comply with treatment regimens; sometimes combined with cataract surgery
- Also called a *filtration procedure*

INDICATIONS

- Glaucoma unresponsive to medications

PROCEDURE

- The patient is given local or possibly topical anesthesia. Mild sedation may also be given if needed.
- The eyelids are held open during the procedure. A small piece of the trabecular tissue in the drainage angle of the eye is resected. A small flap of tissue from the sclera and conjunctiva is formed over the new opening. As the fluid begins to flow through the opening, the covering flap forms a little bubble, called a *bleb*.
- The ophthalmologic surgeon may instill such medications as mitomycin (Mitomycin-C) and fluorouracil (5-FU) at the end of surgery to prevent closure of the opening by scar tissue.
- After surgery, the eyelid is usually taped or held shut with a dressing, and covered with an eye shield.

COMPLICATIONS

- Infection
- Bleeding
- Retinal swelling
- Choroidal detachment
- Retinal detachment
- Droopy eyelid
- Double vision
- Loss of vision
- Loss of eye

NURSING DIAGNOSES

- Acute pain
- Disturbed sensory perception (visual)
- Risk for infection

EXPECTED OUTCOMES

The patient will:
- express feelings of comfort
- regain usual visual function after healing
- demonstrate intact tissue without signs of infection.

PRETREATMENT CARE

- Obtain baseline vital signs and an electrocardiographic rhythm strip if ordered.
- Administer the eye drop regimen as ordered.
- Review the procedure with the patient and describe the nursing care to be given.
- Verify that a consent form has been signed.
- Review medications the patient is taking.

POSTTREATMENT CARE

◆ Assess the exterior of the eye dressing for signs of bleeding initially, but don't remove the shield and dressing unless instructed by the surgeon.
◆ Monitor vital signs, and heart rhythm if ordered.
◆ Assess the patient for pain and administer pain medications as ordered.
◆ Assess for signs of complications, such as infection or changes in vision, after the practitioner has removed the initial dressing.

°PATIENT TEACHING

GENERAL

◆ Review the disorder and treatment plan with the patient.
◆ Tell the patient to modify his environment for safety.
◆ Review prescribed medications and their dosage, administration, and adverse effects with the patient.
◆ Advise the patient to keep follow-up appointments with the ophthalmologist.
◆ Advise the patient that depending on the postoperative pressure in his eye, the surgeon may laser one or two of the flap sutures open to accelerate the filtration process; tell him that this is usually done with a laser in the practitioner's office.
◆ Tell the patient to continue taking antibiotic and anti-inflammatory eye drops as ordered after surgery, and write this schedule down for the patient to use at home.
◆ Inform the patient that numerous follow-up visits are generally required after surgery to assess the adequacy of the fluid drainage and IOP, but will decrease in frequency as healing progresses.
◆ Inform the patient that after the filter site has fully healed, IOP in the eye and visual field testing will determine if his glaucoma medications can be reduced or eliminated.

◆ Instruct that patient to avoid straining activities that might increase the IOP, such as bending, lifting, or straining due to a cough or constipation, for several weeks after surgery.
◆ If the patient is constipated after surgery, tell him to take stool softeners to avoid straining while trying to pass stools.
◆ Inform the patient that he'll experience mild discomfort after the procedure but to report severe pain to the practitioner promptly.

RESOURCES
Organizations
American Academy of Ophthalmology: *www.aao.org*
American Academy of Pediatrics: *www.aap.org*
EyeMDLink, Chris A. Knobbe, MD: *www.eyemdlink.com*

Selected references
Anis, S., et al. "Surgical Reduction of Symptomatic, Circumferential, Filtering Blebs," *Archives of Ophthalmology* 124(6):890-94, June 2006.
Shaw, M.E. "Increasing Compliance with Glaucoma Therapy: 'So, Convince Me I Have Something Wrong With My Eyes,'" *Insight* 30(3):7-9, July-September 2005.
Tham, C.C., et al. "Results of Trabeculectomy With Adjunctive Intraoperative Mitomycin C in Chinese Patients With Glaucoma," *Ophthalmic Surgery, Lasers and Imaging* 37(1):33-41, January-February 2006.

Tracheoesophageal fistula repair

OVERVIEW

- Surgical repair of defects of the trachea and esophagus
- Lower portion of esophagus abnormally connected to trachea by fistula (see *Tracheoesophageal fistula formation*)
- Also known as *TEF*

AGE FACTOR *TEFs commonly occur congenitally, the trachea and upper portion of the digestive tract fail to develop normally during early fetal development. In neonates with esophageal atresia and TEF, the proximal esophagus ends in a blind pouch. In some cases, neonates can't undergo immediate surgery, especially if other congenital anomalies exist, or if the neonate was born prematurely or with a low birth weight. These neonates require intensive medical support before surgical repair.*

- May also be caused by blunt trauma or injuries to the neck and thorax, or by prolonged endotracheal (ET) intubation with a cuffed tube
- Treatment complicated by tumors of the esophagus, lungs, or trachea, or metastatic lymph nodes in the larynx

INDICATIONS
- TEF, congenital or acquired
- Esophageal atresia
- Malignancy

WARNING *TEFs are life-threatening conditions that require immediate intervention. Because saliva and gastric secretions may be aspirated into the lungs through the abnormal opening in the trachea, normal swallowing and digestion of food can't occur.*

PROCEDURE

- The patient is given general anesthesia and positioned on the table with the head elevated to prevent gastric reflux.
- The surgeon makes a right thoracotomy incision, then carefully frees the distal end of the esophagus from surrounding tissue, nerves, and blood vessels below the TEF.
- Next, the surgeon cuts apart the fistula and sutures the ends over the esophageal and tracheal openings.
- The surgeon may reinforce the tracheal and esophageal repair sites with the flaps of the mediastinal pleura. Flaps from the sternohyoid or sternothyroid muscles may also be created between the trachea and esophagus to reinforce the repair. In the lower thorax near the diaphragm, a flap of the pleura, intercostal muscle, and rib periosteum is usually made as further reinforcement of the esophageal tissue.
- When tracheal damage from a large defect is present, the trachea may need to be reconstructed after the damaged areas are removed.
- Large esophageal defects are sutured in two lengthwise layers. A muscle layer is created to cover the esophageal repair, strengthen it, and separate it from the tracheal suture line.
- The surgeon may also use an esophageal stent (endoprosthesis) when the TEF is caused by malignancy.
- When the repairs are complete, a nasogastric (NG) feeding tube is inserted and a chest tube is put in the retropleural space before incisions are closed.

Tracheoesophageal fistula formation

In tracheoesophageal fistula, an abnormal connection exists between the trachea and esophagus. The most common form is a congenital defect where the proximal esophagus ends in a blind pouch, and the distal esophagus forms a fistula with the trachea.

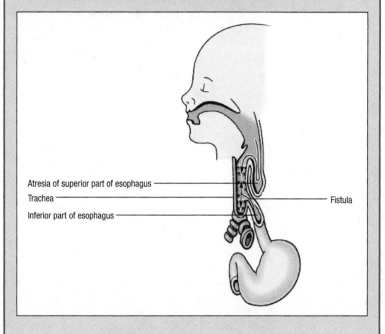

Atresia of superior part of esophagus

Trachea

Inferior part of esophagus

Fistula

COMPLICATIONS

- Pneumonia
- Atelectasis
- Respiratory failure
- Leak at the anastomotic site
- Pneumothorax
- Strictures
- Recurrent TEF
- Apneic spells
- Gastroesophageal reflux
- Laryngospasm
- Infection
- Recurrent pneumonia
- Acute lung injury
- Acute respiratory distress syndrome
- Lung abscess
- Poor nutrition
- Bronchiectasis from recurrent aspiration
- Respiratory failure
- Barrett's esophagus
- Esophageal carcinoma
- Death

NURSING DIAGNOSES

- Impaired gas exchange
- Imbalanced nutrition: Less than body requirements
- Risk for infection

EXPECTED OUTCOMES
The patient will:
- maintain adequate ventilation and lung sounds
- demonstrate no difficulty swallowing and maintaining an adequate nutritional intake
- remain free from infection.

PRETREATMENT CARE

- Obtain thoracic ultrasound, chest radiographs, flexible esophagoscopy or bronchoscopy studies as ordered.
- Provide adequate I.V. hydration and parenteral or enteral nutrition as ordered.
- If the patient develops acute respiratory failure, prepare him and his family to expect ET intubation and mechanical ventilation.
- If the patient develops a lower respiratory tract infection, administer broad-spectrum antibiotics as ordered.
- The practitioner may insert a cuffed ET tube below the fistula site to prevent gastric reflux and aspiration until the surgery can be done.
- If required and possible, a tracheostomy may be done below the TEF to assist ventilation.
- Keep the head of the bed elevated, and suction secretions.
- Esophageal diversion procedures may be needed if the child continues to aspirate.
- If surgery on a child must be delayed for 2 to 4 months, the practitioner may periodically dilate the underdeveloped esophagus.
- Tell the patient and his family what to expect postoperatively.
- Review the procedures and care with the patient and his family and answer questions.
- Verify that a consent form has been signed.

(continued)

- Infants will be in a neonatal intensive care unit preoperatively and postoperatively; adults will be in the intensive care unit (ICU).
- Keep the infant warm and protected from infectious exposure by placing him in an Isolette.
- Assess respiratory function and lung sounds frequently and maintain oxygen therapy or mechanical ventilation as ordered. Suction the patient as indicated. Report deteriorating signs and symptoms to the practitioner.
- Monitor pulse oximetry, arterial blood gas values, and laboratory studies as ordered.
- Monitor drainage and maintain the patency of the chest tube system.
- Maintain I.V. fluids as ordered; monitor intake and output.
- Provide analgesics as indicated and assess for effect.
- Start enteral feedings as soon as ordered and monitor nutritional status.
- Assess for aspiration.
- Obtain a contrast swallowing X-ray on the seventh postoperative day as ordered. If no leak is detected, the practitioner may order oral feedings.
- About 3 weeks postoperatively, the esophagus is dilated up to 24F size to prevent future esophageal stenosis.

- Monitor vital signs regularly.
- Assist with weaning from mechanical ventilation as ordered.
- If the patient has a tracheostomy, make sure a spare tracheotomy tube is at the bedside at all times. Provide tracheostomy care.
- Monitor for bleeding, edema, dehiscence, or infection at the wound site.
- Monitor dressings and drainage while performing wound care as ordered.
- Keep the head of the bed elevated as ordered.
- Assist the patient with turning every 2 hours.
- Maintain the patency of the NG tube, and remove it when sufficient oral intake has been achieved.

⚡ **WARNING** *Don't reposition the NG tube that has been placed intraoperatively; monitor placement of tube with markings. Alert the surgeon if the tube has slipped out of position.*

- Provide emotional support to the patient and his family. Promote bonding between infants and parents by permitting them to hold their child and provide care as they wish under nursing supervision.

GENERAL

- Have the parents or patient and his family speak with the gastroenterologist, pulmonologist, and thoracic surgeon to review the surgery required and aftercare needed.
- Review the ICU environment with the family and prepare them for the appearance of their loved one postoperatively.
- Teach all aspects of care of the infant or child and provide for home health care services as ordered.
- Explain postoperative procedures, such as suctioning, tube feeding; and care of the tracheostomy tube.

RESOURCES
Organizations
American Academy of Pediatrics: *www.aap.org*
American College of Gastroenterology: www.acg.gi.org
American College of Surgeons: *www.facs.org*
American Gastroenterological Association: *www.gastro.org*

Selected references

Aziz, G.A., and Schier, F. "Thoracoscopic Ligation of a Tracheoesophageal H-Type Fistula in a Newborn," *Journal of Pediatric Surgery* 40(6):e35-36, June 2005.

Holcomb, G.W. III, et al. "Thoracoscopic Repair of Esophageal Atresia and Tracheoesophageal Fistula: A Multi-Institutional Analysis," *Annals of Surgery* 242(3):422-30, September 2005.

Krosnar, S., and Baxter, A. "Thoracoscopic Repair of Esophageal Atresia With Tracheoesophageal Fistula: Anesthetic and Intensive Care Management of a Series of Eight Neonates," *Paediatric Anaesthesia* 15(7):541-46, July 2005.

Mariano, E.R., et al. "Successful Thoracoscopic Repair of Esophageal Atresia with Tracheoesophageal Fistula in a Newborn with Single Ventricle Physiology," *Anesthesia and Analgesia* 101(4):1000-1002, October 2005.

Tracheotomy

OVERVIEW

- Surgical creation of an opening into the trachea through the neck
- May be permanent or temporary

INDICATIONS

- Prolonged mechanical ventilation
- Prevent aspiration in an unconscious or paralyzed patient
- Upper airway obstruction caused by trauma, burns, epiglottitis, or tumors
- Remove lower tracheobronchial secretions in patients who can't clear them

PROCEDURE

- The technique varies with the type of tube used.
- If an endotracheal (ET) tube isn't already in place, it's inserted with the patient under general anesthesia.
- A horizontal incision is made in the skin below the cricoid cartilage, and vertical incisions are made in the trachea.
- A tracheostomy tube is placed between the second and third tracheal rings. (See *Comparing types of tracheostomy tubes.*)
- Retraction sutures may be placed in the stomal margins.
- The tube cuff (if present) is inflated.
- Ventilation and suction are performed.
- Oxygen is administered.
- The ET tube is removed.

COMPLICATIONS

- Hemorrhage
- Edema
- Aspiration of secretions
- Pneumothorax
- Subcutaneous emphysema
- Infection
- Airway obstruction
- Hypoxia
- Arrhythmias

(See *Combating complications of tracheotomy.*)

NURSING DIAGNOSES

- Impaired gas exchange
- Ineffective breathing pattern
- Ineffective tissue perfusion: Cardiopulmonary

EXPECTED OUTCOMES

The patient will:

- maintain adequate ventilation with oxygen saturation levels within normal range
- exhibit normal breathing pattern
- maintain vital signs, blood pressure, and respiratory function within normal limits.

PRETREATMENT CARE

- Explain the treatment and preparation to the patient and his family.
- Verify that the patient has signed an appropriate consent form.
- Obtain appropriate supplies or a tracheotomy tray.
- With the patient, devise an appropriate communication system for after the procedure.

Comparing types of tracheostomy tubes

Tracheostomy tubes are made of plastic or metal and are available in cuffed, uncuffed, or fenestrated varieties. Tube selection depends on the patient's condition and the practitioner's preference. Make sure you're familiar with the advantages and disadvantages of these commonly used tracheostomy tubes.

TUBE TYPE	ADVANTAGES	DISADVANTAGES
Uncuffed (plastic or metal) 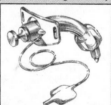	◆ Permits free flow of air around tube and through larynx ◆ Reduces the risk of tracheal damage ◆ Recommended for children because these tubes don't require a cuff ◆ Allows mechanical ventilation in the patient with neuromuscular disease	◆ Lack of a cuff increases the risk of aspiration (in adults) ◆ Adapter may be necessary for ventilation
Plastic cuffed (low pressure and high volume) 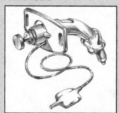	◆ Disposable ◆ Cuff bonded to the tube; won't detach accidentally inside the trachea ◆ Low cuff pressure, which is evenly distributed against the tracheal wall; no need to deflate periodically to lower pressure ◆ Reduces the risk of tracheal damage	◆ May be more costly than other tubes
Fenestrated	◆ Permits speech through the upper airway when the external opening is capped and the cuff is deflated ◆ Allows breathing by mechanical ventilation with an inner cannula in place and the cuff inflated ◆ Inner cannula can be easily removed for cleaning	◆ Fenestration may become occluded ◆ Inner cannula can become dislodged

- Obtain samples for arterial blood gas (ABG) analysis and other required diagnostic tests; report abnormal results.

POSTTREATMENT CARE

- Administer medications as ordered.
- Turn the patient every 2 hours and provide chest physiotherapy.
- Provide oxygen and humidification as ordered.
- Suction the airway as indicated and monitor the amount, color, and consistency of secretions.
- Monitor cuff pressures as ordered (usually less than 25 cm H_2O [18 mm Hg]).
- Provide comfort measures.
- Perform incision site care and dressing changes per facility policy, and monitor the site for infection or inflammation.
- Keep a sterile tracheostomy tube with obturator (including a tube one size smaller) at the bedside.
- Monitor vital signs.
- Assess intake and output.
- Monitor respiratory status and assess breath sounds.
- Observe for abnormal bleeding or other complications.
- Monitor ABG and pulse oximetry values.
- Assess for peritracheal edema.

Combating complications of tracheotomy

COMPLICATION	PREVENTION	DETECTION	TREATMENT
Aspiration	◆ Evaluate the patient's ability to swallow. ◆ Elevate the patient's head a minimum of 45 degrees for 30 minutes after eating to reduce the risk of aspiration. ◆ Inflate the cuff during feedings; keep inflated for 30 minutes after feeding.	◆ Assess for dyspnea, tachypnea, rhonchi, crackles, excessive secretions, and fever.	◆ Obtain chest X-ray, if ordered. ◆ Suction excessive secretions. ◆ Give antibiotics, if necessary.
Bleeding at tracheotomy site	◆ Don't pull on the tracheostomy tube; don't allow the ventilator tubing to do so. ◆ If dressing adheres to wound, wet it with hydrogen peroxide and gently remove it.	◆ Check the dressing regularly; slight bleeding is normal, especially if the patient has a bleeding disorder.	◆ Keep the cuff inflated to prevent edema and blood aspiration. Give humidified oxygen. ◆ Document the character of bleeding. Check for prolonged clotting time. ◆ As ordered, assist with Gelfoam application or ligation of a small bleeder.
Infection at tracheotomy site	◆ Always use strict sterile technique. ◆ Thoroughly clean tubing. ◆ Change nebulizer or humidifier jar and tubing daily. ◆ Collect sputum and wound drainage specimens for culture.	◆ Check for purulent, foul-smelling drainage from the stoma. ◆ Be alert for other signs and symptoms of infection, such as fever, malaise, increased white blood cell count, and local pain.	◆ As ordered, obtain culture specimens and administer antibiotics. ◆ Inflate tracheostomy cuff to prevent aspiration. ◆ Suction the patient frequently; avoid cross-contamination. ◆ Change the dressing whenever soiled.
Pneumothorax	◆ Assess the patient for subcutaneous emphysema, which may indicate pneumothorax. Notify the practitioner if this occurs.	◆ Auscultate for decreased or absent breath sounds. ◆ Check for tachypnea, pain, and subcutaneous emphysema.	◆ If ordered, prepare for chest tube insertion. ◆ Obtain chest X-ray as ordered to evaluate for pneumothorax or to check placement of chest tube.
Subcutaneous emphysema	◆ Make sure the cuffed tube is patent and properly inflated. ◆ Avoid displacement by securing ties and using lightweight ventilator tubing and swivel valves.	◆ Most common in mechanically ventilated patients. ◆ Palpate the neck for crepitus; listen for air leakage around the cuff; and check the site for unusual swelling.	◆ Inflate the cuff correctly or use a larger tube. ◆ Suction the patient and clean the tube to remove blockage. ◆ Document the extent of crepitus.
Tracheal malacia	◆ Avoid excessive cuff pressures. ◆ Avoid suctioning beyond the end of the tube.	◆ Note a dry, hacking cough and blood-streaked sputum when the tube is being manipulated.	◆ Minimize trauma from tube movement. ◆ Keep the cuff pressure below 18 mm Hg.

(Text continues on page 369.)

Caring for your trach tube

Dear Patient:

As part of your laryngectomy, a permanent tracheostomy—a small opening, or stoma—has been created in your throat.

Inserting a tube into the tracheostomy makes breathing easier because the tube keeps your windpipe open. A tracheostomy tube—a "trach" (rhymes with "cake") tube for short—features three parts:

♦ an inner cannula
♦ an outer cannula
♦ an obturator.

The inner cannula fits inside the outer cannula, which you insert with the obturator.

HOW TO CLEAN THE INNER CANNULA

To prevent infection, remove and clean the inner cannula regularly. Follow these steps.

1. Gather your equipment near a sink: a small basin, a small brush, mild liquid dish detergent, a gauze pad, scissors, and clean trach ties (twill tape). Or, open a prepackaged kit that contains the equipment you need.

2. Now wash your hands. Position a mirror so that you can see your face and throat clearly.

3. Unlock the inner cannula and remove it by pulling steadily outward and downward, as shown. (Some cannulas need to be turned counterclockwise to unlock them.)

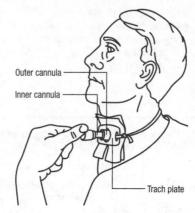

Outer cannula
Inner cannula
Trach plate

4. Prepare to clean the soiled cannula immediately for reinsertion, or put this soiled cannula aside and slip a clean inner cannula inside the outer cannula.

5. If you start to cough, cover your stoma with a tissue, bend forward, and relax until the coughing stops.

6. Next, clean the soiled cannula. Here's how: soak the cannula in mild liquid dish detergent and water (*never* use alcohol or bleach). Then clean it with a small brush. If your cannula is heavily soiled, try soaking it in a basin of hydrogen peroxide solution. You'll see foaming as the solution reacts with the secretions coating the cannula. When the foaming stops, clean the cannula with the brush.

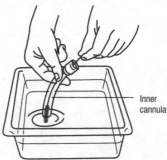

Inner cannula

You can obtain a special trach tube brush at a medical supply company or pharmacy. However, the small brushes used to clean coffee pots work just as well. They're inexpensive and available at hardware stores. Just be sure to use the brush only for your trach tube.

7. Rinse the inner cannula under running water. Make sure you remove all of the cleaning solution. Shake off the excess water and reinsert the clean, moist cannula immediately. Don't dry it; the water drops remaining help lubricate the cannula, making reinsertion easier.

8. After you lock the clean inner cannula in place, replace the soiled trach ties that secure the trach plate. Use scissors to carefully clip and remove one trach tie at a time. Knot the end of each clean trach tie to prevent fraying, then cut a ½" (1.5-cm) slit in each tie. Thread the end that isn't knotted through the opening on the trach plate. Then feed the end through the slit, as shown below, and gently pull the tie taut. Do the same for the other tie.

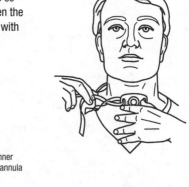

9. Secure the ties at the side of your neck with a square knot. Leave enough room so you can breathe comfortably. You should be able to slip two fingers between the side of your neck and the knot.

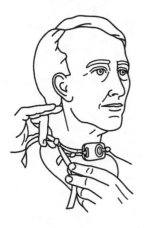

10. Place a 4″ × 4″ gauze bib behind the tube to protect your neck.

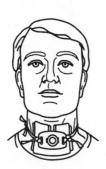

11. Carefully insert the gauze bib under the trach plate. If you have heavy discharge draining from the stoma, you can insert the gauze bib from below. If you don't have a precut bib, fold two 4″ × 4″ gauze pads into triangles and place one on each side of the tube.

HOW TO REINSERT YOUR TRACH TUBE

If you accidentally cough out your trach tube. *Don't panic.* Follow these simple steps to reinsert it:

1. Remove the inner cannula from the dislodged trach tube. Then, if you're using a cuffed tube, make sure you deflate the cuff on the outer cannula.

2. Insert the obturator into the outer cannula. Then use the obturator to reinsert the trach tube into your stoma.

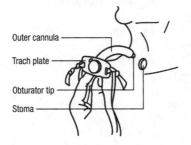

Outer cannula
Trach plate
Obturator tip
Stoma

3. Hold the trach plate in place and immediately remove the obturator, as shown.

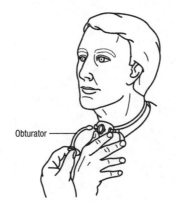

Obturator

4. Insert the inner cannula into the trach tube. Next, turn the inner cannula clockwise until it locks in place. Chances are you'll cough or gag while you're doing this, so be sure to hold onto the trach plate securely.

If you're using a cuffed tube:

5. Next, insert the tip of a syringe into the tube's pillow port. Inflate the cuff, as directed. The inflated cuff will help prevent the tube from accidentally being dislodged again.

6. After inflating the cuff, secure the trach ties and tuck a gauze pad under the trach plate.

Learning a new way to swallow

Dear Patient:

After surgery, you'll need to learn a new way to swallow to prevent food and fluids from flowing the wrong way and entering your trachea (windpipe) and lungs. The nurse or speech therapist will show you how before surgery so you can start practicing. Then she'll review the steps with you after surgery, when you're ready for your first meal.

PRACTICE STEPS

1. To begin, place a small amount of food at the back of your throat.

2. Take a deep breath and hold it. This pulls your vocal cords together and closes the entrance to your trachea.

3. Now use a gulping motion to swallow. Then cough. Repeat this step once or twice to prevent any food left in your throat from entering your trachea.

AFTER SURGERY

You'll have your first meal several days after surgery. It will consist of soft, easy-to-swallow foods such as mashed potatoes. As you get better at swallowing, you'll progress to foods

that are more difficult to swallow until you can swallow liquids.

SWALLOWING TIPS

Here are some tips to help you swallow comfortably:

◆ Eat slowly. It's the best way to avoid choking.

◆ Lean forward slightly as you eat. This position helps prevent food from entering your trachea.

◆ Stay calm. If some food does enter your trachea, the nurse will remove it immediately by suctioning it through your tracheostomy tube.

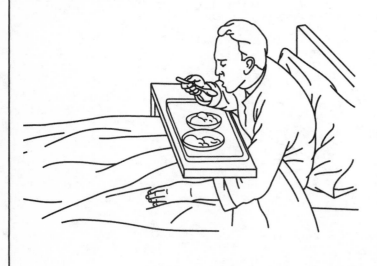

PATIENT TEACHING

GENERAL
◆ Review medications prescribed, their safe use, and possible adverse reactions with the patient.
◆ Teach the patient how to care for the tracheostomy site and tube. (See *Caring for your trach tube*, pages 366 and 367.)
◆ Reinforce the teaching of the speech therapist on how to swallow. (See *Learning a new way to swallow*.)
◆ Remind the patient to protect the stoma from water.
◆ Tell the patient to use a foam filter over the stoma during winter.
◆ Review the signs and symptoms of infection and proper disposal of expelled secretions with the patient.
◆ Review possible complications and when to notify the practitioner.
◆ Advise the patient when to follow-up with the practitioner.

RESOURCES
Organizations
American Academy of Pediatrics: *www.aap.org*
American College of Surgeons: *www.facs.org*
American Medical Association: *www.ama-assn.org*

Selected references
Altman, K.W., et al. "Urgent Surgical Airway Intervention: A 3 Year County Hospital Experience," *Laryngoscope* 115(12):2101-2104, December 2005.
Sidman, J.D., et al. "Tracheotomy and Decannulation Rates in a Level 3 Neonatal Intensive Care Unit: A 12-Year Study," *Laryngoscope* 116(1):136-39, January 2006.
Webber-Jones, J.E. "Tension Pneumocephalus," *Journal of Neuroscience Nursing* 37(5):272-76, October 2005.

Traction, halo-vest

OVERVIEW

- Immobilizes the head and neck after traumatic injury to the cervical vertebrae to prevent further spinal cord injury
- Applied by an orthopedic or neurosurgeon, with nursing assistance, in the emergency department, a specially equipped room, or operating room after surgical reduction of vertebral injuries
- Consists of a metal ring that fits over the patient's head and metal bars that connect the ring to a plastic vest, which distributes the weight of the apparatus around the chest (see *Comparing halo-vest traction devices*)
- Allows greater mobility than traction with skull tongs and has less risk of infection because it doesn't require skin incisions and drilling holes to position skull pins

INDICATIONS
- Cervical spine fractures, especially in the C1-C2 area

PROCEDURE

- Wash your hands; provide privacy.
- Request a second nurse or practitioner to hold the patient's head and neck stable while the practitioner removes the sandbags. This manual support must be maintained until the halo is secure.
- The practitioner measures the patient's head and chest with a tape measure and determines the correct halo-vest unit size.
- The ring should clear the head by ⅝″ (1.6 cm) and fit ½″ (1.3 cm) above the bridge of the nose.
- The practitioner selects four pin sites: ½″ above the lateral one-third of each eyebrow and ½″ above the top of each ear in the occipital area. The temporal bones are not strong enough and aren't used.
- He also considers the degree and type of correction needed to provide proper cervical alignment.
- Trim and shave hair at the pin sites to facilitate subsequent care and help prevent infection, then put on gloves.
- Use gauze pads soaked in povidone-iodine or designated solution to clean the sites.
- Open the halo-vest unit using sterile technique to avoid contamination.
- The practitioner puts on sterile gloves, and then removes the halo and Allen wrench.
- Instruct the patient to close his eyes completely while the pins are inserted, to avoid trapping of the frontalis muscle which can prevent eye closure.
- The surgeon places the halo over the patient's head and inserts the four positioning pins to hold the halo in place temporarily (no anesthetic required).
- Help the surgeon prepare anesthetic. Clean the injection port of a multidose vial of lidocaine with an alcohol pad. Invert the vial so the surgeon can insert a 25G needle attached to the 3-ml syringe and withdraw the anesthetic.
- The surgeon injects the anesthetic at the four permanent pin sites; he may

change needles on the syringe after each injection.
- The surgeon removes four of the five skull pins from the sterile setup and firmly screws in each pin at a 90-degree angle to the skull.
- With the permanent pins in place, he removes the positioning pins.
- He tightens the skull pins with the torque screwdriver.

APPLYING THE VEST
- After the surgeon measures the patient's chest and abdomen, he selects an appropriate-sized vest.
- Place sheepskin liners inside the front and back of the vest for comfort and to help prevent pressure ulcers.
- Help the surgeon carefully logroll or sit up the patient while another practitioner or nurse supports the head and neck; slide the back of the vest under the patient and gently lay him down.
- The surgeon fastens the front of the vest on the patient's chest using Velcro straps and attaches the metal bars to the halo and vest. He tightens each bolt in turn, avoiding tightening completely, which causes maladjusted tension.
- Remove the cervical collar.

⚡ **WARNING** *When the halo-vest traction is in place, lateral cervical spine X-rays must be taken to verify proper alignment.*

COMPLICATIONS
- Loosening of pins
- Infection at pin sites
- Skin breakdown under the vest
- Nerve injury due to spinal cord compression
- Dural penetration of the pins with potential for brain abscess
- Cosmetically apparent scars
- Psychological inability to tolerate being confined in the device
- Respiratory decline in patients with pre-existing severe pulmonary disease
- Treatment failure due to loss of reduction of the spine or failure to develop spinal stability

Comparing halo-vest traction devices

TYPE		DESCRIPTION	ADVANTAGES
Low profile (standard)	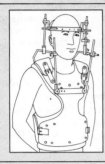	◆ Traction and compression are produced by threaded support rods on either side of the halo ring. ◆ Flexion and extension are obtained by moving the swivel arm to an anterior or posterior position, depending on the location of skull pins.	◆ Immobilizes cervical spine fractures while allowing patient mobility ◆ Facilitates surgery of cervical spine and permits flexion and extension ◆ Allows airway intubation without losing skeletal traction ◆ Facilitates necessary alignment by adjustment at the junction of the threaded support rods and horizontal frame
Mark II (type of low profile)	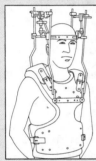	◆ Traction and compression are produced by threaded support rods on either side of the halo ring. ◆ Flexion and extension are obtained by swivel clamps that allow the bars to intersect and hold at any angle.	◆ Enables practitioners to assemble metal framework more quickly ◆ Allows unobstructed access for anteroposterior and lateral X-rays of the cervical spine ◆ Allows patient to wear his usual clothing because uprights are closer to the body
Mark III (update of Mark II)	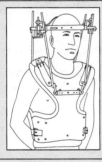	◆ Traction and compression are produced by threaded support rods on either side of the halo ring. ◆ Flexion and extension are accommodated by a serrated split articulation coupling attached to the halo ring, which can be adjusted in 4-degree increments.	◆ Simplifies application while promoting patient comfort ◆ Eliminates shoulder pressure and discomfort by using a flexible padded strap instead of the vest's solid plastic shoulder ◆ Accommodates the tall patient with modified hardware and shorter uprights ◆ Allows unobstructed access for medial and lateral X-rays
Trippi-Wells tongs	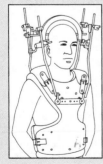	◆ Traction is produced by four pins that compress the skull. ◆ Flexion and extension are obtained by adjusting the midline vertical plate.	◆ Makes it possible to change from mobile to stationary traction without interrupting traction ◆ Adjusts to three planes for mobile and stationary traction ◆ Allows unobstructed access for medial and lateral X-rays

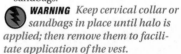

NURSING DIAGNOSES

◆ Disturbed sensory perception (all)
◆ Impaired gas exchange
◆ Impaired skin integrity

EXPECTED OUTCOMES

The patient will:
◆ exhibit no decline in sensory perception
◆ maintain patent airway and adequate oxygenation
◆ remain without change in pin site skin integrity or signs of pressure ulcers under the vest.

PRETREATMENT CARE

◆ Packaged units that include software (jacket and sheepskin liners), hardware (halo, head pins, upright bars, and screws), and tools (torque screwdriver, two conventional wrenches, Allen wrench, and screws and bolts) are commonly used. Obtain a halo-vest traction unit with halo rings and plastic vests in several sizes.
◆ Check for sterility and expiration date of prepackaged tray. Assemble equipment at the patient's bedside.
◆ Check support applied to patient's neck on the way to the hospital. As needed, apply cervical collar or immobilize the head and neck with sandbags.

   WARNING *Keep cervical collar or sandbags in place until halo is applied; then remove them to facilitate application of the vest.*

◆ Explain the basic steps of the procedure to the patient and his family.
◆ Remove the headboard and furniture near the head of the bed to provide ample working space.
◆ Carefully place the patient's head on a board or padded headrest that extends beyond the edge of the bed.
◆ Stand at the head of the bed, and see if the patient's chin lines up with his midsternum, indicating proper alignment.

(continued)

- Verify that an informed consent form has been completed per facility policy.

WARNING *To avoid further spinal cord injury, don't put the patient's head on a pillow before applying the halo.*

- Elevate the bed so the practitioner has access to the front and back of the halo unit.

POSTTREATMENT CARE

- Take routine and neurologic vital signs at least every 2 hours for 24 hours (or every hour for 48 hours), then every 4 hours until stable.

WARNING *Notify the practitioner immediately of any loss of motor function or decreased sensation from baseline, which could indicate spinal cord trauma.*

- Put on gloves and clean the pin sites every 4 hours with cotton-tipped applicators dipped in povidone-iodine or the ordered cleaning solution, to prevent infection and remove debris.
- Rinse the sites with sterile water or normal saline solution to remove excess cleaning solution.
- Watch for signs of infection—a loose pin, swelling or redness, purulent drainage, pain at the site—and notify the practitioner if signs develop.
- Assist the surgeon in retightening the skull pins with the torque screwdriver 24 and 48 hours after the halo is applied.
- If the patient complains of pain after the pins are tightened, obtain an order for an analgesic.

WARNING *If pain occurs with jaw movement, notify the practitioner; this may indicate that the pins have slipped onto the thin temporal plate.*

- Examine the halo-vest every shift to make sure it's secure and the patient's head is centered.
- If the vest fits correctly, you should be able to insert one or two fingers under the jacket at the shoulder and chest when the patient is in a supine position.
- Wash the patient's chest and back daily. Place him on his back, loosening the bottom Velcro straps so you can reach the chest and back.
- Turn the patient on his side (less than 45 degrees) to wash his back. Then close the vest.

WARNING *Don't put stress on the apparatus, which could knock it out of alignment and lead to subluxation of the cervical spine. Never lift or move the patient by the vertical bars because this could strain or tear the skin at the pin sites or misalign the traction.*

- Check frequently for tender areas or pressure spots under the vest that may develop into ulcers.
- If necessary, use a hair dryer to dry damp sheepskin; moisture predisposes the skin to pressure ulcer formation.
- Dust the skin with medicated powder or cornstarch to prevent itching. If itching persists, check to see if patient is allergic to sheepskin or if any drug he's taking might cause skin rash.
- Change the vest lining as necessary, per facility policy.

WARNING *Keep two wrenches available to remove the distal anterior bolts of the vest if cardiac arrest occurs. They may be taped to the halo vest on the chest area. Pull the two upright bars outward, unfasten the chest straps, and remove the front of the vest. Use the back of the vest as a board for cardiopulmonary resuscitation (CPR). Some vests have a hinged front—always know what type of vest the patient is wearing.*

- To prevent subluxating the cervical injury, start CPR with the jaw-thrust maneuver, to avoid hyperextending the neck. Pull the patient's mandible forward, while maintaining proper head and neck alignment. This pulls the tongue forward to open the airway.
- To prevent falls, walk with the ambulatory patient. He may have trouble seeing objects at or near his feet, and the weight of the halo-vest unit (about 10 lb [4.5 kg]) may throw him off balance.
- If the patient's in a wheelchair, lower the leg rests to prevent the chair from tipping backward.
- The vest limits chest expansion; routinely assess pulmonary function, especially in a patient with pulmonary disease.
- Obtain referrals for physical and occupational therapy as needed to evaluate and teach safety precautions and self-care techniques.

GENERAL

- Teach the patient and his family about pin-site care.
- Teach the patient to take three to five deep cleansing breaths every 1 to 2 hours to maintain optimal lung expansion.
- Teach the patient and his family how to shampoo and care for his hair.
- Instruct the patient to turn slowly and incrementally to avoid losing his balance.
- Remind the patient to avoid bending forward; the extra weight of the apparatus may cause him to fall. Instruct him to bend at the knees, not the waist.
- Suggest the patient wear large shirts that button in front to accommodate the halo-vest.

RESOURCES

Organizations

American Academy of Neurology:
  www.aan.com
American Medical Association:
  www.ama-assn.org
American Trauma Society:
  www.amtrauma.org

Selected references

Dickerman, R.D., et al., "Spinal Cord Injury in a 14-Year-Old Male Secondary to Cervical Hyperflexion with Exercise," *Spinal Cord* 44(3):192-95, March 2006.

Shehu, B.B., and Ismail, N.J., "Successful Conservative Management of Traumatic Cervical Spine Fracture-Dislocation," *British Journal of Neurosurgery* 19(1):79, February 2005.

Silva, P., et al., "Two Case Reports of Cervical Spinal Cord Injury in Football (soccer) Players," *Spinal Cord* 44(6): 383-85, June 2006.

Traction, skeletal

- Treatment that exerts a pulling force on part of the body, usually the spine, pelvis, or a long bone of the arm or leg
- Used to reduce fractures, treat dislocations, correct or prevent deformities, improve or correct contractures, or decrease muscle spasms (see *Comparing traction types*)

  AGE FACTOR *The type of mechanical traction used is determined by the orthopedist, based on the patient's condition, age, weight, and skin condition as well as the purpose and expected duration of traction.*

- Involves a pin or wire inserted through the bone; used for longitudinal pulling force (such as fractures of the tibia, femur, or humerus); weight applied is determined by body size and extent of injury
- Applied by an orthopedist

INDICATIONS
- Fracture
- Dislocation
- Deformity
- Contracture
- Muscle spasm

  WARNING *Contraindications to skeletal traction include infections such as osteomyelitis.*

PROCEDURE

- Skeletal traction is applied with the patient under local, general, or spinal anesthesia in an aseptic environment.
- The orthopedist inserts pins, wires, or tongs into or through the affected bone.
- Weights are attached to the pins, wires, or tongs; the usual weight is 25 to 40 lb (11.5 to 18 kg).
- The types of skeletal traction include balanced skeletal, overhead arm, and cervical with tongs.
- Pads, slings, or pushers may be used with traction.

COMPLICATIONS
- Pressure ulcers
- Muscle atrophy
- Weakness
- Contractures
- Osteoporosis
- Urinary stasis and calculi
- Pneumonia
- Thrombophlebitis

- Osteomyelitis
- Nonunion or delayed union of the bone
- Complications of immobility
- Depression

NURSING DIAGNOSES

- Acute pain
- Impaired physical mobility
- Ineffective tissue perfusion: Peripheral

EXPECTED OUTCOMES
The patient will:
- express feelings of increased comfort
- attain the highest degree of mobility possible within the confines of injury
- exhibit adequate tissue perfusion and pulses distally.

Comparing traction types

Traction therapy restricts movement of an affected limb or body part and may confine the patient to bed rest for an extended period. The limb is immobilized by attaching weights that apply pulling force to the affected area. The same level of force—the countertraction—is applied at the opposite end of the limb by attaching additional weights. Countertraction can also be achieved by positioning the patient so that his body weight pulls against the traction force.

SKIN TRACTION
In skin traction, immobilization is accomplished by applying the pulling force directly to the patient's skin. The force may be applied using adhesive or nonadhesive traction tape or skin traction devices, such as a boot, belt, or halter. Adhesive attachment allows more continuous traction, whereas nonadhesive attachment allows easier removal for care.

Skin traction is typically a temporary procedure. It may be applied once or repeatedly applied and removed for an extended period.

SKELETAL TRACTION
Skeletal traction immobilizes a body part by attaching weighted equipment directly to the patient's bones with pins, screws, wires, or tongs. Skeletal traction allows more prolonged traction with heavier weight than skin traction.

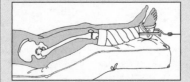

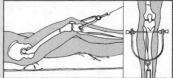

PRETREATMENT CARE

◆ Explain the preparation and treatment to the patient and his family.
◆ Verify that the patient has signed an appropriate consent form.
◆ Set up appropriate traction equipment and a frame according to facility policy.
◆ Emphasize importance of maintaining proper body alignment after traction equipment is set up.

POSTTREATMENT CARE

◆ Administer medications as ordered.
◆ Show the patient how much movement is permitted.
◆ Provide comfort measures.
◆ Maintain the patient in proper body alignment; reposition as necessary.
◆ Provide meticulous skin care.
◆ Administer pin care as ordered. Make sure protruding pin or wire ends are covered with cork. Check pin sites and surrounding skin regularly for signs of infection. Clean pin site and surrounding skin using sterile technique with cotton-tipped applicator dipped in ordered antiseptic. Apply antimicrobial ointment to pin sites, if ordered. Apply sterile gauze pads or petroleum-infused gauze as ordered.
◆ Encourage coughing and deep-breathing exercises.
◆ Assist with ordered range-of-motion exercises for unaffected extremities.
◆ Apply elastic support stockings or compression devices as ordered.
◆ Provide dietary fiber and sufficient fluids.
◆ Administer stool softeners, laxatives, or enemas as needed and ordered.
◆ Inspect traction equipment for kinks, knots, or frays in ropes; make sure the weights hang freely and don't touch the floor.

⚡ *WARNING Maintain traction correctly. At least once per shift, make sure traction equipment connections are tight. Check for impingements such as ropes getting caught between pulleys. Inspect equipment to ensure correct alignment. Inspect the*

ropes for fraying and ensure ropes are positioned properly in the pulley track. Make sure all rope ends are taped above the knot. Inspect traction weights regularly to make sure they hang freely. Weights that touch the floor, bed, or each other reduce traction.

◆ Monitor vital signs.
◆ Monitor intake and output.
◆ Assess skin condition.
◆ If signs of infection occur, notify the practitioner.
◆ Monitor for complications of immobility.
◆ Check neurovascular status of extremities.

PATIENT TEACHING

GENERAL

◆ Review medications and possible adverse reactions with the patient and his family, particularly the use of analgesics.
◆ Inform the patient and his family about the set-up and care of traction equipment.
◆ Show the patient how to use the overhead bed trapeze to reposition without injuring the affected spinal area.
◆ Teach the patient and his family how to care for the pin sites.
◆ Review the signs and symptoms of infection with the patient and his family.
◆ Discuss possible complications with the patient, such as thrombophlebitis or pressure ulcers, and instruct him to notify the practitioner immediately of problems.
◆ Advise the patient how to prevent and manage other complications of immobility.
◆ Tell the patient to follow the diet suggested by the practitioner.
◆ Explain the procedure and why it's needed.
◆ Teach the patient diversional activities within the limits of the traction.
◆ Reinforce the need for bed exercises to prevent muscle atrophy.

◆ Show the patient how much movement he's allowed and instruct him not to adjust the equipment.
◆ Tell him to report pain or pressure from traction equipment.
◆ Stress the need for follow-up care.

RESOURCES
Organizations
American Academy of Orthopaedic Surgeons: *www.aaos.org*
American Academy of Pediatrics: *www.aap.org*
National Foundation for Trauma Care: *www.traumafoundation.org*

Selected references
Holmes, S.B., et al. "Skeletal Pin Site Care: National Association of Orthopaedic Nurses Guidelines for Orthopaedic Nursing," *Orthopaedic Nursing* 24(2): 99-107, March-April 2005.
Patterson, M.M. "Multicenter Pin Care Study," *Orthopaedic Nursing* 24(5): 349-60, September-October 2005.
Talbot, N.J., et al. "A Simple Method of Dressing External Fixator Pin Sites," *Annals of the Royal College of Surgeons of England* 87(3):206-207, May 2005.

Traction, skin

OVERVIEW

- Treatment that exerts a pulling force on a part of the body, usually the spine, pelvis, or a long bone of the arm or leg
- Used to reduce fractures, treat dislocations, correct or prevent deformities, improve or correct contractures, or decrease muscle spasms

  ✿ **AGE FACTOR** *The type of mechanical traction used is determined by the orthopedist, based on the patient's condition, age, weight, and skin condition as well as the purpose and expected duration of traction.*

- Applied directly to the skin (indirectly to the bone)
- Used when a light, temporary, or noncontinuous pulling force is required

INDICATIONS

- Fracture
- Dislocation
- Deformity
- Contracture
- Muscle spasm

  ⚡ **WARNING** *Contraindications to skin traction include severe injury with open wounds, allergy to tape, thrombophlebitis, circulatory disturbances, dermatitis, and varicose veins. Skin traction is used cautiously in patients with diabetes.*

PROCEDURE

- Mechanical traction is applied at the patient's bedside.
- Adhesive or nonadhesive traction tape (or another skin traction device) is used to exert a pulling force (5 to 8 lb [2 to 3.5 kg]) on the skin.
- Types of skin traction include Buck's extension, pelvic (with a pelvic belt), and cervical (with a head halter).

COMPLICATIONS

- Pressure ulcers
- Muscle atrophy
- Weakness
- Contractures
- Osteoporosis
- Urinary stasis and calculi
- Pneumonia
- Thrombophlebitis
- Osteomyelitis
- Nonunion or delayed union of the bone
- Complications of immobility
- Depression

NURSING DIAGNOSES

- Acute pain
- Impaired physical mobility
- Ineffective tissue perfusion: Peripheral

EXPECTED OUTCOMES

The patient will:
- express feelings of increased comfort
- attain the highest degree of mobility possible within the confines of injury
- exhibit adequate tissue perfusion and pulses distally.

PRETREATMENT CARE

- Explain the treatment and preparation to the patient and his family. (See *Learning about pelvic traction.*)
- Verify that the patient has signed an appropriate consent form.
- Set up appropriate traction equipment and a frame according to established facility policy.
- Emphasize importance of maintaining proper body alignment after traction equipment is set up.

POSTTREATMENT CARE

- Administer medications as ordered.
- Show the patient how much movement is permitted.
- Provide comfort measures.
- Unwrap skin traction every shift and assess the skin for redness, warmth, blisters, and other signs of breakdown.
- Maintain the patient in proper body alignment; reposition as necessary.
- Provide meticulous skin care.
- Encourage coughing and deep-breathing exercises.
- Assist with ordered range-of-motion exercises for unaffected extremities.
- Apply elastic support stockings as ordered.
- Provide dietary fiber and sufficient fluids.
- Administer stool softeners, laxatives, or enemas as needed and ordered.

  ⚡ **WARNING** *Maintain traction correctly. At least once per shift, make sure traction equipment connections are tight. Check for impingements such as ropes getting caught between pulleys. Inspect equipment to ensure correct alignment. Inspect the ropes for fraying and make sure ropes are positioned properly in the pulley track. Make sure all rope ends are taped above the knot. Inspect traction weights regularly to make sure they hang freely. Weights that touch the floor, bed, or each other reduce traction.*

- Monitor the patient's vital signs and intake and output.
- Notify the practitioner if signs of pulmonary, skin, or bone infection are observed.
- Monitor for complications of immobility.
- Check neurovascular status of extremities.

Learning about pelvic traction

Dear Patient:

Pelvic traction has been ordered by your health care provider. For about 2 weeks, you'll be spending most of your time in this device. You'll be allowed out of traction for about 4 hours per day to eat meals, use the bathroom, and perform other necessary activities. Here's what to expect.

THE TRACTION SETUP

A beltlike device will be placed around your hipbones over the iliac crests. Make sure you have the correct size belt. It should fit snugly.

Straps on each side of the belt are attach to pulleys, which are attached to weights (8 to 10 lb [3.6 to 4.5 kg] each). Each strap has its own pulley system. Your body weight provides countertraction.

HOW TRACTION WORKS

By exerting a pulling force on your body, traction aligns the lower spine and reduces pressure on the spinal nerve roots. This helps ease back pain and muscle spasms.

PROPER POSITIONING

The head of your bed will be raised 20 to 30 degrees. The traction will hold your lower legs parallel to the floor. Be sure to lie with your hips and knees flexed 30 degrees so your back stays flat against the mattress. However, avoid lying totally flat. This hyperflexes the lumbar spine and may increase your pain.

SOME CAUTIONS

Most patients feel comfortable in pelvic-belt traction. However, if your pain increases, contact the health care provider. The traction may need to be stopped or used intermittently.

Because the traction device is attached directly to the skin, skin breakdown can occur. Remember to check your skin at least twice per day for signs of inflammation, such as redness and swelling.

This patient-teaching aid may be reproduced by office copier for distribution to patients. © 2007 Lippincott Williams & Wilkins.

GENERAL

◆ Review medications and possible adverse reactions with the patient, particularly the use of analgesics.
◆ Inform the patient and his family about the set-up and care of traction equipment.
◆ Show the patient how to use the overhead bed trapeze to reposition without injuring the affected area.
◆ Discuss possible complications with the patient and when to notify the practitioner.
◆ Advise the patient how to prevent and manage complications of immobility.
◆ Tell the patient to follow the diet suggested by the practitioner.
◆ Teach the patient diversional activities within the limits of the traction.
◆ Reinforce the need for bed exercises to prevent muscle atrophy.
◆ Show the patient how much movement he's allowed and instruct him not to adjust the equipment.
◆ Tell the patient to report pain or pressure from traction equipment.
◆ Stress the need for follow-up care.

RESOURCES
Organizations
American Academy of Orthopaedic Surgeons: *www.aaos.org*
American Academy of Pediatrics: *www.aap.org*
National Foundation for Trauma Care: *www.traumafoundation.org*

Selected references
DiFazio, R., and Atkinson, C.C. "Extremity Fractures in Children: When Is It an Emergency?" *Journal of Pediatric Nursing* 20(4):298-304, August 2005.
Kemler, M.A., et al. "Duration of Preoperative Traction Associated with Sciatic Neuropathy after Hip Fracture Surgery," *Clinical Orthopedics and Related Research* 445:230-232, April 2006.
Watters, C.L., et al. "Palliative Care: A Challenge for Orthopaedic Nursing Care," *Orthopaedic Nursing* 24(1):4-7, January-February 2005.

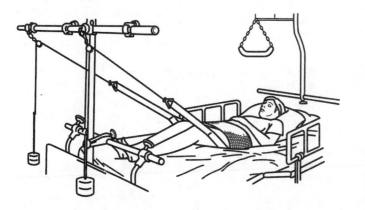

Transcutaneous electrical nerve stimulation

OVERVIEW

- Based on gate control theory of pain (painful impulses pass through a "gate" in the brain)
- Performed with portable battery-powered device that transmits painless electrical current to peripheral nerves or directly to painful area over relatively large nerve fibers
- Changes the patient's perception of pain by blocking painful stimuli traveling over smaller fibers
- Used for postoperative patients and those with chronic pain to reduce the need for analgesics; may allow the patient to resume normal activities
- Usually involves 3 to 5 days of treatment: chronic pain may require intermittent treatments
- May require continuous stimulation for certain conditions, such as phantom limb pain; other conditions, such as a painful arthritic joint, require shorter stimulation periods (3 or 4 hours)
- May be prescribed by a practitioner or registered physical therapist (PT); electrode placement is usually determined initially by the PT
- Also known as *TENS*

INDICATIONS

- Arthritis pain
- Bone fracture pain
- Bursitis pain
- Cancer-related pain
- Musculoskeletal pain
- Myofascial pain
- Pain from neuralgias and neuropathies
- Phantom limb pain
- Postoperative incision pain
- Pain from sciatica
- Whiplash pain

  WARNING Contraindications to TENS include patients with cardiac pacemakers (interferes with function) or dementia and during pregnancy. The unit should also be used cautiously in patients with cardiac disorders. TENS electrodes shouldn't be placed on the head or neck of a patient with a vascular or seizure disorder.

PROCEDURE

- Apply electrode gel to the bottom of each electrode. Electrodes are adhesive and reusable while the adhesive remains intact.
- Place the ordered number of electrodes on the proper skin area, leaving at least 2″ (5 cm) between them. (See *Positioning TENS electrodes*.) Note that some larger patches are designed to contain two electrodes, already separated, in one patch.
- Follow the practitioner's orders about electrode placement. Placement can be over or surrounding the affected area or can be higher in the nerve distribution to block signals to the affected area (as with phantom limb pain). If the patient's skin is moist, a special skin preparation agent can be applied to the skin before the electrodes are applied. Don't use alcohol pads.

  WARNING Incorrect placement of the electrodes results in inappropriate pain control. Never place the electrodes near the patient's eyes or over the nerves that innervate the carotid sinus or laryngeal or pharyngeal muscles to avoid interference with critical nerve function.

- Insert the leadwires into the electrodes. Make sure that the control box controls are off, and then insert the leadwire plug ends into the control box.
- Gradually increase the control settings to within the parameters set by the practitioner. Usually, the pattern and intensity of the stimulation can be set separately.

Positioning TENS electrodes

In transcutaneous electrical nerve stimulation (TENS), electrodes placed around peripheral nerves (or an incisional site) transmit mild electrical pulses to the brain. The current is thought to block pain impulses. The patient can influence the level and frequency of his pain relief by adjusting the controls on the device.

Typically, electrode placement varies even though patients may have similar complaints. Electrodes can be placed in several ways:
- to cover the painful area or surround it, as with muscle tenderness or spasm or painful joints
- to "capture" the painful area between electrodes, as with incisional pain.

In peripheral nerve injury, electrodes should be placed proximal to the injury (between the brain and the injury site) to avoid increasing pain. Placing electrodes in a hypersensitive area also increases pain. In an area lacking sensation, electrodes should be placed on adjacent dermatomes.

These illustrations show combinations of electrode placement (squares) and areas of nerve stimulation (shaded areas) for lower back and leg pain.

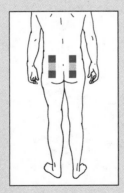
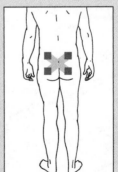
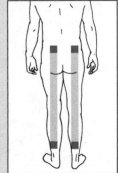

- Set the controls to a level comfortable for the patient; that is, when he feels a comfortable tingling sensation, generally between 60 and 100 Hz.

  ⚡ **WARNING** *Setting the controls too high can cause pain; setting them too low will fail to relieve pain.*

- Attach the TENS control box to part of the patient's clothing, such as a belt, pocket, or bra. Carefully place extra leadwire into clothing so it doesn't dangle loosely.
- To make sure the device is working effectively, monitor for signs of excessive stimulation, such as muscle twitches, and for signs of inadequate stimulation, signaled by the patient not feeling a mild tingling sensation.
- If TENS is used continuously for postoperative pain, remove the electrodes at least daily to check for skin irritation, to provide skin care, and to rotate sites of electrode placement.
- When treatment is completed, turn the controls to OFF and unplug the leadwires from the control box. The electrodes and leadwires may remain on the patient if another treatment will be done soon. The battery should be removed from the unit for charging and the charged battery reinserted.

COMPLICATIONS
- Failure to achieve intended effect
- Skin irritation or allergy to electrode materials

NURSING DIAGNOSES
- Acute pain
- Impaired physical mobility
- Ineffective tissue perfusion: Peripheral

EXPECTED OUTCOMES
The patient will:
- express feelings of increased comfort
- attain the highest degree of mobility possible within the confines of injury
- exhibit adequate tissue perfusion and pulses distally.

PRETREATMENT CARE
- Explain the function of the unit and how it's applied.
- Obtain a commercial TENS kit; this includes the stimulator, leadwires, electrodes, spare battery pack, and battery recharger. Before beginning, always test the battery pack to make sure it's fully charged.
- Provide privacy and demonstrate the procedure to the patient.
- Clean the skin thoroughly where the electrode will be applied with an alcohol pad, then dry.
- If necessary, shave hair at the site where each electrode will be placed, taking care not to break the skin.

POSTTREATMENT CARE
- Turn off the controls and unplug the electrode leadwires, unless another treatment will be given soon, then leave the electrodes in place. If the electrodes must be moved during the procedure, first turn off the controls.
- Clean the electrodes with soap and water, and clean the patient's skin with alcohol pads. Check the patient's skin for reddening or other signs of allergy to the adhesive.
- Don't soak the electrodes in alcohol because it will damage the rubber. Place the electrodes back on the supplied silicone sheet to maintain gel freshness until the next application.

  ⚡ **WARNING** *Replace used electrodes with new ones when the adhesive no longer holds tightly.*

- Remove the battery pack and replace it with a charged battery pack.
- Recharge the used battery pack so it's always ready for use.

(continued)

Learning about TENS

Dear Patient:

Your health care provider has ordered transcutaneous electrical nerve stimulation (TENS) to help relieve your pain.

HOW TENS WORKS

A small, battery-operated device sends safe electrical signals through wires and into your body by way of electrodes, which you attach to your skin.

WHERE TO PLACE THE ELECTRODES

Your TENS therapist will show you where to attach the electrodes. Ask him to label the sites with a marker. If necessary, use a mirror to help you see them. Ask a friend or a family member to note the sites, too. That way he can reassure you if you feel nervous the first few times you use the TENS unit. If needed, he can help you place the electrodes another time.

Placing your electrodes on the wrong sites probably won't harm you, but avoid placing them on your belly if you're pregnant, on the sides of the neck, or on the voice box area.

USING TENS

The knobs on your unit are adjustable:
◆ Set the AMP/A at _____.
◆ Set the rate at _____.
◆ Set the pulse-width at _____.
◆ Turn your TENS unit ON for _____ minutes and OFF for _____ minutes throughout the day.

You should feel a pleasant sensation while the machine is working. If you develop muscle spasms, contact the TENS therapist. The AMP may be set too high, or your may have placed the electrodes in the wrong places.

If your pain increases, follow the directions your TENS therapist gave you to change the settings on your TENS unit.

SAFETY TIPS

Follow your therapist's instructions carefully for the amount of time you should leave your TENS unit on. Don't get into water with the unit on, and don't sleep with it on.

SKIN CARE

Take good care of your skin. Prevent local skin irritation—redness and rash—by cleaning your skin before attaching the electrodes. Watch for signs of irritation.

If your skin becomes irritated, don't place electrodes on those areas. Keep the skin clean and dry until it heals. If it's still irritated after 1 week, contact your health care provider.

If you repeatedly develop local skin irritation from the electrodes, contact your TENS therapist to discuss an alternate wearing schedule or another type of electrode.

CARING FOR THE TENS UNIT

Clean your TENS unit weekly by lightly wiping it with rubbing alcohol.

GENERAL

◆ Review the operator's manual with the patient and reinforce where to locate trouble-shooting information.

◆ Teach the patient how to place the electrodes properly and how to take care of the TENS unit. (See *Learning about TENS.*)

◆ Instruct the patient to report to the practitioner if the treatment becomes ineffective or causes skin irritation.

◆ Teach the patient about medications being taken, including administration and potential adverse reactions.

◆ Instruct the patient to noify the PT or practitioner if the treatment is no longer effective.

RESOURCES

Organizations

American College of Emergency Physicians: *www.acep.org*
American College of Surgeons: *www.facs.org*
American Medical Association: *www.ama-assn.org*

Selected references

Ainsworth, L., et al. "Transcutaneous Electrical Nerve Stimulation (TENS) Reduces Chronic Hyperalgesia Induced by Muscle Inflammation," *Pain* 120(1-2):182-87, January 2006.

Goodstadt, N.M. "Gate Control," *Rehab Management* 18(10):30, 32-33, December 2005.

Khadilkar, A., et al. "Treatment Options for Patients with Osteoarthritis of the Knee," *British Journal of Nursing* 14(18):976-81, October 2005.

Shea, B., and Saginur, M. "Transcutaneous Electrical Nerve Stimulation for the Treatment of Chronic Low Back Pain: A Systematic Review," *Spine* 30(23):2657-66, December 2005.

Transjugular intrahepatic portosystemic shunt

OVERVIEW

- Insertion of small, flexible tube made of medical grade plastic or wire mesh to create a new passageway from the portal vein to the hepatic vein, diverting blood flow away from the liver
- Diverts blood that's returning to the heart from the spleen and intestines, thereby reducing pressure in the portal system within the liver
- Also known as *TIPS*

INDICATIONS

- End-stage portal hypertension
- Active, or recurrent, varices despite treatment
- Ascites unresponsive to other treatments

PROCEDURE

- The patient receives general anesthesia or conscious sedation.
- The procedure is done in a specially equipped suite with emergency equipment and staffing. The patient's electrocardiogram and oxygen status are monitored during the procedure.
- The interventional radiologist threads a catheter through a small incision in the skin near the jugular vein in the neck and guides it through the vena cava to the hepatic vein, using fluoroscopy or ultrasonography.
- With X-ray guidance, the radiologist directs a special needle through the wall of the hepatic vein, across a gap, and into the portal vein.
- Dye is injected to verify catheter placement.
- A balloon is used to dilate the new tract, then one to three stents are inserted and opened to maintain the flow.
- Dye is reinjected to verify correct flow from hepatic vein to portal vein to inferior vena cava.
- The catheter is removed and the incision sutured and bandaged.

COMPLICATIONS

- Bleeding or bruising at the catheter site
- Hematoma of the neck or liver area
- Cardiac arrhythmias
- Liver capsule rupture
- Septicemia
- Hepatic failure
- Encephalopathy
- Shunt failure
- Exsanguination and death

NURSING DIAGNOSES

- Activity intolerance
- Deficient fluid volume
- Risk for infection

EXPECTED OUTCOMES

The patient will:

- carry out activities of daily living without excess fatigue or decreased energy
- maintain adequate blood volume as indicated by hematocrit and pulse oximetry
- remain free from infection.

PRETREATMENT CARE

- Make sure that preliminary evaluation is completed as ordered; this may include liver function testing, angiography, or endoscopy depending on the patient's condition.
- Make sure that diagnostic testing has been completed, including computer tomography, magnetic resonance imaging, ultrasound imaging (such as Doppler ultrasound), and X-rays as indicated.
- Review the procedure with the patient and answer questions.
- Verify that a consent form has been signed.
- Review with the patient what to expect postoperatively.
- Perform a baseline cardiopulmonary and abdominal assessment, including height and weight.
- Make sure that the patient doesn't take anything by mouth after midnight before the procedure.
- Make sure that pre-existing treatments have been performed as ordered.
- Note allergies and medications the patient is taking.

POSTTREATMENT CARE

- Assess vital signs at least every 15 minutes for the first hour, then every 30 minutes for the next hour, and then every hour until the patient is stable.
- Monitor the patient's level of consciousness (LOC), including observing for increased alertness; reorient the patient as necessary. Continue to monitor LOC frequently for changes that may indicate adverse effects of the procedure or possible bleeding.
- Monitor intake and output and daily weight.
- Inspect the catheter insertion site closely for signs and symptoms of bleeding and infection. Change the dressing as ordered.

⚡ **WARNING** *Because of the patient's underlying liver disease, coagulation may be altered. Monitor the dressing at least every 30 minutes initially, and then every 1 or 2 hours. Immediately report bright red drainage on the dressing.*

- Assess cardiopulmonary status at least hourly, noting changes in heart or breath sounds. Institute continuous cardiac monitoring to evaluate for possible arrhythmias secondary to the TIPS procedure or to possible variceal bleeding.
- Monitor hemodynamic values as ordered to evaluate the patient's fluid volume status.
- Assess abdomen for bowel sounds and distention; measure abdominal girth. When bowel sounds return, expect to begin oral feedings.

⚡ **WARNING** *Insertion should cause the patient's abdominal girth to gradually decrease. However, because of the underlying liver disease, bleeding can occur at the catheter insertion site. Be alert to increases in abdominal girth, and notify the practitioner immediately. This increase may indicate bleeding or that the stent isn't functioning.*

- Assess the patient for complaints of abdominal cramping (an expected finding), and administer medication as ordered.
- Check gag reflex, and maintain nothing-by-mouth status until the gag reflex returns.
- Maintain patency of I.V. tubes and provide hydration as ordered.
- Administer medications as ordered, including analgesics as needed.
- Encourage the patient to breathe deeply and cough as indicated; assist with using an incentive spirometer.
- Assist with ambulation as ordered.

⚡ **WARNING** *Report signs of hypovolemic shock, liver failure, sepsis, or cardiac arrhythmia immediately.*

- Before discharge, an ultrasound is done to determine the effectiveness of the shunt. If the shunt appears to be working properly, the patient is allowed to be discharged.
- Monitor the patient's intake and output and daily weight.

PATIENT TEACHING

GENERAL

- Tell the patient about exercise and driving restrictions.
- Review the signs of complications and what to report to the practitioner.
- Review medication administration, dosages, and adverse effects with the patient.
- Inform the patient about dietary restrictions to minimize esophageal or gastric variceal irritation.
- Tell the patient to rest and drink plenty of fluids, except alcoholic beverages.
- Instruct the patient to avoid lifting heavy objects or performing strenuous exercises, and to stop smoking for at least 24 hours. Advise the patient to stop smoking permanently because it's a major cause of atherosclerosis and tissue irritation.
- Inform the patient that 10 to 14 days after discharge, he'll meet with his regular practitioner to evaluate his progress and undergo laboratory testing.
- Tell the patient that 6 weeks after the TIPS procedure (and again at 3 and 6 months) an ultrasound will be done to check shunt function. An angiogram may also be done if the ultrasound indicates a problem. Also, laboratory testing will be done at these visits.
- Inform the patient that at 12 months after the procedure, an ultrasound, angiogram, and laboratory testing will be done to ensure that the shunt is working properly. The patient will also meet with the practitioner during this visit.
- If the shunt is working well, every 6 months after the first year of follow-up appointments the patient will have an ultrasound, undergo laboratory testing, and meet with the practitioner.
- Inform the patient that more frequent follow-up visits may be needed depending on his condition.
- Stress the need for the patient to attend all follow-up appointments to ensure that the shunt is functioning properly.

RESOURCES
Organizations
American College of Surgeons: *www.facs.org*
American Medical Association: *www.ama-assn.org*

Selected references
Cardenas, A., and Gines, P. "Management of Refractory Ascites," *Clinics in Gastroenterology and Hepatology* 3(12): 1187-91, December 2005.
Perkins, J.D. "Indications for Chronic Albumin Infusion," *Liver Transplantation* 12(2):320-23, February 2006.
Wolf, D.C., et al. "Emergent Stent Occlusion for TIPS-Induced Liver Failure," *Digestive Diseases and Sciences* 50(12): 2356-58, December 2005.

Transmyocardial laser revascularization

- Used to treat inoperable cardiac ischemia in patients with persistent angina that's unrelieved by other methods
- Improves blood flow to areas of the heart that can't be treated by angioplasty or coronary artery surgery
- Employs a special carbon dioxide (CO_2) laser creating small channels in poorly perfused but non-necrotic ventricular heart tissue stimulating reperfusion of the muscle through new collateral circulation
- New channels thought to promote angiogenesis (growth of new capillaries)
- Also known as *TMR*

INDICATIONS
- Angina
- Inoperable heart disease

  WARNING *Contraindicated if the heart muscle is severely damaged or necrotic from a myocardial infarction or if the heart muscle has a lot of scar tissue.*

- The patient is given general anesthesia but doesn't require cardiopulmonary bypass or heart stoppage.
- A small incision is made in the left or middle of the chest. The underlying tissues are separated and retracted to expose the heart muscle.
- The laser hand piece is positioned over the poorly perfused ventricular muscle. A special high-energy, computerized CO_2 laser is used to create 20 to 40 1-mm wide channels in the left ventricle. The channels penetrate all layers of the heart but the pericardial holes quickly close. The channels through the myocardium and endocardium remain open. (See *The transmyocardial laser revascularization process.*)
- The laser is guided by a computer that monitors the patient's electrocardiogram so that the laser cuts only between heartbeats, when the ventricle is filled with blood and the heart is relatively still. This helps to prevent arrhythmias.

COMPLICATIONS
- Cardiac tamponade
- Hypovolemic shock
- Arrhythmias

- Activity intolerance
- Decreased cardiac output
- Ineffective tissue perfusion: Cardiopulmonary

EXPECTED OUTCOMES
The patient will:
- carry out activities of daily living without excess fatigue or decreased energy
- maintain adequate cardiac output
- maintain adequate heart rate and rhythm, respiratory rate and depth, and clear lungs.

The transmyocardial laser revascularization process

During transmyocardial laser revascularization (TMR), the laser handpiece is placed on the surface of the heart. The special laser beam is used to create multiple tiny channels through all three layers of the heart muscle. The epicardial channels quickly heal, but the myocardial channels remain open, reperfusing the heart muscle and stimulating creation of new capillaries in the area.

- Endocardium
- Myocardium
- Epicardium
- Blocked vessel
- Laser probe
- Open channel

PRETREATMENT CARE

◆ Tests required before TMR include cardiac catheterization, echocardiogram, positron emission tomography, dobutamine echocardiography, and cardiac magnetic resonance imaging.
◆ Review the disorder and the procedure with the patient and answer questions.
◆ Verify that a consent form has been signed.
◆ Review with the patient what to expect postoperatively.
◆ Perform a baseline assessment and verify pulse quality.
◆ Make sure the patient doesn't take anything by mouth after midnight before the procedure.
◆ Check that treatments have been performed as ordered.
◆ Note allergies and medications the patient is taking.

POSTTREATMENT CARE

◆ Monitor vital signs, peripheral pulses, intake and output, and heart, lung, and abdominal sounds.
◆ Assess hemodynamic status, cardiac monitoring, and pulse oximetry.
◆ Maintain patency of I.V. tubes and provide hydration as ordered.
◆ Administer medications as ordered.
◆ Assess dressings and distal pulses regularly.
◆ Encourage coughing and deep-breathing exercises as indicated; assist with incentive spirometry.
◆ Assist with ambulation as ordered.
◆ Provide wound care as indicated and check for signs and symptoms of infection.

🔺 **WARNING** *Report signs of hypovolemic shock, renal failure, sepsis, or respiratory failure immediately.*

PATIENT TEACHING

GENERAL

◆ Review exercise and driving restrictions with the patient; recommend a supervised cardiac rehabilitation program to help guide recovery and to progress his activity level.
◆ Discuss the signs of complications and what to report to the practitioner.
◆ Review medication administration, dosages, and adverse effects.
◆ Tell the patient about dietary restrictions.
◆ Instruct the patient about the use of an incentive spirometer.
◆ Explain the need for early ambulation, as directed by the practitioner.
◆ Inform the patient that after TMR, some patients have immediate relief from anginal symptoms, whereas for others it is gradual. Also, tell him that some patients don't have improved symptoms, but may have improved tolerance for activity.
◆ Inform the patient that he may still be required to take medications after the procedure to improve blood flow to his heart.
◆ Advise the patient that he'll need to have frequent follow-up visits with the practitioner so that his progress can be evaluated.

RESOURCES
Organizations
American College of Surgeons: *www.facs.org*
American Heart Association: *www.americanheart.org*
American Medical Association: *www.ama-assn.org*

Selected references
Gowdak, L.H., et al. "Mid-Term Results after Thoracoscopic Transmyocardial Laser Revascularization," *Annals of Thoracic Surgery* 80(2):553-68, August 2005.
Krieger, J.E., et al. "Cell Therapy plus Transmyocardial Laser Revascularization for Refractory Angina," *Annals of Thoracic Surgery* 80(2):712-14, August 2005.
Stanik-Hutt, J.A. "Management Options for Angina Refractory to Maximal Medical and Surgical Interventions," *AACN Clinical Issues* 16(3):320-32, July-September 2005.
Yuh, D.D., et al. "Totally Endoscopic Robot-Assisted Transmyocardial Revascularization." *Journal of Thoracic and Cardiovascular Surgery* 130(1):120-24, July 2004.

Transplantation, bone marrow

- Involves infusion of fresh or stored bone marrow into the bloodstream; donated marrow cells migrate to the patient's bone marrow in 10 days to 4 weeks, then begin proliferating
- Performed to replace blood cells destroyed by chemotherapeutic or radiologic destruction of cancerous blood cells
- In *autologous* donation, bone marrow harvested from patient (before chemotherapy or radiation, or during remission) and frozen for use up to 2 weeks later
- In *syngeneic* donation, bone marrow donated by patient's identical twin
- In *allogenic* donation, bone marrow donated by histocompatible individual (see *Understanding your role as a bone marrow donor*)

INDICATIONS
- Aplastic anemia
- Severe combined immunodeficiency diseases
- Acute lymphocytic leukemia
- Myeloid leukemias
- Lymphoma
- Multiple myeloma
- Certain solid tumors
- Sickle cell anemia

- The patient is treated at the bedside. The practitioner inserts a central venous catheter, if none is in place.
- An antihistamine or analgesic is administered as ordered.
- With syngeneic or allogenic donation, marrow is obtained in the operating room the same day as transplantation and is brought to the patient's room immediately.
- For autologous donation, the marrow is allowed to thaw before infusion.
- The practitioner infuses the marrow through the central venous catheter over 2 to 4 hours.
- The nurse obtains vital signs every 15 minutes for 1 hour, every 30 minutes for 2 hours, then every hour for 4 hours. The infusion lasts 2 to 4 hours.
- The patient is monitored for fever, dyspnea, hypotension, bronchospasm, urticaria, chest pain, and back pain throughout the infusion.

COMPLICATIONS
During infusion
- Fluid volume overload
- Anaphylaxis
- Pulmonary fat embolism

After infusion
- Infection
- Abnormal bleeding
- Renal insufficiency
- Venous occlusive disease
- Graft-versus-host disease (GVHD; with allogeneic donation)

- Activity intolerance
- Deficient fluid volume
- Ineffective tissue perfusion: Renal, cardiopulmonary

EXPECTED OUTCOMES
The patient will:
- demonstrate increased ability to perform activities of daily living
- maintain adequate fluid volume
- maintain adequate heart rate and rhythm, pulse amplitude, respiratory rate and oxygen saturation, and intake and output.

Understanding your role as a bone marrow donor

Dear Donor:

As a donor, your healthy bone marrow cells will replace diseased marrow in a patient with leukemia. Here's what to expect.

BEFORE THE PROCEDURE

To make sure you're in the best possible health to donate bone marrow, your health care provider will schedule:

♦ a complete physical examination (you'll also need to answer detailed questions about your health history)
♦ blood and urine tests
♦ a chest X-ray
♦ an electrocardiogram to check your heart.

The night before the procedure, you'll shower using antiseptic soap. This reduces the risk of infection developing during the procedure. Remember, don't eat or drink anything after midnight because your stomach must be empty before you get an anesthetic.

Shortly before the procedure, an I.V. line will be inserted into your hand or arm to provide you with fluids during the procedure. You'll also receive some medicine to make you relax. You may feel sleepy.

DURING THE PROCEDURE

Next, you'll be taken to an operating room, where you'll receive an anesthetic. When the anesthesia takes effect, about 5% of your marrow cells will be collected by placing a needle in your front and back hipbone. The marrow will be filtered to remove fat and bone particles, and then it will be prepared for transplantation.

While you're in the operating room, you may receive 1 unit of blood to help rebuild your bone marrow. The entire procedure takes about 2 to 3 hours. Once it's finished, a pressure dressing will be applied over the area.

AFTER THE PROCEDURE

From the operating room, you'll be moved to the recovery room. When you awaken, you can expect to feel some pain, but you'll receive medicine to relieve it. Your hip area will be covered with tight bandages for about 1 day. When they're removed, the nurse will teach you to keep the area clean and covered for about 3 more days.

In 1 or 2 days, you'll probably be discharged from the hospital. Then you can return to your usual activities. You may experience bone aches and pain for several days to a few weeks.

This patient-teaching aid may be reproduced by office copier for distribution to patients. © 2007 Lippincott Williams & Wilkins.

PRETREATMENT CARE

♦ Explain the treatment and the necessary preparation to the patient. (See *Learning about bone marrow transplantation,* page 388.)
♦ For an allogenic graft, discuss the immunosuppressant drugs that the patient will be taking, and explain their possible adverse effects. Remind the patient that these drugs increase his risk for infection.
♦ Instruct the patient and family members about measures used to control infection and minimize rejection after transplant.
♦ Verify that the patient has signed an appropriate consent form.
♦ Keep diphenhydramine (Benadryl) and epinephrine (Adrenalin) readily available to manage transfusion reactions.
♦ Start an I.V. line, if needed, and administer I.V. fluids as ordered.
♦ Obtain an administration set with a special filter for debris.
♦ Administer medications as ordered.
♦ Obtain baseline vital signs.

WARNING *Be alert for signs and symptoms of bronchospasm, urticaria, erythema, chest pain, and back pain.*

(continued)

Learning about bone marrow transplantation

Dear Patient:

Your health care provider wants you to have a bone marrow transplantation. This procedure will replace diseased bone marrow with healthy cells. Because bone marrow forms blood cells, healthy marrow is essential for life.

OBTAINING THE BONE MARROW

Your bone marrow transplant may come from your brother or sister, mother or father, or another donor whose marrow closely matches your own. In some cases, the transplant may be a sample of your own marrow, which has previously been removed and frozen.

PREPARING FOR TRANSPLANTATION

Before the transplantation, you may receive chemotherapy and total-body radiation to destroy your diseased marrow and to suppress your immune system so that the transplanted marrow can become part of you, or "engraft," with minimal complications.

INFUSING THE BONE MARROW

After the bone marrow has been obtained and processed, it will be infused through I.V. tubing or through a special I.V. catheter that has been placed near your collarbone.

After circulating through your bloodstream, the transplanted cells will eventually lodge in your bone marrow spaces. Here the transplanted cells will grow and produce healthy blood cells in 2 to 4 weeks.

AFTER THE TRANSPLANTATION

Until the donor marrow grafts itself, you'll be especially vulnerable to infection. Hospital precautions may range from careful hand washing to wearing sterile hats, gowns, and shoe covers to minimize contact with germs. For 3 or 4 weeks after the transplantation, you'll also need blood transfusions.

FOLLOW-UP CARE

After you're discharged from the hospital, you'll need regular medical checkups because your immune system needs a long time to recover. Plan to stay away from work or school for 6 months to 1 year after the transplantation.

UNDERSTANDING THE RISKS

The most serious complication of a bone marrow transplant is graft-versus-host disease (GVHD). In this condition, the transplanted bone marrow works against you. The disease may be acute (occurring 1 to 6 weeks after transplantation), or it may be delayed (occurring about 3 months after transplantation).

Protect yourself by learning and reporting suspicious symptoms, including signs of infection (such as breathing problems, dry cough, fatigue, and fever) or bleeding, especially from your nose or gums.

Immediately report abnormally dry eyes, diarrhea, a rash, or skin changes. Follow instructions for medication therapy to help prevent GVHD.

POSTTREATMENT CARE

- Maintain asepsis.
- Institute safety measures.
- Administer transfusions as ordered.
- Obtain blood samples for laboratory analysis as ordered.
- Monitor vital signs and laboratory test results.
- Assess the patient for signs of infection, hemorrhage, and GVHD.

PATIENT TEACHING

GENERAL

- Explain each prescribed medication to the patient, including dosage and possible adverse effects.
- If appropriate, tell the patient that because immunosuppressive medications interfere with his natural immune system, he needs to take the following precautions to avoid infection: wash hands often; keep hands away from face and mouth; stay away from people with colds or other infections; ask friends to visit only when they're well; wash hands before and after dressing changes; wash hands after coughing or sneezing, and throw tissues into the trash immediately; and if a family member has a cold or the flu, have that person follow normal precautions (such as using separate drinking glasses and covering his mouth when coughing).
- Tell the patient how to avoid injury or bleeding.
- Teach the patient to care for his central venous catheter if it's to remain in place for some time.
- Discuss the signs and symptoms of transplant failure and other complications of the procedure.
- Instruct the patient to notify the practitioner at the first sign of complications or rejection or if he has questions.
- Provide the patient with telephone numbers to contact in an emergency.
- Review when the patient should return to the surgeon and hematologist for follow-up care.
  - **AGE FACTOR** *Teach the parents of a pediatric bone marrow recipient how to monitor the child's growth and development.*
- Review with the patient and his family access to support groups and online resources and forums for patients.

RESOURCES

Organizations

American Medical Association: *www.ama-assn.org*
American Society of Clinical Oncologists: *www.plwc.org*
National Marrow Donor Program: *www.marrow.org*

Selected references

Hayashi, T., et al. "Effects of Sarpogrelate Hydrochloride in a Patient with Chronic Graft-Versus-Host Disease: A Case Report," *American Journal of Hematology* 81(2):121-23, January 2006.

Shaiegan, M., et al. "Effect of IL-18 and sIL2R on a GVHD Occurrence after Hematopoietic Stem Cell Transplantation in Some Iranian Patients," *Transplant Immunology* 15(3):223-27, January 2006.

Tamura, K., et al. "Successful Rapid Discontinuation of Immunosuppressive Therapy at Molecular Relapse after Allogeneic Bone Marrow Transplantation in a Pediatric Patient with Myelodysplastic Syndrome," *American Journal of Hematology* 81(2):139-41, January 2006.

Transplantation, cerebral stem cell

- Experimental treatment for Parkinson's disease
- Involves grafting of fetal or adult stem cells into the striatum of affected patients
- Under study: direct modification of existing brain cells by infecting the cells with viruses that carry modified genes for dopamine production or other actions (called a *transfection procedure*)

INDICATIONS

- Neurologic disorders such as Parkinson's disease

PROCEDURE

- The patient is given general anesthesia and his head shaved where the incision will be made.
- The neurosurgeon accesses selected brain tissue, such as in the cortex, hippocampus, or thalamus, with stereotaxic guidance via small burr holes in the skull and dural retraction.
- Genetically engineered cells, adrenal chromaffin cells, fetal neurons, or dopamine-producing tissues have been grafted experimentally.

COMPLICATIONS

- Infection
- Graft rejection
- Increased intracranial pressure (ICP)

NURSING DIAGNOSES

- Disturbed sensory perception (all)
- Ineffective tissue perfusion: Cerebral
- Risk for injury

EXPECTED OUTCOMES

The patient will:
- exhibit improved or normal neurologic status
- maintain ICP within normal limits without negative changes in neurologic vital signs
- remain free from injury.

PRETREATMENT CARE

- Check laboratory values, electrocardiogram, and chest X-rays as ordered, and notify the practitioner of abnormalities.
- Assess the patient's neurologic status and cardiopulmonary status and obtain baseline vital signs.
- Obtain stereotaxic X-rays as ordered for use during the procedure.
- Review the explanation of the planned surgical technique with the patient.
- Verify that the patient has signed a consent form.
- Explain what the patient can expect after he wakens from anesthesia, including the presence of I.V. lines, an indwelling urinary catheter, an arterial line and, possibly, a mechanical ventilator. Describe routine postoperative care, including frequent checks of vital signs, monitoring of intake and output, and respiratory therapy. Prepare him for postoperative pain, and reassure him that analgesics will be available.
- Teach the patient the proper methods for performing coughing, turning, deep breathing and, if ordered, incentive spirometry.
- Discuss the immunosuppressant drugs that the patient will be taking, and explain their possible adverse effects. Remind the patient that these drugs increase his risk for infection.
- Instruct the patient and family members about measures used to control infection and minimize rejection after transplant.
- Tell the patient with Parkinson's disease that he may need adjustment in his medications preoperatively and postoperatively.

POSTTREATMENT CARE

◆ Administer oxygen as indicated, and suction and turn the patient.
◆ Apply elastic stockings or compression boots to reduce the risk of deep vein thrombosis as ordered.
◆ Administer I.V. fluids as ordered.
◆ Assess neurologic status and report changes in trends; monitor for increased ICP.
◆ Monitor intake and output and laboratory test results.

PATIENT TEACHING

GENERAL

◆ Teach the patient and his family how to care for the scalp incisions and to watch for signs and symptoms of infection.
◆ Review medications with the patient and his family, including current doses, expected effects and potential adverse effects.
◆ Review the signs of complications with the patient, such as headache, nausea, vomiting, and changes in level of consciousness or return of previous symptoms or worsening of condition, and tell him to notify the practitioner if these occur.
◆ Tell the patient that because immunosuppressive medications interfere with his natural immune system, he needs to take the following precautions to avoid infection: wash hands often; keep hands away from face and mouth; stay away from people with colds or other infections; ask friends to visit only when they're well; wash hands before and after dressing changes; wash hands after coughing or sneezing, and throw tissues into the trash immediately; and if a family member has a cold or the flu, have that person follow normal precautions (such as using separate drinking glasses and covering his mouth when coughing).
◆ Refer the patient to a home health care service or a rehabilitation center upon discharge, as ordered.

RESOURCES

Organizations

American Academy of Neurology: *www.aan.com*
American Medical Association: *www.ama-assn.org*
National Parkinson Foundation: *www.parkinson.org*

Selected references

Arnhold, S., et al. "Human Bone Marrow Stroma Cells Display Certain Neural Characteristics and Integrate in the Subventricular Compartment After Injection into the Liquor System," *European Journal of Cell Biology* 85(6):551-65, June 2006.

Longhi, L., et al. "Stem Cell Transplantation as a Therapeutic Strategy for Traumatic Brain Injury," *Transplant Immunology* 15(2):143-48, December 2005.

Snyder, B.J., and Olanow, C.W. "Stem Cell Treatment for Parkinson's Disease: An Update for 2005," *Current Opinion in Neurology* 18(4):376-85, August 2005.

Transplantation, corneal

- Damaged portion of cornea replaced with cornea from eye of a donor, available through an eye bank
- Most common type of transplant surgery; has highest success rate
- Surgery considered when corneal damage too severe for treatment with corrective lenses; may be combined with other eye procedures (such as cataract surgery) to resolve multiple eye problems
- May require up to 1 year for healing and full visual correction because corneal tissue is avascular
- Also known as *keratoplasty*

INDICATIONS
- Keratoconus
- Fuchs' dystrophy
- Pseudophakic bullous keratopathy
- Chemical burns to cornea
- Mechanical trauma
- Infection by viruses, bacteria, fungi, or protozoa

WARNING *Although the cornea isn't normally vascular, some corneal diseases cause vascularization into the cornea. In such patients, careful testing of both donor and recipient is done, and repeated surgery may be needed for a successful transplant.*

PROCEDURE
- The patient may receive a local or general anesthetic.
- A disc of tissue is removed from the center of the eye and replaced with a disc from the donor eye. The circular incision is made using a trephine.
- In penetrating keratoplasty—the most common type of corneal transplant—the disc removed is the entire thickness of the cornea as is the replacement disc.
- In lamellar keratoplasty, only the outer layer of the cornea is removed and replaced.
- The donor cornea is attached with fine sutures and an eye patch and shield applied.

COMPLICATIONS
- Infection
- Glaucoma
- Retinal detachment
- Cataract formation
- Rejection of donor cornea
- Photophobia

NURSING DIAGNOSES
- Acute pain
- Disturbed sensory perception (visual)
- Risk for infection

EXPECTED OUTCOMES
The patient will:
- express feelings of comfort
- demonstrate improved visual function
- demonstrate intact tissue without signs of infection.

PRETREATMENT CARE
- Some eye surgeons may request that the patient have a complete physical examination before surgery.
- Ask the patient not to eat on the day of surgery.
- Make sure that active infection or inflammation of the eye is controlled before surgery.
- Review the planned surgical technique with the patient. Tell him that he'll receive a sedative to help him relax.
- Inform the patient that, after surgery, he may have to wear an eye patch and eye shield temporarily to prevent traumatic injury and infection.
- Instruct the patient to call for help when getting out of bed, and tell him that he should sleep on the unaffected side to reduce ocular pressure.
- Explain that he will temporarily experience loss of depth perception and decreased peripheral vision on the operative side.
- If ordered, perform an antiseptic facial scrub to reduce the risk of infection.
- Verify that the patient has signed a consent form.

- After the patient returns to his room, notify the practitioner if severe pain, bleeding, increased drainage, or fever occurs.
- Because of the change in the patient's depth perception, keep the side rails of his bed raised, assist him with ambulation, and observe other safety precautions.
- Maintain the eye patch as instructed by the ophthalmologist, and have the patient wear an eye shield, especially when sleeping. Tell him to continue wearing the shield during sleep for several weeks as ordered.
- Administer corticosteroid and antibiotic eye drops as ordered.

GENERAL

- Explain that an eye shield or glasses must be worn to protect the eye until the surgical wound has healed.
- Teach the patient how to instill the prescribed eye drops for several weeks after surgery.
- Tell the patient that for the first few days after surgery, the eye may feel scratchy and irritated, but to avoid squinting or rubbing it.
- Explain that his vision will be blurry for up to several months until the graft has fully healed.
- Tell the patient that sutures are usually left in place for 6 to 12 months and occasionally for 2 years.

WARNING *Warn the patient to immediately contact the practitioner if sudden eye pain, red or watery eyes, photophobia, or sudden visual changes occur as these are signs of potential graft rejection. If a rejection reaction occurs, it can usually be blocked by treatment with corticosteroids.*

- Inform the patient that rejection reactions may become noticeable within weeks after surgery, but may not occur until 10 or 20 years after the transplant. If full rejection does occur, the surgery will need to be repeated.
- Instruct the patient to avoid activities that raise intraocular pressure; these include heavy lifting, bending, straining during defecation, or vigorous coughing and sneezing. Tell him not to exercise strenuously for 6 to 10 weeks after the surgery.
- Explain that follow-up appointments are needed to monitor the results of the surgery and to detect complications.
- Teach the patient or a family member how to instill eye drops and ointments and how to change the eye patch.
- Suggest that the patient wear dark glasses to relieve glare; photophobia may occur after eye surgery.
- If the patient is wearing eyeglasses, explain that changes in his vision can present safety hazards. To compensate for loss of depth perception, show him how to use up-and-down head movements to judge distances. To overcome the loss of peripheral vision on the operative side, teach him to turn his head fully in that direction to view objects to his side.

RESOURCES
Organizations
American Academy of Ophthalmology: *www.aao.org*

The American Transplant Association: *www.americantransplant.org*

United Organ Transplant Association: *www.uota.org*

Selected references
Coster, D.J. "A Century of Corneal Transplantation," *Clinical and Experimental Ophthalmology* 33(6):557-58, December 2005.

Kuo, I.C., et al. "Is There an Association Between Diabetes and Keratoconus?" *Ophthalmology* 113(2):184-90, February 2006.

Moffatt, S.L., et al. "Centennial Review of Corneal Transplantation," *Clinical and Experimental Ophthalmology* 33(6): 642-57, December 2005.

Nagra, P.K., et al. "Wound Dehiscence after Penetrating Keratoplasty," *Cornea* 25(2):132-35, February 2006.

Transplantation, heart

- Replacement of a damaged heart with a donor heart

INDICATIONS

- End-stage cardiac disease unresponsive to other therapies

PROCEDURE

- The patient receives general anesthesia.
- Orthotopic heart transplantation involves removal of most of the patient's (native) heart, retaining a large portion of the right and left atria. The donor heart is attached to the native atrial cusps, and direct end-to-end anastomoses of the aorta and pulmonary artery are performed.
- The surgeon performs a median sternotomy and uses retractors to access the chest cavity.
- The patient is placed on cardiopulmonary bypass.
- Temporary epicardial pacemaker leadwires are placed because the transplanted heart is denervated and can't respond normally to stimuli from the autonomic nervous system.
- Heterotopic heart transplantation ("piggyback" heart transplantation) is less commonly performed and involves grafting a donor heart to a recipient heart without removing the recipient heart. The donor heart is used to assist the pumping ability of the native heart.

COMPLICATIONS

- Graft rejection
- Infection
- Decreased cardiac output
- Arrhythmias

NURSING DIAGNOSES

- Acute pain
- Decreased cardiac output
- Ineffective tissue perfusion: Cardiopulmonary

EXPECTED OUTCOMES

The patient will:
- verbalize relief from pain
- maintain adequate cardiac output
- maintain vital signs, blood pressure, peripheral pulses, respiratory depth and pattern, and intake and output within normal limits.

PRETREATMENT CARE

- Review necessary diagnostic tests such as antigen typing.
- Reinforce the surgeon's explanation of the surgery, equipment, and procedures used in the cardiac care unit or postanesthesia care unit.
- Explain what the patient can expect after he wakens from anesthesia, including the presence of I.V. lines, an indwelling urinary catheter, and an arterial line. Remind the patient that he'll have a breathing tube in his throat, attached to a ventilator, until he can breathe independently (usually within 6 hours).
- Describe routine postoperative care. Prepare him for postoperative pain, and reassure him that analgesics will be available.
- Teach the patient the proper methods for performing coughing, turning, deep breathing and incentive spirometry.
- Review range-of-motion exercises to be used.
- Discuss the immunosuppressant drugs that the patient will be taking, and their possible adverse effects. Remind the patient that these drugs increase his risk for infection.
- Instruct the patient and family members about measures used to control infection.
- Provide emotional support to the patient and his family, especially because the wait for a donor organ may seem endless.
- Administer immunosuppressant agents as ordered.
- Verify that an appropriate consent form has been signed.
- Maintain oxygenation and hemodynamic stability with pre-existing treatments as ordered.

POSTTREATMENT CARE

- Assess cardiopulmonary and hemodynamic status frequently.
- Explain laboratory testing and diagnostic testing as indicated.

⚡ **WARNING** *Be alert for signs suggestive of rejection, such as a cardiac index less than 2.2, hypotension, atrial or other arrhythmias, fever above 99.5° F (37.5° C), evidence of a third or fourth heart sound, peripheral edema, jugular vein distention, and crackles. Notify the practitioner or transplant coordinator immediately.*

- Resume continuous cardiac monitoring. Keep in mind that the transplanted heart's electrocardiogram (ECG) waveform appears different from that of the patient's native heart. (See *ECG waveform after cardiac transplantation.*)

⚡ **WARNING** *Abnormalities of the donor sinoatrial (SA) node's conduction and automaticity usually occur due to injury to the donor heart during procurement, transportation, or transplantation. If the conduction system is damaged or if the SA node fails to function properly after the heart is transplanted, the ECG will reflect the abnormality.*

- Monitor atrial and ventricular pacing if present, keeping the heart rate greater than 110 beats/minute.
- Institute strict infection control precautions; perform meticulous handwashing.
- Assist with extubating and administer supplemental oxygen as needed. Encourage coughing, deep breathing, incentive spirometry, and splinting, premedicating for pain as necessary.
- Monitor intake and output; nasogastric suction, and chest tube drainage.
- Administer postoperative drugs, such as corticosteroids and immunosuppressants.
- Prepare the patient for myocardial biopsy at about 7 days and 14 days postoperatively, and then as indicated by the surgeon.

PATIENT TEACHING

GENERAL

◆ Review how to use the incentive spirometer and pulse oximeter at home.

◆ Tell the patient to take the following precautions to avoid infection: wash hands often; keep hands away from face and mouth; stay away from people with colds or other infections; ask friends to visit only when they're well; wash hands before and after dressing changes; wash hands after coughing or sneezing, and throw tissues into the trash immediately; and if a family member has a cold or the flu, have that person follow normal precautions (such as using separate drinking glasses and covering his mouth when coughing).

◆ Tell the patient to avoid working in the soil for 6 months after surgery, and to wear gloves thereafter. Also remind him not to handle animal waste or have contact with animals that roam outside. Tell him not to clean bird cages, fish or turtle tanks, or cat litter; the cat litter box should be covered and taken out of the patient's home before it's changed.

◆ Warn the patient to avoid receiving vaccines that consist of live viruses, because the live virus may cause infections. Tell him or family members who intend to receive vaccinations to notify the transplant team or practitioner.

◆ Review the signs of complications and what to report to the practitioner.

◆ Review low-fat, low-cholesterol diet.

◆ Discuss activity restrictions with the patient, including the fact that heart transplants respond more slowly to exercise.

◆ Stress the need for cardiac rehabilitation.

◆ Review medication administration, dosages, and possible adverse effects.

◆ Teach the patient how to care for his incision sites and the signs and symptoms of infection to report to the surgeon.

◆ Advise the patient to brush his teeth twice a day and see the dentist twice a year for cleaning and checkup.

RESOURCES

Organizations

The American Transplant Association: *www.americantransplant.org*
The Transplant Society: *www.transplantation-soc.org*
United Organ Transplant Association: *www.uota.org*

Selected references

D'Amico, C.L. "Cardiac Transplantation: Patient Selection in the Current Era," *Journal of Cardiovascular Nursing* 20(5 Suppl):S4-13, September-October 2005.

Dew, M.A., and DiMartini, A.F. "Psychological Disorders and Distress After Adult Cardiothoracic Transplantation," *Journal of Cardiovascular Nursing* 20(5 Suppl):S51-66, September-October 2005. *Revista Española de Cardiología* 59(Suppl 1):55-65, February 2006.

Haddad, H. "Cardiac Retransplantation: An Ethical Dilemma," *Current Opinion in Cardiology* 21(2):118-19, March 2006.

Patel, J.K., and Kobashigawa, J.A. "Should We be Doing Routine Biopsy After Heart Transplantation in a New Era of Anti-Rejection?" *Current Opinion in Cardiology* 21(2):127-31, March 2006.

Pavie, A. "Heart Transplantation for End-Stage Valvular Disease: Indications and Results," *Current Opinion in Cardiology* 21(2):100-105, March 2006.

ECG waveform after cardiac transplantation

An orthotopic heart transplantation (OHT) leads to characteristic findings on an electrocardiogram (ECG); because the procedure provides the patient with a second functioning heart, the ECG shows two distinct cardiac rhythms—that of the native heart and that of the donor heart. These can be differentiated by analyzing the recipient's preoperative ECG. In addition, the QRS complex of the donor heart usually has a higher amplitude. Remember that in OHT, the sinus node of the native heart remains intact. This accounts for the two P waves commonly seen on the posttransplant ECG. However, only the sinus node of the donor heart conducts through to the ventricles.

Initially, the atrial and ventricular rates are slow, requiring the use of a temporary pacemaker in the immediate postoperative period or therapy with such drugs as theophylline. The patient's native P waves will have a regular rhythm unrelated to the donor heart's QRS complexes. The donor atrial and ventricular rhythms are usually regular. Typically, two separate P waves are seen and the QRS complex may be widened secondary to ventricular conduction defects. Pacemaker activity should appear as long as the patient requires pacemaker support for chronotropic incompetence.

ORTHOTOPIC HEART TRANSPLANTATION

This waveform shows two distinct types of P waves. P waves caused by the native heart's sinoatrial (SA) node are unrelated to the QRS complexes (first shaded area). P waves caused by the donor heart's SA node precede each QRS complex (second shaded area).

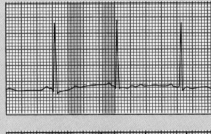

HETEROTOPIC HEART TRANSPLANTATION

This waveform shows the ECG of the recipient's own heart (first shaded area) and the donor heart (second shaded area).

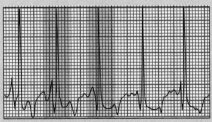

Transplantation, islet cells

- Involves implantation of beta cells of the Islets of Langerhans from a donor pancreas into a patient who doesn't produce insulin; the donor beta cells then make and release insulin
- Islet cells removed from the deceased donor's pancreas using special enzymes; purified in a process that uses a digestive enzyme, heat, and centrifugation; and transplanted soon after
- Allogenic transplants: patients with type 1 diabetes receive islet cells from a donated pancreas
- Autologous transplants: patients with pancreatitis receive infusions of their own cells
- Researchers hoping islet cell transplantation will allow patients with type 1 diabetes to avoid daily injections of insulin
- Researchers attempting to increase the storage time of donated pancreases before islet cell extraction by using a special pump that helps to preserve the tissue
- Investigational: growing insulin-producing cells from stem cells or pancreatic ductal tissue, due to lack of donated islet cells

INDICATIONS
- Type 1 diabetes mellitus
- Severe or intractable pancreatitis

- The patient generally receives a local anesthetic but the surgeon may use general anesthesia in selected patients.
- A small incision is made in the upper abdomen.
- During allogenic transplantation, the surgeon uses ultrasound to guide placement of a catheter through the upper abdomen and into the liver. He then injects the islet cells into the patient's liver through the catheter that's inserted into the portal vein.
- In autologous transplant, the procedure is performed in the operating room after the pancreas has been removed.

COMPLICATIONS
- Rejection of the transplant
- Bleeding or blood clots

- Deficient fluid volume
- Imbalanced nutrition: Less than body requirements
- Risk for infection

EXPECTED OUTCOMES
The patient will:
- maintain adequate fluid volume
- maintain optimum body weight
- remain free from infection.

- Explain the procedure to the patient.
- Explain what the patient can expect after he wakens from anesthesia. Describe routine postoperative care, including frequent checks of vital signs, monitoring of intake and output, and respiratory therapy. Prepare him for postoperative pain, and reassure him that analgesics will be available.
- Teach the patient the proper methods for performing coughing, turning, deep breathing and, if ordered, incentive spirometry.
- Discuss the immunosuppressant drugs that the patient will be taking, and explain their possible adverse effects. Remind the patient that these drugs increase his risk for infection.
- Instruct the patient and family members about measures used to control infection and minimize rejection after transplant.
- Verify that the patient has signed a consent form.

POSTTREATMENT CARE

◆ Monitor the patient's vital signs and intake and output.
◆ Monitor for signs of rejection.
◆ Monitor laboratory test results as indicated.
◆ Administer immunosuppressive drugs, which stop the immune system from rejecting the transplanted islet cells.

PATIENT TEACHING

GENERAL

◆ Review the disorder, diagnostic studies, and treatment with the patient.
◆ Discuss the signs of complications such as rejection.
◆ Review medication administration, dosages, and possible adverse effects with the patient.
◆ Advise the patient about the prescribed meal plan.
◆ Tell the patient that it takes time for the cells to attach to new blood vessels and begin releasing insulin. Inform him that the practitioner may order many tests to check blood glucose levels after the transplant and that insulin may be needed until control is achieved.
◆ Stress the need for continued follow-up care to monitor for transplant rejection.
◆ Tell the patient that because immunosuppressive medications interfere with his natural immune system, he needs to take the following precautions to avoid infection: wash hands often; keep hands away from face and mouth; stay away from people with colds or other infections; ask friends to visit only when they're well; wash hands before and after dressing changes; wash hands after coughing or sneezing, and throw tissues into the trash immediately; and if a family member has a cold or the flu, have that person follow normal precautions (such as using separate drinking glasses and covering his mouth when coughing).

RESOURCES
Organizations
American Academy of Pediatrics: *www.aap.org*
American Medical Association: *www.ama-assn.org*
National Diabetes Clearinghouse Information: *diabetes.niddk.nih.gov/index.htm*

Selected references
Berney, T., and Morel, P. "Islet Transplantation: Steeple Chase and the Next Hurdle," *Transplantation* 80(12):1658-59, December 2005.
Hopkins Tanne, J. "New Technique Improves Safety of Islet Cell Transplantation," *British Medical Journal* 331(7528):1290, December 2005.
Kriz, J., et al. "Magnetic Resonance Imaging of Pancreatic Islets in Tolerance and Rejection," *Transplantation* 80(11):1596-603, December 2005.

Transplantation, kidney

OVERVIEW

- Surgical procedure to implant a healthy kidney from a living donor or a cadaver into a patient with kidney failure
- Represents an alternative to dialysis for patients with otherwise unmanageable end-stage renal disease (ESRD), which commonly results from hypertension, diabetes mellitus, and glomerulonephritis
- Simultaneous transplant of kidney and pancreas may be done; dual organ transplantation suitable for patients with type 1 diabetes and ESRD or renal insufficiency

INDICATIONS

- ESRD
- Traumatic loss of kidney function
- When dialysis is contraindicated

  AGE FACTOR *Patient with severe debilitation, diabetes, human immunodeficiency virus infection, or psychiatric disorders and the elderly aren't good candidates for kidney transplantation.*

  WARNING *Contraindications for kidney transplantation include cardiopulmonary insufficiency, morbid obesity, peripheral and cerebrovascular disease, hepatic insufficiency, and other conditions that increase a patient's overall surgical risk.*

PROCEDURE

- The recipient's kidneys (which secrete erythropoietin fluid) are typically left in place to increase circulating hematocrit, ease dialysis management, and reduce blood transfusion requirements if transplant rejection occurs. They're removed if they're chronically infected, greatly enlarged, cancerous, or causing intractable hypertension.
- Patient receives general anesthesia.
- A curvilinear incision in the right or left lower quadrant, extending from the symphysis pubis to the anterior superior iliac spine, and up to just below the thoracic cage is made.
- The iliac fossa is exposed with a self-retaining retractor, then segmental separation, ligature, and division of perivascular tissue is done.
- The iliac vein and artery are clamped to prepare for anastomosis to the donor kidney's renal vein and artery.
- Meantime, the donor kidney is prepared for transplantation. If a cadaver kidney is being used, it's removed from cold storage or a perfusion preparation machine. Although kidneys can be stored for 72 hours, most transplants are performed within 48 hours. If the kidney is from a living donor, it's removed by laparoscopy or laparoscopy-assisted technique in an adjacent operating room and placed in cold lactated Ringer's solution.
- Before transplantation, the renal artery of the donor kidney is flushed with cold heparinized lactated Ringer's solution to prevent clogging. The surgeon then positions the kidney in a sling over the implantation site. (He never holds the kidney in his hands because this would warm it and possibly cause necrosis.)
- The kidney is implanted in the retroperitoneal area of the iliac fossa, where it's protected by the hip bone. If a donor's left kidney is being used, it's implanted in the recipient's right side; conversely, a donor's right kidney is implanted in the recipient's left side. This allows the renal pelvis to rest anteriorly and enables the new kidney's ureter to rest in front of the iliac artery, where the ureter is more accessible.
- When both kidneys are in place, the renal vein is sutured to the recipient's iliac vein and the renal artery to the recipient's internal iliac artery. (See *Understanding renal transplantation.*)
- The venous and arterial clamps are removed and checked for patency. The donor kidney's ureter is attached to the recipient's bladder, ensuring a watertight closure. A tunneling technique is usually used to connect the ureter to the bladder to prevent urine reflux into the transplanted kidney.
- When the transplantation is complete, the surgeon sutures the incision and applies a sterile dressing.

COMPLICATIONS

- Rejection of donated organ
- Vascular stenosis, leakage, or thrombosis
- Ureteral leakage, fistula, or obstruction
- Calculus formation
- Bladder neck contracture
- Graft rupture
- Cardiovascular complications
- Respiratory complications
- Hepatitis B
- Cirrhosis
- Peptic ulcer disease
- Infection
- Hematomas or abscesses
- Lymphoceles
- Corticosteroid-induced diabetes
- Osteoporosis
- Myopathy
- Aseptic bone necrosis
- Cataracts, glaucoma, and retinitis

NURSING DIAGNOSES

- Deficient fluid volume
- Ineffective gas exchange
- Ineffective tissue perfusion: Cardiopulmonary, renal

EXPECTED OUTCOMES

The patient will:

- maintain adequate fluid volume per intake and output records, skin turgor, and vital signs
- maintain patent airway and adequate oxygenation
- maintain vital signs, blood pressure, cardiac output, and pulmonary artery pressure measurements within normal limits.

PRETREATMENT CARE

- Prepare the patient for transplantation and a prolonged recovery period, and offer him ongoing emotional support.
- Encourage the patient to express his feelings. If he's concerned about rejection of the donor kidney, explain that if this occurs and can't be reversed, he'll resume dialysis and wait for another suitable donor organ.

Reassure him that transplant rejection is common and usually isn't life-threatening.
◆ Describe routine preoperative measures, such as physical examination, laboratory tests, X-rays, electrocardiogram (ECG), bowel preparation, and removal of hair from the operative area if ordered.
◆ Tell the patient that he'll undergo dialysis the day before surgery to clean his blood of unwanted fluid and electrolytes. Indicate that he may need dialysis for a few days after surgery if his transplanted kidney doesn't start functioning immediately.
◆ Review the transplant procedure with the patient and family.
◆ Explain what the patient can expect after he wakens from anesthesia, including the presence of I.V. lines, an indwelling urinary catheter, an arterial line and, possibly, a mechanical ventilator. Describe routine postoperative care. Prepare him for postoperative pain, and reassure him that analgesics will be available.
◆ Teach the patient the proper methods for performing coughing, turning, deep breathing and, if ordered, incentive spirometry.
◆ Discuss the immunosuppressant drugs that the patient will be taking, and their possible adverse effects. Remind the patient that these drugs increase his risk for infection.
◆ Instruct the patient and family members about measures used to control infection.
◆ Provide emotional support to the patient and his family.
◆ Begin giving immunosuppressant drugs and corticosteroids as ordered. Oral azathioprine (Imuran) may be started as early as 5 days before surgery.
◆ Begin slow I.V. infusion of cyclosporine (Neoral) 4 to 12 hours before surgery; closely monitor the patient for anaphylaxis, especially during the first 30 minutes of administration. If anaphylaxis occurs, give epinephrine (Adrenalin) as ordered.
◆ Administer blood transfusions as ordered.
◆ Verify that the patient or a family member has signed an informed consent form.

Understanding renal transplantation

In renal transplantation, the donated organ is implanted in the iliac fossa. The organ's vessels are then connected to the internal iliac vein and internal iliac artery, as shown here. Typically, the patient's own kidneys are left in place.

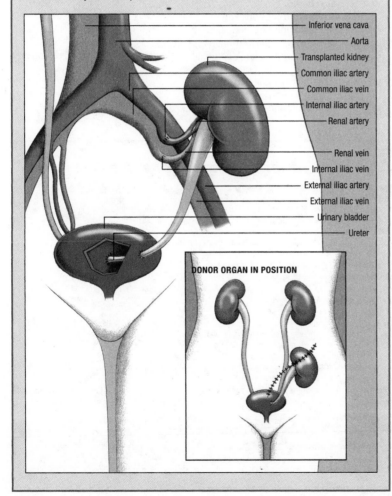

- Inferior vena cava
- Aorta
- Transplanted kidney
- Common iliac artery
- Common iliac vein
- Internal iliac artery
- Renal artery
- Renal vein
- Internal iliac vein
- External iliac artery
- External iliac vein
- Urinary bladder
- Ureter

DONOR ORGAN IN POSITION

POSTTREATMENT CARE

◆ Assess cardiopulmonary and hemodynamic status closely, as indicated by the patient's condition.
◆ Maintain continuous cardiac monitoring, evaluating waveforms for changes in ECG indicative of electrolyte imbalance or ischemia. Watch for signs of hyperkalemia. If these occur, notify the practitioner and administer calcium carbonate I.V. as ordered.

(continued)

- Monitor laboratory blood and urine test results closely.
- Carefully monitor urine output, at least hourly; promptly report output of less than 100 ml/hour.

  ⚡ **WARNING** *In a living donor transplant, urine flow usually begins immediately after revascularization and connection of the ureter to the recipient's bladder. In a cadaver renal transplant, anuria may persist from 2 days to 2 weeks; the patient will need dialysis during this period.*
- Observe urinary catheter function and urine color, which should be slightly blood-tinged for several days and then gradually become clear.
- If the patient is receiving mechanical ventilation, assist with extubating as soon as possible (usually within 4 to 6 hours). Administer supplemental oxygen as needed. Encourage coughing and deep-breathing exercises and use of incentive spirometer after extubation, splinting, and premedicating for pain as needed.

- Assess the patient for incisional and abdominal pain, and provide analgesics as ordered.
- Assess for pain related to bladder spasms, which may continue briefly after catheter removal, and administer analgesics as ordered.
- Assess the patient's fluid and electrolyte balance. Weigh the patient daily, and report rapid gain.
- Maintain nothing-by-mouth status with nasogastric decompression to low intermittent suction (if appropriate) until bowel sounds return. Administer histamine blockers to suppress gastric acid secretion. Begin clear liquids after the patient is extubated and bowel sounds are active. Gradually resume a full diet with restrictions as ordered.
- Institute standard precautions and use strict sterile technique when changing dressings and performing catheter care. Limit the patient's contact with staff, other patients, and visitors, and avoid exposing him to people with an infection. Monitor the patient's white blood cell (WBC)

count; notify the practitioner if it drops precipitously.
- Watch for signs and symptoms of organ rejection. Report suspicious findings immediately. (See *Managing transplant rejection*.)
- Change the patient's position at least every 2 hours, get him out of bed to the chair within 24 hours if his condition is stable. Gradually increase the patient's activity as tolerated.
- To ease emotional stress, allow family members to visit and comfort the patient as much as possible.
- Allow the patient and family members to express their anxiety and fear.

Managing transplant rejection

TYPE OF REJECTION	PATHOPHYSIOLOGIC MECHANISM	ASSESSMENT FINDINGS	TREATMENT MEASURES
Hyperacute	Patient's circulating antibodies attack the donor kidney several minutes to hours after transplantation.	◆ Severe drop in renal perfusion ◆ Ischemia and death of the organ	◆ Immediate removal of the organ
Acute	Antigen-antibody reaction produces acute tubular necrosis that occurs 1 week to 6 months after transplantation of a living-donor kidney, or 1 week to 2 years after transplantation of a cadaver kidney (most common within 7 to 14 days after transplantation).	◆ Infection, including fever, rapid pulse, elevated white blood cell count, and lethargy ◆ Oliguria or anuria ◆ Hypertension ◆ Weight gain of more than 3 lb (1.4 kg) in 24 hours ◆ Kidney enlargement and tenderness ◆ Elevated blood urea nitrogen (BUN) and creatinine levels	◆ Increased dosages of immunosuppressants ◆ Dialysis, if indicated ◆ Removal of the organ, if functioning ceases
Chronic	Long-term antibody destruction of the organ, which may occur from several months to years after transplantation.	◆ Rising BUN and creatinine levels ◆ Declining glomerular filtration rate ◆ Hypertension ◆ Proteinuria	◆ Renal scan, renal biopsy, and other tests to determine the extent of damage ◆ Increased dosages of immunosuppressants ◆ Adjustments in diet and fluid regimen ◆ Dialysis or another transplant, if indicated

PATIENT TEACHING

GENERAL

◆ Advise the patient to monitor his weight and intake and output; include specific parameters for notifying the nephrologist or surgeon.

◆ Teach the patient to check for signs and symptoms of transplant infection or rejection, including redness, warmth, tenderness, or swelling over the kidney; fever exceeding 100° F (37.8° C); decreased urine output; weight gain of more than 3 lb (1.4 kg) in 24 hours; and elevated blood pressure.

◆ Tell the patient to take the following precautions to avoid infection: wash hands often; keep hands away from face and mouth; stay away from people with colds or other infections; ask friends to visit only when they're well; wash hands before and after dressing changes; wash hands after coughing or sneezing, and throw tissues into the trash immediately; and if a family member has a cold or the flu, have that person follow normal precautions (such as using separate drinking glasses and covering his mouth when coughing).

◆ Tell the patient to avoid working in the soil for 6 months after surgery, and to wear gloves thereafter. Also remind him not to handle animal waste or have contact with animals that roam outside. Tell him not to clean bird cages, fish or turtle tanks, or cat litter; the cat litter box should be covered and taken out of the patient's home before it's changed.

◆ Warn the patient to avoid receiving vaccines that consist of live viruses because the live virus may cause infections. Tell him or family members who require vaccinations to notify the transplant team or nephrologist first for instructions.

◆ Remind the patient to watch for fever that continues for more than 2 days; shortness of breath; cough that produces a yellow or green substance; dry cough that continues for more than 1 week; prolonged nausea, vomiting, or diarrhea; inability to take prescribed medication; rash or other skin changes; vaginal discharge or itching; unusual weakness or light-headedness; fluid retention or rapid weight gain; pain or burning during urination; decrease in urine output; blood in the urine; strong odor to the urine; and urgent need to urinate or need to urinate frequently. Instruct the patient to report these symptoms plus exposure to mumps, measles, chicken pox, or shingles or emergency department treatment.

◆ Review the prescribed medication regimens and adverse effects, and stress the need for compliance.

◆ Stress the importance of a program of regular, moderate exercise, beginning slowly and increasing gradually.

◆ Advise the patient to avoid excessive bending, heavy lifting, and contact sports for at least 3 months or until the surgeon permits such activities; also advise him to avoid activities or positions that place pressure on the new kidney—for example, long car trips and lap-style seat belts.

◆ Remind the patient to wait at least 6 weeks before resuming sexual relations. Because pregnancy poses an added risk to a new kidney, provide the female patient with information on birth control.

◆ Stress the importance of regular follow-up visits to the nephrologist and transplant surgeon.

◆ Advise the patient to brush his teeth twice a day and see the dentist twice a year for cleaning and checkup.

AGE FACTOR *Instruct parents of school-age children to ask the school nurse to notify them immediately of communicable diseases (such as, measles or chicken pox) circulating in the school.*

RESOURCES
Organizations
The American Transplant Association: *www.americantransplant.org*
The Transplant Society: *www.transplantation-soc.org*
United Organ Transplant Association: *www.uota.org*

Selected references
Ashwanden, C. "Bridging the Gap Between Patient and Technology," *Nephrology News and Issues* 19(9):61, 63, August 2005.

Lawson, C.A. "Cytomegalovirus after Kidney Transplantation: A Case Review," *Progress in Transplantation* 15(2):157-60, June 2005.

Niu, S.F., and Li, I.C. "Quality of Life of Patients Having Renal Replacement Therapy," *Journal of Advanced Nursing* 51(1):15-21, July 2005.

Transplantation, liver

OVERVIEW

- Removal of a diseased liver and replacement with a healthy liver from a donor

INDICATIONS

- End-stage liver disease secondary to hepatitis B and C, alcoholic cirrhosis, primary sclerosing cholangitis, primary biliary cirrhosis, and metabolic disorders
- Acute fulminant hepatic failure related to drug toxicity
- Hepatitis A
- Autoimmune disorders
- Mushroom poisoning

WARNING *Contraindications to liver transplantation include human immunodeficiency virus infection, spontaneous bacterial peritonitis or other active infection, severely advanced cardiopulmonary disease, extrahepatic malignancy that doesn't meet cure criteria, currently active alcohol or substance abuse, and demonstrated inability to comply with immunosuppression protocols because of psychosocial situations.*

PROCEDURE

- There are four techniques for liver transplantation.
- Orthotopic transplantation is surgical removal of the diseased liver and implantation of a healthy donor liver.
- In an orthotopic liver transplant, the donor liver is removed and transported to the recipient's location.
- The surgeon makes bilateral subcostal incisions and extends the midline incision to the xiphoid process. After the vessels, ligaments, and other attachments are properly severed, the patient is placed on venovenous bypass, and the diseased liver is removed.
- To attach the donor liver, the suprahepatic vena cava is anastomosed, and then the recipient portal vein is cleared and anastomosed to the donor portal vein. Blood flow through these vessels is evaluated, after which the hepatic artery is anastomosed in an end-to-end manner.
- The surgeon then reconstructs the biliary duct by connecting the bile duct of the donor to the recipient's

(with or without T-tube stent brought out to the exterior of the abdomen through a stab wound) or by using a Roux-en-Y anastomosis to the recipient's jejunum (if the recipient's biliary duct is diseased or too small).
- Several drains are placed around the liver and brought out to the exterior abdominal wall to allow for drainage of ascitic fluid and to assess bleeding.
- Alternatively, a reduced-sized liver transplant, split liver transplant, or living donor liver transplant may be done. (See *Alternative liver transplant techniques*.)

AGE FACTOR *Children requiring liver transplants typically receive either living-donor transplants or reduced-sized liver transplants*

AGE FACTOR *To ensure the best possible outcome for the recipient, donors for a split-liver transplant typically meet the following criteria: age older than 50 with normal liver function, hospitalized for fewer than 3 days, with required minimal support with vasopressors, and no evidence of fatty degeneration of the liver.*

Alternative liver transplant techniques

In addition to orthotopic liver transplant, three other techniques may be used. Each of these techniques was developed because of the shortage of donor organs available for the number of candidates requiring a liver transplant.

REDUCED-SIZE LIVER TRANSPLANT

A donor liver from a cadaver is resected to create a right lobe, left lobe, or left lateral segment, which is then anastomosed to the recipient. The remainder of the liver tissue is discarded. This is usually done for pediatric patients because the availability of donors for this population is small.

SPLIT-LIVER TRANSPLANT

With a split-liver transplant, an entire adult donor liver is transected or split into two pieces to provide grafts for two recipients. The liver can be split through the falciform ligament, creating a small (left lateral segment) graft for a

child and a larger (extended right lobe) graft for an adult. The liver may also be split through the main portal fissure and gall bladder bed to create right and left lobe grafts.

LIVING-DONOR TRANSPLANT

With a living-donor transplant, a portion of the liver from a living donor is removed and transplanted to the recipient. This technique was previously used only with children. However, because of its success with children, it's now also used for adults. For transplantation in children, left lateral segments or left lobes are typically used; for adults, right lobe grafts are commonly used.

COMPLICATIONS

◆ Rejection, acute or chronic
◆ Primary graft failure
◆ Biliary malfunction
◆ Hepatic artery thrombosis
◆ Infection
◆ Posttransplant lymphoproliferative disorder
◆ Posttransplant malignancies
◆ Recurrent, metabolic, or autoimmune liver disease

NURSING DIAGNOSES

◆ Deficient fluid volume
◆ Ineffective gas exchange
◆ Ineffective tissue perfusion: Cardiopulmonary, cerebral

EXPECTED OUTCOMES
The patient will:
◆ maintain adequate fluid volume without signs of excessive bleeding
◆ maintain patent airway and adequate oxygenation
◆ maintain vital signs, blood pressure, peripheral pulses, respiratory status, and intake and output within normal limits.

PRETREATMENT CARE

◆ Instruct the patient and his family about the transplant procedure and necessary diagnostic tests such as antigen typing. Reinforce the surgeon's explanation.
◆ Administer medications, including immunosuppressant agents, as ordered.
◆ Explain what the patient can expect after he wakens from anesthesia, including the presence of I.V. lines, an indwelling urinary catheter, an arterial line and, possibly, a mechanical ventilator. Review other equipment, such as continuous cardiac monitoring, nasogastric (NG) tube, an indwelling urinary catheter, arterial lines and, possibly, a pulmonary artery catheter. Tell him that discomfort will be minimal and the equipment will be removed as soon as possible.
◆ Describe routine postoperative care, including frequent checks of vital signs, monitoring of intake and output, and respiratory therapy. Prepare him for postoperative pain, and reassure him that analgesics will be available.
◆ Review range-of-motion exercises with the patient.
◆ Teach the patient the proper methods for performing coughing, turning, deep breathing and, if ordered, incentive spirometry.
◆ Discuss the immunosuppressant drugs that the patient will be taking, and explain their possible adverse effects. Remind the patient that these drugs increase his risk for infection.
◆ Instruct the patient and family members about measures used to control infection and minimize rejection after transplant.
◆ Verify that a consent form has been signed.
◆ Instruct the patient and family members about measures used to control infection and minimize rejection after transplant.
◆ Provide emotional support to the patient and his family, especially because the wait for a donor liver may seem endless.

POSTTREATMENT CARE

◆ Assess cardiopulmonary and hemodynamic status closely at least every 15 minutes for the first 2 hours in the postoperative period, and then hourly or more frequently depending on the patient's condition. Institute continuous cardiac monitoring if not in place, evaluating waveforms frequently. Monitor hemodynamic parameters for changes suggestive of changes in fluid volume status.
◆ Monitor laboratory test results closely, especially liver enzyme and bilirubin levels.

WARNING *Expect liver enzyme levels to be elevated in the immediate postoperative period. Usually, these increases reflect the effects of the donor liver undergoing cold preservation while being transported to the recipient's location. Enzyme and bilirubin levels usually return to normal within 1 week; however, a marked increase in these levels after they begin to decrease suggests possible rejection.*

◆ Other important laboratory tests may include serum electrolyte studies, blood urea nitrogen and creatinine levels, and arterial blood gas analysis.

WARNING *After liver transplantation, the patient is at high risk for bleeding. Monitor appropriate laboratory test results frequently. Be sure to evaluate the results in light of blood component therapy such as fresh frozen plasma that the patient has received. Platelet count usually decreases during the first week after transplantation, but then begins to return to normal during the second week.*

(continued)

- Assess insertion sites, such as I.V. lines and drains, for indications of bleeding. Assess incision site closely for oozing or active bleeding. If the patient has an NG tube, assess color and character of drainage at least every 2 hours.
- Institute strict infection control precautions; perform meticulous hand washing.
- Administer prophylactic antimicrobial agents as ordered.
- Monitor temperature at least every hour initially and then every 2 to 4 hours. If the patient has a fever and an infection is suspected, expect to obtain cultures of all body fluids, X-rays of the chest and abdomen, and a Doppler ultrasound of the hepatic vessels.

⚡ **WARNING** *Sudden onset of high fever and an increase in liver enzyme levels suggests hepatic artery thrombosis. Prepare the patient for a Doppler ultrasound to determine vessel patency.*

- Assist with extubating as soon as possible (usually within 4 to 6 hours), and administer supplemental oxygen as needed, based on mixed venous oxygen saturation or pulse oximetry levels. Encourage coughing and deep-breathing exercises and the use of incentive spirometry after extubation, splinting and premedicating for pain as necessary.
- Monitor intake and output at least hourly and notify the practitioner if output is less than 30 ml/hour. Maintain fluids at 2,000 to 3,000 ml/ day or as ordered to prevent fluid overload.
- Administer postoperative drugs, such as corticosteroids and immunosuppressants, as ordered.
- Maintain nothing-by-mouth status with NG decompression to low intermittent suction until bowel sounds return. Administer histamine blockers to suppress gastric acid secretion. Begin clear liquids after the patient is extubated and bowel sounds are active.
- Change the patient's position at least every 2 hours, getting him out of bed to the chair within 24 hours if his condition is stable. Gradually increase the patient's activity as tolerated.
- Continually assess the patient for signs and symptoms of acute rejection, such as malaise, fever, graft enlargement, and diminished graft function (usually 7 to 14 days after the transplant).

⚡ **WARNING** *Be alert for an increase in bilirubin and transaminase levels with a change in T-tube biliary drainage, which may become thin and lighter in color. Note abdominal pain or tenderness, jaundice, dark yellow or orange urine, and clay-colored stools. Notify the practitioner and prepare the patient for a graft biopsy.*

- To ease emotional stress, plan to allow frequent rest periods and provide privacy. Allow family members to visit and comfort the patient as much as possible.
- Allow family members to express their anger, anxiety, and fear.

PATIENT TEACHING

GENERAL

- Review medication administration, dosages, and possible adverse effects with the patient and family.
- Emphasize the need for follow-up care with the transplant team.
- Refer the patient to appropriate resources and support services.
- Advise the patient to monitor his intake and output and weight; include specific parameters for notifying the practitioner.

⚡ **WARNING** *Remind the patient to take precautions and to watch for signs of infection and rejection that require notifying the practitioner or transplant team immediately. These include a fever that continues for more than 2 days; shortness of breath; cough that produces a yellow or green substance; dry cough that continues for more than 1 week; prolonged nausea, vomiting, or diarrhea; inability to take prescribed medication; rash or other skin changes; vaginal discharge or itching; exposure to mumps, measles, chicken pox, or shingles; unusual weakness or light-headedness; emergency department treatment or hospitalization; pain, redness, tenderness or swelling at the incision site; fluid retention or weight gain (2 lb [1 kg] in 24 hours); decrease in urine output; pain or burning during urination; blood in the urine; strong odor to the urine; and urgent need to urinate or need to urinate frequently.*

- Review his prescribed medication regimens, and stress the need for compliance with immunosuppressant therapy. Remind the patient to use antacids (if ordered) immediately before a corticosteroid to combat its ulcerogenic effects.
- Stress the importance of a program of regular, moderate exercise, beginning slowly and increasing gradually.
- Advise the patient to avoid excessive bending, heavy lifting, and contact sports for at least 3 months or until the practitioner permits such activities; also tell him to avoid activities or positions that place pressure on the abdomen—for example, long car trips and lap-style seat belts.
- Remind the patient to wait at least 6 weeks before resuming sexual relations. Because pregnancy poses an added risk, provide the female patient with information on birth control.
- Stress the importance of regular follow-up with the practitioner to evaluate his liver function and transplant acceptance.
- Tell the patient that because immunosuppressive medications interfere with his natural immune system, he needs to take the following precautions to avoid infection: wash hands often; keep hands away from face and mouth; stay away from people with colds or other infections; ask friends to visit only when they're well; wash hands before and after dressing changes; wash hands after coughing or sneezing, and throw tissues into the trash immediately; and if a family member has a cold or the flu, have that person follow normal precautions (such as using separate drinking glasses and covering his mouth when coughing).

- Tell the patient to avoid working in the soil for 6 months after surgery, and to wear gloves thereafter. Also remind him not to handle animal waste or have contact with animals that roam outside. Tell him not to clean bird cages, fish or turtle tanks, or cat litter; the cat litter box should be covered and taken out of the patient's home before it's changed.
- Warn the patient to avoid receiving vaccines that consist of live viruses, such as Sabin oral polio, measles, mumps, German measles, yellow fever, or smallpox, because the live virus may cause infections. Tell him or family members who intend to receive vaccinations to notify the transplant team or practitioner.
- Advise the patient to take care of his teeth by brushing twice per day and seeing the dentist twice per year for cleaning and checkup.

AGE FACTOR *Instruct parents of school-age children to ask the school nurse to notify them immediately of communicable diseases (such as measles or chicken pox) circulating in the school.*

RESOURCES
Organizations
The American Transplant Association: *www.americantransplant.org*
The Transplant Society: *www.transplantation-soc.org*
TransWeb: *www.transweb.org*
United Organ Transplant Association: *www.uota.org*

Selected references
del Barrio, M., et al. "Liver Transplant Patients: Their Experience in the Intensive Care Unit. A Phenomenological Study," *Journal of Clinical Nursing* 13(8):967-76, November 2004.

Jacob, M., et al. "Functional Status of Patient Before Liver Transplantation as a Predictor of Posttransplant Mortality," *Transplantation* 15:80(1):52-57, July 2005.

Pfadt, E., and Carlson, D.S. "Transfusion-Associated Graft-Versus-Host Disease," *Nursing* 35(2):88, February 2005.

Taylor, R., et al. "A Critical Review of the Health-Related Quality of Life of Children and Adolescents after Liver Transplantation," *Liver Transplantation* 11(1):51-60; discussion 7-9, January 2005.

Transplantation, lung

OVERVIEW

- Replacement of one or both of the lungs with those from a donor
- Sometimes, only one lobe transplanted

INDICATIONS

- Single-lung transplantation considered for patients with end-stage restrictive or obstructive pulmonary disease
- Double-lung transplantation considered for patients with cystic fibrosis (CF) or septic pulmonary diseases

  🌼 **AGE FACTOR** *CF is a common reason for lung transplantation in children, adolescents, and young adults. Other diseases affecting this age-group that may require lung transplantation include bronchopulmonary dysplasia, pulmonary hypertension, and pulmonary fibrosis.*

  ⚡ **WARNING** *A patient must meet certain criteria to be a candidate for lung transplantation; these include forced vital capacity of less than 40%; amount of air exhaled in first second of expiration less than 30% of predicted value; partial pressure of arterial oxygen less than 60 mm Hg on room air at rest; evidence of major pulmonary complications; and demonstration of increased antibiotic resistance.*

  ⚡ **WARNING** *Contraindicated in patients with major organ dysfunction, especially involving the renal or cardiovascular system; human immunodeficiency virus infection; active malignancy; positive for antigen to hepatitis B; hepatitis C with biopsy positive for liver damage; active infection; and progressive neuromuscular disease. Other conditions, such as symptomatic osteoporosis or need for invasive ventilation, are relative contraindications for lung transplantation.*

PROCEDURE

- The patient is given general anesthesia. If a single lung is to be transplanted, the patient is intubated with double lumen endotracheal (ET) tube to allow the other lung to be ventilated during the surgery.
- The surgeon makes a lateral thoracotomy incision and removes the patient's lung via a posterolateral approach.
- The donor lung is implanted and anastomosed to the patient's bronchus, pulmonary artery, and cuff of the left atrium. Typically, cardiopulmonary bypass isn't used unless the patient can't be supported with ventilation of a single lung.
- For a double-lung transplantation, the surgeon makes bilateral anterior thoracotomy incisions along with a transverse sternotomy incision. Intubation is accomplished with a double lumen ET tube.
- After removal of the patient's lungs, the donor lungs are implanted with anastomoses at the same sites as for a single lung transplant.
- Cardiopulmonary bypass is commonly used during a double-lung transplant.

COMPLICATIONS

- Rejection, leading to fibrosis and scar formation on the transplanted lung
- Infection
- Hemorrhage
- Reperfusion edema
- Obliterative bronchiolitis and post-transplant lymphoproliferative disorder, which may result in death

NURSING DIAGNOSES

- Decreased cardiac output
- Ineffective gas exchange
- Ineffective tissue perfusion: Cardiopulmonary, cerebral

EXPECTED OUTCOMES

The patient will:
- maintain adequate cardiac output
- maintain patent airway and adequate oxygenation
- maintain vital signs, blood pressure, peripheral pulses, respiratory status, and intake and output within normal limits.

◆ Instruct the patient and his family about the transplant procedure and necessary diagnostic tests such as antigen typing.

◆ Reinforce the surgeon's and anesthesiologist's explanation of the procedure.

◆ Explain what the patient can expect after he wakens from anesthesia, including the presence of I.V. lines, an indwelling urinary catheter, an arterial line and, possibly, a mechanical ventilator. Review other equipment, such as continuous cardiac monitoring, nasogastric (NG) tube, an indwelling urinary catheter, arterial lines and, possibly, a pulmonary artery catheter. Tell him that discomfort will be minimal and the equipment will be removed as soon as possible.

◆ Describe routine postoperative care, including frequent checks of vital signs, monitoring of intake and output, and respiratory therapy. Prepare him for postoperative pain, and reassure him that analgesics will be available.

◆ Discuss the immunosuppressant drugs that the patient will be taking, and explain their possible adverse effects. Remind the patient that these drugs increase his risk for infection.

◆ Instruct the patient and family members about measures used to control infection and minimize rejection after transplant.

◆ Provide emotional support to the patient and his family, especially because the wait for a donor organ may seem endless.

◆ Administer immunosuppressant agents as ordered.

◆ Review techniques of incentive spirometry, coughing and deep-breathing, and range-of-motion (ROM) exercises with the patient and his family.

◆ Verify that a consent form has been signed.

◆ Instruct family members in measures used to control infection and minimize rejection after transplant.

◆ Assess cardiopulmonary and hemodynamic status closely at least every 15 minutes in the immediate postoperative period and then hourly or more frequently as indicated by the patient's condition.

⚡ *WARNING Watch for a cardiac index less than 2.2, increased pulmonary artery wedge pressure or central venous pressure, decreased hematocrit, hypotension, temperature above 99.5° F (37.5° C), increased white blood cell count, crackles or rhonchi, decreased oxygen saturation, shortness of breath, dyspnea, malaise, and increased sputum production. These signs and symptoms suggest acute rejection, infection, or bleeding. Notify the practitioner or transplant coordinator immediately.*

◆ If the patient becomes hemodynamically unstable, expect to administer vasoactive and inotropic agents as ordered and titrate them until the desired response is achieved.

◆ Assess ET tube placement, patency, and function, and mechanical ventilation; administer supplemental oxygen as necessary. Monitor oxygen saturation and arterial blood gas (ABG) values as ordered.

⚡ *WARNING Remember that for the patient undergoing a single-lung transplant, the newly implanted lung is denervated, but his original lung continues to send messages to the brain indicating poor oxygenation. Be alert that the patient may complain of shortness of breath and dyspnea even with oxygen saturation levels above 90%.*

◆ Suction as necessary.

(continued)

◆ Monitor chest tubes attached to suction (usually for the first 24 hours or until drainage is less than 100 ml in 8 hours). When chest tubes are in place, expect to administer antibiotics as ordered. Assess drainage amount, color, and characteristics. Assess for bleeding. Notify the practitioner if chest tube drainage is greater than 200 ml in 1 hour, appears increasingly bloody, or suddenly stops, or an air leak develops or increases.

◆ **WARNING** *Encourage the patient to cough and breathe deeply, and to splint the incision for comfort. Know that such patients have difficulty with airway clearance because of denervation, loss of the cough reflex below the tracheal suture line, and slowing of the mucociliary clearance.*

◆ Institute continuous cardiac monitoring, evaluating waveforms frequently for arrhythmias that may result from hypoxemia, electrolyte imbalance, or hemorrhage.

◆ Administer analgesics for pain relief as ordered.

◆ In the immediate postoperative period, monitor laboratory test results including complete blood count, hemoglobin level, hematocrit, platelet count, serum chemistry, serum electrolyte levels, blood urea nitrogen (BUN) levels and creatinine levels, ABG values, and 12-lead electrocardiogram. Anticipate the following tests daily: serum electrolytes, liver and renal function studies, coagulation studies, chest X-ray, urine and sputum cultures, BUN and creatinine, cultures such as for cytomegalovirus (CMV) and toxoplasmosis, and immunosuppressant drug levels.

◆ Institute strict infection control precautions; perform meticulous handwashing.

◆ **WARNING** *The postoperative transplant patient is continuously trying to balance the risk for infection with that of rejection. CMV is a major cause of morbidity and mortality with transplant patients. Expect to administer ganciclovir (Cytovene) prophylactically and as treatment for CMV.*

◆ Assist with extubating as soon as possible and administer supplemental oxygen as needed, based on mixed venous oxygen saturation or pulse oximetry levels. Encourage coughing and deep breathing and use of an incentive spirometer after extubation, splinting and premedicating for pain as necessary.

◆ Assess intake and output at least hourly and notify the practitioner if output is less than 30 ml/hour. Maintain fluids at 2,000 to 3,000 ml/day or as ordered.

◆ Administer postoperative drugs, such as corticosteroids and immunosuppressants. Check blood glucose levels as ordered because corticosteroids may cause transient or sustained hyperglycemia even in patients who aren't diabetic.

◆ Maintain nothing-by-mouth status with NG decompression to low intermittent suction until bowel sounds return. Administer histamine blockers to suppress gastric acid secretion. Begin clear liquids after the patient is extubated, gag reflex is present, and bowel sounds are active. Consult with a dietitian for adequate nutritional intake.

◆ Change the patient's position at least every 2 hours, getting him out of bed to the chair within 24 hours if his condition is stable. Gradually increase the patient's activity as tolerated.

◆ Prepare the patient for transbronchial biopsy to rule out rejection and infection. Explain the procedure to the patient and his family.

◆ Monitor pulmonary function tests to determine lung function; obtain sputum cultures as ordered to evaluate for infection.

◆ Inspect incision site, chest tube insertion site, and other entry sites for signs and symptoms of infection or formation of hematoma.

◆ To ease emotional stress, plan to allow frequent rest periods and provide privacy. Allow family members to visit and comfort the patient as much as possible.

◆ Allow family members to express their anger, anxiety, and fear.

GENERAL

◆ Instruct the patient about the signs and symptoms of infection to report to the practitioner. Teach the patient and his family about infection control measures.

◆ **WARNING** *Remind the patient to take precautions and to watch for signs of infection and rejection that require notifying the practitioner or transplant team immediately. These signs include a fever that continues for more than 2 days; shortness of breath; cough that produces a yellow or green substance; dry cough that continues for more than 1 week; prolonged nausea, vomiting, or diarrhea; inability to take prescribed medication; rash or other skin changes; vaginal discharge or itching; exposure to mumps, measles, chicken pox, or shingles; unusual weakness or light-headedness; emergency department treatment or hospitalization; pain, redness, tenderness or swelling at the incision site; fluid retention or weight gain (2 lb [1 kg] in 24 hours); decrease in urine output; pain or burning during urination; blood in the urine; strong odor to the urine; and urgent need to urinate or need to urinate frequently.*

◆ Review medication administration, dosages, and possible adverse effects, with the patient. Stress the need for compliance with immunosuppressant therapy. Remind the patient to use antacids (if ordered) immediately before a corticosteroid to combat its ulcerogenic effects.

◆ Stress the importance of a program of regular, moderate exercise, beginning slowly and increasing gradually.

◆ Remind him of the need to wait at least 6 weeks before resuming sexual relations. Because pregnancy poses an added risk, provide the female patient with information on birth control.

◆ Stress the importance of regular follow-up visits to the practitioner to evaluate the patient's renal function and transplant acceptance.

◆ Tell the patient that because immunosuppressive medications interfere with his natural immune system, he needs to take the following precautions to avoid infection: wash hands often; keep hands away from face and mouth; stay away from people with colds or other infections; ask friends to visit only when they're well; wash hands before and after dressing changes; wash hands after coughing or sneezing, and throw tissues into the trash immediately; and if a family member has a cold or the flu, have that person follow normal precautions (such as using separate drinking glasses and covering his mouths when coughing).

◆ Tell the patient to avoid working in the soil for 6 months after surgery, and to wear gloves thereafter. Also remind him not to handle animal waste or have contact with animals that roam outside. Tell him not to clean bird cages, fish or turtle tanks, or cat litter; the cat litter box should be covered and taken out of the patient's home before it's changed.

◆ Warn the patient to avoid receiving vaccines that consist of live viruses, such as Sabin oral polio, measles, mumps, German measles, yellow fever, or smallpox, because the live virus may cause infections. Tell him or his family members who intend to receive vaccinations to notify the transplant team or practitioner.

◆ Advise the patient to take care of his teeth by brushing twice per day and seeing the dentist twice per year for cleaning and checkup.

◆ Refer the patient to appropriate resources and support services.

AGE FACTOR *Instruct parents of school-age children to ask the school nurse to notify them immediately of communicable diseases (such as, measles or chicken pox) circulating in the school.*

RESOURCES
Organizations
The American Transplant Association: *www.americantransplant.org*
The Transplant Society: *www.transplantation-soc.org*
TransWeb: *www.transweb.org*
United Organ Transplant Association: *www.uota.org*

Selected references
Dew, M.A., and DiMartini, A.F. "Psychological Disorders and Distress after Adult Cardiothoracic Transplantation," *Journal of Cardiovascular Nursing* 20(5 Suppl):S51-66, September-October 2005.

Finkelstein, S.M., et al. "Decision Support for the Triage of Lung Transplant Recipients on the Basis of Home-Monitoring Spirometry and Symptom Reporting," *Heart Lung* 34(3):201-208, May-June 2005.

Teets, J.M., et al. "Pediatric Thoracic Organ Transplants: Challenges in Primary Care," *Pediatric Nursing* 30(1).23-30, January-February 2004.

Transplantation, pancreas

OVERVIEW

- Replacement of a diseased pancreas with a donor pancreas
- Aims to restore blood glucose levels to normal and limit the progression of complications in patients with type 1 diabetes
- Most commonly occurs simultaneously with renal transplantation (called *simultaneous pancreas-kidney [SPK] transplant*)
- Can also be done after renal transplantation (termed *pancreas-after-kidney [PAK] transplant*) or as a single transplant procedure (termed *pancreas transplant alone [PTA]*)
- Usually involves transplanting the entire pancreas; however, when a living donor is used, only a segment of the organ is transplanted

INDICATIONS

- End-stage pancreatic disease, primarily type 1 diabetes mellitus

   ⚡ **WARNING** *Contraindicated in patients with heart disease that can't be controlled; active infection, positive serology for human immunodeficiency virus or hepatitis B surface antigen, malignancy within the past 3 years, current and active substance abuse, history of noncompliance or psychiatric illness, active untreated peptic ulcer disease, irreversible liver or lung dysfunction, and other systemic illness that would delay or prevent recovery.*

PROCEDURE

- The patient is given general anesthesia.
- In a PTA, the donor pancreas is placed in the right iliac fossa. With SPK or PAK transplant, the donor kidney may be placed in the right iliac fossa or intraperitoneal space and the donor pancreas may be placed in the left iliac fossa or on the side opposite the kidney transplant.
- In the systemic bladder technique, the pancreas and a segment of the donor's duodenum are placed in the iliac fossa. In an SPK or PAK transplant, this side is opposite that of the transplanted kidney.
- The superior mesenteric and splenic arteries of the donor are connected to the patient's iliac artery. The donor's portal vein is attached to the patient's iliac vein.
- The segment of duodenum at the head of the donor pancreas is then anastomosed to the patient's bladder (duodenocystostomy) to allow drainage of pancreatic secretions and enzymes. Thus, urine amylase levels can be used to monitor for graft rejection. (See *SPK transplantation.*)
- In the portal enteric technique, the arterial and venous anastomoses are the same as that for the systemic bladder technique. However, instead of the duodenal segment being attached to the bladder, the segment is anastomosed to a portion of the patient's small bowel, usually the jejunum. Thus, pancreatic secretions drain directly into the GI tract for reabsorption, allowing carbohydrates and lipids to be metabolized as normal.

COMPLICATIONS

- Graft thrombosis (arterial or venous)
- Infection
- Pancreatitis
- Intrapancreatic abscess
- Cystitis, urethritis, or urinary tract infection (with systemic bladder technique)
- Leakage at the anastomosis
- Rejection

SPK transplantation

This illustration depicts simultaneous pancreas-kidney (SPK) transplant, in which the donor pancreas is anastomosed using the systemic bladder technique.

- Ineffective tissue perfusion: GI
- Risk for imbalanced fluid volume
- Risk for infection

EXPECTED OUTCOMES
The patient will:
- demonstrate resumption of pancreatic hormone production by return to normal blood glucose levels without exogenous insulin
- maintain balanced intake and output and stable central venous pressure
- exhibit no signs of infection.

- Prepare the patient for transplantation and a prolonged recovery period; offer him ongoing emotional support.
- Encourage the patient to express his feelings. If he's concerned about rejection, explain what will occur if this happens. Explain that transplant rejection is common.
- Describe routine preoperative measures, such as a physical examination and several laboratory tests to detect infection, electrolyte studies, abdominal X-rays, an electrocardiogram (ECG), an enema, and removal of hair from the operative area, if ordered.
- If the patient is scheduled for a simultaneous kidney transplant, tell him that he'll undergo dialysis the day before surgery to clean his blood of unwanted fluid and electrolytes. Point out that he may need dialysis for a few days after surgery if the transplanted kidney doesn't start functioning immediately.
- Review the transplant procedure.
- Explain what the patient can expect after he awakens from anesthesia, including the presence of I.V. lines, an indwelling urinary catheter, an arterial line and, possibly, a mechanical ventilator. Describe routine postoperative care, including frequent checks of vital signs, monitoring of intake and output, and respiratory therapy. Prepare him for postoperative pain, and reassure him that analgesics will be available.
- Teach the patient the proper methods for performing coughing, turning, deep breathing, and if ordered, incentive spirometry.
- Discuss the immunosuppressant drugs that the patient will be taking, and explain their possible adverse effects. Remind him that these drugs increase his risk for infection.
- Instruct the patient and family members about measures used to control infection and minimize rejection after transplant.
- As ordered, begin giving immunosuppressant drugs; expect to administer low-dose aspirin or, possibly, dipyridamole (Persantine) to prevent thrombosis.
- Verify that a consent form has been signed.

- Assess vital signs and cardiopulmonary and hemodynamic status closely at least every 15 minutes in the immediate postoperative period and then hourly or more frequently as indicated by the patient's condition.
- Maintain continuous cardiac monitoring, evaluating waveforms frequently for ECG changes indicative of electrolyte balance or ischemia.
- Administer fluid replacement therapy, as ordered. Keep in mind that some patients may require I.V. fluid replacement of 1 to 2 L/day, necessitating insertion of a long-term I.V. access device.
- Obtain serial arterial blood gas values, as ordered, to evaluate oxygenation and acid-base status.

WARNING *Watch for metabolic acidosis in the patient who has undergone transplantation with systemic bladder technique; pancreatic secretions are highly alkaline and are eliminated with urine. Some patients increase their respiratory rate to compensate for this imbalance. If metabolic acidosis occurs, expect to administer bicarbonate I.V.*

- In the immediate postoperative period, monitor laboratory test results closely, especially blood urea nitrogen (BUN) and creatinine levels, and serum and urine amylase levels (especially if systemic bladder technique was used or a SPK or PAK transplant was performed). If the patient has a wound drain in place, monitor amylase level in the wound drainage.

(continued)

- Monitor serial blood glucose levels and glycosylated hemoglobin and C peptide levels to evaluate graft function.

  WARNING *In the immediate postoperative period, monitor blood glucose levels every 2 hours to evaluate endocrine function of the pancreas. Also anticipate administering insulin as ordered. Usually, blood glucose levels begin to decline in 12 to 24 hours; the patient is euglycemic within several days of the transplant.*

  WARNING *Watch for an acute increase in pain with significant tenderness and swelling at the operative site and a marked increase in blood glucose and amylase levels. These findings suggest venous graft thrombosis, which is rarely reversible.*

- Carefully monitor intake and output, including urine and drainage from a nasogastric (NG) tube or wound, at least hourly; maintain urinary catheter drainage for at least 5 days after use of the systemic bladder technique.
- Administer anticoagulation therapy as ordered, such as subcutaneous or I.V. heparin therapy, for patients who have had a PTA transplant. Administer prophylactic antibiotic, antifungal, and antiviral agents as ordered; expect the patient to continue taking these after discharge.
- Weigh the patient daily, and report rapid gain (a possible sign of fluid retention).
- Maintain nothing-by-mouth status with NG decompression to low intermittent suction (if appropriate) until bowel sounds return. Administer histamine blockers to suppress gastric acid secretion. Periodically auscultate for bowel sounds, and notify the practitioner when they return. Begin clear liquids after the patient is extubated and bowel sounds are active. Institute measures to prevent constipation, which can lead to reflux pancreatitis.

  WARNING *Know that the patient's immune system has been suppressed by medication and is, therefore, at high risk for infection. Institute standard precautions and use strict sterile technique when changing*

dressings and performing catheter care; limit the patient's contact with staff, other patients, and visitors; and avoid exposing him to people with known infection. Monitor the patient's white blood cell (WBC) count; if it drops precipitously, notify the practitioner.

- Assess the patient for pain, and provide analgesics as ordered. Look for a significant decrease in pain after 24 hours.
- If the patient has an endotracheal tube in place and is receiving mechanical ventilation, assist with extubating as soon as possible (usually within 4 to 6 hours) and administer supplemental oxygen, as needed, based on mixed venous oxygen saturation or pulse oximetry levels. Encourage coughing and deep breathing and the use of an incentive spirometer after extubation, splinting, and premedicating for pain as necessary.
- Change the patient's position at least every 2 hours, getting him out of bed to the chair within 24 hours if his condition is stable. Gradually increase the patient's activity as tolerated; assess him for signs and symptoms of complications related to immobility.
- Monitor the patient for signs and symptoms of rejection, including low-grade fever, elevated WBC count, swelling of the graft area, and increasing serum amylase, lipase, and glucose levels (late appearing).

  WARNING *Elevations in serum amylase and lipase may also suggest pancreatitis and thus aren't specific indicators for rejection. However, when the systemic bladder technique is used, watch for a decrease in urinary amylase levels. This decline usually occurs before hyperglycemia occurs and can be a useful marker for identifying acute rejection. The only true way to confirm rejection is by performing a pancreatic biopsy.*

  WARNING *In the patient who has had SPK transplantation, monitor serum creatinine and BUN levels because rejection of the kidney and pancreas occur simultaneously and kidney function begins to deteriorate*

before pancreatic function does.

- To ease emotional stress, plan to allow frequent rest periods and provide privacy. Allow family members to visit and comfort the patient as much as possible.
- Allow family members to express their anxiety and fear.

GENERAL

- Review the signs and symptoms of infection or transplant rejection with the patient.
- Discuss the prescribed medication regimens and stress the need for compliance with immunosuppressant therapy.
- Tell the patient that because immunosuppressive medications interfere with his natural immune system, he needs to take the following precautions to avoid infection: wash hands often; keep hands away from face and mouth; stay away from people with colds or other infections; ask friends to visit only when they're well; wash hands before and after dressing changes; wash hands after coughing or sneezing, and throw tissues into the trash immediately; and if a family member has a cold or the flu, have that person follow normal precautions (such as using separate drinking glasses and covering his mouths when coughing).
- Tell the patient to avoid working in the soil for 6 months after surgery, and to wear gloves thereafter. Also remind him not to handle animal waste or have contact with animals that roam outside. Tell him not to clean bird cages, fish or turtle tanks, or cat litter; the cat litter box should be covered and taken out of the patient's home before it's changed.
- Warn the patient to avoid receiving vaccines that consist of live viruses, such as Sabin oral polio, measles, mumps, German measles, yellow fever, or smallpox, because the live virus may cause infections. Tell him or his family members who intend to

receive vaccinations to notify the transplant team or practitioner.

- Tell the patient to take an antacid (if ordered) immediately before a corticosteroid to combat its ulcerogenic effects; also tell him to take his prophylactic anti-infective therapy.
- Stress the importance of regular follow up to evaluate pancreatic function (and renal function, if appropriate) and acceptance of transplant.
- Inform the patient that after successful pancreas transplantation, no dietary restrictions are needed.
- Tell the patient that there are few activity restrictions. Advise him to avoid extreme contact sports to prevent accidental trauma to the newly placed intra-abdominal organ.
- Inform the patient that all pancreas transplant recipients require life-long immunosuppression to prevent a T-cell alloimmune rejection response.
- Encourage the patient to keep follow-up appointments with the transplant team. Tell him that the typical visit schedule is two or three visits in the first week, two visits in the second week, one visit in the third week, then monthly thereafter, until 6 months posttransplantation when visits are every 3 months through the first year, every 6 months through the second year, and annually thereafter.
- Tell the patient to keep laboratory follow-up studies as ordered. These may occur in the transplantation clinic and at a local laboratory near the patient's home. A typical schedule is every Monday, Wednesday, and Friday in month 1; every Monday and Thursday in month 2; every Monday in months 3 to 6; every other week in months 7 to 24; and monthly after 24 months. Typical laboratory evaluation includes complete blood count, electrolytes, BUN, creatine, glucose, serum amylase, and immunosuppression blood levels.
- Review the immunosuppression medication schedule; tell him that immunosuppressants need to be taken for as long as the patient's transplanted organs are functioning; if stopped, rejection of the organs will result.

- Advise the patient to take care of his teeth by brushing twice per day and seeing the dentist twice per year for cleaning and checkup.

RESOURCES

Organizations

The American Transplant Association: *www.americantransplant.org*
The Transplant Society: *www.transplantation-soc.org*
TransWeb: *www.transweb.org*
United Organ Transplant Association: *www.uota.org*

Selected references

Malek, S.K., et al. "Percutaneous Ultrasound-Guided Pancreas Allograft Biopsy: A Single-Center Experience," *Transplantation Proceedings* 37(10):4436-37, December 2005.

Melcher, M.L., et al. "Antibody-Mediated Rejection of a Pancreas Allograft," *American Journal of Transplantation* 6(2):423-28, February 2006.

Takahashi, H., et al. "Organ-Specific Differences in Acute Rejection Intensity in a Multivisceral Transplant," *Transplantation* 81(2):297-99, January 2006.

Transplantation, peripheral blood stem cell

OVERVIEW

- Also known as *PBSCT;* restores blood stem cells destroyed by high doses of chemotherapy and radiation therapy
- Patients less likely to develop graft-versus-host disease (GVHD) if stem cells of donor and patient match closely
- Most hematopoietic stem cells found in bone marrow, but some peripheral blood stem cells (PBSCs) occur in blood; umbilical cord blood also contains hematopoietic stem cells—cells from these sources can be used in transplants
- Three types of transplants: autologous (patients receive their own stem cells), syngeneic (patients receive stem cells from their identical twin), and allogeneic (patients receive stem cells from a histocompatible individual)
- Transplanted stem cells restoring bone marrow's ability to produce new blood cells
- To minimize adverse effects, practitioners use transplanted stem cells that match the patient's as closely as possible
- Stem cells used in PBSCT come from the blood; apheresis or leukapheresis used to obtain PBSCs for transplantation
- For 4 or 5 days before apheresis: donor may be given a granulocyte-colony stimulating factor to increase the number of white stem cells released into the bloodstream
- In apheresis: blood is removed through a large vein in the arm or a central venous catheter; it then goes through a machine that removes the stem cells; the blood is then returned to the donor and the collected cells are stored (The stem cells are then frozen until they're given to the recipient.)
- In autologous transplant: stem cells are removed; patient undergoes chemotherapy or radiation therapy to kill cancer cells

INDICATIONS

- Leukemia
- Lymphoma
- Neuroblastoma
- Multiple myeloma

PROCEDURE

- The patient is treated at the bedside. The practitioner inserts a central venous catheter if none is in place.
- A mild sedative or antiemetic may be administered.
- The frozen stem cell infusion is thawed, then administered over 10 minutes. Several infusions are required; so, treatment takes 4 to 6 hours.
- A nurse obtains baseline vital signs just before each infusion.

COMPLICATIONS
During infusion
- Garlic smell and odor
- Nausea and vomiting
- Cough and shortness of breath
- Fever
- Generalized edema
- Abdominal cramps or diarrhea
- Increased blood pressure and decreased pulse

After infusion
- Infection
- Bleeding
- Secondary cancers
- Damage to liver, kidneys, lungs, or heart

NURSING DIAGNOSES

- Activity intolerance
- Deficient fluid volume
- Risk for infection

EXPECTED OUTCOMES
The patient will:
- demonstrate increased ability to perform activities of daily living
- maintain adequate fluid volume
- remain free from infection.

PRETREATMENT CARE

- Review the treatment and preparation with the patient.
- Verify that an appropriate consent form has been signed.
- Discuss the immunosuppressant chemotherapeutic drugs that the patient took; remind him that these drugs increase his risk for infection.
- Instruct the patient and family members about measures used to control infection.
- Provide emotional support to the patient and his family.

- Start an I.V. line and administer I.V. fluids as ordered.
- Obtain an administration set without a filter for infusion.
- Perform a baseline focused nursing assessment.
- Tell the patient to expect his urine to be red for a few days, that he'll experience a garlic taste in his mouth for several hours, and that he'll emit a garlic odor for 2 to 3 days.

POSTTREATMENT CARE

- Maintain asepsis.
- Institute safety precautions.
- Administer ordered transfusions of blood cells, platelets, anti-infectives, or fluids.
- Obtain blood samples for laboratory analysis as ordered.
- Monitor vital signs and laboratory test results.
- Assess for signs of infection, hemorrhage, and end-organ damage.

PATIENT TEACHING

GENERAL

- Review medications and possible adverse reactions.
- Tell the patient of measures to decrease exposure to infection such as avoiding crowded shopping areas or people with known infections.
- Tell the patient that because immunosuppressive medications interfere with his natural immune system, he needs to take the following precautions to avoid infection: wash hands often; keep hands away from face and mouth; stay away from people with colds or other infections; ask friends to visit only when they're well; wash hands before and after dressing changes; wash hands after coughing or sneezing, and throw tissues into the trash immediately; and if a family member has a cold or the flu, have that person follow normal precautions (such as using separate drinking glasses and covering his mouths when coughing).
- Warn the patient to avoid receiving vaccines that consist of live viruses, such as Sabin oral polio, measles, mumps, German measles, yellow fever, or smallpox, because the live virus may cause infections. Until ordered by the practitioner (usually 6 months after transplant), tell his family members who intend to receive vaccinations to notify the transplant team or practitioner.
- Tell the patient of measures to take to avoid injury and risk of bleeding such as use of seat belts in cars, and proper use of knives when cooking.
- Teach the patient how to care for the central venous catheter.
- Review the signs and symptoms of transplant complications.
- Tell the patient to expect peak effects of chemotherapy 1 to 2 weeks after completion, to call the practitioner promptly if he develops a fever greater than 100.5° F (40.8° C), and to expect hospitalization for supportive care.
- Provide the patient with telephone numbers to contact in an emergency.
- Stress the need for follow-up care.
- Explain that engraftment usually occurs 2 to 4 weeks after transplantation; explain what the term means if he's unclear.
- Advise the patient that complete recovery of immune function takes several months for autologous transplant recipients and 1 or 2 years for allogeneic or syngeneic transplant recipients.
- Inform the patient that the practitioner will continue to evaluate him to ensure that new blood cells are being produced and that the cancer hasn't recurred.

RESOURCES
Organizations
American Society of Clinical Oncologists: *www.plwc.org*
National Marrow Donor Program: *www.marrow.org*

Selected resources
Burt, R.K., et al. "Nonmyeloablative Hematopoietic Stem Cell Transplantation for Systemic Lupus Erythematosus," *JAMA* 295(5):527-35, February 2006.
Ljungman, P., et al. "Allogeneic and Autologous Transplantation for Haematological Diseases, Solid Tumours and Immune Disorders: Definitions and Current Practice in Europe," *Bone Marrow Transplantation* 37(5):439-49, January 2006.
Weinstock, D.M., et al. "Preemptive Diagnosis and Treatment of Epstein-Barr Virus-Associated Post Transplant Lymphoproliferative Disorder after Hematopoietic Stem Cell Transplant: An Approach in Development," *Bone Marrow Transplantation* 37(6):539-46, February 2006.

Transplantation, small intestine

- Surgical replacement of major portions of the jejunum and ileum with donated small intestines
- Other organs may be transplanted at the same time, depending on the disease process: liver, stomach, pancreas
- Sources of donated tissue: cadaveric intestines; intestines from living, compatible relatives; or cadaveric multivisceral multi-organ tissue

INDICATIONS

- Short-bowel syndrome
- Irreversible intestinal failure or dysfunction
- Severe absorptive disorders unresponsive to total parenteral nutrition
- End-stage liver disease with bowel dysfunction (combined liver and small-bowel transplantation)
- Major abdominal trauma
- Abdominal malignancy
- Intractable Crohn's disease

   AGE FACTOR *Transplant indications for children include intestinal atresia, gastroschisis, microvillous involution disease, necrotizing enterocolitis, midgut volvulus, chronic intestinal pseudo-obstruction, and Hirschsprung's disease.*

   Children may develop pseudo-obstruction that requires urologic assessment because up to one-third of them may also have a dysfunctional urinary tract. Children with necrotizing enterocolitis and pseudo-obstruction will require neurologic and pulmonary workups to exclude such other causes as intraventricular cerebral hemorrhage or bronchopulmonary dysplasia.

   WARNING *Contraindications to transplantation include patients with congenital immunodeficiency syndromes (risk of graft-versus-host disease [GVHD]); transplantation of cytomegalovirus (CMV) or Epstein-Barr virus (EBV)-positive donor organs to patients who are CMV- or EBV-negative; and possibly critically ill patients.*

PROCEDURE

- The patient is given general anesthesia.
- The patient's gut is decontaminated with antibiotic and antifungal preparations administered via a nasogastric tube along with standard I.V. antibiotic prophylaxis. The new graft is flushed in situ as well.
- Grafts must be 150 to 200 cm long, including the distal jejunum and a portion of the ileum to ensure sufficient tissue for nutrient absorption.
- Living donors retain the distal ileum, ileocecal valve, and cecum, and the descending branch of the right colic artery is carefully protected.
- The surgeon carefully preserves the donated ileocolic artery and vein with the ileum. These vessels are attached end-to-side to the recipient's infrarenal aorta and vena cava. If a cadaveric graft is used, the arteries are attached to the infrarenal aorta, but venous drainage may be done through the inferior vena cava or through the patient's portal vein.

   AGE FACTOR *A small-bowel transplantation accompanied by grafting of a portion of donated liver can help secure more size-matched donor organs for infants and small children.*

- A gastrostomy or jejunostomy is typically done to allow continuous enteral feeding. Graft ileostomy permits frequent endoscopic and histologic postoperative monitoring.

COMPLICATIONS

- Infection
- Sepsis
- EBV-associated lymphoproliferative disease
- Acute and chronic allograft rejection

   WARNING *Intestinal rejection signs and symptoms include fever, abdominal pain, increased bowel output through the ostomy, abdominal distention, and acidosis. Rejection may also be seen with malabsorption and electrolyte abnormalities. Final diagnoses is by endoscopic intestinal biopsy through the ileostomy.*

- GVHD
- Anastomotic leaks
- Hepatic artery thrombosis

NURSING DIAGNOSES

- Imbalanced nutrition: Less than body requirements
- Ineffective tissue perfusion: GI
- Risk for infection

EXPECTED OUTCOMES
The patient will:

- regain functional bowel transit time and excretion and maintain or increase body weight without excess edema
- remain free from signs and symptoms of graft rejection or GVHD
- exhibit no signs of infection.

PRETREATMENT CARE

- Perform cardiopulmonary, vascular, and abdominal nursing assessment.
- Obtain baseline vital signs and monitor intake and output.
- Verify that preoperative urine and blood testing results are in the patient's chart, and assess for coagulation abnormalities and seropositive viral or bacterial disorder. Notify practitioner of findings if appropriate.
- Make sure that ordered X-rays and other imaging studies are in the chart.
- Administer ordered ongoing medications and bowel preparation or antibiotic drugs as ordered.
- Explain what the patient can expect after he wakens from anesthesia, including the presence of I.V. lines, an indwelling urinary catheter, an arterial line and, possibly, a mechanical ventilator. Describe routine postoperative care, including frequent checks of vital signs, monitoring of intake and output, and respiratory therapy. Prepare him for postoperative pain, and reassure him that analgesics will be available.
- Teach the patient the proper methods for performing coughing, turn-

ing, deep breathing and, if ordered, incentive spirometry.
◆ Discuss the immunosuppressant drugs that the patient will be taking, and explain their possible adverse effects. Remind the patient that these drugs increase his risk for infection.
◆ Instruct the patient and family members about measures used to control infection and minimize rejection after transplant.
◆ Provide emotional support to the patient and his family.
◆ Verify that the patient has signed a consent form.

POSTTREATMENT CARE

◆ Monitor the patient's vital signs and intake and output.
◆ Assess patency of gastrostomy and jejunostomy or ileostomy as indicated.
◆ Monitor respiratory status; assess breath sounds and pulse oximetry.
◆ Assess cardiovascular and hemodynamic status closely.
◆ Suction the patient as indicated; maintain patency of the endotracheal tube while it's in place.
◆ Assist with extubating and administer supplemental oxygen as needed, based on mixed venous oxygen saturation or pulse oximetry levels. Encourage coughing, deep breathing, incentive spirometry, and splinting, and premedicate the patient for pain as needed.
◆ Monitor laboratory and other test values and notify practitioner of abnormalities.

⚡ **WARNING** *High levels of immunosuppression are usually done early in the postoperative period when the risk of rejection is greatest, then it's followed with a lower dose for maintenance therapy. Also, multiple immunosuppressive agents are used (as with other organ transplants) to minimize toxicity and to maximize therapeutic effects. Monitor the patient carefully for signs of rejection and complications.*

◆ Monitor fluid status, stool losses, and serum electrolytes.

◆ Institute strict infection control precautions; perform meticulous handwashing.
◆ Administer postoperative drugs, such as corticosteroids (to suppress T- and B-cell function, to reduce or prevent edema, promote normal capillary permeability, and prevent vasodilation) and immunosuppressants (to prevent rejection).
◆ Explain laboratory testing and diagnostic testing ordered.

PATIENT TEACHING

GENERAL
◆ Review how to use the incentive spirometer and pulse oximeter.
◆ Tell the patient that because immunosuppressive medications interfere with his natural immune system, he needs to take the following precautions to avoid infection: wash hands often; keep hands away from face and mouth; stay away from people with colds or other infections; ask friends to visit only when they're well; wash hands before and after dressing changes; wash hands after coughing or sneezing, and throw tissues into the trash immediately; and if a family member has a cold or the flu, have that person follow normal precautions (such as using separate drinking glasses and covering his mouth when coughing).
◆ Tell the patient to avoid working in the soil for 6 months after surgery, and to wear gloves thereafter. Also remind him not to handle animal waste or have contact with animals that roam outside. Tell him not to clean bird cages, fish or turtle tanks, or cat litter; the cat litter box should be covered and taken out of the patient's home before it's changed.
◆ Warn the patient to avoid receiving vaccines that consist of live viruses, such as Sabin oral polio, measles, mumps, German measles, yellow fever, or smallpox, because the live virus may cause infections. Tell him or family members who intend to receive vaccinations to notify the transplant team or practitioner.

◆ Review the signs of complications and what to report to the surgeon.
◆ Review dietary changes with the patient.
◆ Instruct the patient in incision and ostomy care and signs and symptoms of infection or bleeding to report to the transplant team.
◆ Discuss activity restrictions with the patient.
◆ Review medication administration, dosages, and possible adverse effects.
◆ Explain the continued need for follow-up care with the transplant team.
◆ Advise the patient to take care of his teeth by brushing twice per day and seeing the dentist twice per year for cleaning and checkup.

RESOURCES
Organizations
The American Transplant Association: *www.americantransplant.org*
The Transplant Society: *www.transplantation-soc.org*
TransWeb: *www.transweb.org*
United Organ Transplant Association: *www.uota.org*

Selected references
Chen, H.X., et al. "Abdominal Cluster Transplantation and Management of Perioperative Hemodynamic Changes," *Hepatobiliary and Pancreatic Diseases International* 5(1):28-33, February 2006.
Gupte, G.L., et al. "Current Issues in the Management of Intestinal Failure," *Archives of Disease in Childhood* 91(3):259-64, March 2006.
Kelly, D.A. "Intestinal Failure-Associated Liver Disease: What Do We Know Today?" *Gastroenterology* 130(2S):S70-77, February 2006.
Siirtola, A., et al. "Cholesterol Absorption and Synthesis in Pediatric Kidney, Liver, and Heart Transplant Recipients," *Transplantation* 81(3):327-34, February 2006.

Transurethral microwave thermotherapy

OVERVIEW

- Also known as *TUMT;* used to treat benign prostatic hyperplasia (BPH)
- Eliminates excess prostate cells with minimal patient risk
- Uses controlled heat (above 113° F [45° C]) via microwave energy to target areas of an enlarged prostate
- Poor candidates for treatment: patients with prostate glands smaller than 30 g or heavier than 100 g, prostatic urethral length of less than 3 cm, or a prominent median prostatic bar

INDICATIONS

- Benign prostatic hyperplasia (BPH)
- Moderate-to-severe obstructive or irritative voiding symptoms
- Patients in whom medical therapy has failed
- Patients who choose not to be treated medically

⚡ **WARNING** *Contraindications include untreated urinary tract infection or known or suspected prostate or urothelial cancer. Other contraindications include patients with metallic implants or a penile prosthesis, artificial urinary sphincters, severe urethral stricture disease prohibiting proper probe placement, severe peripheral vascular disease with claudication, or Leriche syndrome. Patients who want to preserve fertility should be warned about the risk for retrograde ejaculation and erectile dysfunction.*

PROCEDURE

- The procedure can be done in the urologist's office or a short procedure unit.
- The patient is given an oral analgesic before the procedure.
- Lidocaine (Xylocaine) gel is injected into the urethral meatus. The treatment catheter is then inserted. A rectal probe is used to monitor the temperature of the tissues during treatment.
- Intraoperative details vary based on type of TUMT machine used. The protocol for specific equipment is followed per the manufacturer's guidelines.
- Essentially, microwave (heat) energy is directed at the excess prostatic tissue while a special cooling fluid circulates through the probe to prevent damage from overheating. If the safe temperature level is exceeded with the rectal probe, the unit shuts down. Prostate tissue temperatures of 140° to 176° F (60° to 80° C) are used during therapy with the urethral coolant circulating at 46.4° F (8° C) to maintain the overall urethral temperature at 102.2° to 105.8° F (39° to 41° C). The manufacturer may vary the specific temperature, coolant, and timing of treatment. A dilating balloon may be available on some models to facilitate the process.
- The patient may experience mild perineal warmth, mild pain, and a sense of urinary urgency during the treatment.

COMPLICATIONS

- Urine retention
- Infection
- Postoperative pain
- Changes in sexual function
- Erectile dysfunction
- Myocardial infarction, especially more than 2 years after therapy
- Cardiovascular disease
- Urethrorectal fistula
- Bladder perforation
- Bowel irradiation
- Chronic pain
- Urethral injury
- Prostatitis
- A "pressure" sensation
- Urinary urgency
- Urethral tear
- Anal irritation
- Urethral stricture
- Infertility
- Retrograde ejaculation

NURSING DIAGNOSES

- Acute pain
- Impaired urinary elimination
- Risk for infection

EXPECTED OUTCOMES

The patient will:
- demonstrate signs of comfort
- demonstrate normal elimination patterns
- not develop signs of an infection.

PRETREATMENT CARE

- Make sure the history and physical examination has been completed.
- The practitioner's clinical evaluation determines the presence and degree of voiding dysfunction and the potential role of BPH.
- Verify that the patient with a pacemaker has received written clearance from his cardiologist before undergoing TUMT because the pacemaker may need to be turned off during therapy.
- Evaluate laboratory studies before treatment; these may include complete blood count, serum chemistries, and prostate-specific antigen levels.
- Pretreatment imaging studies may include transrectal ultrasonography and renal ultrasonography; for patients with hematuria, renal ultrasonography may be needed, especially if I.V. pyelography or computer tomography scanning is contraindicated.
- The voiding velocity test may be done to evaluate urinary flow rate. The postvoid residual (PVR) is done by ultrasound to measure the volume

of urine remaining in the bladder immediately after micturition.
- Other diagnostic procedures may include cystourethroscopy, pressure-flow study, cystometrography, or urethral pressure profile test; video urodynamics is usually done in patients with complex conditions or in those who need to have the specific site of obstruction identified.
- Reinforce the practitioner's explanation of the risks, benefits, alternatives, and expected results of therapy.
- Administer ordered antibiotics to the patient with a urinary catheter still in place or who has had recent urinary tract manipulation.
- Verify that the patient has taken nothing by mouth for 6 hours before therapy.

POSTTREATMENT CARE

- Maintain a patent airway and adequate oxygenation.
- Provide adequate hydration.
- Assess for pain and administer medications as ordered.
- Monitor vital signs, fluid status, and intake and output.
- Be aware that prostatic edema may occur after therapy, leading to a risk for urine retention, especially with higher energy protocols; therefore, a catheter may be left in place for a few days to 2 weeks.

PATIENT TEACHING

GENERAL
- Review the administration, dosage, and possible adverse reactions of medications with the patient.
- Tell the patient that urinary flow may gradually improve over a few months posttreatment as the coagulated tissue is absorbed by the body, and the treated area heals.
- Inform the patient that medications, such as alpha-adrenergic blockers, may eventually be decreased or stopped after full healing has been achieved.
- Tell the patient that a temporary prostatic bridge catheter may be placed for 3 to 7 days to prevent prostatic obstruction immediately after the procedure.
- Stress the need to return to the clinic for follow-up care.
- If a catheter has been placed, teach the patient care of the catheter and drainage system, and how to remove the catheter when permitted by the practitioner.
- Instruct the patient to call the practitioner promptly for an inability to void, painful voiding, high fever, abdominal pain, or other problems.
- Refer the patient and his family for follow-up care.

RESOURCES

Organizations
American College of Emergency Practitioners: *www.acep.org*
American Urological Association: *www.auanet.org*

Selected references
Disantostefano, R.L., et al. "The Long-Term Cost Effectiveness of Treatments for Benign Prostatic Hyperplasia," *Pharmacoeconomics* 24(2):171-91, 2006.
Miner, M., et al. "Treatment of Lower Urinary Tract Symptoms in Benign Prostatic Hyperplasia and its Impact on Sexual Function," *Clinical Therapeutics* 28(1):13-25, January 2006.
Wright, J.L., et al. "Virtual Reality as an Adjunctive Pain Control During Transurethral Microwave Thermotherapy," *Urology* 66(6):1320, December 2005.

Trigger point injection

- Used to treat extremely painful areas of muscle
- Pathophysiology: Muscle spasms and knotting may trap or irritate and inflame the surrounding nerves, causing referred pain to other areas of the body and, possibly, scar tissue, loss of range of motion (ROM), and weakness from disuse
- Manifested as a knot or tight, ropy band of muscle that forms when muscle fails to relax properly; can be felt under the skin and may twitch involuntarily when touched ("jump sign")
- Relief usually achieved with a brief course of treatment: injection of medication inactivates the trigger point and alleviates the pain
- Also known as *TPI*

INDICATIONS

- Myofascial pain syndrome unresponsive to other treatment
- Pain in muscle groups
- Fibromyalgia
- Tension headaches
- Muscle spasm in back or neck
- Focal areas of muscle hyperactivity

- An orthopedist, physiatrist, pain specialist, or neurologist can administer TPI. Injections are given in the practitioner's office and take about 30 minutes.
- Before performing TPI, the practitioner may give the patient a nerve block to prevent pain from needle penetration.
- A small needle is inserted into the trigger point and a local anesthetic and often a corticosteroid is injected.
- The injection may cause a twitch or pain that lasts a few seconds to a few minutes. The corticosteroid reduces swelling and inflammation in the area as the anesthetic blocks the pain receptors that prevent relaxation.
- TPI may also be done by electromagnetically-guided (EMG) injection. The needle used for injection is electronically connected to an EMG machine that can interpret signals about nerve reactions in muscle tissue. First, the practitioner feels for the trigger point. He then inserts the needle into the area. The needle relays information back to a monitor, which the practitioner uses to further guide the needle directly into the trigger point.

COMPLICATIONS

- Puncture of a lung or pleura when a muscle near the rib cage receives a trigger point injection
- Infection
- Light-headedness
- Tingling or burning (as the anesthetic begins to take effect)
- Bruising around the injection site
- Pain around the injection site

- Acute pain
- Impaired physical mobility
- Ineffective tissue perfusion: Peripheral

EXPECTED OUTCOMES

The patient will:
- express feelings of increased comfort
- attain the highest degree of mobility possible within the confines of injury
- exhibit adequate tissue perfusion and pulses distally.

PRETREATMENT CARE

◆ Explain the procedure to the patient.
◆ Verify that a consent form has been signed.
◆ Answer questions the patient may have.

POSTTREATMENT CARE

◆ Monitor the patient's vital signs.
◆ Provide care to the site as indicated.
◆ Monitor neurologic and pain status.
◆ Monitor response to analgesics.
◆ Monitor mobility and ROM.
◆ Monitor for complications.

PATIENT TEACHING

GENERAL

◆ Explain prescribed medications.
◆ Stress the importance of follow-up examination.
◆ Inform the patient about required restrictions in activity and changes in lifestyle until the treatment takes effect.
◆ Tell the patient that numbness from the anesthetic may last about 1 hour and that a bruise may form at the injection site.
◆ Inform the patient that pain can be relieved by alternately applying moist heat and ice for 1 or 2 days.
◆ Tell the patient that physical therapy is recommended after TPI; stretching exercises enhance the effects of the injection by keeping the muscle fibers limber.
◆ Review signs of infection that should be reported to the practitioner, such as redness or swelling.
◆ Tell the patient that the injections may be repeated on an as-needed basis.
◆ Refer the patient for follow-up care.
◆ Refer the patient for physical and occupational therapy as indicated.

RESOURCES

Organizations

American College of Rheumatology: *www.rheumatology.org*
Arthritis Foundation: *www.arthritis.org*

Selected references

Friedberg, F., et al. "Do Support Groups Help People With Chronic Fatigue Syndrome and Fibromyalgia? A Comparison of Active and Inactive Members," *Journal of Rheumatology* 32(12):2416-20, December 2005.
O'Sullivan, J., and McCabe, J.T. "Migraine Development, Treatments, Research Advances, and Anesthesia Implications," *American Association of Nurse Anesthetists Journal* 74(1):61-69, February 2006.
Yousefi, P., and Coffey, J. "For Fibromyalgia, Which Treatments are the Most Effective?" *Journal of Family Practice* 54(12):1094-95, December 2005.

Turbinectomy

- Surgical procedure that opens up the nasal passages
- May be performed with other nasal surgeries, such as septoplasty, rhinoplasty, or sinus surgery

INDICATIONS

- Deviated nasal septum
- Swelling of the turbinate due to allergy, chronic inflammation, or chronic sinusitis
- Nasal polyps or other tumors obstructing the nose
- Swelling of the adenoids
- Snoring
- Obstructive sleep apnea

- The patient receives general anesthesia.
- There are many types of turbinectomy, depending on the patient's anatomy. The surgeon may remove bone only or bone and soft tissue by cauterization, electrocautery, or microdebrider.
- A microdebrider is a tiny, high-speed device that shaves soft tissue. It may be inserted through a tiny tube so that nasal surgeries can be performed with minimal incisions. The microdebrider is inserted into the turbinate through a tiny incision in the nose using a computer tomography (CT)–guided imaging system. The practitioner removes the desired tissue, leaving adjacent tissues intact.
- The nose is packed after completion of the procedure, or a stasis agent is used to reduce incidence of bleeding.

COMPLICATIONS

- Bleeding
- Swelling
- Bruising

- Impaired gas exchange
- Ineffective breathing pattern
- Ineffective tissue perfusion: Cardiopulmonary

EXPECTED OUTCOMES

The patient will:

- maintain adequate ventilation
- exhibit normal breathing pattern
- maintain tissue perfusion.

PRETREATMENT CARE

- Review the procedure with the patient and answer questions.
- Make sure that a history and physical examination has been completed.
- Verify that a consent form has been signed.
- Verify that the patient hasn't had anything by mouth for 6 to 12 hours before surgery.

POSTTREATMENT CARE

- Maintain a patent airway and provide oxygenation and humidification as ordered.
- Monitor for bleeding and signs of infection.
- Observe nasal packing, if present, and monitor drainage.
- Monitor the patient's vital signs and intake and output.
- Monitor for swelling and bruising.
- Monitor neurologic status and pain level.
- Administer medications as ordered.
- Position the patient for comfort and to facilitate breathing.
- Monitor pulse oximetry.

PATIENT TEACHING

GENERAL

- Inform the patient that nasal packing may remain in place for several days after surgery and will be removed in the practitioner's office.
- Review the signs of infection with the patient and to call the practitioner if these signs are seen.
- Stress the importance of follow-up care.

RESOURCES

Organizations
American Academy of Otolaryngology—Head and Neck Surgery: *www.entnet.org*
American College of Surgeons: *www.facs.org*
American Medical Association: *www.ama-assn.org*

Selected references

Barbosa Ade, A., et al. "Assessment of Pre and Postoperative Symptomatology in Patients Undergoing Inferior Turbinectomy," *Revista Brasileira de Otorrinolaringologia (English ed)* 71(4):468-71, July-August 2005.

Harsten, G. "How We Do It: Radiofrequency-Turbinectomy for Nasal Obstruction Symptoms," *Clinical Otolaryngology* 30(1):64-66, February 2005.

Wexler, D., and Braverman, I. "Partial Inferior Turbinectomy Using the Microdebrider," *Journal of Otolaryngology* 34(3):189-93, June 2005.

Ultraviolet light therapy

OVERVIEW

- Ultraviolet (UV) light: causes profound biological changes in the skin, including temporary suppression of epidermal basal cell division, an increase in cell turnover, and UV light-induced immune suppression
- UV spectrum (emitted by the sun): subdivided into A (UVA), B (UVB), and C (UVC) subband; each affects the skin differently
- UVA radiation (wavelength 320 to 400 nm): rapidly darkens preformed melanin pigment, augments UVB in causing sunburn and skin aging, and induces phototoxicity in the presence of certain drugs
- UVB radiation (wavelength 280 to 320 nm): causes sunburn and erythema
- UVC radiation (wavelength 200 to 280 nm): normally absorbed by the earth's ozone layer without reaching the ground; kills bacteria and is used in operating-room germicidal lamps
- Combination treatment of UVA and a photosensitizing agent, such as methoxsalen: enhances therapeutic effect and is called psoralen plus UVA (PUVA) or photochemotherapy; given before a UV light treatment
- Other photochemotherapeutic drugs used with PUVA: acitretin (Soriatane)—an oral vitamin A derivative—and methotrexate (Rheumatrex)
- Topical preparations, such as coal tar, also possibly used with UVB (Goeckerman treatment)

INDICATIONS

- Psoriasis
- Mycosis fungoides
- Atopic dermatitis
- Uremic pruritus

WARNING *Contraindications to PUVA and UVB therapy include a history of photosensitivity diseases, skin cancer, arsenic ingestion, or cataracts or cataract surgery; current use of photosensitivity-inducing drugs; and previous skin irradiation (which can induce skin cancer). UV light therapy is also contraindicated in patients who have undergone previous ionizing chemotherapy and in those using photosensitizing or immunosuppressant drugs.*

PROCEDURE

- The patient can undergo UV light therapy in the hospital, a practitioner's office, or at home. Typically set into a reflective cabinet, the light source consists of a bank of high-intensity fluorescent bulbs. (At home, the patient may use a small fluorescent sunlamp.)
- The practitioner calculates the UVB dose based on skin type or by determining a minimal erythema dose—the least amount of UV light needed to produce mild erythema.
- To begin therapy, bring the patient to the phototherapy unit. Instruct him that he may keep his hospital gown on (to protect vulnerable skin areas) and to expose just the area needing treatment.
- Provide the patient with goggles to protect his eyes.

WARNING *All male patients receiving PUVA must wear protection over the groin area.*

- If the patient is having local UVB treatment, position him at the correct distance from the light source. For example, for facial treatment with a sunlamp, position the patient's face about 12″ (30.5 cm) from the lamp. For body treatment, position the patient's body about 30″ (76 cm) from either the sunlamp or the hot quartz lamp.
- If the patient must stand for the treatment, ask him to report dizziness.
- Prevent eye damage by using gray or green polarized lenses during UVB therapy or UV-opaque sunglasses during PUVA therapy. The patient undergoing PUVA therapy should wear these glasses for 24 hours posttreatment because methoxsalen can cause photosensitivity.

COMPLICATIONS

- Erythema (major adverse effect of UVB therapy)
- Marked edema, swelling, or blistering
- Erythema, nausea, and pruritus (major short-term adverse effects of PUVA)

Long-term adverse effects

- Premature aging (xerosis, wrinkles, and mottled skin)
- Lentigines
- Telangiectasia
- Increased risk of skin cancer
- Ocular damage if eye protection isn't used

NURSING DIAGNOSES

- Anxiety
- Impaired tissue integrity
- Risk for infection

EXPECTED OUTCOMES

The patient will:

- exhibit signs of comfort and decreased anxiety
- demonstrate skin that's intact and healing
- remain free from infection.

PRETREATMENT CARE

- Check the practitioner's orders to confirm the light treatment type and dose. For PUVA, the initial dose is based on the patient's skin type and is increased based on the treatment protocol and patient tolerance.
- Review the patient's history for contraindications to UV light therapy.
- Ask the patient if he's taking photosensitizing drugs, such as anticonvulsants, certain antihypertensives, phenothiazines, salicylates, sulfonamides, tetracyclines, tretinoin (Avita), and certain cancer drugs.
- If coal tar is to be applied to the patient's skin before UV light therapy, be sure to remove it completely with mineral oil before treatment begins to allow the light penetrate the skin.
- If the patient is to have PUVA therapy, make sure he took methoxsalen (with food) 1½ hours before treatment.
- Before giving methoxsalen or etretinate (Tegison), check that baseline liver function studies have been done.

WARNING *Keep in mind that methoxsalen and etretinate are hepatotoxic agents and shouldn't be given together. Liver function and blood lipid studies are required before treatment with acitretin and at regular intervals during treatment. Liver function studies and a complete blood count are required before and during methotrexate treatment.*

POSTTREATMENT CARE

- After delivering the prescribed UVB dose, help the patient out of the unit and instruct him to shield exposed areas of skin from sunlight for 8 hours after therapy.
- Overexposure to UV light (sunburn) can result from prolonged treatment, an inadequate distance between the patient and light sources, use of photosensitizing drugs, or from overly sensitive skin.
- Tell the patient to look for marked erythema, blistering, peeling, or other signs of overexposure 4 to 6 hours after UVB therapy and 24 to 48 hours after UVA therapy; mild erythema should disappear within 24 hours.
- If the practitioner prescribes tar preparations with UVB treatment, monitor for signs of sensitivity, such as erythema, pruritus, and eczema.

(continued)

Caring for your skin

Dear Patient:

Your health care provider has recommended that you receive ultraviolet light treatment for your condition. Follow the skin care tips below to protect your skin from injury:

◆ Use emollients and drink plenty of fluids to combat dry skin and maintain adequate hydration. Also, avoid hot baths or showers and use soap sparingly because heat and soap promote dry skin.

◆ Notify your health care provider before taking any medication, including aspirin, to prevent heightened photosensitivity.

◆ If you're receiving PUVA therapy, follow your dosage schedule to prevent burns or ineffective treatment. Wear appropriate sunglasses outdoors for at least 24 hours after taking methoxsalen. Have your eyes examined yearly to detect cataracts.

◆ If you're using a sunlamp at home, let the lamp warm for 5 minutes before beginning treatment. Expose your skin to the light for the exact amount of time prescribed by your health care provider. Remember to protect your eyes with goggles and to use a dependable timer or have someone else time your therapy. Never use the sunlamp when you're tired because you could sustain a burn if you fall asleep under the lamp.

◆ Know how to apply first aid for a local burn: Apply cool-water soaks for 20 minutes or until the skin temperature cools. For more extensive burns, notify the health care provider and then use tepid tap water baths. After bathing, use an oil-in-water moisturizing lotion (not a petroleum-based product, which can trap radiant heat).

◆ Limit your exposure to natural light. Also, use a sunscreen when you're outdoors, and notify your physician immediately if you notice unusual skin lesions.

◆ Avoid using harsh soaps and chemicals, such as paints and solvents, and find ways to manage physical and psychological stress, which may exacerbate skin disorders.

PATIENT TEACHING

GENERAL

◆ Review prescribed medications with the patient, including dosage and potential adverse reactions.

◆ Teach the patient how to care for the skin properly.

◆ Stress the importance of follow-up care.

◆ Inform the patient that it's normal for UV light treatments to produce a mild sunburn.

◆ Tell the patient that mild dryness and desquamation will occur in 1 or 2 days; teach him appropriate skin care measures. (See *Caring for your skin.*)

◆ Advise the patient to notify the practitioner if overexposure occurs. The practitioner will stop treatment for a few days and then starting over at a lower exposure level.

◆ Tell the patient to minimize the effects of UV exposure by using emollients, sunscreens, and cover-ups.

◆ Refer the patient for resource and support services.

RESOURCES

Organizations

American Academy of Dermatology: *www.aad.org*

American Association of Pediatrics: *www.aap.org*

American Medical Association: *www.ama-assn.org*

Selected references

Lebwohl, M.G. "Advances in Psoriasis," *Archives in Dermatology* 141(12):1589-90, December 2005.

Moss, F.M. "New Insights into the Mechanism of Action of Extracorporeal Phototherapy," *Transfusion* 46(1):6-8, January 2006.

Yoon, T.Y., and Kim, Y.G. "Infant Alopecia Universalis: Role of Topical PUVA (psoralen ultraviolet A) Radiation," *International Journal of Dermatology* 44(12):1065-67, December 2005

Urethral dilation and internal urethrotomy

- Treat symptomatic strictures of the anterior portion of the urethra in men (strictures are rare in women but may also be treated with these methods)
- Symptomatic strictures: caused by scar tissue; affect the urinary pattern, eventually leading to urine retention and risk for infection
- Urethral dilation: minimally invasive technique to progressively dilate a narrowed area
- Internal urethrotomy: minimally invasive technique to surgically release scar tissue; may include permanent stent placement
- If these measures fail repeatedly or cause further strictures or major damage to the urethra, open surgical urethral reconstruction possibly required

INDICATIONS
- Urethral stricture

- Depending on the procedure, the patient receives local or general anesthesia.

URETHRAL DILATION
- The patient is treated in the urologist's office using local anesthetic gel.
- Have the patient lie in a supine position on the treatment table.
- The urologist uses sterile technique to clean the glans penis.
- A small sterile guide wire is inserted into the urethra just past the area of stricture.
- A series of progressively larger dilators are threaded over the guide wire to stretch the narrowed area to an adequate degree of opening, then all the tools are gently removed and the patient may wash himself and dress.
- The procedure is repeated at scheduled intervals (usually several months) to maintain the opening.
- If the stricture is prone to reclose rapidly, the patient may be taught self-catheterization with an appropriately sized catheter to perform every month between visits. However, he'll most likely undergo urethrotomy because of the stricture's tendency to reclose so quickly after catheterization.

INTERNAL URETHROTOMY
- The patient is treated in an outpatient surgery center or inpatient hospital setting, usually under general anesthesia but possibly with local anesthesia and some sedation.
- Position the patient on his back with his legs spread widely and either flat or in a lithotomy position.
- The urologist inserts a cystoscope with a knife, laser, or electrocautery tool attachment into the urethra until the stricture is easily seen.
- The scar tissue is then cut or heated by laser or cautery, releasing the source of the narrowing.

- A small metal stent may be placed in the newly opened area by a cystoscopic attachment in selected patients.

⚡ **WARNING** *Care must be taken not to injure the corpora cavernosa in a male, which may lead to erectile dysfunction.*

- An indwelling urinary catheter is placed.

COMPLICATIONS
- Recurrence of stricture
- Postoperative bleeding
- Urinary tract infection
- Formation of new strictures by damaging the urethra with repeated catheterizations or treatments
- Pain with sitting or intercourse with distal stent migration
- Hypertrophic reaction around the stent

NURSING DIAGNOSES

◆ Acute pain
◆ Impaired urinary elimination
◆ Risk for infection

EXPECTED OUTCOMES
The patient will:
◆ verbalize feelings of increased comfort
◆ demonstrate adequate urinary output based on intake, lack of urinary retention, and return of normal elimination patterns after catheter removal
◆ remain free from infection.

PRETREATMENT CARE

◆ Review the procedure with the patient and describe pretreatment and posttreatment nursing or self-care.
◆ Verify that an appropriate consent form has been signed.
◆ Verify that all ordered pretreatment studies have been completed, including urinalysis to rule out current urinary tract infection (UTI) and tests to eliminate a neoplastic cause of the dysfunction.
◆ Verify that the patient has completed previously ordered treatment for UTI.
◆ Ask the patient to void before the procedure.

POSTTREATMENT CARE

◆ After internal urethrotomy, assess the urinary catheter drainage for color, turbidity, and odor and the urinary meatus for signs of irritation or bleeding.
◆ Assess the patient's pain level and give medications as needed.
◆ Monitor the patient's vital signs and intake and output.
◆ Provide instructions on managing the urinary catheter when turning or getting out of bed.

PATIENT TEACHING

GENERAL
◆ Discuss the administration, dosage, and possible adverse reactions of any medications with the patient, particularly analgesics or antibiotics if ordered.
◆ Tell the patient with a urinary catheter to schedule an appointment with the practitioner for the fifth day after the procedure to be evaluated and have the catheter removed.
◆ Teach the patient care of the urinary catheter and drainage bags to prevent backflow of urine or urinary tract infection; provide written instructions on care after discharge.
◆ For patients who will perform periodic self-catheterization after dilation or healed urethrotomy, teach the procedure based on clean technique.

RESOURCES
Organizations
American Urological Association:
www.urologyhealth.org
U.S. National Library of Medicine:
www.nlm.nih.gov/medlineplus

Selected references
Kamp, S., et al., "Low-power Holmium: YAG Laser Urethrotomy for Treatment of Urethral Strictures: Functional Outcome and Quality of Life," *Journal of Endourology* 20(1):38-41, January 2006.
Naude, A.M., and Heyns, C.F., "What is the Place of Internal Urethrotomy in the Treatment of Urethral Stricture Disease?" *Nature Clinical Practice: Urology* 2(11):538-45, November 2005.
Schwender, C.E., et al. "Technique and Results of Urethroplasty for Female Stricture Disease," *The Journal of Urology* 175(3 Pt 1):976-80, March 2006.

Urinary diversion surgery

OVERVIEW

- Provides an alternative route for urine excretion when disease impedes normal urine flow through the bladder
- Incontinent diversion: used when urine flow is constant and patient requires an external collection device permanently; types include ileal conduit, ureterosigmoidostomy, and nephrostomy
- Continent diversion: used when an external collection bag isn't needed; types include the Kock pouch (continent internal ileal reservoir), Indiana pouch, Mainz reservoir, and Camey procedure (orthotopic bladder replacement (see *Reviewing selected types of urinary diversion*)

INDICATIONS

- Cystectomy
- Congenital urinary tract defect
- Severe, unmanageable urinary tract infection that threatens renal function
- Chronic cystitis
- Injury to the ureters, bladder, or urethra
- Obstructive malignancy
- Neurogenic bladder

PROCEDURE

- The patient is given general anesthesia.
- The surgeon makes a midline or paramedial abdominal incision.

ILEAL CONDUIT

- The surgeon excises a segment of the ileum measuring 6″ to 8″ (15 to 20.5 cm).
- The remaining ileal ends are anastomosed to maintain intestinal integrity.
- The ureters are dissected from the bladder and implanted in the ileal segment.
- The surgeon sutures one end of the ileal segment closed.
- The other end of the segment is brought through the abdominal wall to form a stoma.

NEPHROSTOMY

- The surgeon inserts a catheter into the renal pelvis percutaneously or through a flank incision.

Reviewing selected types of urinary diversion

Types of urinary diversion include ileal conduit, Camey procedure (orthotopic bladder replacement), and Kock pouch (continent internal ileal reservoir).

ILEAL CONDUIT

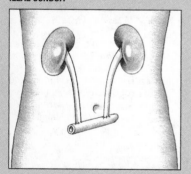

Both ureters are anastomosed to a small segment of ileum, one end of which is brought to the surface of the lower abdomen to form a stoma.

CAMEY PROCEDURE

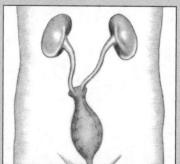

An internal pouch is created from the small bowel or small and large bowel. The urethral stump is anastomosed to the pouch. The patient voids through the urethra. This procedure is performed in males only. The patient commonly experiences nocturnal incontinence.

KOCK POUCH

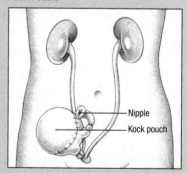

An internal pouch is created from a segment of ileum. The ureters are implanted into the pouch's sides, and nipple valves are intussuscepted to them. One valve prevents urine backflow; the other valve is used to form a stoma.

Nipple
Kock pouch

◆ This procedure is usually palliative because it carries a high risk for infection and renal calculus formation.

KOCK POUCH
◆ Segments of the small bowel and colon are used.
◆ The surgeon excises 24″ to 32″ (61 to 81 cm) of ileum and anastomoses the remaining ileal ends.
◆ The isolated ileum segment is shaped into a pocket to serve as a bladder.
◆ The Kock pouch is connected to the urethra, or an intussuscepted nipple valve is used to connect the pouch to the external skin of the anterior abdominal wall.
◆ A second nipple valve is constructed at the other end of the pouch.
◆ The ureters are then implanted at the site of the second nipple valve.
◆ Temporary ureteral stents may be placed. These originate in the pelvis of the kidneys and extend through the ureter into the pouch and out through the abdominal opening or separate stab wounds.
◆ One or two drainage tubes are inserted into the reservoir and remain until healing has occurred and pouch integrity is confirmed.

CAMEY PROCEDURE
◆ The surgeon creates a pouch from both the small and large bowels and connects it to the urethral stump.
◆ An indwelling catheter is inserted and remains in place for about 3 weeks.
◆ After the catheter is removed, the patient voids through the urethra by abdominal straining.

COMPLICATIONS
◆ Skin breakdown
◆ Infection
◆ Urinary extravasation
◆ Ureteral obstruction
◆ Small-bowel obstruction
◆ Peritonitis
◆ Hydronephrosis
◆ Stomal stenosis
◆ Pyelonephritis
◆ Renal calculi
◆ Psychological problems

NURSING DIAGNOSES
◆ Acute pain
◆ Impaired urinary elimination
◆ Risk for infection

EXPECTED OUTCOMES
The patient will:
◆ verbalize feelings of comfort
◆ demonstrate adequate urine output in relation to intake
◆ remain free from infection.

PRETREATMENT CARE
◆ Explain the treatment and preparation to the patient and his family. Try using a simple anatomic diagram to enhance the discussion, and provide printed information from the United Ostomy Association or other sources, if possible and appropriate. Explain that the patient will receive a general anesthetic and may have a nasogastric tube in place after surgery.
◆ If appropriate, prepare the patient for the appearance and general location of the stoma. For example, if he's scheduled for an ileal conduit, explain that the stoma will be located somewhere in the lower abdomen, probably below the waistline.
◆ Ensure that the patient having a continent internal ileal reservoir understands that his "new bladder" won't function identically to the natural bladder. If the reservoir will be attached to the external skin, explain that the stoma will be flush with the skin of the anterior abdominal wall, and that the exact location of the stoma is usually determined during surgery.
◆ Review the enterostomal therapist's explanation of the urine collection device or catheterization procedure to be used after surgery. Reassure the patient that he'll be trained on how to manage urine drainage after surgery.
◆ If possible, arrange for a visit by a well-adjusted patient who has undergone the same type of urinary diversion. He can provide a firsthand account of the surgery and offer some insight into the realities of ongoing care of urinary drainage. Also, as appropriate, be sure to include the patient's family members in all aspects of preoperative teaching—especially if they'll be providing much of the care after discharge.
◆ Verify that the patient or a legally authorized representative has signed an appropriate consent form.
◆ Explain postoperative care.
◆ Initiate referrals if the patient needs assistance with stoma management.

(continued)

- Prepare the bowel as ordered (such as with a low-residue or clear liquid diet, an enema, antimicrobial drugs, total parenteral nutrition (TPN), or fluid replacement therapy).

POSTTREATMENT CARE

- Administer medications as ordered.
- Provide comfort measures.
- Observe urine drainage for pus and blood; report findings.
- Maintain patency of drainage catheters, as ordered, and report urine leakage from the drain or suture line.

WARNING *Watch for signs and symptoms of peritonitis (such as fever, abdominal distention, and pain), which can develop from intraperitoneal urine leakage. Notify the practitioner if urine leaks from the drain or suture line; such leakage may indicate developing complications such as hydronephrosis.*

- Perform surgical wound care and dressing changes as ordered.
- Continue I.V. replacement therapy and TPN.
- Monitor the patient's vital signs and intake and output.
- Assess the surgical wound and dressings.
- Monitor drainage and urine characteristics.
- Monitor for complications, such as abnormal bleeding and infection.
- Assess the patient's bowel sounds.
- Perform routine ostomy maintenance as indicated. Make sure the collection device fits tightly around the stoma. Regularly check the appearance of the stoma and peristomal skin. The stoma should appear bright red; notify the practitioner if it appears deep red or blue, indicating a problem with blood flow. The stoma should also be smooth; report dimpling or retraction, which suggests stenosis. Check the peristomal skin for irritation or breakdown. The primary cause of irritation is urine leakage around the edges of the collection device's faceplate. If leakage occurs, change the device, taking care to properly apply the skin sealer to ensure a tight fit.
- If the patient has a continent internal ileal reservoir, irrigate the drainage tube as ordered (usually every 2 to 8 hours) with about 60 ml of normal saline solution to maintain patency. To avoid abdominal distention during the postoperative period and allow suture lines to heal, perform irrigations gently.
- If skin breakdown occurs, clean the area with warm water and pat it dry; then apply a light dusting of karaya gum powder and a thin layer of protective dressing. If you detect severe excoriation, notify the practitioner promptly.
- Provide emotional support during the recovery period to help the patient adjust to the stoma and collection pouch or to self-catheterization as appropriate. Assure the patient that the pouch shouldn't interfere with his lifestyle and that he can eventually resume all of his former activities.

PATIENT TEACHING

GENERAL

- Review medications, including dosage and adverse reactions with the patient.
- Make sure the patient and his family understand and can properly perform stoma care and change the urostomy pouch.
- Teach the patient with a continent internal ileal reservoir how to care for the pouch drainage tube, which is usually removed 3 weeks after the procedure. Tell the patient to empty the pouch correctly (using either passive emptying or intermittent self-catheterization) and irrigate the pouch as needed.
- Refer the patient for home care as indicated. (See *Caring for your urinary stoma.* See also *Caring for your nephrostomy tube,* page 435.)
- Instruct the patient and his family to watch for and report signs and symptoms of complications, such as fever, chills, flank or abdominal pain, and pus or blood in the urine. Describe the appearance of a healthy stoma, and review stoma changes that the practitioner should assess.
- Inform the patient that he should be able to return to work soon after discharge; however, if his job requires heavy lifting, tell him to talk to his practitioner before resuming work. Explain that he can safely participate in most sports, even such strenuous ones as skiing, skydiving, and scuba diving. Do, however, suggest that he avoid contact sports, such as football and wrestling.
- If the patient expresses doubts or insecurities about his sexuality related to the stoma and collection device, refer him for sexual counseling. Assure the female patient that pregnancy should cause her no special problems; however, urge her to consult her practitioner before she becomes pregnant.

(continued)

Caring for your urinary stoma

Dear Patient:

The surgeon has constructed a new passageway for your urine. This passageway leads directly to the outside of your body through an opening on your abdomen called a *stoma*. You'll wear a baglike appliance called an *ostomy bag* to collect the urine that drains from the stoma.

LEARNING ABOUT YOUR OSTOMY BAG

Most ostomy bags can be worn from 3 to 5 days—sometimes for as long as 7 days. To prevent infection, you'll need to change the bag at least weekly. If the bag begins to leak, change it immediately to prevent infection.

To keep the weight of the bag from loosening its seal against the stoma, empty the bag whenever it becomes one-third to one-half full.

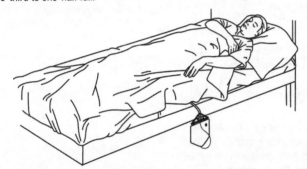

At bedtime, consider connecting the bag to a larger urine-collection container. This will keep the urine from stagnating in the bag and will minimize the risk of infection.

Also, when the urine drains into another container, the weight of the urine won't loosen the bag's seal.

The best time to change the bag is usually in the morning when urine output is less. To control leakage while your bag is off, you may want to insert a thin gauze roll, a tampon, or a rolled paper towel into the stoma.

GATHERING THE EQUIPMENT

To make changing your ostomy bag easier, gather all the equipment that you'll need. Whether your ostomy bag is permanent, temporary, disposable, or reusable, you'll need the following supplies:

◆ adhesive tape and scissors
◆ a skin barrier—either a paste or a solid seal—to protect the skin around your stoma (types include karaya gum, gelatin wafers, or paste)
◆ ostomy cement or spray adhesive

◆ an odorproof ostomy bag with an opening at the bottom for draining urine
◆ a mounting ring (called a *faceplate*) for attaching the bag
◆ cleaning supplies, such as soap and water
◆ gauze pads and a soft, clean towel
◆ an electric razor (optional).

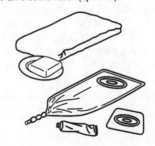

CARING FOR THE STOMA

After you remove the ostomy bag, use warm water and a clean, soft white washcloth or paper towel to wash off any crystal deposits on or around the stoma.

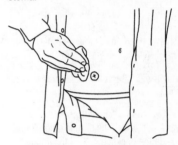

Soap can leave a residue and lead to skin irritation, but if you must use soap, choose a nondrying, nonalkaline soap, such as Basis, Dove, or castile.

Next, rinse the area thoroughly and pat your skin dry with a towel. Soap or moisture remaining on your skin may keep the ostomy bag from adhering.

If you notice hairs growing around the stoma, carefully trim them with scissors or an electric razor. Don't risk cutting your skin with a razor blade.

Take meticulous care of your stoma to prevent irritation. Poor skin care may lead to a urinary tract or yeast infection. Avoid changing the ostomy bag too frequently because this can also irritate the skin, and don't rub the skin around the stoma.

APPLYING THE ADHESIVE

If you use ostomy cement, apply a thin layer around the stoma and allow it to dry.

If you use a spray adhesive, *cover the stoma,* and spray the adhesive onto the surrounding skin. Alternatively, you may spray the adhesive onto a gauze pad and then dab the adhesive around the stoma.

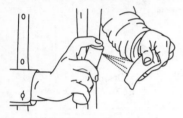

If you use a skin barrier, measure your stoma with the cutting guide found inside the package. Select the flange size that's ¼" (0.6 cm) larger than your stoma.

Next, trace the right size onto the adhesive paper backing. Now, cut out a skin barrier wafer. Peel off the backing and place the wafer over your stoma. Press the skin barrier wafer against your skin for 30 seconds to form a seal. For more security, you may also wish to apply adhesive tape around the barrier.

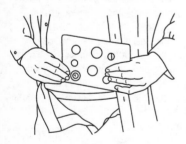

ATTACHING THE OSTOMY BAG

Remove the gauze roll, tampon, or paper towel that you placed in your stoma to control leakage.

If you use adhesive, attach the ostomy bag when the adhesive becomes tacky. Center the bag over the stoma and leave a small amount of skin exposed around the stoma.

If you use a skin barrier, attach the ostomy bag by placing the flange on the wafer and pressing firmly, as shown below. You should feel the flanges snap together.

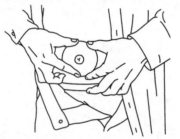

Finally, if you use an adhesive bag system, trace a circle that's ⅛" (0.3 cm) larger than your stoma onto the adhesive backing. Cut around the tracing and remove the backing. Next, check to make sure that the bottom drainage valve is closed.

Starting at the bottom, press the adhesive firmly but gently around the stoma. Be careful not to wrinkle the material. You may also wish to apply adhesive tape around the faceplate.

If you want to wear an ostomy belt to secure the bag, be sure to wear the belt at the level of the stoma. Wear it loose enough so it doesn't irritate the skin and leave red marks. (You should be able to slip two fingers between your skin and the belt.)

CONTROLLING ODOR

Try drinking cranberry or apple juice or taking vitamin C tablets to help acidify urine and decrease odor.

You can also add a few drops of vinegar or commercially available ostomy deodorizer directly to the ostomy bag to eliminate odors.

BATHING WITH AN OSTOMY BAG

You may take a bath or shower with your ostomy bag on or off, whichever makes you feel most comfortable. With the bag off, of course, urine will flow into the bath water.

Caring for your nephrostomy tube

Dear Patient:

A nephrostomy tube allows urine to drain from your kidney into a drainage bag. This bag is attached to the tube's free end with a length of tubing. Because the nephrostomy tube goes directly into your kidney, you'll need to take proper care of the tubing and bag each day to prevent infection.

HOW TO CHANGE THE TUBING AND DRAINAGE BAG

1. Gather your equipment: a clean drainage bag, connecting tube, and alcohol swabs. Wash your hands. *Important:* Always keep the drainage bag lower than the nephrostomy tube.
2. Disconnect the nephrostomy tube from the used tubing and drainage bag. Don't use your fingernails to disconnect the tubing. Clean the end of the nephrostomy tube with an alcohol swab. Also clean the end of the tubing that connects the new drainage bag to the nephrostomy tube.
3. Attach the ends of the nephrostomy tube and the connecting tube securely. Don't touch the end of either tube. Check the tubing periodically for kinks.

HOW TO CLEAN THE BAG AND TUBING

1. Wash the used bag and tubing with a weak detergent solution daily. Avoid a biodegradable or chlorine product because it may erode the bag.
2. Twice weekly, wash the bag and tubing with a weak vinegar solution (one part vinegar and three parts water) to prevent crystalline buildup. Rinse the bag and tubing with plain water and hang them on a clothes hanger to air-dry.

HOW TO CHANGE THE DRESSING

Change the dressing daily as your health care provider orders.
1. Gather the necessary equipment: absorbent powder, sterile gauze pads, and adhesive tape. Then wash your hands and remove the old dressing.
2. Gently wash around the tube with soap and water. Inspect the skin around the tube. Is redness present? If so, apply absorbent powder.

If you notice white, yellow, or green drainage, with or without odor, suspect infection, and report it to your practitioner. If you see drainage that looks or smells like urine, the tube may be displaced. Report this to your health care provider.
3. Next, fold several sterile gauze pads in half and place them around the tube's base. Cover with an unfolded gauze pad. Apply adhesive tape to secure the gauze pads to your skin. If your skin is sensitive, you can use a protective barrier wipe or a skin preparation under the tape.

This patient-teaching aid may be reproduced by office copier for distribution to patients. © 2007 Lippincott Williams & Wilkins.

◆ Stress the importance of keeping scheduled follow-up appointments with the practitioner and enterostomal therapist to evaluate reservoir function and stoma care and make necessary changes in equipment. For instance, stoma shrinkage, which normally occurs within 8 weeks after surgery, may require a change in pouch size to ensure a tight fit.
◆ Instruct the patient to expect a call from the home health care service, if ordered, and write down the agency's name and telephone contact information.
◆ Instruct the patient how to access support groups such as the United Ostomy Association.

RESOURCES
Organizations
American Academy of Pediatrics: *www.aap.org*
American Urological Association: *www.urologyhealth.org*
United Ostomy Association: *www.uoa.org*

Selected references
Brewster, L. "The Implications of Nurse Prescribing in Stoma Care," *Nursing Times* 101(19):56-57, May 2006.
Burch, J. "The Pre- and Postoperative Nursing Care for Patients with a Stoma," *British Journal of Nursing* 14(6):310-18, March-April 2005.
Gomez, M. "Promising New Suprapubic Catheter," *Urologic Nursing* 25(4):288, 291-92, August 2005.

Vacuum-assisted closure pressure therapy

OVERVIEW

- Used to enhance delayed or impaired wound healing
- Applies localized subatmospheric pressure to draw the edges of the wound toward the center
- Dressing placed in wound or over a graft or flap and therapy applied; wound packing removes fluids from the wound, stimulating growth of healthy granulation tissue (see *Understanding vacuum-assisted closure therapy*)
- Should be used cautiously in patients with active bleeding, those taking anticoagulants, and when achieving wound hemostasis has been difficult
- Also known as *negative pressure wound therapy*

INDICATIONS

- Acute and traumatic wounds
- Pressure ulcers
- Chronic open wounds (such as diabetic ulcers, dehisced surgical wounds, meshed grafts, and skin flaps)

⚡ **WARNING** *Vacuum-assisted closure pressure therapy is contraindicated in patients with fistulas tht involve organs or body cavities, necrotic tissue with eschar, untreated osteomyelitis, and malignant wounds.*

PROCEDURE

- Attach the 19G catheter to the 35-ml piston syringe and irrigate the wound thoroughly using the normal saline solution.
- Clean the area around the wound with normal saline solution; wipe intact skin with a skin protectant wipe and allow it to dry well.
- Remove and discard your gloves. Put on sterile gloves.
- Using sterile scissors cut the foam to the shape and measurement of the wound. More than one piece of foam may be needed if the first piece is cut too small.
- Carefully place the foam in the wound.
- Place the fenestrated tubing into the center of the foam; this delivers negative pressure to the wound.
- Place the transparent occlusive air permeable drape over the foam, enclosing the foam and the tubing together. Remove and discard gloves.
- Connect the free end of the fenestrated tubing to the tubing that's connected to the evacuation canister.
- Turn on the vacuum unit.

COMPLICATIONS

- Increased pain (temporary)
- Increased risk for infection

NURSING DIAGNOSES

- Deficient fluid volume
- Impaired skin integrity
- Ineffective tissue perfusion: Peripheral

EXPECTED OUTCOMES

The patient will:

- maintain adequate fluid volume
- demonstrate healing of affected areas
- maintain adequate peripheral warmth, color, and pulsations.

Understanding vacuum-assisted closure pressure therapy

Vacuum-assisted closure pressure therapy may be used when a wound fails to heal in a timely manner. It encourages healing by applying localized subatmospheric pressure at the site of the wound. This reduces edema and bacterial colonization and stimulates the formation of granulation tissue.

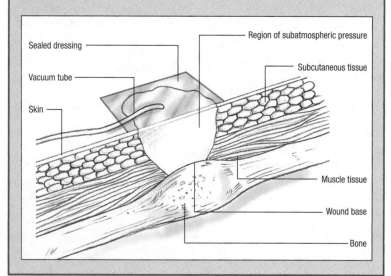

Labels: Sealed dressing, Vacuum tube, Skin, Region of subatmospheric pressure, Subcutaneous tissue, Muscle tissue, Wound base, Bone

---

PRETREATMENT CARE

◆ Assemble the vacuum-assisted closure device at the bedside per manufacturer's instructions.
◆ Set the negative pressure according to the practitioner's order (25 to 200 mm Hg).
◆ Check the practitioner's order, and assess the patient's condition.
◆ Explain the procedure to the patient and provide privacy.
◆ Premedicate the patient for pain as needed.
◆ Wash your hands and, if necessary, put on a gown and goggles to protect yourself from wound drainage and contamination.
◆ Place a linen-saver pad under the patient to catch spills and avoid linen changes.
◆ Position the patient to allow maximum wound exposure.
◆ Place the emesis basin under the wound to collect drainage.
◆ Remove the soiled dressing and discard it in the waterproof trash bag.

POSTTREATMENT CARE

◆ Make sure the patient is comfortably repositioned.
◆ Properly dispose of drainage, solution, linen-saver pad, and trash bag, and clean and dispose of soiled equipment and supplies according to facility policy and guidelines from the Centers for Disease Control and Prevention.
◆ Change the dressing every 48 hours. Try to coordinate dressing change with the practitioner's visit so he can inspect the wound.
◆ Measure the amount of drainage every shift.
◆ Use audible and visual alarms to alert you if the unit is tipped greater than 45 degrees (acute care model), the canister is full, the dressing has an air leak, or the canister becomes dislodged.
◆ Administer medications as ordered.
◆ Provide adequate hydration.
◆ Provide skin care.
◆ Provide emotional support.
◆ Monitor the patient's vital signs, intake and output, and peripheral pulses.
◆ Assess the patient for signs of decreased tissue perfusion and new or increasing infection.

PATIENT TEACHING

GENERAL
◆ Review medication administration, dosage, and possible adverse effects, with the patient, particularly pain medications and antibiotics ordered.
◆ Review the signs and symptoms of infection to report to the practitioner.
◆ If the patient will be discharged with the home care version of the device, teach him the correct procedures for caring for the device and his wound.
◆ Refer the patient to resources and support services.
◆ Refer the patient to home care, as indicated, and a wound care specialist follow up, as indicated.

RESOURCES
Organizations
American Academy of Pediatrics: *www.aap.org*
American Medical Association: *www.ama-assn.org*
Wound, Ostomy and Continence Nurses Society: *www.wocn.org*

Selected references
Clubley, L., and Harper, L. "Using Negative Pressure Therapy for Healing of a Sternal Wound," *Nursing Times* 101(16):44-46, April 2005.
Gibson, K. "Vacuum-Assisted Closure," *AJN* 104(12):16, December 2004.
Malli, S. "Keep a Close Eye on Vacuum-Assisted Wound Closure," *Nursing* 35(7):25, July 2005.
Smith, N. "The Benefits of VAC Therapy in the Management of Pressure Ulcers," *British Journal of Nursing* 13(22):1359-65, December 2004.

Vagal maneuvers

OVERVIEW

- Include Valsalva's maneuver and carotid sinus massage
- Can slow the patient's heart rate
- Work by stimulating nerve endings that send messages to brain stem, which then stimulates the autonomic nervous system to increase vagal tone and decrease heart rate
- Valsalva's maneuver: raises intrathoracic pressure, which initially decreases venous return, stroke volume, and systolic blood pressure; within seconds, baroreceptors cause peripheral vasoconstriction, which then stimulates the vagus nerve and decreases the heart rate
- Carotid sinus massage: manual pressure slows heart rate

⚡ **WARNING** *Vagal maneuvers are contraindicated in patients with severe coronary artery disease (CAD), acute myocardial infarction, and hypovolemia. Carotid sinus massage is contraindicated in patients with digoxin (Lanoxin) toxicity or cerebrovascular disease and in those who have had carotid surgery.*

INDICATIONS

- Sinus, atrial, or junctional tachyarrhythmias

PROCEDURE

VALSALVA'S MANEUVER

- Obtain a rhythm strip before the procedure
- The practitioner will ask the patient to take a deep breath and bear down, as if he were trying to defecate.
- If the patient doesn't feel light-headed or dizzy, and if no new arrhythmias occur, he will be told to hold his breath and bear down for 10 seconds.
- If the patient feels dizzy or light-headed, or if a new arrhythmia is noted on the monitor—asystole for more than 6 seconds, frequent premature ventricular contractions (PVCs), or ventricular tachycardia or ventricular fibrillation—he will be instructed to exhale and stop bearing down.
- After 10 seconds, he will be instructed to exhale and breathe quietly.
- If the maneuver is successful, the monitor will show his heart rate slowing before he exhales.
- Obtain a rhythm strip after the procedure.

CAROTID SINUS MASSAGE

- Obtain a rhythm strip, using the lead that shows the strongest P waves.
- The practitioner will auscultate both carotid sinuses for bruits.
- Assist with positioning the patient for massage as ordered. (See *Location and technique for carotid sinus massage*.)

Location and technique for carotid sinus massage

Before the practitioner applies manual pressure to the patient's right carotid sinus, she'll locate the bifurcation of the carotid artery on the right side of the neck. The patient will be asked to turn his head slightly to the left and hyperextend his neck, bringing the carotid artery closer to the skin and moving the sternocleidomastoid muscle away from the carotid artery.

Using a circular motion, the practitioner will massage the right carotid sinus between her fingers and the transverse processes of the spine for 3 to 5 seconds. Massage shouldn't be done for more than 5 seconds, to avoid risking life-threatening complications.

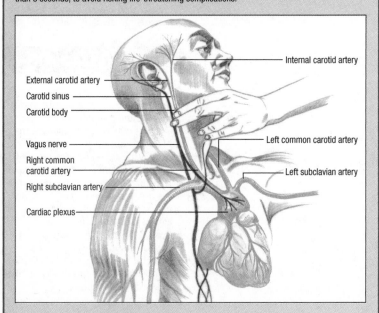

- Internal carotid artery
- External carotid artery
- Carotid sinus
- Carotid body
- Vagus nerve
- Right common carotid artery
- Right subclavian artery
- Cardiac plexus
- Left common carotid artery
- Left subclavian artery

◆ Monitor the electrocardiogram (ECG) during the procedure.

⚡ **WARNING** *The practitioner will stop massaging the carotid sinus when the ventricular rate slows sufficiently to permit diagnosis of the rhythm. Alternatively, she may stop as soon as evidence of a rhythm change appears. Have the crash cart handy to perform emergency treatment if a dangerous arrhythmia occurs.*

◆ If the procedure doesn't have an effect within 5 seconds, the practitioner will stop massaging the right carotid sinus and may begin to massage the left sinus. Assist the patient with positioning himself correctly for this maneuver as needed.

◆ If this also fails, administer cardiotonic drugs as ordered.

⚡ **WARNING** *Remember that a brief period of asystole — 3 to 6 seconds — and several PVCs may precede conversion to normal sinus rhythm.*

◆ If the vagal maneuver succeeds in slowing the patient's heart rate and converting the arrhythmia, print a rhythm strip and continue monitoring him for several hours.

COMPLICATIONS

◆ Decreased arterial blood pressure in patients taking a cardiac glycoside and in those with heart block, hypertension, CAD, diabetes mellitus, or hyperkalemia

✿ **AGE FACTOR** *Elderly patients with heart disease are especially susceptible to the adverse effects of vagal maneuvers.*

◆ Bradycardia or complete heart block

NURSING DIAGNOSES

◆ Activity intolerance
◆ Decreased cardiac output
◆ Ineffective tissue perfusion: Cardiopulmonary

EXPECTED OUTCOMES
The patient will:
◆ carry out activities of daily living without excess fatigue or decreased energy
◆ maintain adequate cardiac output

◆ maintain adequate heart rate and rhythm, respiratory rate and depth, skin color and temperature, and peripheral pulses.

PRETREATMENT CARE

◆ Review the procedure with the patient to ease his fears and promote cooperation. Ask him to let the practitioner know if he feels light-headed during the procedure.

◆ Place the patient in a supine position.

◆ Insert an I.V. line if necessary. Then administer dextrose 5% in water at a keep-vein-open rate as ordered; use this line if emergency drugs become necessary.

◆ Prepare the patient's skin, and attach ECG electrodes

◆ Adjust the leads monitored and the size of the ECG complexes on the monitor so that the arrhythmia can be seen clearly.

POSTTREATMENT CARE

◆ Monitor the patient's cardiac rhythm continuously for return of arrhythmia.

◆ Report signs of complications.

◆ Monitor the patient's vital signs and intake and output.

◆ Administer supplemental oxygen as ordered.

◆ Assist with treatments, such as pacemaker insertion or cardiopulmonary resuscitation, as indicated.

◆ Administer medications and monitor for effect.

◆ Maintain the patient's hydration.

◆ Monitor the patient's mental status and level of consciousness.

◆ Assess hemodynamic monitoring if in place.

◆ Monitor the patient for abnormal heart and breath sounds; report changes immediately.

◆ Assess the results of ordered laboratory test.

PATIENT TEACHING

GENERAL
◆ Review medication administration, dosage, and possible adverse effects with the patient.
◆ Review with the patient the signs and symptoms of recurrent arrhythmia and when to notify the practitioner.
◆ Stress the importance of follow-up care.

RESOURCES
Organizations
American College of Cardiology: *www.acc.org*
American Heart Association: *www.americanheart.org*

Selected references
Barutcu, I., et al. "Cigarette Smoking and Heart Rate Variability: Dynamic Influence of Parasympathetic and Sympathetic Maneuvers," *Annals of Noninvasive Electrocardiology* 10(3):324-29, July 2005.
Carrasco-Sosa, S., et al. "Baroreflex Sensitivity Assessment and Heart Rate Variability: Relation to Maneuver and Technique," *European Journal of Applied Physiology* 95(4):265-75, October 2005.
Gowda, R.M., et al. "Cardiac Arrhythmias in Pregnancy: Clinical and Therapeutic Considerations," *International Journal of Cardiology* 88(2-3):129-33, April 2003.

Vagotomy

OVERVIEW

- Surgery to sever the vagus nerve to reduce secretion of acid within the stomach
- Usually done in emergency situations, such as with stomach perforation and excessive bleeding
- May be accompanied by other stomach surgery, such as partial resection of the stomach or enlargement of the pyloric sphincter
- Truncal (or total abdominal) vagotomy: cuts the vagus nerve at the base of the esophagus where it enters the abdomen before splitting into several branches; requires additional surgery to further open the pyloric sphincter (pyloroplasty)
- Highly selective vagotomy (also called *parietal cell* or *proximal gastric vagotomy*): cuts only the branches of the vagal nerve that go to stomach cells that secrete acid; most commonly performed procedure

INDICATIONS

- Excessive acid production that can't be controlled by other means, such as antibiotics for *Helicobacter pylori*, histamine-2 blockers, or proton pump inhibitors
- Nonhealing or frequently recurring ulcers in the stomach and duodenum

PROCEDURE

- Vagotomy is performed by a surgeon on an inpatient basis, either by an open abdominal procedure or, more commonly, a laparoscopic procedure.
- The patient is given general anesthesia.
- For an open abdominal procedure, a midline incision is made in the abdomen. For a laparoscopic procedure, the laparoscope is usually inserted through a small incision near the umbilicus; an additional four (small) incisions are made over the upper abdomen for instruments.
- The vagus nerve and its abdominal branches are carefully located and isolated.
- The trunk or the proximal branches leading to the stomach are then electrocauterized or ligated.
- The damaged portion of the stomach may be removed, or a drainage procedure, which further opens the pyloric valve, may be performed as needed.
- The abdominal layers are sutured closed, and the skin incisions are closed with sutures or staples.

COMPLICATIONS

- Excessive bleeding
- Infection
- Perforation of nearby organs or structures
- Dumping syndrome
- Diarrhea

WARNING *Patients at higher risk for complications include those who use alcohol excessively, smoke, are obese, or who are very young or very old.*

NURSING DIAGNOSES

- Acute pain
- Impaired tissue integrity
- Risk for infection

EXPECTED OUTCOMES

The patient will:
- verbalize or demonstrate feelings of comfort
- demonstrate healing of wounds
- remain free from infection.

PRETREATMENT CARE

- Review the procedure with the patient and answer questions.
- Verify that an appropriate consent form has been signed.
- Verify that a gastroscopy and X-rays of the GI system have been completed as ordered.
- Make sure that laboratory, urine, and electrocardiogram testing has been completed as ordered.
- Complete a nursing history and physical examination, including medication history.
- Notify the surgeon and anesthesiologist of the patient's use of drugs or herbs that may contribute to bleeding.
- Tell the patient that he will likely stay in the hospital for up to 7 days and that nasogastric (NG) suctioning may be required for the first 3 or 4 days.

POSTTREATMENT CARE

◆ Monitor the NG suctioning device for amount and type of drainage.
◆ Monitor the patient's vital signs and intake and output.
◆ Assess abdominal sounds and bowel function for return of activity and signs of complications, such as perforation and peritonitis.
◆ Assess the patient for pain and medicate as ordered.
◆ Inspect the incision sites and provide care as required; report signs of infection to the practitioner.
◆ Assist the patient with ambulating as soon as possible and performing leg exercises to prevent thrombophlebitis.
◆ Start the patient on a clear liquid diet after the GI tract is functioning again. Instruct him to avoid spicy and acidic foods as he progresses to a regular diet.

PATIENT TEACHING

GENERAL

◆ Review with the patient medication administration, dosage, and possible adverse effects.
◆ Tell the patient that it takes about 6 weeks to fully recover from the surgery.
◆ Inform the patient that the sutures may be removed in 7 to 10 days.
◆ Encourage the patient to be mobile soon after the procedure to prevent the formation of deep vein clots.
◆ Inform the patient that pain medication, stool softeners, and antibiotics may be prescribed following the surgery.
◆ Advise the patient with a truncal vagotomy that the stomach's emptying patterns will be slowed and peristalsis throughout the GI tract will be reduced. Instruct him to report bloating, feelings of excessive fullness, and changes in bowel habits to the practitioner promptly.
◆ Review the signs of dumping syndrome (palpitations, sweating, nausea, cramps, vomiting, and diarrhea shortly after eating), which may occur particularly with truncal vagotomy. Teach him ways to avoid this condition.
◆ Stress the importance of follow-up care for ulcer disease.
◆ Refer the patient for home health care services as needed.

RESOURCES
Organizations
American College of Surgeons: *www.facs.org*
American Medical Association: *www.ama-assn.org*
Society of American Gastrointestinal and Endoscopic Surgeons: *www.sages.org*

Selected references
de la Fuente, S.G., et al. "Comparative Analysis of Vagotomy and Drainage Versus Vagotomy and Resection Procedures for Bleeding Peptic Ulcer Disease: Results of 907 Patients from the Department of Veterans Affairs National Surgical Quality Improvement Program Database," *Journal of the American College of Surgeons* 202(1):78-86, January 2006.

Smith, L., et al. "Acute and Long-Term Effect of Alpha-Glucosidase Inhibitor on Dumping Syndrome in a Patient after a Vagotomy and Pyloric Surgery," *Australia and New Zealand Journal of Surgery* 75(12):1124-26, December 2005.

Sokolis, D.P., et al. "Post-Vagotomy Mechanical Characteristics and Structure of the Thoracic Aortic Wall," *Annals of Biomedical Engineering* 33(11):1504-16, November 2005.

Vagus nerve stimulation

OVERVIEW

- Increases seizure threshold by causing widespread release of gamma-aminobutyric acid and glycine in the brain
- Improves mood by stimulating serotonin and norepinephrine neurotransmitters and possibly specific brain structures involved in mood regulation
- Composed of a pulse generator; a bipolar vagal nerve stimulator lead; a programming wand, with accompanying computer software; a tunneling tool for implantation of the lead; and handheld magnets
- Placed on the left vagus nerve, due to the higher risk of cardiac arrhythmias with stimulation of the right vagus nerve
- Also called *VNS*

INDICATIONS
- Partial seizures
- Treatment resistant depression

PROCEDURE

- In an outpatient or inpatient setting, the patient is generally given general anesthesia.
- The left vagus nerve is isolated through a small incision, and a stimulating electrode is attached to it.
- The pulse generator with battery pack is positioned in the anterior chest wall through a small incision. (See *Vagus nerve stimulator placement.*)
- The tunneling tool forms a channel under the subcutaneous tissue to thread the stimulating lead from the neck to the chest where the lead is hooked to the pulse generator.
- The tissues and incisions are replaced, sutured, and dressed.
- Generally, the pulse generator is then externally programmed using the magnetic wand. The pulse amplitude (maximum of 14 volts), pulse width, pulse frequency, and pulse on and off times are then set. Sometimes, how-

ever, the device is left off until the first postoperative day.
- Usually, the current output is adjusted to the patient's tolerance, and a pattern of 30 seconds "on" time and 5 minutes "off" time is set.

COMPLICATIONS
- Hoarseness, throat pain, or voice alteration
- Difficulty swallowing and aspiration risk
- Coughing or dyspnea
- Paresthesia
- Muscular pain or nonspecific pain
- Chest pain or irregular heart rhythm
- Nausea, dyspepsia, or vomiting
- Infection at incision sites

NURSING DIAGNOSES

- Disturbed sensory perception (all)
- Risk for impaired swallowing
- Risk for infection

EXPECTED OUTCOMES
The patient will:
- exhibit decreased seizure activity
- demonstrate no signs or symptoms of aspiration from swallowing difficulties
- remain free from infection.

PRETREATMENT CARE

- Make sure that presurgery medical evaluation and testing has been completed as ordered; this may include monitoring seizures and performing electroencephalography, magnetic resonance imaging, or positron emission tomography.
- Verify that an appropriate consent form has been signed.
- Review with the patient the procedure, nursing preparation, and post-surgical care, and answer any questions that he may have.

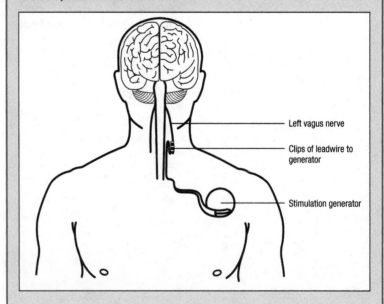

Vagus nerve stimulator placement

The vagus nerve stimulator is placed on the left side during the procedure to minimize the risk of cardiac arrhythmias.

Left vagus nerve

Clips of leadwire to generator

Stimulation generator

- Tell the patient that part of his head and chest may be shaved in the operating room.
- Explain to the patient that he'll be in the intensive care unit postoperatively and review the equipment he'll see when he awakens.
- Perform a baseline neurologic and mental status nursing assessment.

POSTTREATMENT CARE

- Position the patient on his side with the head of the bed elevated 15 to 30 degrees; assist the patient with turning every 2 hours.
- Ensure a quiet, calm environment.
- Maintain seizure precautions.
- Monitor the patient's vital signs, intake and output, level of consciousness, respiratory status, heart rate and rhythm, and mental status.
- Monitor drainage and the surgical wound and dressings.
- Administer medications, including antiseizure or antidepressant drugs and analgesics, as ordered.
- Monitor for complications, particularly throat and voice changes, swallowing or breathing difficulties, and pain during stimulation; notify practitioner promptly.
- Reinforce to the patient that the vagus nerve stimulator can begin working immediately, or as soon as the practitioner programs it, but that full effects develop over time.
- As a measure to prevent seizure or modify its severity, initiate teaching on use of the handheld magnet to stimulate a pulse when seizure aura is felt; instruct the patient to call the nurse for assistance as needed.
- Initiate teaching about the use of the handheld magnet; instruct the patient to stop stimulation if it becomes painful or triggers significant coughing, swallowing, or heart rate problems, and to call the nurse immediately if this occurs.

PATIENT TEACHING

GENERAL

- Review medications, including dosage and possible adverse reactions with the patient. Reinforce that some medications, prescribed for the original diagnosis, may be continued indefinitely or discontinued, based on response to the VNS therapy over time.
- Teach the patient how to care for the surgical wounds and the signs and symptoms of infection to report to the practitioner.
- Tell the patient that he may notice a slight bulge in the area under his collarbone (where the device is) and that the surgery will leave small scars on the side of his neck where the wire lead was placed and on his chest where the device was implanted.
- Stress the importance of appropriate psychiatric or neurologic follow-up care.
- Inform the patient that the VNS system isn't affected by microwave transmission, cellular phones, small electrical appliances, or airport security systems.
- Tell the patient that he must notify every health care provider or facility that he has an implanted VNS device because certain procedures may affect the device's functioning or aren't allowed, including:
  - any type of diathermy (special heat-based procedures) although diagnostic ultrasound is safe
  - use of certain electrical instruments, as in surgery
  - certain types of magnetic resonance imaging (check with the imaging physician for safety)
  - external defibrillators
  - extracorporeal shockwave lithotripsy.
- Tell the patient that it may take several weeks to tune the pulse parameters to effective settings and up to two years to reach full benefit.
- Show the patient and his family how to use the supplied handheld magnet to activate a pulse at the onset of a seizure or aura by passing the magnet over the generator for a few seconds. Reinforce that keeping the magnet over the generator actually turns the generator off.
- Teach the patient that continuous stimulation with the magnet over a 4-hour period could damage his vagus nerve.
- Tell the patient that the battery needs to be replaced surgically every 1 to 16 years (depending on patient physiologic characteristics and usage), and to check it daily by activating one magnet stimulation each morning.
- Refer the patient to appropriate resources and support services.

RESOURCES
Organizations
American Academy of Neurology: *www.aan.com*
American Psychiatric Association: *www.psych.org*
Epilepsy Foundation: *www.efa.org*
Epilepsy Therapy Development Project: *www.epilepsy.com*

Selected references
Dunn, D. "Preventing Perioperative Complications in Special Populations," *Nursing* 35(11):36-45, November 2005.
Gallo, B.V. "Epilepsy, Surgery, and the Elderly," *Epilepsy Research* 68(Suppl 1):83-86, January 2006.
Khoury, J.S., et al. "Predicting Seizure Frequency after Epilepsy Surgery," *Epilepsy Research* 67(3):89-99, December 2005.
Nahas, Z., et al., "Two-year Outcome of Vagus Nerve Stimulation (VNS) for Treatment of Major Depressive Episodes," *The Journal of Clinical Psychiatry* 66(9):1097-104, September 2005.

Varicose vein excision and stripping

- Removes or blocks the circulation in leg veins that have become stretched and weakened so that the valves permit backflow of blood and vein engorgement
- Relieves pain, achiness, burning, tiredness, and swelling in the legs as well as improves appearance
- Newer procedure using radiofrequency energy: involves only one small incision, the threading of an electrocautery device to the origin of the affected vessel, and the closing of the vessel by tissue destruction

INDICATIONS

- Vessels damaged by an arteriosclerotic or thromboembolic disorder
- Vessel trauma, infection, or congenital defect
- Vascular disease unresponsive nonsurgical treatments

- The patient usually receives general anesthesia.
- A small incision is made near the groin and the upper end of the great saphenous vein is located.
- The vein is separated from the femoral vein and the femoral vein is then tied or cauterized closed. A special wire is then inserted into the saphenous vein, the end is tied to the wire, and the wire is moved down the vein to just below the knee or above the ankle. A second incision is made at the end to allow the wire out, which also pulls the diseased vein with it.
- The wounds are sutured and dressings and compression bandages are applied along the length of the leg.

COMPLICATIONS

- Vessel trauma
- Thrombus formation
- Embolism
- Hemorrhage
- Infection

- Acute pain
- Risk for impaired gas exchange
- Risk for infection

EXPECTED OUTCOMES

The patient will:

- verbalize relief of pain
- exhibit no signs or symptoms of pulmonary emboli
- remain free from infection.

PRETREATMENT CARE

- Explain the treatment and nursing care before and after the procedure to the patient and his family.
- Verify that the patient has signed an appropriate consent form.
- Perform a complete cardiovascular and pulmonary assessment.
- Obtain baseline vital signs.
- Evaluate pulses, noting bruits.
- Restrict food and fluids as ordered.
- Insert an I.V. access device as ordered

POSTTREATMENT CARE

- Administer medications as ordered.
- Position the patient as ordered.
- Provide comfort measures and medicate for pain as needed.
- Use Doppler ultrasonography if peripheral pulses aren't palpable.
- Encourage frequent coughing, turning, and deep breathing.
- Assess the operative sites for drainage or other signs of infection.
- Change dressings and compression bandages and provide incision care as ordered.
- Monitor the patient's vital signs, intake and output, heart rate and rhythm, and neurovascular and cardiopulmonary status.
- Assess the patient for complications and report changes to the practitioner.
- Monitor the patient for signs of excessive bleeding.

PATIENT TEACHING

GENERAL

- Review medications, including dosage and possible adverse reactions with the patient.
- Instruct the patient to observe his extremities for changes in temperature, sensation, and motor ability, and to report such problems to the practitioner.
- Teach the patient how to care for the incisions and the signs and symptoms of infection.
- Review possible complications with the patient, and instruct him to notify the practitioner promptly if he develops heat, swelling, pain, and redness in the leg, or acute shortness of breath.
- Advise the patient to modify his risk factors, such as stopping smoking, maintaining a healthy weight, and eating a well-balanced diet low in fat and cholesterol.
- Stress the importance of follow-up care and complying with compression therapy as prescribed.

RESOURCES
Organizations
American College of Cardiology:
  www.acc.org
American Heart Association:
  www.americanheart.org
The Society for Vascular Surgery:
  www.vascularweb.org

Selected references
Galvan, L. "Assessing Venous Ulcers and Venous Insufficiency," *Nursing* 35(11): 70, November 2005.
Galvan, L. "Using Compression Therapy for Venous Insufficiency," *Nursing* 35(12):24-25, December 2005.
Lin, S.D., et al. "Management of the Primary Varicose Veins With Venous Ulceration With Assistance of Endoscopic Surgery," *Annals in Plastic Surgery* 56(3):289-94, March 2006.

Vasectomy

- Procedure in which the vas deferens (bilaterally) are surgically altered so that sperm can't be released
- Can be performed in the practitioner's office (surgeon, family practitioner, or urologist)

INDICATIONS

- Voluntary surgical sterilization

- The patient lies in a supine position and the groin area is thoroughly cleaned; a local anesthetic is given by injection or by jet injection spray.
- One of the vas deferens is located manually, then a small incision is made in the scrotum or a tiny forceps is used to create a punctuate opening over the vas (no scalpel technique).
- The vas is lifted up and cut, then the two ends are cauterized, tied, or clipped before being returned to the scrotum.
- The same technique is then applied to the opposite vas deferens. The incisions are closed with sutures in a traditional vasectomy, or allowed to close naturally in the no scalpel technique.

COMPLICATIONS

- Bleeding
- Infection
- Prolonged pain due to inflammation

- Acute pain
- Impaired urinary elimination
- Risk for infection

EXPECTED OUTCOMES

The patient will:
- verbalize feelings of comfort after the procedure
- demonstrate normal elimination patterns
- remain free from infection.

PRETREATMENT CARE

- Tell the patient to wash thoroughly and wear clean, snug underwear or an athletic supporter to the appointment.
- Tell the patient that the practitioner may shave the front portion of the scrotum before the procedure.
- Instruct the patient to stop taking aspirin or other anti-inflammatory drugs for 10 days before the procedure to reduce the risk of bleeding.
- Review the procedure with the patient and answer questions.
- Verify that an appropriate consent form has been signed.

POSTTREATMENT CARE

- Monitor the patient for bleeding and edema.
- Monitor the patient's vital signs.
- Make sure that the patient can void without difficulty.
- Administer pain medication, if needed, and assess its effect.

PATIENT TEACHING

GENERAL

- Explain the administration, dosage, and possible adverse reactions to ordered pain or antibiotic medications.
- Inform the patient that discomfort is usually mild, and that he can use over-the-counter pain relievers as needed.
- Instruct the patient to wrap an ice pack in a towel and to apply it the scrotum for the first 24 to 48 hours after the procedure to minimize edema.
- Instruct the patient to avoid prolonged standing and walking for a few days to minimize swelling, and to avoid heavy lifting or exercising for at least 1 week after the procedure.
- Encourage the patient to wear snug cotton briefs or an athletic supporter to help apply pressure against the affected area and to support the scrotum for 1 or 2 weeks after surgery.
- Instruct the patient to wait at least 1 week before resuming sexual activity and to also use contraception until an examination of his semen reveals that no sperm are present (about 4 to 8 weeks after surgery).
- Instruct the patient to call his practitioner if fever, chills, a large black-blue area, increased pain, drainage, a growing mass, or excessive swelling of the scrotum occurs.

RESOURCES
Organizations
American Medical Association: *www.ama-assn.org*
American Urological Association: *www.auanet.org*
ProMedical Alliance LLC: *www.vasectomy.com*

Selected references
Labrecque, M., et al. "Re: How Little is Enough? The Evidence for Post-Vasectomy Testing," *Journal of Urology* 175(2):791-92; author reply 792, February 2006.
Parekattil, S.J., et al. "Multi-Institutional Validation of Vasectomy Reversal Predictor," *Journal of Urology* 175(1):247-49, January 2006.
Seenu, V., and Hafiz, A. "Routine Antibiotic Prophylaxis Is Not Necessary for No Scalpel Vasectomy," *International Urology and Nephrology* 37(4):763-65, December 2005.

Vena cava filter placement

- Placement of a filter in the inferior vena cava to trap clots and prevent pulmonary embolism (PE)
- Used for prophylaxis and for treatment of thromboemboli

INDICATIONS

- Deep vein thrombosis (DVT) or PE in patients unable to take or unresponsive to anticoagulants
- Frequently recurring thromboses
- Extension of a thromboembolism while on appropriate doses of anticoagulants
- Patients undergoing pulmonary embolectomy
- Prophylaxis for certain patients scheduled for elective orthopedic surgery, patients with major trauma, selective patients with malignancies or who are pregnant, and certain patients with serious heart or lung conditions

- Techniques vary based on type of filter chosen (for example, Greenfield filter, Bird's Nest filter, Vena Tech filter, or Simon Nitinol filter).
- Generally, a local anesthetic is administered at the site where the catheter containing the filter will be inserted—either the femoral or jugular vein.
- A small incision is made over the selected site, and the catheter is inserted. Using X-ray equipment and fluoroscopy or ultrasound, the catheter is guided to the desired location in the vena cava.
- The filter is released from the catheter allowing it to open and attach to the wall of the vena cava.
- The catheter is removed and the incision closed and dressed.

COMPLICATIONS

- Bleeding at the insertion site
- Damage to the vein during insertion
- Partial blockage of the vena cava

- Decreased cardiac output
- Impaired gas exchange
- Ineffective tissue perfusion: Cardiopulmonary

EXPECTED OUTCOMES

The patient will:

- maintain adequate cardiac output
- maintain clear lung sounds and adequate pulse oximetry
- maintain heart rate and rhythm, respiratory rate and rhythm, and blood pressure within normal limits.

- Verify that a venacavogram report is available in the chart.
- If ordered, check that computed tomography scanning or magnetic resonance imaging of the trunk have been completed.
- Review the procedure and nursing care with the patient and answer questions that he may have.
- Verify that an appropriate consent form has been signed.
- Check that preoperative laboratory studies, particularly bleeding studies, and an electrocardiogram have been completed if ordered.
- Administer preoperative sedation or muscle relaxant as ordered.
- Complete a cardiovascular, pulmonary, and neurologic assessment and obtain baseline vital signs.

POSTTREATMENT CARE

◆ Place the patient in a comfortable position and give supplemental oxygen as indicated.
◆ Assess the incision site for bleeding or signs or symptoms of infection.
◆ Monitor peripheral pulses and check for adequacy of circulation.
◆ Administer medications, including analgesics, and monitor for effects.
◆ Maintain the patency of I.V. tubes; maintain fluid restriction if ordered.
◆ Monitor the patient's vital signs, intake and output, and perform cardiac monitoring if ordered.
◆ Monitor the patient's hemodynamic status if ordered.
◆ Assess the patient for abnormal heart and breath sounds, and report changes immediately.
◆ Monitor the results of ordered laboratory studies.

PATIENT TEACHING

GENERAL

◆ Explain that annual checkups will be scheduled (after postoperative recovery is complete) to evaluate the filter's function and to retest for recurrence of clots or other problems.
◆ Instruct the patient to watch for signs of ongoing venous insufficiency, such as edema, darkened skin, tissue loss, and skin ulceration of the legs, notifying the practitioner immediately.
◆ Instruct the patient to call the practitioner promptly if new swelling of both legs occurs; this is a sign of a thrombus trapped in the filter or in the vena cava.
◆ Teach the patient about anticoagulant therapy, precautions, and monitoring if prescribed.
◆ Advise the patient to continue to use compression stockings as long as instructed by the practitioner.
◆ Reinforce basic precautions to prevent DVT, such as avoiding crossed legs or ankles when sitting, alternating sitting with brief standing and walking every 1 to 2 hours, and keeping the legs elevated above heart level when lying or resting in a chair.
◆ Encourage the patient to perform regular exercise and leg exercises as directed by the practitioner.
◆ Advise the patient to maintain a healthy diet and body weight and to stop smoking.
◆ Advise the patient to regularly check the legs for signs of DVT.

RESOURCES
Organizations
American College of Cardiology: *www.acc.org*
American Heart Association: *www.americanheart.org*
American Venous Forum: *www.venousinfo.com*

Selected references
Ignotus, P., et al. "CT Fluoroscopic Guided Insertion of Inferior Vena Cava Filters," *British Journal of Radiology* 79(939):258-60, March 2006.
Kaskarelis, I.S., et al. "Clinical Experience with Gunther Temporary Inferior Vena Cava Filters," *Clinical Imaging* 30(2):108-13, March-April 2006.
Seinturier, C., et al. "More on: Clinical Experience with Retrievable Vena Cava Filters—Results of a Prospective Observational Multicenter Study," *Journal of Thrombosis and Haemostasis* 4(3):708-709, March 2006.

Ventricular assist device

- Provides support to a failing heart as well as provides systemic and pulmonary support
- Also called *VAD*
- In a surgical procedure, an artificial pump is implanted to divert blood from a ventricle to an artificial pump; pump synchronizes to the patient's electrocardiogram (ECG) and functions as the ventricle
- Right VAD (RVAD): provides pulmonary support by diverting blood from the failing right ventricle to the VAD, which then pumps blood to the pulmonary circulation via the VAD connection to the pulmonary artery
- Left VAD (LVAD): blood flows from left ventricle to the VAD, which then pumps blood back to the body via the VAD connection to the aorta (see *Ventricular assist device: Help for the failing heart*)
- When RVAD and LVAD are used, biventricular (BiVAD) support provided

INDICATIONS

- Ventricular failure
- Cardiac transplantation
- Refractory cardiogenic shock
- Cardiopulmonary bypass

PROCEDURE

- The patient is given general anesthesia.
- An incision is made through the breastbone to expose the heart; heparin is administered to keep the blood from clotting.
- Cardiopulmonary bypass is initiated.
- An incision is made to form a pocket for the LVAD in the abdominal wall.
- Small incisions are placed through the diaphragm to allow placement of the tubes, which are used to channel blood from the ventricle to the LVAD and connect the pump to the aorta.

- An incision is also made through the abdominal wall to connect the VAD to an external power source.
- The surgeon cannulates the left ventricle with the inflow tube and the aorta with the outflow tube.
- When the pump is adequately supporting the heart, the patient is removed from the heart-lung machine.
- All incisions are sutured and dressings are applied.

COMPLICATIONS

- Hemorrhage
- Air embolus
- Thrombus
- Infection
- Lethal arrhythmias

- Activity intolerance
- Decreased cardiac output
- Ineffective tissue perfusion: Cardiopulmonary

EXPECTED OUTCOMES

The patient will:

- carry out activities of daily living without excess fatigue or decreased energy
- maintain adequate cardiac output
- maintain heart rate and rhythm, respiratory rate and rhythm, and blood pressure within normal limits.

Ventricular assist device: Help for the failing heart

A ventricular assist device (VAD) functions like an artificial heart. The major difference is that the VAD assists the heart instead of replacing it. The VAD can aid one or both ventricles. The pumping chambers themselves aren't usually implanted in the patient.

A permanent VAD is implanted in the patient's chest cavity, although it still provides only temporary support. The device receives power through the skin by a belt of electrical transformer coils (worn externally as a portable battery pack). It can also operate off an implanted, rechargeable battery for up to 1 hour at a time.

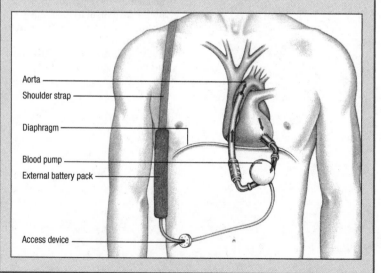

PRETREATMENT CARE

- Review the purpose of the VAD and what to expect after its insertion.
- Verify that an appropriate consent form has been signed.
- Provide emotional support.
- Monitor ECG, pulmonary artery and hemodynamic status, and intake and output.
- Administer ongoing medications as ordered.
- Before surgery, restrict food and fluid intake, and monitor cardiac function.

POSTTREATMENT CARE

- Assess cardiovascular status; monitor blood pressure, hemodynamic parameters, including cardiac output and input, ECG, and peripheral pulses.
- Inspect incision and dressings; monitor urine output; maintain I.V. fluid therapy as ordered, and monitor for fluid overload or decreasing urine output.
- Keep the patient immobile to prevent accidental extubation, contamination, or disconnection of the VAD.
- Maintain cardiac output at 5 to 8 L/ minute, central venous pressure at 8 to 16 mm Hg, pulmonary artery wedge pressure at 10 to 20 mm Hg, mean arterial pressure at greater than 60 mm Hg, and left atrial pressure between 4 and 12 mm Hg.

⚡ **WARNING** *Monitor the patient for signs and symptoms of poor perfusion and ineffective pumping, including arrhythmias, hypotension, low capillary refill, cool skin, oliguria or anuria, confusion, anxiety, and restlessness.*

- Assess chest tube drainage and function. Notify the practitioner if drainage is greater than 150 ml/hour over 2 hours. Auscultate breath sounds, and monitor oxygen saturation or mixed venous oxygen saturation.
- Obtain laboratory test results; assess for bleeding.

- When stable, turn the patient every 2 hours and begin range-of-motion (ROM) exercises.
- Administer antibiotics prophylactically if ordered.
- Give heparin, as ordered, to prevent clotting in the pump head and formation of thrombus.
- Check for bleeding, especially at the operative sites.
- Assess the incisions and the cannula insertion sites for signs of infection. Monitor the white blood cell count and differential daily, and take rectal or core temperatures every 4 hours.
- Use sterile technique in dressing changes. Change the dressing site over the cannula sites daily or according to facility policy.
- Provide supportive care, including ROM exercises and oral and skin care.

⚡ **WARNING** *If ventricular function fails to improve within 4 days, the patient may need a transplant. Provide psychological support for the patient and his family as they endure referral.*

PATIENT TEACHING

GENERAL

- Instruct the patient to perform coughing and deep-breathing exercises.
- Tell the patient to use an incentive spirometer.
- Advise the patient about dietary and activity restrictions.
- Stress the need for regular follow-up care with his cardiologist.
- Explain medication administration, dosage, and possible adverse effects.
- Instruct the patient in wound care and the signs and symptoms of infection to report to his practitioner.
- Review with the patient the signs and symptoms of increasing heart failure, bleeding, pulmonary embolism, or cerebral embolism, and instruct him to call the practitioner promptly.
- Teach the patient how to care for the exit port and battery pack.

- Arrange for home care referral for follow-up care and teaching as indicated.

RESOURCES
Organizations
American College of Cardiology:
www.acc.org
American Heart Association:
www.americanheart.org

Selected references
Havemann, L., et al. "Rapid Ventricular Remodeling with Left Ventricular Unloading Postventricular Assist Device Placement: New Insights with Strain Imaging," *Journal of the American Society of Echocardiography* 19(3):355.e9-355.e911, March 2006.

Newcomb, A.E., et al. "Successful Left Ventricular Assist Device Bridge to Transplantation after Failure of a Fontan Revision," *Journal of Heart and Lung Transplantation* 25(3):365-67, March 2006.

Yoda, M., et al. "Permanent Use of a Ventricle Assist Device for Dilated Cardiomyopathy in Friedreich's Ataxia," *Journal of Heart and Lung Transplantation* 25(2):251-52, February 2006.

Ventriculoperitoneal shunt placement

- Relieves intracranial pressure (ICP) caused by hydrocephalus
- Drains excess cerebrospinal fluid from lateral ventricles of the brain into the abdominal cavity or, in rare cases, into the right atrium

INDICATIONS
- Hydrocephalus

PROCEDURE

- The patient is given general anesthesia.
- The patient's hair is clipped or shaved in the area for opening into the brain.
- A scalp incision and small hole is made in the front or back of the skull to allow access to the brain and lateral ventricles.
- A special stylet is used to thread the proximal portion of the draining catheter into the lateral ventricles.
- The one-way valve and the distal portion of the catheter are joined to the end of the proximal catheter and secured together with sutures, then observed and tested to ensure all pieces are functioning properly.
- A small incision is made in the upper abdomen to access the peritoneum where the distal catheter will be placed.
- Using a special tunneling tool, the surgeon then passes the distal catheter and valve section through the skull opening and under the skin of the neck and chest to the incision in the peritoneum.
- Surgical staples or sutures are used to close the incisions and dressings are applied.

VENTRICULOATRIAL SHUNT PLACEMENT

- The procedure is similar except that the second incision is made in the neck to allow clearer access to the internal jugular or common facial vein.
- The distal catheter and valve segment are tunneled under the skin of the scalp and upper neck to the second incision site.
- Using a special needle, a guide wire with a vessel dilator is inserted into the vein and the distal catheter is guided into the right atrium of the heart.

   AGE FACTOR *In an infant, the facial vein or internal jugular vein will need to be exposed to insert the shunt.*

- Fluoroscopy is done to verify that the tip of the catheter is in the right atrium.
- The incisions are closed with surgical staples or sutures and dressings applied.

COMPLICATIONS
- Shunt malfunction
- Blockage
- Infection
- Brain tissue passing into the shunt catheter
- Neurologic deficit
- Air embolism
- Respiratory compromise
- Increased ICP

   AGE FACTOR *As an infant or child grows, the shunt will need to be replaced with longer catheters.*

NURSING DIAGNOSES

- Disturbed sensory perception (all)
- Ineffective breathing pattern
- Risk for infection

EXPECTED OUTCOMES
The patient will:
- exhibit improved or normal neurologic status
- maintain adequate ventilation
- remain free from infection.

PRETREATMENT CARE

- Make sure that all preoperative testing has been completed as ordered.
- Review the treatment and nursing care with the patient and his family.
- Verify that an appropriate consent form has been signed.
- Tell the patient and his family that at least part of his head will be shaved in the operating room.
- Explain the intensive care unit and equipment that the patient will see postoperatively.
- Perform a complete neurologic and cardiopulmonary assessment, including baseline vital signs.

POSTTREATMENT CARE

- Position the patient on his side with the head of the bed elevated 15 to 30 degrees; assist the patient with turning every 2 hours, as needed.
- Encourage careful deep breathing and coughing.
- Ensure a quiet, calm environment.
- Maintain seizure precautions.
- Monitor vital signs, intake and output, level of consciousness, respiratory and neurologic status, heart rate and rhythm, and hemodynamic status (if being monitored).
- Assess for pain and medicate, as ordered.
- Monitor the surgical incisions and provide care, as ordered.
- Maintain a patent airway; administer prescribed oxygen, if required.
- Protect the patient's safety.
- Administer medications, as ordered.
- Provide support to the parents of infants and children undergoing surgery.
- Monitor for signs and symptoms of bleeding, increased ICP, or infection.

⚡ **WARNING** *Notify the practitioner immediately if the patient develops a decreasing level of alertness, confusion, pupillary changes, or increasing weakness in an arm or leg—these are signs of increased ICP and shunt failure.*

PATIENT TEACHING

GENERAL
- Review medications and possible adverse reactions with the patient and his family.
- Teach the patient and his family how to care for the incisions.
- Review with the patient and his family the signs and symptoms of infection and complications, such as increased ICP, and to call the practitioner promptly if these occur.
- Stress the importance of regular follow-up care to check that the shunt continues to drain properly.
- Refer patients and families, particularly those of children, to support groups or web resources for patients with hydrocephalus.

RESOURCES
Organizations
American Academy of Neurology: *www.aan.com*
American Academy of Pediatrics: *www.aap.org*
Epilepsy Therapy Development Project: *www.epilepsy.com*

Selected references
Dunn, D. "Preventing Perioperative Complications in Special Populations," *Nursing* 35(11):36-45, November 2005.
Sarguna, P., and Lakshmi, V. "Ventriculoperitoneal Shunt Infections," *Indian Journal of Medical Microbiology* 24(1):52-54, January-March 2006.
Simpkins, C.J. "Ventriculoperitoneal Shunt Infections in Patients with Hydrocephalus," *Pediatric Nursing* 31(6):457-62, November-December 2005.

Wound care: burns

- Aims to maintain physiologic stability, repair skin integrity, prevent infection, and maximize functionality and psychosocial health; care given immediately after a burn improves success of treatment
- Burn severity determined by the depth and extent of the burn and other factors, such as age, complications, and coexisting illnesses; a patient with burns involving more than 20% of his total body surface area usually needs fluid resuscitation to support his compensatory mechanisms without overwhelming them
- Infection: increases wound depth, rejects skin grafts, slows healing, worsens pain, and prolongs hospitalization; death may result
- Careful positioning and regular exercise necessary for burned extremities: to help maintain joint function, prevent contractures, and minimize deformity
- Skin integrity repaired by aggressive wound debridement and maintenance of clean wound bed until wound heals or is covered with skin graft
- Full-thickness burns and certain deep partial-thickness burns: need debridement and grafting in operating room; occurs promptly after fluid resuscitation
- Most wounds managed with twice-daily dressing changes and topical antibiotics
- Dressings: encourage healing by barring germ entry and removing exudate, eschar, and other debris that host infection
- After thorough wound cleaning, topical antibacterial agents applied and wound covered with absorptive, coarse mesh gauze
- Roller gauze used to top dressing; secured with elastic netting or tape

INDICATIONS
- Burn injury

PROCEDURE

- Pour warmed normal saline solution into a sterile bowl on the sterile field.

REMOVING A DRESSING WITHOUT HYDROTHERAPY
- Put on a gown, a mask, and sterile gloves.
- Remove the dressing layers to the innermost layer by cutting the outer dressings with blunt sterile scissors.
- Lay open these dressings.
- Remove the inner dressing with sterile tissue forceps or a sterile gloved hand; if the inner layer appears dry, soak it with warm normal saline solution to ease removal.
- Dispose of soiled dressings carefully in an impervious plastic trash bag according to facility policy; these dressings harbor infection.
- Dispose of gloves and wash hands.
- Put on a new pair of sterile gloves.
- Using gauze pads moistened with normal saline solution, gently remove exudate and old topical drug.
- Carefully remove loose eschar with sterile forceps and scissors if ordered.
- Assess wound condition: it should appear clean, with no debris, loose tissue, purulence, inflammation, or darkened margins.
- Before applying a new dressing, remove your gown, gloves, and mask.
- Discard them properly; put on a clean mask, surgical cap, gown, and sterile gloves.

APPLYING A WET DRESSING
- Soak a fine-mesh gauze dressing and elastic gauze dressing in a large sterile basin containing the ordered solution.
- Wring out the fine-mesh gauze dressing until it's moist but not dripping, and apply it to the wound.
- Warn the patient that he may feel transient pain when the dressing is applied.
- Wring out the elastic gauze dressing and position it to hold the fine-mesh gauze dressing in place.
- Roll the elastic gauze dressing over the fine-mesh gauze dressing to keep it intact.
- Cover the patient with a cotton bath blanket to prevent chills.
- Change the blanket if it becomes damp.
- Use an overhead heat lamp, if necessary.
- Change the dressings frequently, as ordered, to keep the wound moist, especially if silver nitrate is being used; if the dressings become dry, silver nitrate becomes ineffective, and its silver ions may damage tissue.
- To maintain moist dressings, some protocols call for irrigating the dressing with solution at least every 4 hours through small slits cut into the outer dressing.

APPLYING A DRY DRESSING WITH A TOPICAL DRUG
- Remove old dressings and clean the wound (as described previously).
- Apply the drug to the wound in a thin layer—about 2 to 4 mm thick—with a sterile gloved hand or sterile tongue blade.
- Apply several layers of burn gauze over the wound to contain the drug but allow exudate to escape.
- Cut the dressing to fit only the wound areas.
- Don't cover unburned areas.
- Cover the entire dressing with roller gauze and secure it with elastic netting or tape.

PROVIDING ARM AND LEG CARE

◆ Apply the dressings from the distal to the proximal area to stimulate circulation and prevent constriction.
◆ Wrap the burn gauze once around the arm or leg so the edges overlap slightly.
◆ Continue wrapping until the gauze covers the wound.
◆ Apply dry roller gauze dressing to hold bottom layers in place.
◆ Secure with elastic netting or tape.

PROVIDING HAND AND FOOT CARE

◆ Wrap each finger separately with a single gauze pad to allow the patient to use his hands and to prevent webbing contractures.
◆ Place the hand in a functional position and secure using a dressing.
◆ Apply splints if ordered.
◆ Put gauze between each toe, as appropriate, to prevent webbing contractures.

PROVIDING CHEST, ABDOMEN, AND BACK CARE

◆ Apply the ordered drug to the wound in a thin layer.
◆ Cover the entire burned area with sheets of burn gauze.
◆ Wrap with roller gauze or apply a specialty vest dressing to hold the burn gauze in place.
◆ Secure the dressing with elastic netting or tape.
◆ Make sure the dressing doesn't restrict respiratory motion, especially in very young or elderly patients, or in those with circumferential injuries.

PROVIDING SCALP AND FACIAL CARE

◆ If the patient has scalp burns, clip or shave the hair around the burn as ordered.
◆ Clip other hair until it's about 2″(5 cm) long to prevent contamination of burned scalp areas.
◆ Shave facial hair if it contacts burned areas.
◆ Typically, facial burns are managed with milder topical agents (such as triple antibiotic ointment) and are left open to air.
◆ If dressings are required, make sure they don't cover the eyes, nostrils, or mouth.

PROVIDING EAR CARE

◆ Clip or shave hair around the affected ear.
◆ Remove exudate and crusts with cotton-tipped applicators dipped in normal saline solution.
◆ Place a layer of gauze behind the auricle to prevent webbing.
◆ Apply the ordered topical drug to gauze pads and place them over the burned area.
◆ Before securing the dressing with a roller bandage, position the patient's ears normally to avoid damaging the auricular cartilage.
◆ Assess the patient's hearing ability.

PROVIDING EYE CARE

◆ Clean the area around the patient's eyes and eyelids with a cotton-tipped applicator and normal saline solution every 4 to 6 hours, or as needed, to remove crust and drainage.
◆ Give ordered eye ointments or drops.
◆ If the patient's eyes can't be closed, apply topical lubricating ointments or drops as ordered.
◆ Be sure to close the patient's eyes before applying eye pads to prevent corneal abrasion.

PROVIDING NASAL CARE

◆ Check the patient's nostrils for evidence of inhalation injury, such as an inflamed mucosa, a singed vibrissae, and soot.
◆ Clean the patient's nostrils with cotton-tipped applicators dipped in normal saline solution.
◆ Remove crust.
◆ Apply the ordered ointments.
◆ If the patient has a nasogastric tube, use tracheostomy ties to secure the tube. Check the ties frequently for tightness caused by swelling facial tissue.
◆ Clean the area around the tube every 4 to 6 hours.

COMPLICATIONS

◆ Infection (most common)
◆ Sepsis
◆ Allergic reaction to ointments or dressings
◆ Renal failure
◆ Multisystem organ dysfunction
◆ Hypothermia
◆ Hypovolemia

(continued)

- Deficient fluid volume
- Impaired gas exchange
- Risk for infection

EXPECTED OUTCOMES
The patient will:

- maintain adequate fluid volume
- maintain a patent airway and adequate oxygenation
- remain free from wound or systemic infection.

- Open equipment packages using sterile technique and arrange supplies on a sterile field in the order of use.
- Dress the cleanest areas first and the most contaminated areas last to prevent cross-contamination.
- Dress in stages to avoid exposing all wounds at the same time and to help prevent excessive pain or cross-contamination.
- Give the ordered analgesic about 20 minutes before beginning wound care to maximize patient comfort and cooperation.
- Explain the procedure and provide privacy.
- Turn on overhead heat lamps to keep the patient warm, but without overheating.
- Provide adequate I.V. hydration as ordered (See *Fluid replacement: The first 24 hours after a burn.*)

Fluid replacement: The first 24 hours after a burn

Use the Parkland formula as a general guideline for the amount of fluid replacement. Administer 4 ml/kg of crystalloid × % total burn surface area; give half of the solution over the first 8 hours (calculated from time of injury) and the balance over the next 16 hours. Vary the specific infusions according to the patient's response, especially his urine output.

- Maintain patent airway; administer oxygen as indicated.
- Administer medications (including analgesics) as ordered.
- Prepare the patient for surgery or other follow-up therapies as indicated.
- Assist with diagnostic testing and other treatments as indicated (such as splinting or treatment of concurrent injuries).
- Provide emotional support to the patient and his family.
- Monitor the patient's vital signs, intake and output, peripheral pulses, and pulse oximetry.
- Monitor for signs of decreased tissue perfusion.
- Assess the patient for complications.
- Monitor the patient's level of pain; provide an analgesic and assess its effect.
- Assess the results of ordered laboratory studies.
- Arrange to transport the patient to a burn care facility as ordered.
- Thoroughly assess and document the wound's appearance because this is essential to detect infection and other complications.

WARNING *A purulent wound or green-gray exudate indicates infection, an overly dry wound suggests dehydration, and a wound with a swollen, red edge suggests cellulitis. Suspect a fungal infection if the wound is white and powdery.*

- Know that healthy granulation tissue appears clean, pinkish, faintly shiny, and free from exudate.
- Because blisters protect underlying tissue, leave them intact unless they impede joint motion, become infected, or cause discomfort.
- Make sure to meet the increased nutritional needs of the patient with healing burns; extra protein and carbohydrates are needed to accommodate an almost doubled basal metabolism.

- If the burn is being managed with topical drugs, fully exposure to air, and watch for such problems as wound adherence to bed linens, poor drainage control, and partial loss of topical drugs.

PATIENT TEACHING

GENERAL

- Review medication administration, dosages, and possible adverse effects with the patient and his family.
- To encourage therapeutic compliance, inform the patient and his family to expect scarring, but advise that following the proper therapies can minimize it.
- Teach the patient and his family wound management and pain control, and encourage him to do the prescribed exercises.
- Arrange for home care services as ordered.
- Refer the patient and his family to appropriate resources and support services, such as burn survivor support groups and web resources.

RESOURCES
Organizations
American Medical Association:
www.ama-assn.org
The Burn Foundation:
www.burnfoundation.org

Selected references
Cubison, T.C., and Gilbert, P.M. "So Much for Percentage, but What About the Weight?" *Emergency Medicine Journal* 22(9):643-45, September 2005.
Laskowski-Jones, L. "First Aid for Burns," *Nursing* 36(1):41-43, January 2006.
Nowlin, A. "The Delicate Business of Burn Care," *RN* 69(1):52-54, 56-57, January 2006.
"Patient Information. How to Care for Your Burn Wound," *RN* 69(1):55, January 2006.

Wound care: dehiscence and evisceration

- Dehiscence: edges of a surgical wound fail to join or later separate, although the wound appears to be healing normally; may lead to evisceration
- Evisceration: part of the viscera (usually a bowel loop) protrudes through the opened incision, possibly leading to peritonitis and septic shock (see *Recognizing dehiscence and evisceration*)
- Dehiscence and evisceration most likely occurring 6 or 7 days postoperatively after sutures are removed
- Contributing factors: poor nutrition; chronic pulmonary or cardiac disease or metastatic cancer; localized wound infection; stress on the incision from coughing, vomiting, straining, or obesity; and location of incision (midline abdominal incision at higher risk of wound dehiscence)

INDICATIONS
- Dehiscence
- Evisceration

PROCEDURE

- Place a linen-saver pad under the patient to keep the sheets dry when the exposed viscera is moistened.
- Using sterile technique, unfold a sterile towel to create a sterile field.
- Open the package containing the irrigation set, and place the basin, solution container, and 50-ml syringe on the sterile field.
- Open the bottle of normal saline solution and pour about 400 ml into the solution container. Also pour about 200 ml into the sterile basin.
- Open several large abdominal dressings and place them on the sterile field.
- Put on sterile gloves and place one or two of the large abdominal dressings into the basin to saturate them with saline solution.
- Place the moistened dressings over the exposed viscera.
- Then place a sterile, waterproof drape over the dressings to prevent the sheets from getting wet.
- Moisten the dressings every hour by withdrawing saline solution from the container through a syringe and then gently squirting the solution onto the dressings.

  ⚡ **WARNING** *If the eviscerated tissue appears dusky or black, notify the practitioner immediately. With its blood supply interrupted, a protruding organ may quickly become ischemic and necrotic.*

- Keep the patient on absolute bed rest in low Fowler's position (no more than 20 degrees' elevation) with his knees flexed; this prevents further injury and reduces stress on an abdominal incision.
- Don't allow the patient to have anything by mouth to decrease the risk of aspiration if surgical repair is ordered.
- Assist the practitioner in closure of less severe dehisced wounds, by obtaining supplies for the sterile procedure and medications for local anesthesia as ordered.

- In patients with eviscerated wounds, monitor the patient's pulse, respirations, blood pressure, and temperature every 15 minutes to detect signs of shock.
- If necessary, prepare the patient to return to the operating room. After gathering the appropriate equipment, start an I.V. infusion as ordered.
- Insert a nasogastric (NG) tube and connect it to continuous or intermittent low suction as ordered.

  ⚡ **WARNING** *Because NG intubation may make the patient gag or vomit, causing further evisceration, the practitioner may choose to have the tube inserted in the operating room with the patient under anesthesia.*

- Continue to reassure the patient while you prepare him for surgery.

Recognizing dehiscence and evisceration

In wound dehiscence, the layers of the surgical wound separate. With evisceration, the viscera (in this case, a bowel loop) protrude through the surgical incision.

WOUND DEHISCENCE

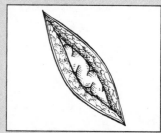

EVISCERATION OF BOWEL LOOP

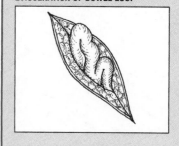

- Verify that an appropriate consent form has been signed and the operating room staff has been informed about the procedure.
- Also administer preoperative medications to the patient as ordered.

COMPLICATIONS
- Infection
- Peritonitis
- Septic shock
- Necrosis of the affected organ

NURSING DIAGNOSES

- Deficient fluid volume
- Ineffective tissue perfusion: Cardiopulmonary, renal, cerebral
- Risk for infection

EXPECTED OUTCOMES
The patient will:
- maintain adequate fluid volume
- maintain adequate heart rate and rhythm, blood pressure, respiratory rate and pulse oximetry, urine intake and output, and level of consciousness
- remain free from wound infection or peritonitis.

PRETREATMENT CARE

- Provide support and an explanation of what measures will be taken immediately by the nurse, to ease the patient's anxiety.
- Instruct the patient to stay in bed and attempt not to move the affected area.
- If possible, stay with him while someone else notifies the practitioner and collects the necessary equipment to dress the wound until the practitioner arrives.

POSTTREATMENT CARE

- Maintain a patent airway; administer oxygen as indicated.
- Provide adequate I.V. hydration as ordered.
- Administer medications (including analgesics) as ordered.
- Provide emotional support.
- Monitor the patient's vital signs, intake and output, peripheral pulses, and pulse oximetry.
- Observe the patient for signs of decreased tissue perfusion.
- Assess the patient for complications.
- Assess the results of laboratory studies or other tests ordered.
- Frequently assess the wound's appearance and drainage or signs of infection, and provide care as ordered.

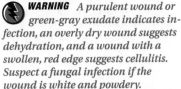 **WARNING** *A purulent wound or green-gray exudate indicates infection, an overly dry wound suggests dehydration, and a wound with a swollen, red edge suggests cellulitis. Suspect a fungal infection if the wound is white and powdery.*

- Explain to a patient whose dehisced wound will be allowed to heal by secondary intention that healthy granulation tissue appears clean, pinkish, faintly shiny, and free from exudate.
- When changing wound dressings, always use sterile technique.
- If local secondary infection develops, clean the wound, as needed, to eliminate a buildup of purulent drainage, and notify the practitioner immediately.

PATIENT TEACHING

GENERAL
- Review what dehiscence and evisceration mean, the treatment given, and the practitioner's follow-up instructions with the patient and his family.
- Review medication administration, including dosage and possible adverse effects, with the patient.
- Teach the patient and his family how to care for the wound as well as review signs of infection or recurrent

dehiscence to report to the practitioner immediately.
- Instruct the patient and his family about measures to achieve pain control, including analgesics ordered.
- Arrange referral to home care services as appropriate.

RESOURCES
Organizations
American Academy of Pediatrics: *www.aap.org*
American Medical Association: *www.ama-assn.org*
American Society of Colon and Rectal Surgeons: *www.fascrs.org*

Selected references
Ekmektzoglou, K.A., and Zografos, G.C. "A Concomitant Review of the Effects of Diabetes Mellitus and Hypothyroidism in Wound Healing," *World Journal of Gastroenterology* 12(17):2721-29, May 2006.
Heller, L., et al. "Management of Abdominal Wound Dehiscence Using Vacuum Assisted Closure in Patients with Compromised Healing," *American Journal of Surgery* 191(2):165-72, February 2006.
Moz, T. "Wound Dehiscence and Evisceration," *Nursing* 34(5):88, May 2004.

Wound care: irrigation

OVERVIEW

- Cleans tissues and flushes cell debris and drainage from an open wound
- Commercial wound cleanser: helps wound heal properly from the inside tissue layers outward to the skin surface; also helps prevent premature surface healing over an abscess pocket or infected tract
- Requires strict sterile technique
- Open wounds usually packed to absorb additional drainage

INDICATIONS

- Open wound

PROCEDURE

- Place the linen-saver pad under the patient to catch spills and avoid linen changes.
- Place the emesis basin below the wound so the irrigating solution flows from the wound into the basin.
- Wash hands thoroughly.
- If necessary, wear a gown to protect your clothing from wound drainage and contamination.
- Put on clean gloves.
- Remove the soiled dressing; then discard the dressing and gloves in the trash bag.
- Establish a sterile field with the equipment and supplies needed for irrigation and wound care.
- Pour the prescribed amount of irrigating solution into a sterile container so as not to contaminate the sterile gloves later by picking up unsterile containers.
- Put on sterile gloves, gown, and goggles, if indicated.
- Fill the syringe with the irrigating solution; then connect the catheter to the syringe.
- Gently instill a slow, steady stream of irrigating solution into the wound until the syringe is empty. (See *Irrigating a deep wound.*)
- Make sure the solution flows only from the clean to the contaminated area of the wound to prevent contamination of clean tissue by exudate. Also, make sure the solution reaches all areas of the wound.
- Refill the syringe, reconnect it to the catheter, and repeat the irrigation.
- Continue to irrigate the wound until the prescribed amount of solution is administered or until the solution returns clear.
- Note the amount of solution administered.
- Remove and discard the catheter and syringe in the waterproof trash bag.
- Keep the patient positioned to allow further wound drainage into the basin.
- Clean the area around the wound with normal saline solution; wipe intact skin with a skin protectant wipe

and allow it to dry well to help prevent skin breakdown and infection.
- Pack the wound, if ordered, and apply a sterile dressing.
- Remove and discard gloves and gown.

COMPLICATIONS

- Infection
- Hypovolemia
- Pain

WARNING *Wound irrigation increases the risk of infection and may cause excoriation and increased pain. Pressure over 15 psi causes trauma to the wound and directs bacteria back into the tissue.*

Irrigating a deep wound

When preparing to irrigate a wound, attach a 19G needle or catheter to a 35-ml piston syringe. This setup delivers an irrigation pressure of 8 psi, which is effective in cleaning the wound and reducing the risk of trauma and wound infection. To prevent tissue damage or, in an abdominal wound—intestinal perforation, avoid forcing the needle or catheter into the wound.

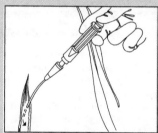

Irrigate the wound with gentle pressure until the solution returns clean. Position the emesis basin under the wound to collect remaining drainage.

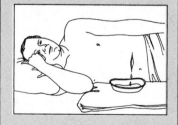

◆ Deficient fluid volume
◆ Ineffective tissue perfusion: Cardio-pulmonary, renal, cerebral
◆ Risk for infection

EXPECTED OUTCOMES
The patient will:
◆ maintain adequate fluid volume
◆ maintain vital signs, blood pressure, neurologic signs, intake and output, and respiratory status within normal limits
◆ remain free from infection.

◆ Assemble all equipment in the patient's room.
◆ Check the expiration date on each sterile package, and inspect for tears.
◆ Check the sterilization date and the date that each bottle of irrigating solution was opened; don't use solution that has been open longer than 24 hours.
◆ Using sterile technique, dilute the prescribed irrigant to the correct proportions with sterile water or normal saline solution, if necessary.
◆ Let the solution stand until it reaches room temperature, or warm it to 90° to 95° F (32.2° to 35° C).
◆ Open the waterproof trash bag, and place it near the patient's bed.
◆ Position the bag to avoid reaching across the sterile field or the wound when disposing of soiled items.
◆ Form a cuff by turning down the top of the trash bag to provide a wide opening, thus preventing contamination by touching the bag's edge.
◆ Check the practitioner's order, and assess the patient's condition.
◆ Identify the patient's allergies, especially to povidone-iodine or other topical solutions or medications.
◆ Explain the procedure to the patient, provide privacy, and position the patient correctly for the procedure.

◆ Make sure the patient is comfortable.
◆ Properly dispose of drainage, solutions, and the trash bag; clean or dispose of soiled equipment and supplies according to facility policy and guidelines from the Centers of Disease Control and Prevention (CDC).

⚡ **WARNING** *To prevent contamination of other equipment, don't return unopened sterile supplies to the sterile supply cabinet.*

◆ Provide adequate I.V. hydration as ordered.
◆ Administer medications (including analgesics) as ordered.
◆ Provide emotional support.
◆ Monitor the patient's, vital signs, intake and output, peripheral pulses, and pulse oximetry.
◆ Monitor the patient for signs of decreased tissue perfusion.
◆ Check the patient for complications.
◆ Monitor the patient's level of pain; provide an analgesic and assess its effect.
◆ Assess the results of ordered laboratory studies.
◆ Thoroughly assess and document the wound's appearance as this is essential to detect infection and other complications.

⚡ **WARNING** *A purulent wound or green-gray exudate indicates infection, an overly dry wound suggests dehydration, and a wound with a swollen, red edge suggests cellulitis. Suspect a fungal infection if the wound appears white and powdery*

◆ Healthy granulation tissue appears clean, pinkish, faintly shiny, and free from exudate.
◆ Try to coordinate wound irrigation with the practitioner's visit so that he can inspect the wound.
◆ Use only the irrigant specified by the practitioner because other solutions may be erosive or harmful to the patient.
◆ Remember to follow the facility's policy and CDC guidelines concerning wound and skin precautions.

(continued)

Applying a special wound-cleaning agent

Dear Caregiver:

Follow these steps to apply a special wound-cleaning agent.

ASSEMBLE THE EQUIPMENT

You'll need several 4" × 4" sterile gauze pads, a 5" × 9" sterile dressing, hypoallergenic tape, linen-saver pads, irrigation syringe, irrigating solution (usually sterile water) and a container in which to pour it, a container to catch irrigation runoff, a wound-cleaning agent (beads or paste) prepared as directed, sterile disposable gloves, and a disposable bag.

CHECK THE WOUND

Place a linen-saver pad under the patient in the area where care will be performed. Remove the old dressing and check it for drainage or pus. Then fold its sides together with the soiled side in, and put it in the disposable bag. Carefully inspect the wound for signs of infection, such as redness, swelling, drainage, or pus. *Don't touch the wound.* Write down a description of the wound, including the color and amount of drainage.

IRRIGATE THE WOUND

1. Pour the irrigating solution into its container and wash your hands. Draw about 1 oz (30 ml) of the solution into a bulb syringe or a large syringe with a plunger.

2. After placing the irrigation-runoff container against the skin below the base of the wound, hold the syringe with its tip about 2" (5 cm) from the wound, and squirt all the solution into the wound as shown. Be sure to remove *all* the old paste and debris from the wound; if necessary, irrigate the wound again. Don't touch the wound with the syringe tip; if you do so, the syringe tip will be contaminated and unusable for future dressing changes.

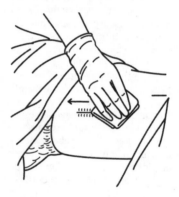

3. Put on the sterile gloves. Then wrap a sterile gauze pad around your finger and gently pat dry the area around the wound. But leave the wound itself moist to stimulate the action of the beads or paste. Then throw the pad in the disposable bag.

PUT ON THE CLEANING AGENT

1. If you're using wound-cleaning paste, apply it with a sterile gauze pad into the wound—at least ¼" (0.5 cm) deep. If you're using wound-cleaning beads, pour the beads into the wound—at least ¼" deep.

2. Cover the wound with a sterile dressing. Tape the dressing down on all four sides. Finally, take off the sterile gloves, throw them away in the disposable bag, and wash your hands thoroughly.

3. Check every 8 hours to see if the wound cleaning agent has changed color. If it has, remove the beads or paste by irrigating again. If it hasn't, change the beads or paste every 12 hours.

◆ Irrigate with a bulb syringe only if a piston syringe is unavailable. However, use a bulb syringe cautiously because it doesn't deliver enough pressure to adequately clean the wound. If the wound is small or shallow, use the syringe for irrigation.

PATIENT TEACHING

◆ If the wound must be irrigated at home, teach the patient or a family member how to perform it using sterile technique.
◆ Ask for a return demonstration of the proper technique. (See *Applying a special wound-cleaning agent.*)
◆ Include written instructions for the irrigation procedure with the discharge information.
◆ Arrange for home health services as appropriate.
◆ Teach the patient the signs and symptoms of infection to report to his practitioner immediately.

RESOURCES
Organizations
American Medical Association: *www.ama-assn.org*
Wound, Ostomy and Continence Nursing Society: *www.wocn.org*

Selected references
Draeger, R.W., and Dahners, L.E. "Traumatic Wound Debridement: A Comparison of Irrigation Methods," *Journal of Orthopedic Trauma* 20(2):83-88, February 2006.
Ichioka, S., et al. "Benefits of Surgical Reconstruction in Pressure Ulcers with a Non-Advancing Edge and Scar Formation," *Journal of Wound Care* 14(7):301-305, July 2005.
Moore, Z.E., and Cowman, S. "Wound Cleansing for Pressure Ulcers," *Cochrane Database System Review* 19(4):CD004983, October 2005.

Wound care, pressure ulcer

OVERVIEW

- Involves relieving pressure, restoring circulation, promoting adequate nutrition, and resolving or managing related disorders; other care measures: decreasing risk factors, use of topical treatments, wound cleaning, debridement, and use of dressings to support moist wound healing
- May require special pressure-reducing devices, such as beds, mattresses, mattress overlays, and chair cushions
- Effectiveness and duration of treatment dependent on characteristic of ulcer

INDICATIONS

- Pressure ulcer

PROCEDURE

- Provide privacy.
- Use standard precaution guidelines from the Centers for Disease Control and Prevention (CDC).

CLEANING THE PRESSURE ULCER

- Position the patient for comfort and easy access to the site.
- Cover bed linens with a linen-saver pad to prevent soiling.
- Open the normal saline solution container and the piston syringe.
- Pour solution carefully into a clean or sterile irrigation container.
- Put the piston syringe into the opening of the irrigation container.
- Open the packages of supplies.
- Put on gloves before removing the old dressing and exposing the pressure ulcer.
- Discard the soiled dressing in the impervious plastic trash bag.
- Inspect the wound, noting color, amount, and odor of drainage or necrotic debris.
- Measure the wound perimeter with a disposable wound-measuring device.
- Apply full force of the piston syringe to irrigate the ulcer, remove necrotic debris, and decrease bacteria in the wound.
- For nonnecrotic wounds, use less pressure to prevent damage.
- Remove and discard soiled gloves and put on a clean pair.
- Insert a gloved finger or sterile cotton swab into the wound to assess wound tunneling or undermining.
- Assess and note condition of clean wound and surrounding skin.
- Notify a wound care specialist if there's remaining adherent necrotic material.
- Apply the appropriate topical dressing.

APPLYING A MOIST SALINE GAUZE DRESSING

- Irrigate the ulcer with normal saline solution. Blot surrounding skin dry.
- Moisten the gauze dressing with normal saline solution.
- Gently place the dressing over the surface of the ulcer.
- To separate surfaces within the wound, gently place a dressing between opposing wound surfaces. Don't pack the gauze tightly.
- Change the dressing often enough to keep the wound moist.

APPLYING A HYDROCOLLOIDAL DRESSING

- Irrigate the ulcer with normal saline solution. Blot surrounding skin dry.
- Choose a clean, dry, presized dressing, or cut one to overlap the pressure ulcer by about 1″ (2.5 cm).
- Remove the dressing from its package, remove the release paper and apply the dressing to the wound. Carefully smooth wrinkles when applying the dressing.
- If using tape to secure the dressing, apply a skin sealant to the intact skin around the ulcer.
- When dry, tape the dressing to the skin. Avoid tension or pressure.
- Remove and discard gloves and other refuse.
- Wash your hands.
- Change a hydrocolloid dressing every 2 to 7 days.
- Discontinue if signs of infection are present.

APPLYING A TRANSPARENT DRESSING

- Irrigate the ulcer with normal saline solution. Blot surrounding skin dry.
- Clean and dry the wound as described above.
- Select a dressing to overlap the ulcer by 2″ (5 cm).
- Gently lay the dressing over the ulcer, taking care not to stretch it.
- Press firmly on the edges of the dressing to promote adherence.
- Tape edges to prevent them from curling.
- If necessary, aspirate accumulated fluid with a 21G needle and syringe.

- Clean the site with an alcohol pad and cover it with a transparent dressing.
- Change the dressing every 3 to 7 days, depending on drainage.

APPLYING AN ALGINATE DRESSING

- Irrigate the ulcer with normal saline solution. Blot surrounding skin dry.
- Apply alginate dressing to the ulcer surface. Cover with a second dressing (such as gauze pads). Secure with tape or elastic netting.
- If drainage is heavy, change the dressing once or twice daily for the first 3 to 5 days.
- As drainage decreases, change the dressing less frequently—every 2 to 4 days or as ordered.
- When drainage stops or the wound bed looks dry, stop using alginate dressing.

APPLYING A FOAM DRESSING

- Irrigate the ulcer with normal saline solution. Blot surrounding skin dry.
- Lay the foam dressing over the ulcer.
- Use tape, elastic netting, or gauze to hold the dressing in place.
- Change the dressing when the foam no longer absorbs the exudate.

APPLYING A HYDROGEL DRESSING

- Irrigate the ulcer with normal saline solution. Blot surrounding skin dry.
- Apply gel to the wound bed.
- Cover the area with a second dressing.
- Change the dressing, as needed, to keep the wound bed moist.
- If you're using a sheet form dressing, cut it to match the wound base.
- Hydrogel dressings also come in a prepackaged, saturated gauze to fill "dead space." Follow the manufacturer's directions.

COMPLICATIONS

- Infection
- Cellulitis
- Septicemia

- Deficient fluid volume
- Ineffective tissue perfusion: Cardiopulmonary, renal, cerebral
- Risk for infection

EXPECTED OUTCOMES

The patient will:
- maintain adequate fluid volume
- maintain vital signs, blood pressure, neurologic signs, intake and output, and respiratory status within normal limits
- remain free from infection.

- Explain the procedure to the patient to ease fear and promote cooperation.
- Assemble all of the equipment at the patient's bedside.
- Attach an impervious plastic trash bag to the overbed table.
- Cut the tape into strips.
- Loosen the lids on cleaning solutions and drugs.
- Loosen the existing dressing edges and tapes.
- Wash your hands and put on gloves.

- Make sure the patient is comfortable.
- Properly dispose of drainage, solutions, and trash bag, and clean or dispose of soiled equipment and supplies according to facility policy and CDC guidelines.

⚡ **WARNING** *To prevent contamination of other equipment, don't return unopened sterile supplies to the sterile supply cabinet.*

- Provide adequate I.V. hydration as ordered.
- Administer medications (including analgesics) as ordered.
- Provide emotional support.
- Monitor the patient's vital signs, intake and output, peripheral pulses, and pulse oximetry.
- Observe the patient for signs of decreased tissue perfusion.
- Assess the patient for complications.
- Monitor the patient's level of pain; provide an analgesic and assess its effect.
- Assess the results of ordered laboratory studies.
- Thoroughly assess and document the wound's appearance as this is essential to detect infection and other complications.

⚡ **WARNING** *A purulent wound or green-gray exudate indicates infection, an overly dry wound suggests dehydration, and a wound with a swollen, red edge suggests cellulitis. Suspect a fungal infection if the wound appears white and powdery.*

- Healthy granulation tissue appears clean, pinkish, faintly shiny, and free of exudate.
- Try to coordinate wound irrigation with the practitioner's visit so that he can inspect the wound.
- Turn and reposition the patient every 1 or 2 hours unless contraindicated.
- Use an air, gel, or foam mattress for patients who can't turn themselves or for those who are turned on a schedule. Low- or high-air-loss therapy may be indicated.
- Implement active or passive range-of-motion exercises.

(continued)

- Lift rather than slide the patient when turning. Use a turning sheet and get help from coworkers as necessary.
- Use pillows to position the patient and increase his comfort. Eliminate sheet wrinkles.
- Post a turning schedule at the patient's bedside.
- Avoid the trochanter position. Instead, position the bed at a 30-degree angle.
- Avoid raising the bed more than 30 degrees for long periods.
- Adjust or pad appliances, casts, or splints, to ensure proper fit.
- Gently apply lotion after bathing to keep skin moist.
- Clean and dry soiled skin. Apply a protective moisture barrier.

PATIENT TEACHING

GENERAL

- Teach the patient and his family the importance of prevention, position changes, and treatment. Teach proper methods and encourage participation. (See *Care and prevention of leg ulcers.*)
- Encourage the patient to follow a diet with adequate calories, protein, and vitamins.
- Direct the patient in a chair or wheelchair to shift his weight every 15 minutes.
- Instruct the paraplegic patient to shift his weight by doing push-ups.
- Tell the patient to avoid heat lamps and harsh soaps.
- Instruct the patient to avoid using elbow and heel protectors with a single narrow strap or artificial sheepskin.
- Advise the patient and his family to explore the use of gel cushions and special mattresses if prolonged immobility is expected, and refer them to appropriate resources for information on the varyious products available.
- Teach the patient and his family about medications prescribed, particularly analgesics, including correct administration, frequency of use, and possible adverse effects.
- Refer the patient to home health care services.

RESOURCES
Organizations
American Medical Association: *www.ama-assn.org*
Wound, Ostomy and Continence Nursing Society: *www.wocn.org*

Selected references
Draeger, R.W., and Dahners, L.E. "Traumatic Wound Debridement: A Comparison of Irrigation Methods," *Journal of Orthopedic Trauma* 20(2):83-88, February 2006.
Ichioka, S., et al. "Benefits of Surgical Reconstruction in Pressure Ulcers with a Non-Advancing Edge and Scar Formation," *Journal of Wound Care* 14(7):301-305, July 2005.
Moore, Z.E., and Cowman, S. "Wound Cleansing for Pressure Ulcers," *Cochrane Database of Systematic Reviews* 19(4):CD004983, October 2005.

Care and prevention of leg ulcers

Dear Patient:

You can help your leg ulcer heal and prevent new ulcers from forming by learning about your condition and its required care.

WHAT IS A LEG ULCER?

A leg ulcer is an area of dying skin. An ulcer can form wherever an artery becomes blocked or constricted. When this happens, not enough blood gets to the skin and the tissue beneath it to nourish the area. Instead, blood tends to pool in your leg veins—sometimes from a condition called *venous insufficiency.*

Pressure then builds up in these congested leg vessels, and the blood supply to the tissues decreases. As the condition worsens, the skin becomes fragile, and an infection may develop from injury, pressure, and irritation. As a result, leg ulcers may develop.

IMPROVING YOUR CIRCULATION

To improve circulation in your legs, wear elastic support stockings. Called *antiembolism stockings*, these hose will help to return blood to your heart. They'll improve circulation to your existing ulcer and may help to keep new ones from forming.

Put your feet up. Rest and elevate your legs for as long and as often as your health care provider directs. This will reduce your legs' needs for nutrients and oxygen and help to promote healing. Always raise your lower leg above heart level. Don't cross your legs.

PROMOTING HEALING

Follow these measures to help your ulcer heal:

◆ Keep your ulcer clean to prevent infection. Always wash your hands before and after changing your dressing or touching the wound. This keeps the area germ-free.

◆ Follow instructions exactly when changing your dressing and applying ointments or other medications.

◆ Be patient. Your ulcer may take 3 months to 1 year to heal.

◆ Inform your health care provider if your ulcer grows larger, feels increasingly painful, or becomes foul-smelling.

PREVENTING ULCERS

Follow these measures to prevent ulcers:

◆ Watch for signs and symptoms of new ulcers. These signs include leg swelling, pain, and discolored skin that looks brownish or dark blue.

◆ Wear support stockings to help prevent ulcers and to help heal existing ones.

◆ Be careful to avoid injury to your leg, which can lead to ulcer development. For example, avoid activities that involve rugged physical contact such as roughhousing with children or dogs.

◆ Prevent falls by installing safety rails or a grab bar and placing a nonskid mat in your bathtub.

◆ Wear low, nonskid footwear whenever possible.

Wound care, surgical

- Helps prevent infection by stopping pathogens from entering the wound
- Protects skin surface from maceration and excoriation caused by contact with irritating drainage
- Allows measurement of wound drainage to monitor healing and fluid and electrolyte balance
- Two primary methods used: dressing and pouching
- Lightly-seeping wounds with drains and wounds with minimal purulent drainage: managed with packing and gauze dressings
- Certain wounds, including chronic ones: may require occlusive dressings
- Wounds with copious, excoriating drainage: need pouching to protect surrounding skin
- Type of dressing to apply dependent on wound color (see *Tailoring wound care to wound color*)

PROCEDURE

REMOVING THE OLD DRESSING

- Check the practitioner's order for specific wound care and medication instructions. Note the location of surgical drains to avoid dislodging them during the procedure.
- Assess the patient's condition.
- Identify the patient's allergies, especially to adhesive tape, povidone-iodine or other topical solutions, or medications.
- Provide the patient with privacy, and position him as necessary.

> **WARNING** *To avoid chilling the patient, expose only the wound site.*

- Wash your hands thoroughly; put on a gown and a face shield, if necessary. Put onclean gloves.
- Loosen the soiled dressing by holding the patient's skin and pulling the tape or dressing toward the wound.

This protects the newly formed tissue and prevents stress on the incision.

- Moisten the tape with acetone-free adhesive remover, if necessary, to make the tape removal less painful (particularly if the skin is hairy).

> **WARNING** *Don't apply solvents to the incision because they could contaminate the wound.*

- Slowly remove the soiled dressing. If the gauze adheres to the wound, loosen the gauze by moistening it with sterile normal saline solution.
- Observe the dressing for the amount, type, color, and odor of drainage.
- Discard the dressing and gloves in the impervious trash bag.

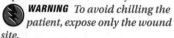

Tailoring wound care to wound color

If your patient has an open wound, you can assess how well it's healing by inspecting its color, which you can then use to guide management of the wound.

RED WOUNDS

Red indicates normal healing. When a wound begins to heal, a layer of pale pink granulation tissue covers the wound bed. As it thickens, it becomes beefy red.

Cover a red wound, keep it moist and clean, and protect it from trauma. Use a transparent dressing (such as Tegaderm or Op-site), a hydrocolloidal dressing (such as DuoDerm), or a gauze dressing moistened with sterile normal saline solution or impregnated with petroleum jelly or an antibiotic.

YELLOW WOUNDS

Yellow is the color of exudate produced by microorganisms in an open wound. Exudate usually appears whitish-yellow, creamy yellow, yellowish-green, or beige. Water content influences shade; dry exudate appears darker.

If the wound is yellow, clean it and remove exudate, using high-pressure irrigation; then cover it with a moist dressing. Use absorptive products (for example, Debrisan beads and

paste) or a moist gauze dressing with or without an antibiotic. You may also use hydrotherapy with whirlpool or high-pressure irrigation.

BLACK WOUNDS

Black, the least healthy color, signals necrosis. Dead, avascular tissue slows healing and provides a site for microorganisms to proliferate.

You should debride a black wound. After removing dead tissue, apply a dressing to keep the wound moist and guard against external contamination. As ordered, use enzyme products, surgical debridement, hydrotherapy with whirlpool or high-pressure irrigation, or a moist gauze dressing.

MULTICOLORED WOUNDS

You may note two or even all three colors in a wound. In this case, classify the wound according to the least healthy color present. For example, if the patient's wound is red and yellow, classify it as a yellow wound.

CARING FOR THE WOUND

♦ Wash your hands.
♦ Establish a sterile field with the equipment and supplies needed for suture-line care and the dressing change, including a sterile dressing set and povidone-iodine swabs.
♦ If the practitioner has ordered ointment, squeeze the needed amount onto the sterile field.
♦ Pour the antiseptic cleaning agent into a sterile container and place on a sterile field. Then put on clean gloves.
♦ Saturate the sterile gauze pads with the prescribed cleaning agent.

⚡ **WARNING** *Avoid using cotton balls because they may shed fibers in the wound, causing irritation, infection, or adhesion.*

♦ If ordered, obtain a wound culture; then proceed to clean the wound.
♦ Pick up the moistened gauze pad or swab, and squeeze out the excess solution.
♦ Working from the top of the incision, wipe once to the bottom and then discard the gauze pad.
♦ With a second moistened pad, wipe from top to bottom in a vertical line next to the incision; always wipe from the clean area toward the less clean area (usually from top to bottom).
♦ Continue to work outward from the incision in lines running parallel to it.
♦ Use each gauze pad or swab for only one stroke to avoid tracking wound exudate and normal body flora from surrounding skin to the clean areas.
♦ Use sterile cotton-tipped applicators for efficient cleaning of tight-fitting wire sutures, deep and narrow wounds, or wounds with pockets. Because the cotton on the swab is tightly wrapped, it's less likely than a cotton ball to leave fibers in the wound. Remember to wipe only once with each applicator.
♦ If the patient has a surgical drain, clean the drain's surface last. Because moist drainage promotes bacterial growth, the drain is considered the most contaminated area. Clean the skin around the drain by wiping in half or full circles from the drain site outward.

♦ Clean all areas of the wound to wash away debris, pus, blood, and necrotic material. Try not to disturb sutures or irritate the incision.
♦ Clean to at least 1″ (2.5 cm) beyond the end of the new dressing. If new dressing isn't being applied, clean to at least 2″ (5 cm) beyond the incision.
♦ Check to ensure that the edges of the incision are lined up properly, and check for signs of infection (such as heat, redness, swelling, induration, and odor), dehiscence, or evisceration. If such signs are observed or if the patient reports pain at the wound site, notify the practitioner.
♦ Irrigate the wound as ordered.
♦ Wash the skin surrounding the wound with soap and water, and pat dry using a sterile 4″ × 4″ gauze pad.

⚡ **WARNING** *Avoid oil-based soap because it may interfere with pouch adherence. Apply prescribed topical medication.*

♦ Apply a skin protectant if needed.
♦ If ordered, pack the wound with gauze pads or strips folded to fit, using sterile forceps.
♦ Pack the wound using the wet-to-damp method. Soaking the packing material in solution and wringing it out so it's slightly moist provides a moist wound environment that absorbs debris and drainage. However, removing the packing won't disrupt new tissue.

⚡ **WARNING** *Don't pack the wound tightly because the pressure exerted may damage the wound granulation tissue.*

APPLYING A FRESH GAUZE DRESSING

♦ Gently place sterile 4″ × 4″ gauze pads at the center of the wound, and move progressively outward to the edges of the wound site.
♦ Extend the gauze at least 1″ beyond the incision in each direction, and cover the wound evenly with enough sterile dressings (usually two or three layers) to absorb all drainage until the next dressing change.
♦ Use large absorbent dressings to form outer layers, if needed, to provide greater absorbency.
♦ Secure the dressing's edges to the patient's skin with strips of tape to maintain the sterility of the wound site or secure the dressing with a T-binder or Montgomery straps to prevent skin excoriation, which may occur with repeated tape removal necessitated by frequent dressing changes.
♦ If the wound is on a limb, secure the dressing with a fishnet tube elasticized dressing support.
♦ Make sure that the patient is comfortable.
♦ Properly dispose of the solutions and the trash bag, and clean or discard soiled equipment and supplies according to your facility's policy.

⚡ **WARNING** *If the patient's wound has purulent drainage, don't return unopened sterile supplies to the sterile supply cabinet because this could cause cross-contamination of other equipment.*

(continued)

DRESSING A WOUND WITH A DRAIN

◆ Prepare a drain dressing by using sterile scissors to cut a slit in a sterile 4" × 4" gauze pad. Fold the pad in half; then cut inward from the center of the folded edge. Don't use a cotton-lined gauze pad because cutting the gauze opens the lining and releases cotton fibers into the wound. Prepare a second pad the same way, or use commercially precut gauze.

◆ Gently press one folded pad close to the skin around the drain so that the tubing fits into the slit. Press the second folded pad around the drain from the opposite direction so that the two pads encircle the tubing.

◆ Layer as many uncut sterile 4" × 4" gauze pads or large absorbent dressings around the tubing as needed to absorb expected drainage. Tape the dressing in place, or use a T-binder or Montgomery straps.

POUCHING A WOUND

◆ If the patient's wound is draining heavily or if drainage may damage surrounding skin, apply a pouch.

◆ Measure the wound. Cut an opening ⅜" (0.3 cm) larger than the wound in the facing of the collection pouch.

◆ Apply a skin protectant as needed. (Some protectants are incorporated within the collection pouch and also provide adhesion.)

◆ Before applying the pouch, keep in mind the patient's usual position. Then plan to position the pouch's drainage port so that gravity facilitates drainage.

◆ Make sure that the drainage port at the bottom of the pouch is closed firmly to prevent leaks.

◆ Then gently press the contoured pouch opening around the wound, starting at its lower edge, to catch drainage.

◆ To empty the pouch, put on gloves and a face shield or a mask and goggles to avoid splashing.

◆ Then insert the pouch's bottom half into a graduated biohazard container, and open the drainage port.

◆ Note the color, consistency, odor, and amount of fluid.

◆ If ordered, obtain a culture specimen and send it to the laboratory immediately.

◆ Remember to follow the guidelines from the Centers of Disease Control and Prevention (CDC) when handling infectious drainage.

◆ Wipe the bottom of the pouch and the drainage port with a gauze pad to remove drainage that could irritate the patient's skin or cause an odor.

◆ Then reseal the port.

◆ Change the pouch only if it leaks or fails to adhere. More frequent changes are unnecessary and only irritate the patient's skin.

◆ If the patient has two wounds in the same area, cover each wound separately with layers of sterile 4" × 4" gauze pads. Then cover each site with a large absorbent dressing secured to the patient's skin with tape. Don't use a single large absorbent dressing to cover both sites because drainage quickly saturates a pad, promoting cross-contamination.

◆ When packing a wound, don't pack it too tightly because this compresses adjacent capillaries and may prevent the wound edges from contracting. Avoid overlapping damp packing onto surrounding skin because it macerates the intact tissue.

◆ To save time when dressing a wound with a drain, use precut tracheostomy pads or drain dressings instead of custom-cutting gauze pads to fit around the drain.

◆ If the patient is sensitive to adhesive tape, use paper or silk tape because it's less likely to cause a skin reaction and will peel off more easily than adhesive tape.

◆ Use a surgical mask to cradle a chin or jawline dressing; this provides a secure dressing and avoids the need to shave the patient's hair.

◆ If ordered, use a collodion spray or similar topical protectant instead of a gauze dressing. Moisture- and contaminant-proof, this covering dries in a clear, impermeable film that leaves the wound visible for observation and avoids the friction caused by a dressing.

◆ If a sump drain isn't adequately collecting wound secretions, reinforce it with an ostomy pouch or another collection bag.

◆ Use waterproof tape to strengthen a spot on the front of the pouch near the adhesive opening; then cut a small "X" in the tape. Feed the drain catheter into the pouch through the "X" cut. Seal the cut around the tubing with more waterproof tape; then connect the tubing to the suction pump. This method frees the drainage port at the bottom of the pouch so you don't have to remove the tubing to empty the pouch. If more than one collection pouch for a wound or wounds is used, record drainage volume separately for each pouch. Avoid using waterproof material over the dressing because it reduces air circulation and promotes infection from accumulated heat and moisture.

◆ Because many practitioners prefer to change the first postoperative dressing themselves to check the incision, don't change the first dressing unless directed. If there's no instruction and drainage penetrates the dressings, reinforce the dressing with fresh sterile gauze. Request an order to change the dressing, or ask the practitioner to change it as soon as possible. A reinforced dressing shouldn't remain in place longer than 24 hours because it's an optimum medium for bacterial growth.

◆ For the recent postoperative patient or the patient with complications, check the dressing every 15 to 30 minutes or as ordered. For the patient with a properly healing wound, check the dressing at least once every 8 hours.

◆ If the dressing becomes wet from the outside (for example, from spilled drinking water), replace it as soon as possible to prevent wound contamination.

COMPLICATIONS

◆ Allergic reaction to an antiseptic cleaning agent, a prescribed topical medication, or adhesive tape
◆ Excoriation
◆ Infection

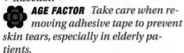 **AGE FACTOR** *Take care when removing adhesive tape to prevent skin tears, especially in elderly patients.*

NURSING DIAGNOSES

◆ Deficient fluid volume
◆ Deficient knowledge (postoperative wound care)
◆ Risk for infection

EXPECTED OUTCOMES

The patient will:
◆ maintain adequate fluid volume
◆ verbalize and demonstrate an understanding of how to assess and treat his wound
◆ remain free from infection.

PRETREATMENT CARE

◆ Explain the procedure to the patient to allay his fears and ensure his cooperation.
◆ Ask the patient about allergies to tapes and dressings.
◆ Assemble all equipment in the patient's room.
◆ Check the expiration date on each sterile package, and inspect for tears.
◆ Open the waterproof trash bag, and place it near the patient's bed.
◆ Position the bag to avoid reaching across the sterile field or the wound when disposing of soiled articles.
◆ Form a cuff by turning down the top of the trash bag to provide a wide opening and to prevent contamination of instruments or gloves by touching the bag's edge.

POSTTREATMENT CARE

◆ Make sure the patient is comfortable.
◆ Properly dispose of drainage, solutions, and trash bag, and clean or dispose of soiled equipment and supplies according to facility policy and CDC guidelines.

⚡ **WARNING** *To prevent contamination of other equipment, don't return unopened sterile supplies to the sterile supply cabinet.*

◆ Provide adequate I.V. hydration as ordered.
◆ Administer medications (including analgesics) as ordered.
◆ Provide emotional support.
◆ Monitor the patient's vital signs, intake and output, peripheral pulses, and pulse oximetry.
◆ Observe the patient for signs of decreased tissue perfusion.
◆ Assess the patient for complications.
◆ Monitor the results of ordered laboratory studies.
◆ Thoroughly assess and document the wound's appearance because this is essential to detect infection and other complications.
◆ If the patient will need wound care after discharge, demonstrate the procedure and explain each step.

PATIENT TEACHING

GENERAL

◆ Encourage the patient to follow a diet with adequate calories, protein, and vitamins.
◆ Teach the patient how to care for the wound himself and change the dressings, stress the importance of using clean technique at home, and teach him how to examine the wound for signs of infection and other complications. Give him written instructions for these homecare procedures. (See *Changing a dry dressing*.)
◆ Stress the importance of keeping all supplies in a clean area and of meticulous hand washing before and after procedures.
◆ Refer the patient to appropriate resources and support services.
◆ Arrange for home health care services if required.

RESOURCES
Organizations
American Medical Association: *www.ama-assn.org*
Wound, Ostomy and Continence Nursing Society: *www.wocn.org*

Selected references
Jones, M.J. "M0488: Status of Surgical Wound," *Home Health Nurse* 23(10): 673-76, October 2005.
Millsaps, C.C. "Pay Attention to Patient Positioning!" *RN* 69(1):59-63, January 2006.
Zorrilla, P., et al. "Shoelace Technique for Gradual Closure of Fasciotomy Wounds," *Journal of Trauma* 59(6): 1515-17, December 2005.

(continued)

Changing a dry dressing

Dear Patient or Caregiver:

Changing a dry dressing at least once per day keeps the wound clean, allows you to see how well it's healing, and lets you apply medication. If dressing changes are recommended, here's how to proceed.

GATHER YOUR SUPPLIES

You'll need a new dressing, several 4″ × 4″ gauze pads, sterile saline, cleaning solution, special ointment or powder if ordered, baby oil, surgical tape, waterproof disposal bag for soiled supplies, and two pairs of disposable gloves.

REMOVE THE OLD TAPE

1. Wash your hands, and put on disposable gloves.
2. To remove the tape, hold the skin taut, and pull the old tape strips toward the wound. Be sure to remove *all* the old tape. If the tape sticks, use baby oil to soften it and make removal easier. Then proceed as follows.

REMOVE THE OLD DRESSING

1. Slowly remove the old dressing. If it sticks to the wound, stop. To help prevent infection, moisten the dressing with sterile saline solution or lukewarm water that has been boiled for 5 minutes and then cooled. Remove the dressing when it's loose.
2. Remove and discard the gloves in the disposal bag.

CLEAN THE WOUND

1. Before you clean the wound, check it for signs of infection: puffiness or swelling, redness, yellow or green drainage or pus, or a foul odor. If the wound looks infected, report the condition immediately.
2. Put on another pair of disposable gloves. Saturate one of the gauze pads with cleaning solution. Then fold the pad into quarters.
3. Pinching the pad between your thumb and first two fingers, gently wipe from the top of the wound to the bottom in one motion. Then discard the pad in the disposal bag.

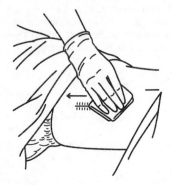

4. Saturate another gauze pad, fold it in half and then into quarters.
5. Wipe the wound again, this time on one side first and then on the other. Do this several times to clean the entire wound area that the dressing will cover.

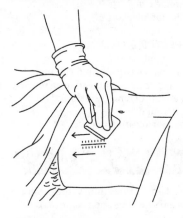

6. Finally, use another clean gauze pad to pat the wound dry.

Changing a dry dressing *(continued)*

APPLY OINTMENT OR POWDER

1. Remove the cap from the ointment or powder container.

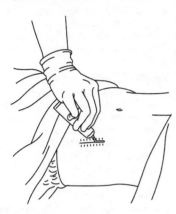

2. If you're using special ointment, squeeze a generous strip of it along the wound's outline (shown above). Don't let the tube touch the wound. This helps to prevent germs from gathering on the tube and creating a source of infection.

If you're using a special powder, dust the wound with a fine layer of it.

APPLY THE NEW DRESSING

1. Open the new dressing carefully, taking care to make sure it touches only the wound. Center the dressing over the wound and apply it.

2. Secure the edges of the dressing to the skin around the wound with strips of surgical tape. Make sure the strips overlap and create a tight seal against germs.

3. When you're finished, remove and discard your gloves and wash your hands.

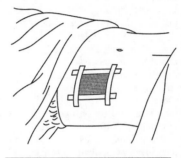

Wound care, traumatic

- Traumatic injuries: include abrasions, lacerations, puncture wounds, and amputations
- Abrasions: skin is scraped, with partial loss of the skin surface
- Lacerations: skin is torn, causing jagged, irregular edges; severity of a laceration dependent on its size, depth, and location
- Puncture wound: occurs when a pointed object, such as a knife or glass fragment, penetrates the skin
- Amputation: removal of part of the body or a limb

INDICATIONS
- Traumatic wound

PROCEDURE

- Use appropriate protective equipment, such as a gown, gloves, a mask, and goggles, if spraying or splashing of body fluids is possible.

    ⚡ **WARNING** *Hydrogen peroxide should never be instilled into a deep wound because of the risk of embolism from the evolving gases. Moreover, solutions such as hydrogen peroxide or sodium hypochlorite may damage tissue and delay healing.*

    ⚡ **WARNING** *Avoid cleaning a traumatic wound with alcohol because it causes pain and dehydrates tissue. Also, avoid using antiseptics for wound cleaning because they can impede healing. In addition, never use a cotton ball or cotton-filled gauze pad to clean a wound because cotton fibers left in the wound can cause contamination.*

ABRASION
- Flush the scraped skin with normal saline solution.
- Remove dirt or gravel with a sterile 4″ × 4″ gauze pad moistened with normal saline solution. Rub in the opposite direction from which the dirt or gravel became embedded.
- If the wound is extremely dirty, use a surgical brush to scrub it.
- With a small wound, allow it to dry and form a scab. With a larger wound, cover it with a nonadherent pad or petroleum gauze and a light dressing. Apply antibacterial ointment if ordered.

LACERATION
- Moisten a sterile 4″× 4″ gauze pad with normal saline solution.
- Clean the wound gently, working outward from its center to about 2″ (5 cm) beyond its edges.
- Discard the soiled gauze pad and use a fresh one as necessary.
- Continue until the wound appears clean.
- If the wound is dirty, irrigate it with a 50-ml catheter-tip syringe and normal saline solution.
- Assist the practitioner in suturing the wound edges using the suture kit, or apply sterile strips of porous tape.
- Apply the prescribed antibacterial ointment to help prevent infection.
- Apply a dry sterile dressing over the wound to absorb drainage and help prevent bacterial contamination.

PUNCTURE WOUND
- If the wound is minor, allow it to bleed for a few minutes before cleaning it.
- For a larger puncture wound, irrigate it before applying a dry dressing.
- Stabilize an embedded foreign object until the practitioner can remove it.
- After the practitioner removes the object and bleeding is stabilized, clean the wound similar to that for a laceration or deep puncture wound.

AMPUTATION
- Apply a gauze pad moistened with normal saline solution to the amputation site. Elevate the affected part, and immobilize it for surgery.
- Recover the amputated part, and prepare it for transport to a facility where microvascular surgery is performed.
- When irrigating an amputation, avoid using more than 8 psi of pressure. High-pressure irrigation can seriously interfere with healing, kill cells, and allow bacteria to infiltrate the tissue.
- To clean the wound, use normal saline or hydrogen peroxide; its foaming action facilitates debris removal. Be sure to rinse your hands well after using hydrogen peroxide.

COMPLICATIONS
- Temporarily increased pain
- Disrupt tissue integrity

- Deficient fluid volume
- Ineffective tissue perfusion: Cardio-pulmonary, renal, cerebral
- Risk for infection

EXPECTED OUTCOMES

The patient will:
- maintain adequate fluid volume
- maintain vital signs, blood pressure, neurologic signs, intake and output, and respiratory status within normal limits
- remain free from infection.

PRETREATMENT CARE

⚡ WARNING *When caring for a patient with a traumatic wound, first assess his ABCs — airway, breathing, and circulation. Once the patient's ABCs are stabilized, turn to the traumatic wound. Initial management focuses on controlling bleeding — usually by applying firm, direct pressure and elevating the extremity. If bleeding continues, compress a pressure point. Assess the condition of the wound. Management and cleaning technique usually depend on the type of wound and degree of contamination.*

- Place a linen-saver pad under the area to be cleaned.
- Remove clothing covering the wound.
- If necessary, cut hair around the wound with scissors to promote cleaning and treatment.
- Assemble needed equipment at the patient's bedside.
- Fill a sterile basin with normal saline solution.
- Make sure the treatment area has enough light to allow close observation of the wound.
- Depending on the nature and location of the wound, wear sterile or clean gloves to avoid spreading infection.

- Check the patient's medical history for previous tetanus immunization and, if needed and ordered, arrange for immunization.
- Administer an analgesic if ordered.

POSTTREATMENT CARE

- After a wound has been cleaned, the practitioner may want to debride it to remove dead tissue and reduce the risk of infection and scarring. Pack the wound with gauze pads soaked in normal saline solution until debridement.
- Observe for signs and symptoms of infection, such as warm red skin at the site or purulent discharge. Know that infection of a traumatic wound can delay healing, increase scar formation, and trigger systemic infection, such as septicemia.
- Observe all dressings. If edema is present, adjust the dressing to avoid impairing circulation to the area.
- Make sure the patient is comfortable.
- Properly dispose of drainage, solutions, and the trash bag, and clean or dispose of soiled equipment and supplies according to facility policy and the Centers of Disease Control and Prevention guidelines.
- Provide adequate I.V. hydration as ordered.
- Administer medications (including analgesics) as ordered.
- Provide emotional support.
- Monitor the patient's vital signs, intake and output, peripheral pulses, and pulse oximetry.
- Observe the patient for signs of decreased tissue perfusion.
- Assess the patient for complications.
- Monitor the patient's level of pain; provide an analgesic and assess its effect.
- Assess the results of ordered laboratory studies.

PATIENT TEACHING

GENERAL

- Encourage the patient to follow a diet with adequate calories, protein, and vitamins.
- Teach the patient how to check the wound for infection and other complications.
- Show the patient how to change dressings, and have him repeat the procedure to demonstrate his understanding.
- Give the patient written instructions for procedures to be performed at home.
- Refer the patient to appropriate resources and support services.
- Arrange for home health care services if required.

RESOURCES

Organizations
American Medical Association: *www.ama-assn.org*
Wound, Ostomy and Continence Nursing Society: *www.wocn.org*

Selected references

Naylor, W.A., "A Guide to Wound Management in Palliative Care," *International Journal of Palliative Nursing* 11(11): 572, 574-79, November 2005.
Nowlin, A. "The Delicate Business of Burn Care," *RN* 69(1):52-57, January 2006.
Posnett, J. "Making Cost Effectiveness the Basis of Product Selection," *Journal of Wound Care* 15(1):S14-15, January 2006.

Appendices

ALTERNATIVE AND COMPLEMENTARY TREATMENTS

The National Institutes of Health through the National Center for Complementary and Alternative Medicine (NCCAM) defines these treatments as "a group of diverse medical and health care systems, practices, and products that aren't presently considered to be a part of conventional medicine. Five domains of treatments are listed by NCCAM: alternative medical systems, mind-body interventions, biologically based therapies, manipulative and body-based methods, and energy therapies. The chart below lists several popular alternative and complementary treatments, their domains, uses, and special considerations for patient teaching.

TREATMENT AND DESCRIPTION	REPORTED USES	SPECIAL CONSIDERATIONS
Acupressure		
◆ Form of Chinese medicine that uses finger pressure on key points (acupoints) on the surface of the skin to stimulate the body's natural self-curative ability. ◆ Alternative medical systems	◆ Tension reduction ◆ Circulation improvement ◆ Body relaxation ◆ Pain relief	◆ Pressure shouldn't be applied to areas of inflammation or to wounds. ◆ Certain points must not be used in pregnant women because stimulation can cause premature contractions.
Acupuncture		
◆ Form of traditional Chinese medicine that uses thin needles inserted at designated points on the body to restore health. The needles are believed to work by enhancing the flow of energy (qi) in the body. ◆ Alternative medical systems	◆ Pain relief ◆ Nausea and vomiting relief ◆ Drug and alcohol abuse treatment ◆ Smoking cessation	◆ Needles are fine and not hollow, so the patient feels relatively little pain, compared with insertion of tunneling needles used in Western injections. ◆ Life-threatening reactions, such as pneumothorax, can occur in some types of acupuncture.
Alexander technique		
◆ Form of body work aimed at correcting poor habits of posture and movement that are believed to strain the body and result in various ailments. This technique focuses on proper alignment of the head, neck, and trunk. ◆ Manipulative and body-based methods	◆ Neck and back pain relief ◆ Chronic disorders (postural disorder, myalgia, breathing problems, hypertension, and anxiety) treatment ◆ Repetitive stress injury prevention	◆ The patient should consult with his physician first to make sure that this technique won't exacerbate his condition or interfere with treatment. ◆ The patient must follow the technique closely because it can be misapplied.
Aromatherapy		
◆ Therapeutic use of plant oils to treat specific ailments. Oils can be inhaled, massaged into the skin, or placed in bath water for specific therapeutic purposes. Specific oils are believed to have either relaxing or stimulating effects. ◆ Mind-body interventions	◆ Tension reduction ◆ Anxiety relief ◆ Body relaxation ◆ Pain relief	◆ Some oils can cause irritation with sensitive skin or even nonlethal poisoning. ◆ Many essential oils are toxic to children younger than age 5 and should be used with caution. ◆ Essential oils should be kept away from the eyes and mucous membranes.
Ayurveda (Ayurvedic medicine)		
◆ Ancient traditional Indian system of medicine that focuses on establishing and maintaining balance of the life energies within the body and stresses the importance of metabolic body type (dosha) in determining health, personality, and susceptibility to disease. ◆ Alternative medical systems	◆ Disorder management ◆ Wellness enhancement ◆ Disease prevention	◆ The patient needs to cooperate in making the recommended changes in diet and lifestyle. ◆ The patient's medication history must be obtained to make sure that herbal compounds don't interact with other prescribed herbs or drugs. ◆ The patient shouldn't share Ayurvedic compounds with others.
Biofeedback		
◆ A method of promoting relaxation by consciously controlling body functions, such as blood pressure, heart and respiratory rates, temperature, and perspiration. This method involves the use of an electronic device that informs the patient when changes in these functions occur. ◆ Mind-body interventions	◆ Disease prevention ◆ Health restoration ◆ Stress reduction ◆ Muscle contraction headaches	◆ Skin irritation may develop from the electrodes used in monitoring. ◆ It's contraindicated in patients with low blood pressure, psychiatric disorders, impaired attention or memory, or mental handicaps such as dementia. ◆ The patient should continue to take medications (such as antihypertensive drugs) while receiving biofeedback training.

TREATMENT AND DESCRIPTION	REPORTED USES	SPECIAL CONSIDERATIONS
Chiropractic medicine		
◆ A manual healing therapy based on the belief that many medical problems are caused by vertebral misalignment and can be corrected by manipulating the spine. ◆ Alternative medical systems	◆ Pain relief ◆ Spinal or vertebral malfunction ◆ Nerve impingement	◆ It's contraindicated in patients with conditions that might worsen as the result of a spinal adjustment, such as osteoporosis and advanced degenerative joint disease.
Herbalism		
◆ The use of plants for healing purposes. ◆ Biologically based therapies	◆ Disease prevention ◆ Health restoration	◆ The patient should check with his physician or pharmacist to make sure that the herbal therapy doesn't interact with his present medication or make his present condition worse.
Hypnotherapy (hypnosis)		
◆ Therapy that applies suggestion and altered levels of consciousness to affect positive changes in behavior or to treat a health condition. ◆ Mind-body interventions	◆ Enhanced physiological well-being ◆ Pain relief ◆ Anxiety relief ◆ Substance abuse relief	◆ Patients with psychosis, organic psychiatric conditions, or antisocial personality disorders shouldn't be treated with hypnosis. ◆ Some patients may experience light-headedness or psychological reactions after hypnosis.
Magnet therapy (magnetic field therapy, biomagnetic therapy, magnetotherapy)		
◆ Involves the use of magnetic fields in the prevention and treatment of disease and first-aid treatment for injuries with a goal to restore a person's internal bioelectromagnetic balance. ◆ Energy therapies	◆ Pain relief ◆ Bone healing ◆ Stress reduction ◆ Sprain and strain relief	◆ Positive (biosouth) magnetic energy should only be used under medical supervision because overstimulation of the brain may occur, producing seizures, hallucinations, insomnia, hyperactivity, and magnetic addiction. ◆ A bedridden patient who uses a magnetic bed 24 hours per day risks suppressed adrenal function and slowed energy recovery. ◆ Therapy isn't recommended for pregnant women or those younger than age 5 because of its experimental nature. ◆ Patients with pacemakers or defibrillators shouldn't use magnetic beds; no magnet should be closer than 6″ (15 cm) to such devices.
Massage therapy		
◆ Manipulation of muscles and tissues by rubbing, kneading, tapping, or stroking. ◆ Manipulative and body-based methods	◆ Stress relief ◆ Relaxation promotion ◆ Pain relief ◆ Circulation improvement	◆ It's contraindicated in patients with diabetes, varicose veins, phlebitis or other blood vessel problems, or swollen limbs.
Nutritional therapy		
◆ Consuming or eliminating certain dietary components to heal the body and maintain optimum health. ◆ Biologically based therapies	◆ Disease prevention ◆ Health restoration	◆ Before considering a dietary change, the patient should consult with his physician to make sure that it complements his condition and doesn't exacerbate it.
Qigong		
◆ An ancient Chinese health discipline consisting of breathing exercises, deep concentration, and physical exercises aimed at balancing qi (the flow of energy) to maintain health and prevent disease. ◆ Energy therapies	◆ Relaxation response enhancement ◆ Chronic illness treatment	◆ Patients with respiratory problems may not be able to perform the breathing exercise aspect of qigong. ◆ Patients with serious illnesses should be aware that qigong may be beneficial as a complementary therapy, but it isn't a substitute for conventional treatment.

Reflexology

- Form of body work involving the application of pressure to specific points on the feet or hands. These points are believed to be connected to, and have a therapeutic effect on, specific body parts or organs.
- Manipulative and body-based methods

- Stress reduction
- Muscle tension relaxation
- Disorder management

- Treatment may produce a healing crisis consisting of fever, rash, diaphoresis or urinary changes, or worsening of the condition as toxins are released.
- The patient should check with his physician first if he has diabetes, peripheral vascular disease, or vascular problems of the legs (thrombosis or phlebitis).
- Pregnant women need to get their physician's consent before trying this therapy.

Reiki

- A Japanese technique using prayers, herbal remedies, crystals, and other implements administered by "laying on hands." It's thought to be best applied to the whole body to clean and revitalize the complete system because disease impacts the whole body.
- Energy therapies

- Stress reduction
- Pain relief
- Muscle relaxation

- The patient should consult with his physician to make sure that the therapy doesn't interact negatively with his condition or present medications. (Herbal remedies may be used.)

Tai chi chuan

- Ancient Chinese exercise program based on the teachings of Taoism and the theory and practice of traditional Chinese medicine. It's practiced today as a physical culture regimen to promote health and longevity. It includes meditation and breathing exercises.
- Mind-body interventions

- Balance, posture, coordination, flexibility, and endurance improvement
- Stress reduction

- Stretching before exercises can help prevent strains and sprains.
- The patient should stop exercising if he experience pain or shortness of breath.
- The patient should wear appropriate footwear to reduce the risk of slipping and falling.

Yoga

- Ancient Hindu exercise and health maintenance program that consists of assuming specific positions combined with deep breathing and meditation.
- Mind-body interventions

- Stress reduction
- Health promotion

- The patient should consult with his physician before undertaking a yoga program because some postures can be stressful if he has certain health problems, such as glaucoma, acute abdominal diseases, and during acute flare-ups of arthritis.

The chart below lists several common cosmetic treatments, a brief description of how they are done, and important nursing considerations.

TREATMENT	DESCRIPTION	NURSING CONSIDERATIONS
Abdominoplasty (tummy tuck)	◆ This is a major procedure that removes skin and fat from the abdomen as well as tightens the abdominal wall muscles. ◆ The procedure can dramatically reduce the appearance of a protruding abdomen, but produces a large, permanent scar.	◆ Tell the patient that recovery may take several months as this is major abdominal surgery. ◆ The better physical condition that the patient is in before surgery, the faster recovery will be after surgery.
Blepharoplasty (eyelid surgery)	◆ This procedure corrects droopy eyelids and puffiness and bags under the eyes. ◆ Fat, muscle, and skin may be removed in the affected areas to enhance appearance and, in the case of drooping eyelids, to improve vision.	◆ The procedure can't improve dark circles, wrinkles, and fine lines around the eyes or sagging eyebrows. ◆ Infection and scarring are general risks. ◆ Removal of too much skin can make eye closure difficult or show tissues underlying the lower lid, requiring surgical repair. ◆ Dry eye syndrome is a potential risk and can lead to corneal abrasions and vision loss if untreated with artificial tears. ◆ Although rare, retrobulbar hematoma may also develop.
Botox injection	◆ Botulinum toxin injections temporarily reduce or eliminate crow's feet near the eyes, creases and frown lines in the forehead, and thick bands in the neck. ◆ The toxin blocks the nerve impulses, which temporarily paralyzes the muscles that cause wrinkles, helping to give the skin a smoother appearance. ◆ It may also relieve excessive sweating, migraine headaches, and muscle spasms in the neck and eyes.	◆ The effects from one treatment last 3 to 4 months. ◆ Possible adverse effects include a burning sensation during injection, and local numbness, swelling, or bruising after the injection. Some patients may have a temporary headache and nausea.
Breast augmentation (augmentation mammoplasty)	◆ This is a surgical procedure to increase the size and shape of a woman's breast; the surgeon inserts an implant behind each breast, increasing breast size by one or more cup sizes.	◆ Capsular contracture occurs if the scar or capsule around the implant begins to tighten, causing the breast to feel hard. This is treated in several ways, including removing or "scoring" of the scar tissue, or removal or replacement of the implant. ◆ Excessive bleeding may cause some swelling and pain. Depending on the amount of bleeding, a second operation may be necessary to control the bleeding and remove the hematoma (if present). ◆ Infection may occur, which may necessitate removal of the implant for several months until the infection clears. A new implant can then be inserted. ◆ Inform the patient that her nipples may become oversensitive, undersensitive, or even numb; small patches of numbness may appear near the incisions. These symptoms usually disappear with time, but may be permanent in some patients. ◆ The breast implants may break or leak.
Breast reduction (reduction mammoplasty)	◆ This procedure involves removing fat, glandular tissue, and skin from the breasts, resulting in breasts that are smaller and firmer and more in proportion to the patient's body. ◆ The size of the areola may also be reduced.	◆ Complications may occur, including reaction to the anesthesia, bleeding, or infection. ◆ If a small sore develops around the nipple area, it's treated with antibiotic cream. ◆ Tell the patient she'll have a noticeable, permanent scar. ◆ The patient may have unevenly positioned nipples or slightly mismatched breasts. The patient may not be able to breast-feed because the surgery removes many of the milk ducts leading to the nipples. ◆ Some patients may experience a permanent loss of feeling in their nipples or breasts. ◆ Rarely, the nipple and areola may lose their blood supply, causing tissue death. If this happens, the nipple and areola can usually be rebuilt using skin grafts from elsewhere on the body.

TREATMENT	DESCRIPTION	NURSING CONSIDERATIONS
Brow-lift (forehead-lift)	◆ This procedure is done to restore a more refreshed, youthful look to the area above the eyes. ◆ The procedure can improve horizontal lines and furrows and correct drooping brows that often make a person appear sad, angry, or tired. ◆ By removing or altering the muscles and tissues that cause the drooping or furrowing, the forehead is smoother, the eyebrows are raised, and frown lines minimized.	◆ An injury to the nerves that control eyebrow movement may occur, resulting in an inability to wrinkle the forehead or raise the eyebrows. Additional surgery can correct the problem. ◆ If a broad scar occurs, removing it will result in a smaller, thinner scar. ◆ Some patients may have hair loss along the scar edges. ◆ The patient may have loss of sensation along or just beyond the incision line, especially after a classic forehead-lift. It's usually temporary, but may be permanent in some patients. ◆ Infection and bleeding are common complications.
Chemical peel	◆ Phenol, trichloroacetic acid (TCA), and alphahydroxy acids (AHAs) are used to improve and smooth the texture of the facial skin by removing damaged outer layers. ◆ This procedure is best for patients with wrinkles, facial blemishes, and uneven skin pigmentation.	◆ After an AHA peel, flaking, scaling, redness, and dryness of the skin may occur but should disappear as the skin adjusts to treatment. ◆ After a phenol or TCA peel, a mild pain medication may be prescribed to relieve tingling or throbbing. Remove any tape covering the face after 1 to 2 days. A crust or scab will then form on the treated area. To ensure proper healing, the patient must follow the specialist's postoperative instructions closely. ◆ Depending on the strength of the peel used, a TCA peel may cause significant swelling. ◆ If the patient had a phenol peel, the face may become quite swollen and the eyes may even be swollen shut temporarily. Depending on the extent of swelling, the patient be limited to a liquid diet and advised not to talk much during the first few days of recovery.
Chin surgery (mentoplasty)	◆ This procedure reshapes the chin either by enhancement or reduction surgery on the bone. ◆ It may be done for cosmetic reasons or to repair dental malocclusion or other functional problems. ◆ Augmentation can involve extending the jawbone with an alloplastic implant placed in a pocket of connective tissue. ◆ Sliding genioplasty (cutting of the jawbone and then sliding the distal portion out to the correct position and holding it with a metal plate) may also be done when more complicated repairs and dental surgery are involved.	◆ Complications may include infection. ◆ A scar may form at the incision line. ◆ Implants may dislocate over time or erode the bone. ◆ Injury to the trigeminal nerve may cause numbness or paralysis of jaw muscles. ◆ Roots of the teeth can be damaged. ◆ Bone segments in genioplasty may not reunite properly. ◆ A hematoma may form, causing pressure that distorts the final shape of the chin after surgery.
Collagen and injectable fillers	◆ This procedure involves injecting Zyderm and Zyplast, natural substances obtained from purified cow collagen, under the skin. This helps replace the natural collagen that's lost over time. (Human collagen injections are also available.) ◆ This procedure is useful in treating crow's feet, frown lines, and nasolabial folds (smile lines). ◆ There are also filler materials available, such as soft ePTFE (expanded polytetrafluoro-ethylene) that are surgically implanted to help decrease deep creases or to enhance the fullness of the lips.	◆ Treatments are needed every 3 to 6 months ◆ There may be some slight bruising at the injection site. ◆ The patient should be pretested for an allergic reaction. Itching and redness are signs of an allergic reaction.
Dermabrasion	◆ Dermabrasion and dermaplaning help "refinish" the top layers of the skin through controlled surgical scraping. ◆ These treatments help give the skin a smoother appearance by softening the sharp edges of surface irregularities. ◆ It's often used to improve the look of facial skin scarred by deep acne or previous surgery or trauma, to remove precancerous growths, called *keratoses,* and to smooth out fine facial wrinkles.	◆ A change in skin pigmentation is the most common risk. Some patients may have permanent darkening of the skin caused by exposure to the sun after surgery; others may have lighter or blotchy skin at the treated area. ◆ If tiny whiteheads occur, tell the patient they may disappear on their own, or to use an abrasive pad or soap. In extreme cases, they may have to be removed by the practitioner. ◆ Immediately after the procedure, the patient may have enlarged pores; they should shrink back to normal size after the swelling has diminished. ◆ Infection and scarring are possible complications, although rare. Some patients develop excessive scar tissue, which is treated with steroid medication to soften the tissue.

TREATMENT	DESCRIPTION	NURSING CONSIDERATIONS
Dermagraphics (permanent makeup, or micropigmentation)	◆ With this procedure, a trained specialist injects iron oxide pigment into the middle layer of skin for results that last longer. ◆ It may be done to improve the appearance of thin eyebrows or lips, fix an uneven hairline, or for someone who's allergic to make-up or who has physical limitations (making it easier to apply cosmetics).	◆ Tell the patient to expect swelling in the treated region. The practitioner should instruct the patient on how often to ice the area and what type of ointment to apply. ◆ If the procedure is performed in the eye region, someone should drive the patient home. Tearing may also occur (normal). ◆ Pigmentation typically appears darker in the weeks after the procedure but fades over time. ◆ The practitioner should instruct the patient about what to avoid, such as peroxide and sunlight, either of which can damage the new look.
Electrolysis	◆ Electrolysis removes individual hairs from the face or body by using medical electrolysis devices, called *epilators*, to destroy the growth center of the hair with a short-wave radio frequency. ◆ A very fine probe is inserted into the hair follicle at the surface of the skin and the hair is then removed harmlessly with forceps.	◆ Because many factors influence hair growth, the patient needs to return for several visits. The total number of sessions will vary from patient to patient. ◆ Each treatment session lasts between 15 and 60 minutes. ◆ A slight reddening of the skin may occur during or immediately after treatment, but is temporary.
Face-lift (rhytidectomy)	◆ A face-lift helps diminish visible signs of aging by tightening underlying muscles, removing excess fat, and redraping the skin of the face and neck. ◆ This procedure can be done alone or with other procedures, such as eyelid surgery, nose reshaping, or a forehead-lift.	◆ Complications include reactions to the anesthesia, hematoma, infection, and injury to the nerves that control facial muscles (usually temporary). ◆ Patients who smoke are more likely to have poorer healing. ◆ Tell the patient to report severe or persistent pain, or if there's a sudden swelling of the face. There will be some numbness of the skin, but it should disappear within a few months. ◆ To minimize swelling after surgery, keep the patient's head elevated and limit movement as much as possible. ◆ If present, remove the drainage tube 1 to 2 days after surgery. Remove the bandages after 1 to 5 days, preparing the patient for the fact that the face will initially be bruised, pale, and puffy. ◆ Most stitches are removed after about 5 days. Because the scalp may take longer to heal, the stitches or metal clips in the hairline may be left in an additional few days.
Laser resurfacing	◆ Areas of damaged or wrinkled skin are removed layer by layer with a laser. ◆ It's most commonly used to decrease the appearance of fine lines around the mouth and eyes, but may also be used to treat facial scars or areas of uneven pigmentation. ◆ It may be performed on the entire face or in specific regions. ◆ The procedure is usually done in combination with another procedure, such as eyelid surgery or a face lift.	◆ Risks associated with laser resurfacing include burns or other injuries from the heat of the laser energy, scarring, and obvious lightening or darkening of the treated skin. ◆ Laser resurfacing can activate herpes virus infections and, rarely, other types of infection, so carefully assess the patient's immune status. ◆ If healing is delayed or abnormal or if there's scarring or abnormal pigmentation, additional corrective measures may be required. ◆ Ice packs and medication can help reduce swelling and discomfort. ◆ The practitioner should instruct the patient to replace the initial bandage with a fresh one after 1 or 2 days. After 1 week, the bandage may be removed and a thin layer of ointment may be applied to the skin. The patient must follow the practitioner's instructions on how to wash and care for the skin. ◆ Instruct the patient not to pick the crusts off the treated area because scarring may result. Usually, the patient is free from crusts 10 days postoperatively; however, redness may persist for several weeks.
Lip augmentation	◆ This procedure involves injecting a natural or synthetic biocompatible material, or the patient's own fat, into the lips. ◆ It helps to create plumper, fuller lips and reduce the appearance of fine lines around the mouth.	◆ Collagen and fat injections are procedures that produce temporary results in the form of a fuller-lipped look. ◆ If the procedure was nonsurgical, the patient can return to normal activities immediately. If the procedure was done surgically, the recovery period may be up to 1 week. ◆ Complications include bleeding, lip asymmetry, migration and extrusion of the implant, and allergic reactions. Allergic reactions can range from prolonged redness, swelling, or itching to firmness at the injection site. Normal swelling and bruising lasts from 3 days to 1 week.

TREATMENT	DESCRIPTION	NURSING CONSIDERATIONS
Lipoplasty (liposuction or suction lipectomy)	◆ This procedure helps sculpt the body by removing unwanted fat from specific areas, including the abdomen, buttocks, cheeks, chin, hips, knees, neck, thighs, and upper arms. ◆ Newer techniques, including ultrasound-assisted lipoplasty, the tumescent technique, and the superwet technique, help provide more specific results and faster recovery times. ◆ Liposuction can remove stubborn areas of fat that don't respond to traditional weight-loss methods; however, it isn't a substitute for diet and exercise.	◆ Complications include infection, delays in healing, the formation of fat or blood clots that may migrate to the lungs and cause death, excessive fluid loss leading to shock, fluid accumulation, friction burns, damage to the skin or nerves, perforation injury to vital organs, or unfavorable drug reactions. ◆ The scars from liposuction are small and strategically placed to be hidden from view, but the patient may still have imperfections in the skin afterwards. A baggy skin appearance is common in older patients. ◆ Some patients may need additional surgery to help remove excess skin.
Neck-lift	◆ This set of procedures is used to improve the appearance of the neck. The removal of excess skin is cervicoplasty, and the removal or alteration of neck muscles is platysmaplasty. ◆ Neck liposuction may also be performed. ◆ If fullness or "bands" are present, Botox injections may be used.	◆ Swelling and bruising can last for several days. ◆ Tightness or tingling, burning or pulling, and numbness can occur in the first few weeks after surgery and shouldn't be cause for concern. ◆ As with any surgery, infection can occur.
Otoplasty	◆ This procedure is usually done to set prominent ears back closer to the head or to reduce the size of large ears. The operation is typically performed on children ages 4 to 14. ◆ An incision is made in the back of the ear, the skin is removed, and stitches are used to fold the cartilage back on itself to reshape the ear; or, cartilage is removed to reshape the ear.	◆ A blood clot may form in the ear, which may dissolve naturally or be removed by the practitioner. ◆ Occasionally, an infection in the cartilage may develop and cause scar tissue to form. Such infections are usually treated with antibiotics; rarely, surgery may be required to drain the infected area.
Rhinoplasty	◆ This procedure shortens, lengthens, or reshapes the nasal bone and cartilage to improve appearance or breathing. ◆ Small incisions are made inside the nostrils or to the columnar skin between the nares to allow access to the nasal structures. ◆ Cartilage and bone are then manipulated to achieve the desired effects. ◆ Synthetic or allographic bone or cartilage may be used in remodeling.	◆ Complications include infection at the site, excess bleeding, or allergy to the anesthetic. ◆ Scarring may occur. ◆ Small capillaries on the nose may break, causing tiny but permanent reddened marks.
Tattoo removal	◆ Lasers are used to remove tattoos by emitting pulses of light that are then absorbed by the tattoo pigment. ◆ Certain colors of light are absorbed by specific colors of the tattoo ink. ◆ The pigment breaks up and is then destroyed by the immune system.	◆ Ice may be applied to the area to help relieve pain and swelling. ◆ In many cases, the tattoo may be removed completely; however, the ink used in tattooing isn't regulated. ◆ Not knowing which ink, how deep, or how much was used can make the tattoo difficult to completely remove.

Index

i refers to an illustration; t refers to a table.

i refers to an illustration; t refers to a table.

i refers to an illustration; t refers to a table.

---

i refers to an illustration; t refers to a table.

i refers to an illustration; t refers to a table.

i refers to an illustration; t refers to a table.

i refers to an illustration; t refers to a table.

i refers to an illustration; t refers to a table.

i refers to an illustration; t refers to a table.

i refers to an illustration; t refers to a table.

i refers to an illustration; t refers to a table.

i refers to an illustration; t refers to a table.

i refers to an illustration; t refers to a table.

i refers to an illustration; t refers to a table.

i refers to an illustration; t refers to a table.

Pressure ulcer *(continued)*
   wound care for, 464-467
      posttreatment care for, 465-466
      pretreatment care for, 465
      procedure for, 464-465
PRK. *See* Photoreactive keratectomy.
Prostatectomy, 292-293
   indications for, 292
   patient-teaching aid for, 293
   posttreatment care for, 292
   pretreatment care for, 292
   procedure for, 292
Prostate surgery, recovery after, 293
Prothrombin complex, transfusing, 26-29
Proton beam therapy, 294-295
   indications for, 294
   posttreatment care for, 295
   pretreatment care for, 294-295
   procedure for, 294
Proximal gastric vagotomy, 440
Psoralen plus UVA, 424
Psoriasis, ultraviolet light therapy for, 424-427
PTCA. *See* Angioplasty, percutaneous transluminal coronary.
PTK. *See* Phototherapeutic keratectomy.
Pulmonary disease, thoracentesis for, 346-349
Puncture wound, caring for, 474, 475
PUVA, 424

Q
Qigong, 479t

R
Radiation
   external, 296-297
   hair and scalp care during, 64i
   internal, 298-301
Radical neck dissection, 302-303
   indications for, 302
   posttreatment care for, 303
   pretreatment care for, 303
   procedure for, 302
Radioactive iodine therapy, 304-305
   indications for, 304
   patient-teaching aid for, 305
   posttreatment care for, 304
   pretreatment care for, 304
   procedure for, 304
Radiofrequency ablation
   for arrhythmias, 6-7

Radiofrequency ablation *(continued)*
   of tumors, 306-307
      posttreatment care of, 307
      pretreatment care of, 307
      procedure for, 306, 307i
Radiolabeled antibodies, 298
Range of motion, passive. *See* Continuous passive motion.
Rectocele, surgical repair of, 84-85
Reduction mammoplasty, 481t
Red wounds, caring for, 468
Reflexology, 480t
Reiki, 480t
Renal cell carcinoma, nephrectomy for, 250-251
Renal obstruction, lithotripsy for, 222-225
Replacement heart valves, 150-151
   indications for, 150
   posttreatment care for, 150
   pretreatment care for, 150
   procedure for, 150
   types of, 151i
Residual limb, above-the-knee, wrapping, 13i
Respiratory failure
   extracorporeal membrane oxygenation for, 126-127
   noninvasive positive airway pressure for, 254-257
Restrictive gastric surgeries, 308-309
   indications for, 308
   posttreatment care for, 309
   pretreatment care for, 308
   procedure for, 308
   types of, 308i
Retinal detachment, scleral buckling for, 310-311
Retropubic prostatectomy, 292-293
Rhinoplasty, 484t
Rhytidectomy, 483t
Rod implantation, 328-329
   indications for, 328
   posttreatment care for, 329
   pretreatment care for, 328
   procedure for, 328
   types of spinal instrumentation for, 328
Rotator cuff repair, continuous passive motion for, 88-89
Roux-en Y bypass. *See* Gastric bypass.

S
Salpingectomy, 258-259
   indications for, 258
   posttreatment care for, 259
   pretreatment care for, 259
   procedure for, 258
Salpingo-oophorectomy, 258-259

i refers to an illustration; t refers to a table.

i refers to an illustration; t refers to a table.

i refers to an illustration; t refers to a table.

i refers to an illustration; t refers to a table.

Turbinectomy, 422-423
  indications for, 422
  posttreatment care for, 423
  pretreatment care for, 423
  procedure for, 422
TURP. *See* Transurethral resection of the prostate.
Twin transfusion syndrome, therapeutic amniocentesis
      for, 10
Tympanostomy tubes, 248

U

Ulcerative colitis
  continent ileostomy for, 178-180
  conventional ileostomy for, 182-183
  ileoanal reservoir for, 176-177
Ultraviolet light therapy, 424-427
  indications for, 424
  patient-teaching aid for, 426
  posttreatment care for, 425
  pretreatment care for, 425
  procedure for, 424
  subdivision of spectrum in, 424
Umbilical hernia repair, 168-169
  posttreatment care for, 168
  pretreatment care for, 168
  procedure for, 168
Upper airway obstruction, tracheotomy for, 364-368
Upper gastrointestinal bleeding, gastric lavage for, 134-135
Urethral dilation, 428-429
  indications for, 428
  posttreatment care for, 429
  pretreatment care for, 429
  procedure for, 428
Urethrocele, surgical repair of, 84-85
Urethrotomy, internal, 428-429
  indications for, 428
  posttreatment care for, 429
  pretreatment care for, 429
  procedure for, 428
Urinary diversion. *See* Cystectomy *and* Cystostomy.
Urinary diversion surgery, 430-435
  indications for, 430
  patient-teaching aid for, 433-434i
  posttreatment care for, 432
  pretreatment care for, 431-432
  procedure for, 430-431
  types of, 430, 430i
Urinary incontinence, bladder retraining for, 22-25
Urinary stoma, caring for, 433-434i

Urinary tract disorders, urinary diversion surgery for,
      430-435
Uterine fibroids, removal of, 4-5
Uterus, removal of, 174-175
UVA radiation, 424
UVB radiation, 424
UVC radiation, 424

V

Vacuum-assisted closure pressure therapy, 436-437
  indications for, 436
  posttreatment care for, 437
  pretreatment care for, 437
  procedure for, 436, 436i
VAD. *See* Ventricular assist device.
Vagal maneuvers, 438-439
  indications for, 438
  location and technique for, 438i
  posttreatment care for, 439
  pretreatment care for, 439
  procedure for, 438-439
Vaginal wall defect, repairing, 84-85
Vagotomy, 440-441
  indications for, 440
  posttreatment care for, 441
  pretreatment care for, 440
  procedure for, 440
Vagus nerve stimulation, 442-443
  indications for, 442
  placement of, 442i
  posttreatment care for, 443
  pretreatment care for, 442-443
  procedure for, 442
Valsalva's maneuvers, 438-439
Varicose vein excision and stripping, 444-445
  indications for, 444
  posttreatment care for, 445
  pretreatment care for, 445
  procedure for, 444
Vascular access sites for hemodialysis, 156i
Vasectomy, 446-447
  indications for, 446
  posttreatment care for, 447
  pretreatment care for, 447
  procedure for, 446
Vena cava filter placement, 448-449
  indications for, 448
  posttreatment care for, 449
  pretreatment care for, 448
  procedure for, 448

i refers to an illustration; t refers to a table.

Ventilator alarms, responding, to, 238t
Ventral hernia repair, 168-169
   posttreatment care for, 168
   pretreatment care for, 168
   procedure for, 168
Ventricular assist device, 450-451
   indications for, 450
   mechanics of, 450i
   posttreatment care for, 451
   pretreatment care for, 451
   procedure for, 450
Ventricular drainage system for cerebrospinal fluid, 60, 60i
Ventriculoatrial shunt placement, 452
Ventriculoperitoneal shunt placement, 452-453
   indications for, 452
   posttreatment care for, 453
   pretreatment care for, 453
   procedure for, 452
Vertebroplasty, 330-331
   indications for, 330
   posttreatment care for, 331
   pretreatment care for, 330
   procedure for, 330
Vesicant drugs, administration guidelines for, 63
Vision correction, laser eye surgery for, 214-217
Volume-cycled ventilator, 238

WX

Wavefront-guided LASIK, 214
Wedge resection, 350i, 351
Wet dressing, applying, in burn care, 454
Wet-to-dry dressings as debridement method, 108
Whipple procedure. *See* Pancreaticoduodenectomy.
White blood cells, transfusing, 26-29
Whole blood transfusion, 26-29
Wound care
   for burns, 454-457
   for dehiscence and evisceration, 458-459
   irrigation in, 460-463
   for pressure ulcer, 464-467
   surgical, 468-473
   tailoring, to wound color, 468
   traumatic, 474-475
Wound-cleaning agent, applying, 462i
Wound healing, vacuum-assisted closure pressure therapy
     for, 436-437
W-pouch. *See* Ileoanal reservoir.
Wrapping above-the-knee residual limb, 13i

YZ

Yellow wounds, caring for, 468
Yoga, 480t

---

i refers to an illustration; t refers to a table.